Humoral Immunity
in Neurological Diseases

NATO ADVANCED STUDY INSTITUTES SERIES

A series of edited volumes comprising multifaceted studies of contemporary scientific issues by some of the best scientific minds in the world, assembled in cooperation with NATO Scientific Affairs Division.

Series A: Life Sciences

Recent Volumes in this Series

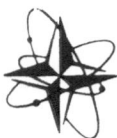

The series is published by an international board of publishers in conjunction with NATO Scientific Affairs Division

A Life Sciences	Plenum Publishing Corporation
B Physics	New York and London
C Mathematical and Physical Sciences	D. Reidel Publishing Company Dordrecht and Boston
D Behavioral and Social Sciences	Sijthoff International Publishing Company Leiden
E Applied Sciences	Noordhoff International Publishing Leiden

Humoral Immunity in Neurological Diseases

Edited by

D. Karcher and A. Lowenthal

Universitaire Instelling Antwerpen, Neurochemie
Wilrijk, Belgium

and

A. D. Strosberg

Vrije Universiteit Brussel
St. Genesius-Rode, Belgium
and Université Paris VII
Paris, France

PLENUM PRESS ● NEW YORK AND LONDON
Published in cooperation with NATO Scientific Affairs Division

Library of Congress Cataloging in Publication Data

Nato Advanced Study Institute on Humoral Immunity in Neurological Diseases,
Antwerp, 1978.
Humoral immunity in neurological diseases.

(NATO Advanced study institutes series: Series A, Life sciences; v. 24)
"Lectures presented at the NATO Advanced Study Institute on Humoral Immunity
in Neurological Diseases, held in Antwerp, Belgium, September 10-22, 1978."
Includes index.
1. Multiple sclerosis—Immunological aspects—Congresses. 2. Virus diseases, Slow—
Immunological aspects—Congresses. 3. Immunopathology—Congresses. 4. Immuno-
globulins—Congresses. I. Karcher, Denise. II. Lowenthal, Armand. III. Strosberg, A. D.
IV. Title. V. Series. [DNLM: 1. Nervous system diseases—Immunology—Congresses.
WL100.3 N106h 1978]
RC377.N36 1978   616.8'34'079   79-15096
ISBN 978-1-4684-1005-1   ISBN 978-1-4684-1003-7 (eBook)
DOI 10.1007/978-1-4684-1003-7

Lectures presented at the NATO Advanced Study Institute on Humoral Immunity
in Neurological Diseases, held in Antwerp, Belgium, September 10—22, 1978

© 1979 Plenum Press, New York
Softcover reprint of the hardcover 1st edition 1979
A Division of Plenum Publishing Corporation
227 West 17th Street, New York, N.Y. 10011

FOREWORD

The Nato Advanced Study Institute on Humoral Immunity in
Neurological Diseases became possible thanks to the active help of
many people. I will not mention our colleagues at the neurochemical laboratory of the Born-Bunge Foundation : it was our common
job. But I wish to thank :

- the Nato and Dr. Kester for their aid, support and gene-
  rosity,
- the Belgian Ministry of Foreign Affairs and Secretary-ge-
  neral Mr. Grandry for their help and assistance in establishing valuable contacts with many foreign countries,
- the Belgian Ministry of Culture for their grant,
- the National Fund for Scientific Research and the Belgian
  Society of Neurology for their financial support.

Substantial help came from the Universitaire Instelling Antwerpen : not only financially but by allowing members of their
staff to assist us in many ways.

The Belgian Friends of the Weizmann Institute and the Belgian
Medical Care for Israel helped invite some participants, and
many firms made a contribution to our organization.

To all of them our warmest thanks.

A. Lowenthal

CONTENTS

Introduction
    A. Lowenthal

PART I SPONTANEOUS AND EXPERIMENTAL DISEASES

A. Multiple Sclerosis

CONTENTS

TOPIC III   THERAPEUTIC CONSIDERATIONS

INTRODUCTION

        The reasons for suggesting the organization of this meeting
also constitute its justification.

        First we will say that we have been encouraged to do so in
September 1977 at the International Neurological Congress in
Amsterdam. In answer to a question, it was said that as in the
case of subacute sclerosing panencephalitis, multiple sclerosis
could be a disease with hyperimmunisation, but that the relationship between the disease and the immunological phenomena would
have to be further defined.

        Research, in the field of humoral immunological reactions in
neurological diseases, came to the forefront with the demonstration
of the oligoclonal pattern of γ globulins (fig. 1) first described
by us 20 years ago. It was generally accepted by everyone as the
only known biological result which could confirm the clinical
diagnosis of multiple sclerosis.

        This oligoclonal pattern is not specific : therefore various
questions have to be asked :

1) what is the relationship of the oligoclonal reaction to slow
   viral diseases? Why has it only been observed in one of the
   groups of slow viral diseases : visna, subacute sclerosing
   panencephalitis, distemper and multiple sclerosis, and not,
   in the group of spongiform encephalopathies?

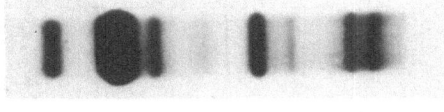

Fig. 1 : Agar gel electrophoresis of the cerebrospinal fluid
        proteins with IgG oligoclonal reaction in a case of
        multiple sclerosis.

2) how can this reaction be demonstrated? Should one confine oneself to the electrophoretic techniques? Do other methods directly or indirectly reveal the reaction?

3) what is the significance of this reaction? Does it really lead to the formation of homogeneous antibodies? Should one go on calling it oligoclonal reaction?

4) is this reaction a generalized physiological phenomenon, existing in many organisms and which can be brought about by numerous and various antigens? Does it develop really in the central nervous system? Does it induce a particular reaction of the central nervous system?

5) or does this reaction imply the presence of immunological anomalies and can it therefore, on this basis, only be observed in very definite conditions, maybe genetically linked?

6) can one modify or influence this phenomenon? Will immunochemical studies enable us to envisage practical therapeutic conclusions?

These are some of the questions we have been asking ourselves for many years whilst examining our electrophoretic patterns and reporting to the clinicians that the γ globulins of the cerebrospinal fluid which they entrusted to us, were fractionated. For a long time, we had to be satisfied with this purely contemplative attitude.

First described in neurology and in the cerebrospinal fluid, the oligoclonal reaction had been later found experimentally by immunologists and studied immunochemically. Virologists have tried to reproduce it experimentally, and clinicians reported comparable phenomena in myeloma and in certain collagenoses, or in autoimmune diseases. It therefore became clear that in order to better understand the significance of this oligoclonal reaction, so that the young and active researchers, which of course is one and the same thing, can make new comparisons, have new ideas, one had to try to bring together clinicians, immunologists, biochemists, virologists and all those concerned with the problem. This is what was tried during the NATO Advanced Study Institute on humoral immunity in neurological diseases.

Many papers were read. We hope they will help define the terminology, the required methods, the avenues for research and indicate eventually a practical application.

A. Lowenthal

CELLULAR IMMUNOLOGY IN MULTIPLE SCLEROSIS

INTRODUCTION AND HISTORY

J.L. Sever, D.L. Madden and W.C. Wallen

National Institutes of Health, NINCDS
Bethesda, Maryland, U.S.A.

INTRODUCTION

Studies of the cellular immune responses of patients with multiple sclerosis (MS) have received increasing attention in recent years. Numerous investigations have involved studies of general immunocompetence of patients during various phases of the disease while others have tested specific cell-mediated immune reactions with viral or other antigens. We will present reports on these studies in three parts: 1) Introduction and History; 2) Current Studies; and 3) Studies on Regulatory Cells.

The investigations reported, to date, can be divided into eight main types (Table 1). These, in turn, involve three main approaches: A) Intradermal Tests; B) In Vitro Tests; and C) Clinical Trials with various drugs and antigenic reagents. Each approach has certain advantages and limitations.

A. Intradermal Tests

1. Skin Tests. Skin tests are the oldest and best known methods for assessing cell-mediated responsiveness. A variety of antigens have been used in MS patients. The literature prior to 1960 included references to "positive" tests with "homologous cerebral antigens"; rabies vaccine; "encephalogenic factor"; tuberculin; mumps virus; Candida albicans; streptococci; and equine serum proteins (1,2). There was considerable disagreement in these reports, however, as well as many claims and counter-claims regarding detection of immune reactivity and their significance. The problems in analysis of these studies related to: 1) the validity of the diagnosis of MS;

Table 1. Multiple Sclerosis - Tests of Cellular Immunity

A. INTRADERMAL

   1. Skin Tests

B. IN VITRO

   1. T- and B-Lymphocyte Distributions
   2. Lymphocyte Stimulation
      a. General mitogens
      b. Specific antigens
   3. Leukocyte Migration Inhibition
   4. Cytotoxicity

C. CLINICAL TRIALS

   1. Immunosuppression
   2. Immunostimulation
   3. Desensitization

2) the type and time of skin reactions; 3) the adequacy of the control groups; and 4) the appearance of the reactions after a second injection of antigen.

Since 1960, several "brain" antigens have been studied in some detail. First, "encephalogenic factor" was tested in 17 patients with MS (1,2). A water soluble extract from human brain was used. This material was similar to that prepared for investigations with experimental allergic encephalomyelitis (EAE). Second, suspensions of lyophilized human white matter were given to 28 MS patients. Most patients failed to have skin reactions with these antigens. The authors concluded that the findings contradicted the hypothesis that MS is a primary autoimmune disease. In a separate study, one additional MS patient was tested with "encephalogenic factor". This patient also failed to have a skin reaction (3).

In a study of a variety of common skin test antigens, 24 MS patients, were tested; some were receiving the immunosuppressive drug 6-MP (4). The antigens included monilia, dermatophytin "O", streptokinase-streptodornase, tuberculin and histoplasmin. All patients had the expected normal skin responses to at least one of the five antigens.

Finally, we used several measles virus antigens, a mumps virus antigen and control antigens intradermally in a study of 20 MS and 40 control patients (5). We were not able to show a significant increase or decrease in dermal reaction toward any of these antigens by the MS patients when compared with appropriate controls.

In summary, using skin tests, the majority of MS patients reported did not respond to "encephalogenic factor" nor to human white matter. In addition, MS patients had normal responses to common skin test antigens as well as to measles and mumps viral antigens.

B. In Vitro Tests

1. T-Cell to B-Cell Ratios. Several groups of investigators have determined T- and B-lymphocyte distributions in MS patients (6). Some authors have reported that T-cells are decreased during exacerbations and "avid" T-rosettes are also decreased. In addition, B-cells have been reported to be increased in MS patients. There are contradicting studies by other investigators, however, which have found normal levels of T-cells but a reduction in lymphocytes with C3 and Fc receptors. In addition, one study of 40 MS patients and a similar number of controls showed a significant increase in T-cells in the MS group (6). B-cells in this study were tested for surface immunoglobulin and there was a slight increase in the IgG positive cells in the MS groups. The patients in this latter study were in a stable phase of their disease. The apparent differences in these studies may be due to fluctuations in the distributions of lymphocytes which occur during various phases of the disease.

These investigations suggest that T-cells may be decreased during exacerbations of MS but are probably normal or increased during remission. It will be important to document the time course of the change in T-cells, if present, in relation to exacerbations and to determine T-cell levels in the CSF as well as to correlate these distributions with alterations in general immunocompetence to determine their significance. It is possible that the decrease in T-cells follows rather than precedes the exacerbations.

2. Lymphocyte Stimulation. A large number of studies have been conducted with lymphocytes from MS and control patients using various agents to test responsiveness. These studies may be subdivided into two subgroups: 1) those in which general mitogens were used; and 2) those in which specific antigens were employed. Here we will review only selected reports from a much larger literature.

a. Response to general mitogens. In a study of 19 MS patients and six normal adults, lymphocyte stimulation was measured by tritiated thymidine (^{3}H-TdR) incorporation into cellular DNA (7). Cultures were stimulated using phytohemagglutinin (PHA) M. There was no difference in the reactivity between the patients and controls. In addition, spontaneous DNA synthesis by activated lymphocytes was measured from these patients using ^{3}H-TdR incorporation. No abnor-

malities were noted between the patients and controls regarding
spontaneous lymphoproliferative activity.

The second study involved 40 MS patients and 42 controls who
were hospital staff (6). Lymphocyte stimulation was measured in
response to PHA-P. No significant differences were noted for the
patients when compared to the controls in this study either.

These reported studies, thus, have failed to show any differences in the response of lymphocytes from MS patients compared to
controls when PHA stimulation was used. In addition, no abnormalities were found in the proportion of spontaneously activated lymphocytes among MS patients compared to controls.

b. Antigenic reactivity. Studies of specific and recall
antigen stimulation have been performed with a variety of materials.
First, in an investigation of 24 MS patients and 21 controls, the
lymphocyte blastogenic response was measured using streptolysin O,
SK-SD and KLH (7). No differences were found between the patient
groups and controls. In a second study with 40 patients and 42
normal controls, the antigens included PPD, Candida albicans,
Staphylococcus aureus and Escherichia coli (6). Here again there
was no significant difference between the MS and control patients
in their frequency of positive reactivity. Lastly, a recent study
of 12 patients and 16 healthy controls showed no significant difference between the groups when tested with measles virus, para-
influenza virus and vaccinia virus (8).

A number of investigators have used various brain extracts for
studies of lymphocyte responsiveness. One investigation of 28 MS
patients and 21 neurological controls used bovine intact basic
protein, bovine fragment protein and human basic protein (7). This
study did not find any significant difference in the response of
peripheral blood lymphocytes from the patients when compared with
controls. A second study with 153 MS patients and 59 patients with
other neurological diseases was conducted with human basic protein
(9). The authors reported that both MS and control patients showed
"hypersensitization" to basic protein in about 1/3 of the cases.
More of the "positive reactors" were found in MS patients with a
short duration of illness and oligoclonal IgG in the cerebrospinal
fluid (CSF). They considered the possibility that the results were
influenced by a lymphoblastic inhibitory factor which may be present
in patients during exacerbations and in patients with significant
disability. In a third study of 19 MS patients in various stages
of disease and 14 normal controls, both peripheral blood lymphocytes
and CSF lymphocytes were tested using human myelin basic protein
(10). These authors reported that when employing peripheral blood
lymphocytes there was a significant increase in reactivity by
patients with progressive MS. However, there were only five patients

in this group and the overall effect was primarily due to the results
of one patient. Using CSF lymphocytes, the authors found significant
increases in activity with lymphocytes from patients with acute and
progressive MS. The authors point out that this increased responsiveness to acute demyelinization is consistent with previous reports
of increased basic protein in the CSF of patients during these
stages of the disease. It would be important to learn if the increased reactivity of the lymphocytes in the CSF preceded or followed
the exacerbations of MS.

One recent study partially addressed this question of the timing
of the response but only for peripheral lymphocytes. The authors
tested serial samples from 72 MS patients and 11 controls (11).
Myelin A protein was used to stimulate the cultures. Increased
responses of lymphocytes were found one to three weeks after exacerbations of disease, but not in later specimens. Unfortunately,
test data was not available just prior to exacerbations.

In summary, the studies of brain extracts for lymphocyte stimulation have generally failed to show significant differences for
MS patients compared to controls when peripheral blood was used
and the activity of disease was not considered. In one study, however, increased responses were reported with peripheral blood samples
taken shortly after exacerbations. Also, using CSF lymphocytes,
increased reactivity was reported with specimens from patients with
acute and progressive MS. For these studies, the question of the
timing of the increased responsiveness remains unanswered since
none of the patients were tested prior to, during and after an
exacerbation. It is possible, therefore, that increased lymphocyte
activity, if present, may simply be a response to the presence of
myelin breakdown products known to occur in the central nervous
system at the time of exacerbations and thus not central to the
cause of the disease.

Research has been reported on lymphocyte response to autologous
and homologous CSF (7). One study indicated that CSF from normal
individuals as well as MS patients contained an antigen to which
only lymphocytes from MS patients were sensitive. This work was
not confirmed by later investigations (7).

Interest in the increased measles antibody levels found in MS
patients stimulated studies of the cell-mediated immune responses
of lymphocytes to measles antigens. In a study of 8 MS patients
with relapses and 10 normal controls, peripheral lymphocytes were
tested using measles and control antigens (12). There was no significant difference in the reponse to measles or control antigen
between the MS and normal individuals.

3. Leukocyte migration inhibition. Several studies have been
reported in which the inhibition due to leukocyte sensitization has

been studied for MS patients and controls using various myelin basic protein preparations. In one investigation, human, bovine and guinea pig basic proteins were used (13). A total of 40 MS patients were studied along with 34 patients with other neurological diseases. Both acute and chronic MS patients were included. Guinea pig macrophages were used as responder cells for the tests. There was no evidence of antigenic recognition of basic proteins by MS patients' compared to the controls using the indirect macrophage migration inhibition test. In a second study, however, using direct migration of the patients' leukocytes, 24 MS patients were tested along with six controls (14). For stimulation, myelin basic protein preparations from a normal brain and a MS patient were used. Initial tests were performed without serum. These authors reported significant inhibition of migration for the MS patients with partial disability. They suggested their findings correlated with the presence of active disease. The effects were most marked when 10% CSF was added to the test, but when autologous serum was added, the migration results tended to return to normal levels. A third group published several reports involving 100 MS patients and a similar number of controls (11,15). They included MS patients in various stages of disease as well as several groups of patients with other central or peripheral nervous system diseases and normal controls. Utilizing the indirect test with guinea pig macrophages and myelin A protein as antigen they reported significant inhibition of migration for specimens taken from patients within four weeks of exacerbation. Migration became more normal within 5-12 weeks after an attack and was only slightly depressed with chronic MS. Increased inhibition was also found in some patients with thrombotic cerebral infarctions, encephalitis associated with small pox vaccination or mumps, alcoholic neuropathy, myasthenia gravis and polyneuritis. The authors suggested that lymphocyte sensitization might be expected in some patients with these illnesses since a degree of myelin breakdown would occur with most of these diseases. They also reported three patients from whom they had taken blood samples a few days prior to exacerbations of MS. In these cases, there was significant inhibition of migration prior to and immediately following the acute attack. They concluded that "cellular hypersensitivity may play a major role in the disease process, but only in combination with other factors lacking in other disease processes". It is obviously important to know the time of development of the inhibition before exacerbations and its relation to the appearance of basic protein and antibody to basic protein in the CSF. These authors have also published on the direct migration inhibition test with results similar to those they obtained with the indirect tests (16).

In summary, reports on leukocyte migration inhibition with various myelin preparations have differed in their findings. Some investigators have failed to find any difference between MS patients and controls while others report significant cellular immune reac-

tivity in patients with acute MS. The recognition of myelin basic
proteins as antigens capable of inducing cell-mediated immune responses may represent a reaction which follows the increased breakdown of myelin and not necessarily contributing to pathogenesis.
One group has reported that in three cases they found significant
inhibition just before exacerbations. Extension of this work to
include CSF basic protein levels and antibody to basic protein is
needed to determine whether cellular responses to brain proteins
contribute to pathogenesis or monitor levels of demyelination.

Reports on leukocyte migration inhibition with specific viral
antigens will be considered in the second paper of this three part
series.

4. Cytotoxicity. The tests of complement-mediated serum cytotoxicity (CMC) and direct lymphocyte-mediated cytotoxicity (LMC)
have been studied for MS patients and controls using several viral
infected cells as target antigens (17). These tests will be discussed in detail in the second part of this three part presentation.

C. Clinical Trials

Many "clinical trials" have been conducted with MS patients.
Some of these have involved drugs purported to produce immunosuppression, immunostimulation or "desensitization". Several of
these studies have been selected for consideration in this report.

1. Immunosuppression. There is a general impression that
exacerbations of MS often improve more rapidly when steroids are
given. This has lead to trials with a variety of steroids and
other drugs which would be expected to suppress cellular immunity
(18). The initial studies of the treatment of MS patients with
various combinations of thoracic duct drainage, anti-lymphocyte
globulin, azathioprine, and cortisone seem quite heroic and potentially quite dangerous (19). The authors, however, reported that
most of their patients with progressive MS either improved (9
patients) or showed no further deterioration (5 patients). The
periods of treatment were one month to 2-1/4 years. Studies by
other investigators using Azathioprine alone or ACTH and anti-lymphocyte globulin, with similar MS patients showed no evidence of beneficial effects (20,21).

The original investigators continued to use the combination
therapy and reported clinical improvement in about half of their
20 MS patients over a period of one to five years (22). Another
study group used a combined regimen of anti-lymphocyte globulin,
azathioprine and steroids (23). They reported a significant reduction in relapse rate among patients while on treatment. They also
found depression of lymphocyte reactivity in vitro during intensive

treatment (24). With some patients, the in vitro changes were somewhat variable (25).

The studies of combination therapy were conducted primarily
with patients who had fulminant disease and who had failed to respond to steroids alone. Further studies with patients in a less
severe state of disease are necessary to evaluate this approach to
treatment.

2. _Imunostimulation_. Stimulation of the immune response with
levamisole was studied in seven MS patients (26). Five of the
patients had increased signs or symptoms of their disease. When
the drug was stopped, one of the five improved but the other four
did not. They were then given immunosuppressive drugs and some
showed signs of clinical improvement. In a second study with this
drug, 15 MS patients remained unchanged, two were worse and two
improved (27). Therefore, the significance of this drug remains
undetermined but treatment of MS patients with it does not seem to
be beneficial.

Transfer factor has also been used to "improve the immune
response" of MS patients. Initial reports were encouraging and it
seemed to increase cellular responses to measles antigens (28). In
a recent study, however, 16 MS patients who participated in a 13-
month double blind clinical trial did not have evidence for arrest
of the progression of their disease (29). There was only some
temporary improvement of the in vitro responses to measles antigens.

3. _Desensitization_. Because of the possible relation between
experimental allergic encephalomyelitis (EAE) and MS, clinical
trials have been proposed in which "desensitization", similar to
that used for EAE would be tried for MS patients. There has always
been concern about such trials since many investigators do not feel
that EAE is a valid model for MS. In addition, there is a potential
risk of increased sensitization of patients with the encephalogenic
material. A study was recently reported in which bovine basic protein (5 mg) was given weekly to 35 MS patients for three to eleven
months (mean 7.5 months) (30). The patients were followed for a
minimum of two years. No deleterious effects were observed, but
the annual relapse rate was not changed. The authors concluded that
"basic protein therapy does not influence the course of MS". The
amount of basic protein used, however, may have been too small for
evaluation of therapeutic benefit.

CONCLUSIONS

The findings for the various tests of cellular immunity are
summarized in Table 2. It should be recognized that in this paper

Table 2. Multiple Sclerosis - Tests of Cellular Immunity

Tests	Findings
A. INTRADERMAL	
Skin Tests	
Brain Extracts	Most patients do not react.
Common Skin Test Antigens, Measles and Mumps Virus Antigens	Normal.
B. IN VITRO	
1. T- to B-Cell Distributions	Possible T-cells reduction during exacerbations. Timing important.
2. Lymphocyte Stimulation	
General mitogens	Normal.
Specific and Common antigens	Normal.
Brain cell antigens	Blood - normal but possibly up after exacerbations.
	CSF - possibly up with active disease. Timing important.
CSF fluid and measles	Normal.
3. Leukocyte Migration	
Brain cell antigens	Variable results. Possible increased reactivity with exacerbations. Timing may be important.
C. CLINICAL TRIALS	
1. Immunosuppression	
Multiple treatments	Possible benefit.
Azathioprine alone	No benefit.
ACTH and antilymphocyte globulin	Probably no benefit.
2. Immunostimulation	
Levamisole	Some worse, others unchanged.
Transfer factor	No value.
3. Desensitization	
Basic protein	No value.

we have only referred to selected studies. Some of the reports are subject to interpretation, extension and further confirmation. The Findings then represent our analysis of the current state of published information in the field.

The reports which do not favor a direct pathologic relationship between cellular immune responses and MS include:

1. No abnormal skin reactions to brain antigens, recall antigens or measles or mumps viral antigens.

2. Some studies find no abnormal T-cell distributions.

3. No general loss of immunocompetence as measured by lymphocyte responses to nonspecific mitogens and common recall antigens.

4. Some reports of a lack of specific cellular responsiveness to brain cell antigens.

5. Some data for no altered migration of leukocytes in response to brain cell antigens.

6. Some clinical trials employing immunosuppressive drugs have failed to show beneficial effects on the outcome of disease.

7. Desensitization with low doses of basic protein was of no value.

8. Treatment with transfer factor was of no value.

The findings which support cellular immunity as a contributor to the clinical course of MS include:

1. Reports of decreased T-cell levels concommittant with exacerbations of MS.

2. Some reports of increased lymphocyte responses to brain antigens just before and for a few weeks after exacerbations.

3. Clinical benefit from use of intensive multiple immunosuppressive treatments.

4. Worsening of patients given immunostimulation with levamisole.

Before the true role of cellular immunity in MS can be established it will be necessary to determine if it is possible to confirm and extend the types of studies noted above. In particular, the several findings which support cellular immunity as a contributor to the clinical course of MS need careful confirmation and then possible extension.

SUMMARY

Cellular immunity has been studied using intradermal tests, in vitro methods and clinical trials with MS patients. Skin tests have generally been normal and there has been no evidence of significant sensitization to brain antigens. In some studies, T-cells have been decreased following attacks. In vitro lymphocyte responses to brain antigens have been increased in some investigations following exacerbations of diseases. There has been one report that these changes preceded the exacerbations. Clinical trials have shown some benefit from multiple drug immunosuppression. Immune stimulation, however, has caused worsening of the disease in some patients.

Unfortunately, both "stimulation" with transfer factor and "desensitization" with basic protein has been of no value under the conditions which they were used for treatment of this disease.

While a number of studies do not support a central role for cellular immunity in MS, several in vitro and clinical reports indicate leads which may be important in demonstrating some role for cellular immunity in the progression of MS. These include: possible decreased levels of T-cells; increased lymphocyte reactivity with exacerbations, as well as clinical studies which seem to have shown some benefit from massive immunosuppression while there was worsening of MS with immunostimulation. Research is needed to determine if these studies can be confirmed and extended.

REFERENCES

1. Cendrowski, W., 1966, Concerning the reaction to encephalito-genic factor in familial multiple sclerosis, *Archivum Immunologiae et Therapiae Experimentalis* 14:491.

2. Cendrowski, W., and Murawski, K., 1966, Skin reactions to myelin antigen and purified encephalitogenic factor in multiple sclerosis, *Archivum Immunologiae et Therapiae Experimentalis* 14:164.

3. Field, E.J., 1965, Some observations on the clinical immunology of multiple sclerosis. In Slow, Latent and Temperate Virus Infections, Monograph 2, pp. 187-192, National Institute of Neurological Diseases and Blindness, Washington, D.C.

4. Davis, L.E., Hersh, E.M., Curtis, J.E., Lynch, R.E., Ziegler, D.K., Neumann, J.W., and Chin, D.Y., 1972, Immune status of patients with multiple sclerosis: analysis of primary and established immune responses in 24 patients, *Neurology* 22:989.

5. Sever, J.L., and Kurtzke, J.F., 1969, Delayed dermal hypersen-
    sitivity to measles and mumps antigens among multiple sclerosis
    and control patients, *Neurology* 19:113.

6. Platz, P., Fog, T., Morling, N., Svejgaard, A., Sonderstrup, G.,
    Ryder, L.P., Thomsen, M., and Jersild, C., Immunological in
    vitro parameters in patients with multiple sclerosis and in
    normal individuals, *Acta. Path. Microbiol. Scand.* 84:501.

7. Kibler, R.F., Paty, D.W., and Sherr, V., 1971, Immunology of
    multiple sclerosis, *Res. Publ. Assoc. Res. Nerv. Ment. Dis.*
    49:95.

8. Symington, G.R., and Mackay, I.R., 1978, Cell-mediated immunity
    to measles virus in multiple sclerosis: correlation with dis-
    ability, *Neurology* 28:109.

9. Gosseye-Lissoir, F., Delmotte, P., and Carton, H., 1977, Bio-
    chemical findings in multiple sclerosis. V. Transformation
    of lymphocytes from patients with multiple sclerosis by human
    basic protein, *J. Neurol.* 216:197.

10. Lisak, R.P., and Zweiman, B, 1977, In vitro cell-mediated
    immunity of cerebrospinal fluid lymphocytes to myelin basic
    protein in primary demyelinating diseases, *N. Engl. J. Med.*
    207:350.

11. Colby, S.P., Sheremata, W., Bain, B., and Eylar, E.H., 1977,
    Cellular hypersensitivity in attacks of multiple sclerosis.
    1. A comparative study of migration inhibitory factor produc-
    tion and lymphoblastic transformation in response to myelin
    basic protein in multiple sclerosis, *Neurology* 27:132.

12. Knowles, M., and Saunders, M., 1970, Lymphocyte stimulation
    with measles antigen in multiple sclerosis, *Neurology* 20:700.

13. Behan, P.O., Behan, W.M.H., Feldman, R.G., and Kies, M.W.,
    1972, Cell-mediated hypersensitivity to neural antigens:
    occurrence in human patients and nonhuman primates with neuro-
    logical diseases, *Arch. Neurol.* 27:145.

14. Day, M.P., Day, J.H., and Mann, P.L., 1976, Direct leukocyte
    migration inhibition in multiple sclerosis - a possible assess-
    ment of activity, *Le Journal Canadien des Sciences Neurologiques*
    3:99.

15. Sheremata, W., Cosgrove, J.B.R., and Eylar, E.H., 1976, Multiple
    sclerosis and cell-mediated hypersensitivity to myelin A protein,
    J. Neurol. Sci. 27:413.

16. Sheremata, W., Triller, H., Cosgrove, J.B.R., and Eylar, E.H.,
    1977, Direct leukocyte migration inhibition by myelin basic
    protein in exacerbations of multiple sclerosis, *CMA Journal*
    116:985.

17. Fuccillo, D.A., Madden, D.L., Castellano, G.A., Uhlig, L.,
    Traub, R.G., Mattson, J., Krezlewicz, A., and Sever, J.L.,
    1978, Multiple sclerosis: cellular and humoral immune re-
    sponses to several viruses, *Neurology* 28:613.

18. Ellison, G.W., and Myers, L.W., 1978, A review of systemic
    nonspecific immunosuppressive treatment of multiple sclerosis,
    Neurology 28:132.

19. Brendel, W., Seifert, J., and Lob, G., 1972, Effect of 'maximum
    immune suppression' with thoracic duct drainage, ALG, azathio-
    prine and cortisone in some neurological disorders, *Proc. Roy.
    Soc. Med.* 65:531.

20. Silberberg, D., Lisak, R., and Zweiman, B., 1973, Multiple
    sclerosis unaffected by azathioprine in pilot study, *Arch.
    Neurol.* 28:210.

21. MacFadyen, D.J., Reeve, C.E., Bratty, P.J.A., and Thomas, J.W.,
    1973, Failure of antilymphocytic globulin therapy in chronic
    progressive multiple sclerosis, *Neurology* 23:592.

22. Ring, J., Lob, G., Angstwurm, H., Brass, B., Backmund, H.,
    Seifert, J., Coulin, K., Frick, E., Mertin, J., and Brendel,
    W., 1974, Intensive immunosuppression in the treatment of
    multiple sclerosis, *The Lancet,* pp. 1093.

23. Lance, E.M., Kremer, M., Abbosh, J., Jones, V.E., Knight, S.,
    and Medawar, P.B., Intensive immunosuppression in patients
    with disseminated sclerosis. I. Clinical response, *Clin.
    Exp. Immunol.* 21:1.

24. Knight, S.C., Lance, E.M., Abbosh, J., Munro, A., and O'Brien,
    J., 1975, Intensive immunosuppression in patients with dissemi-
    nated sclerosis. III. Lymphocyte response in vitro, *Clin.
    Exp. Immunol.* 21:23.

25. Knight, S.C., Abbosh, J., and Lance, E.M., 1976, The effect of
    intensive immunosuppression on the in vitro activity of lympho-
    cytes from multiple sclerosis patients, *Postgraduate Medical
    Journal* 52:S131.

26. Dau, P.C., Johnson, K.P., and Spitler, L.E., 1976, The effect
     of levamisole on cellular immunity in multiple sclerosis, *Clin.
     Exp. Immunol.* 26: 302.

27. Cendrowski, W., and Czionkowska, A., 1978, Levamisole in multi-
     ple sclerosis with special reference to immunological parameters.
     A pilot study, *Acta. Neurol. Scandinav.* 57:354.

28. Zabriskie, J.B., Utermohlen, V., Espinoza, L.R., Plank, C.R.,
     and Collins, R.C., 1975, Immunologic studies with transfer
     factor in multiple sclerosis patients, *Neurology* p. 490, May.

29. Fog, T., Raun, N.E., Pedersen, L., Kam-Hansen, S., Mellerup,
     E., Platz, P., Ryder, L.P., Jakobsen, B.K., and Grob, P., 1978,
     Long-term transfer-factor treatment for multiple sclerosis,
     The Lancet pp. 851.

30. Gonsette, R.E., Delmotte, P., and Demonty, L., 1977, Failure
     of basic protein therapy for multiple sclerosis, *J. Neurol.*
     216:27.

CELLULAR IMMUNOLOGY IN MULTIPLE SCLEROSIS

RESPONSE TO SEVERAL VIRUSES

D.L. Madden, W.C. Wallen and J.L. Sever

National Institutes of Health, NINCDS
Bethesda, Maryland, U.S.A.

INTRODUCTION

In the past few years a number of studies have been conducted
on possible altered immune responses to viruses in patients with
multiple sclerosis (MS). Several groups, including our own, have
found slightly increased measles antibody levels in MS patients
(1,2). Recently, altered cellular immune responses to measles
have been reported (5). Other studies have suggested the association of measles and an unidentified agent with MS (3,4,5,6,7,8).

Our present studies focused on specific immune responses to
viruses in patients with MS and carefully matched controls. We
also looked for possible cellular immune stimulatory or inhibitory
factors in the sera and cerebrospinal fluids (CSF) of another group
of MS patients and controls. A variety of techniques were used to
test for changes in humoral and cellular immunity. For detection
of humoral immunity, we used the complement fixation (CF) and hemagglutination inhibition (HI) tests as well as the complement mediated cytotoxicity (CMC) assay. A comparison of the humoral response
and HLA antigen was made. For cellular immunity studies we employed
direct migration inhibition (DMI), lymphocyte-mediated cytotoxicity
(LMC) and lymphocyte rosetting on measles infected cells.

MATERIALS AND METHODS

Patients

Sera and lymphocytes were obtained from 108 patients and their paired controls from the Milwaukee, Wisconsin area. Diagnosis of MS was based upon history, clinical signs, symptoms and laboratory findings. The following criteria were used for matching of controls: a) same sex; b) age ± 12 years; c) born and lived in the same general location (within a 50 mile radius) for the first 15 years of life; and d) have known each other for the past 10 years. Ten of the patients were on steroid treatment. Blood was collected from both groups on the same day. Samples from 12 MS patients and pal controls were collected, immediately taken to our laboratory and tested within five hours. An aliquot of each of these samples was also tested after being held for 18 hours. These tests showed no significant differences and all other paired specimens were shipped to our laboratory and tested within 18 hours after collection.

CSF samples from 13 MS patients were obtained from Dr. Boines of Wilmington, Delaware. Control CSF were obtained from three patients diagnosed as migraine, one as Influenza B encephalitis, two as cerebrovascular accidents and one as herniated disc.

Humoral Immune Tests

1. <u>Virus Antibodies</u>. Measles antibody was determined by the CF and HI techniques. Antibody to Herpes Simplex virus, types I and II (HSVI and II) and cytomegalovirus (CMV) was determined by indirect hemagglutination (IHA). The methods used have been reported previously (9).

2. <u>Complement-Mediated Cytotoxicity (CMC)</u>. The technique used for the determination of complement-mediated ^{51}Cr release was with slight modification similar to the test previously described (10). The target cells were frozen human prostate (MA-160) cells chronically infected (90% membrane antigen positive) with the Mantooth strain of Subacute Sclerosing Panencephalitis (SSPE) measles virus (MA-72046). Frozen control target cells consisting of the parent MA-160 cells were also used. Radiolabeled (^{51}Cr) target cells (1 X 10^4 cells) were added to test serum and unheated adult guinea pig serum (complement source) in microtiter plate wells. After 18 hours incubation at 37°C in a 5% CO_2 atmosphere incubator, the plates were centrifuged at 1500 g for 20 minutes and aliquots of supernatant fluid were removed and the release of ^{51}Cr was determined with a Packard Auto-gamma counter. The percentage of Specific

Immune Release (SIR) as determined by the Kibler and ter Meulen formula (10) was used as an index of immune cytolysis of the test serum:

$$\% \text{ SIR} = \frac{\begin{array}{l}\text{counts per minute from} \\ \text{complement and serum}\end{array} - \begin{array}{l}\text{counts per minute for} \\ \text{spontaneous release}\end{array}}{\begin{array}{l}\text{counts per minute} \\ \text{total}\end{array} - \begin{array}{l}\text{counts per minute} \\ \text{spontaneous release}\end{array}} \text{ X } 100$$

Cellular Immune Tests

1. Direct Migration Inhibition (DMI). The DMI assay of peripheral blood leukocytes as originally described by Bendixen and modified by Utermohlen and Zabriskie was used (12). The leukocytes were obtained from gelatin sedimentation of peripheral blood, washed once in saline, treated with 0.83% ammonium chloride and resuspended in RPMI-1640 medium with 10% heat inactivated fetal calf serum at 2 X 10^7 leukocytes per ml. Capillary tubes were loaded, sealed with clay and centrifuged at 300 g for 10 minutes. The tubes were cut at the medium-cell interface and placed in planchettes (York Scientific, Ogdensburg, N.Y.). Measles antigen (Flow No. M-44034), Edmonston strain measles virus CF antigen (3-5878) and a vaccinia hemagglutination (HA) antigen (3-5503) produced by Microbiological Associates were used in this test. In addition, soluble cell pack antigens of Herpesvirus I and II and CMV were prepared as described by Fuccillo et al. (9) for the IHA test. Control antigen was prepared from the same lot of tissue in the same manner as the virus infected antigen. The planchettes were incubated at 37°C for 18 hours in a 5% CO_2 atmosphere. The resultant fans (migration of lymphocytes) were measured with a planimeter. The migration index was calculated as:

$$\text{MI} = \frac{\text{area of migration with antigen}}{\text{area of migration without antigen}} \text{ X } 100$$

The figure obtained from the above calculation was substracted from 100% to determine the precentage migration inhibition.

2. Lymphocyte-Mediated Cytotoxicity (LMC). The technique used for determination of lymphocyte-mediated cytotoxicity was similar to that described by Steel et al. (11). Cells persistently infected with SSPE measles virus (MA-72046) and controls as previously described for the CMC assay were used in these studies. Frozen human foreskin (MA-184) infected with CMV (50% antigen positive) and control target cells consisting of parent MA-184 cells were labeled with ^{51}Cr as previously described and resuspended to a final concentration of 1 X 10^5 cells/ml.

Approximately 20 ml of peripheral blood was collected and the lymphocytes were separated by Ficoll-Hypaque centrifugation at 1000 g for 45 minutes. The cells were washed once and counted in a cytograph. In each test, 0.05 ml of target or control cells (5×10^3 cells) was placed in microtiter plate wells with five dilutions of lymphocytes (2.5×10^4 to 4.0×10^5 per 0.1 ml media). For each patient studied, 0.1 ml of each dilution of lymphocytes was added to six wells of infected and six wells of control cells. After incubation for 18 or 24 hours at 37°C in a 5% CO_2 incubator, the plates were centrifuged at 430 g for 20 minutes and aliquots of supernatant fluid were removed and counted for released ^{51}Cr. The percentage SIR was determined as follows:

$$\% \text{ SIR} = \frac{(I^L - I) - (C^L - C)}{(Ti - I) - (Tc - C)} \times 100$$

I^L = ^{51}Chromium released by labeled infected target cells and lymphocytes.

I = ^{51}Chromium released by labeled infected cells spontaneously.

Ti = Total amount of ^{51}Chromium attached to infected cells divided by the percent of the total volume.

C^1 = ^{51}Chromium released by labeled control cells and lymphocytes.

C = ^{51}Chromium released by labeled control cells spontaneously.

Tc = Total amount of ^{51}Chromium attached to control cells divided by the percent of the total volume.

3. <u>Stimulation or Blocking Factors</u>. The technique used was similar to the one described by Steel et al. (13). In each test 0.05 ml of media containing 5×10^3 cells was placed in microtiter plate wells. To each well 0.05 ml of diluted test serum (1:10) or CSF (1:3) was added and incubated at 37°C for one hour. Lymphocytes from a person with a positive response to measles virus were added at 4×10^5 per 0.15 ml. Percent blocking (13) or stimulation (14) was calculated by subtracting the SIR of the serum or CSF from the SIR of the donor lymphocytes and dividing by the SIR of the donor lymphocytes.

4. <u>Rosette Technique</u>. The lymphocyte rosette technique described by Levy et al. (5) was used. Briefly, lymphocytes from 38 MS and matched controls were obtained and resuspended to a concentration of 4×10^6 cells/ml. The MA-72046 measles infected cell line and MA-106 parent cells were resuspended to 4×10^5 cells/ml. One ml of lymphocytes and one ml of tissue culture cells were mixed,

centrifuged and gently resuspended. Triplicate samples were examined in a hemacytometer for rosette formation. Cells with three or more lymphocytes attached were considered positive and expressed as percent of the specific measles rosettes using the following formula:

$$\frac{\text{Mean of rosette counted}}{\begin{array}{l}\text{Mean of measles infected}\\\text{cells counted}\end{array}} - \frac{\text{Mean of rosette counted}}{\begin{array}{l}\text{Mean of control cells}\\\text{counted}\end{array}} \times 100$$

HLA and DW$_2$ Determination. The HLA and DW$_2$ antigen types were determined by Dr. Paul Terasaki, UCLA, Los Angeles, California as previously described (20).

Statistical Analysis. The difference between MS patients and matched "pal" controls were analyzed by the Student's two-tailed "t" test or χ^2 using the Yates correction factor for small numbers.

RESULTS

Humoral Immune Tests

1. Virus Antibodies. Antibody levels of the 108 pairs of MS patients and matched controls are presented in Table 1. There was a slight but significant increase in the level of the measles CF and HI titers in the MS patients as compared to controls ($p<0.01$). However, there was no difference in the level of HSV-I and II and CMV antibody titers between MS patients and controls.

2. Complement-Mediated Cytotoxicity. The mean amount of SIR obtained using 1:10 dilution of serum was 44.6% for MS patients and 47.7% for "pal" controls. Patients receiving steroids were not significantly different from those not on steroids ($p = 0.1$). The mean titer, log 2, for MS patients was 7.40 and for "pal" controls 6.68 (significant difference at $p<0.02$) (Table 2). Inclusion of titer from patients on steroids only slightly depressed the cytotoxic mean titer of the MS patients and removal of these titers from the analysis increased the significance in their differences to $p<0.001$. The mean titer, log 2 by CF test was 3.9 for MS patients and 2.8 for "pal" controls (significant at the $p<0.001$ level).

Cellular Immune Tests

1. Direct Migration Inhibition. A comparison of the amount of DMI of lymphocytes obtained from 12 MS patients and "pal" controls when tested 5 and 18 hours after collection showed no significant difference observed in response between MS and "pal" controls.

Table 1. Serological Responses of MS Patients and Matched Controls

Antigen	Patient Pairs	Mean Titer Log 2 MS Patient/ Control	Standard Error of the Means MS Patient/ Control
Measles			
HI	108[a]	3.56/3.13*	1.61/1.48
	98[b]	3.58/3.10*	1.62/1.48
	10[c]	3.4 / 3.5	1.65/1.51
CF	108	3.91/2.94**	1.89/1.91
	98	3.93/2.85**	1.92/1.91
	10	3.7 / 3.8	1.57/1.75
Herpes I (IHA)	97	6.44/6.38	3.02/3.21
	89	6.49/6.46	3.0 /3.16
	8	5.87/5.5	3.40/3.80
Herpes II (IHA)	93	4.56/4.59	2.2 /2.58
	85	4.54/4.65	2.15/2.59
	8	4.75/4.0	2.82/2.56
CMV (IHA)	89	4.43/5.07	2.82/2.75
	80	4.62/5.26	2.79/2.69
	9	2.67/3.33	2.55/2.78

 * = Significant difference at the $p = <0.05$ level.
** = Significant difference at the $p = <0.0001$ level.
 a = Total number of patients studied.
 b = Number of patients studied that had not been treated with
     steroids for the past 6 months.
 c = Number of patients presently being treated with steroids.

     The results obtained using the DMI test are presented in
Table 3. No significant difference between the reaction of lymphocytes from MS and "pal" controls was observed for any of the six
antigens tested except for the Microbiological Associates measles
antigen at a 1:1000 dilution. The difference in the mean percent
DMI at this dilution was significant at the $p = <0.05$ level, indicating that the measles antigen at this level caused an increase
in the stimulation of the lymphocytes. No correlation could be
found between cellular immune activity for measles as measured with
DMI and humoral immunity as measured by the CF tests (Figure 1).
There was also no correlation between DMI results for any of the
viruses tested and humoral immunity as measured by the HI or IHA
tests.

Table 2. Cytotoxic Antibody Response of MS and Matched Controls
          to Measles Virus Antigen

	No. of Pairs	Mean Titer Log 2 MS Patient/Control	Standard Error of Mean
All MS Patients	60	7.40/6.68*	.19/.19
MS Patients No Steroids	53	7.50/6.60**	.20/.20
MS Patients Steroids	7	6.57/7.28	.56/.57

  * = Significant at the p = <0.02 level.
 ** = Significant at the p = <0.001 level.

2. Lymphocyte Mediated Cytotoxicity. The cytotoxicity of
lymphocytes from MS patients and "pal" controls on cells infected
with measles and CMV are presented in Table 5. The amount of SIR,
using a lymphocyte:target cell ratio of 200:1 was 31.2% for the MS
patient and 30.49% for the "pal" controls. Although a higher ratio
of lymphocytes to target cells was required to effect a response
with the CMV infected cells, the amount of SIR produced was 13.53%
for MS patients and 16.62% for "pal" controls at a ratio of 80:1.
Regardless of the ratio used for both antigens, no significant
difference in SIR were detected between the response of MS patients
and controls. Elimination of MS patients treated with steroids did
not significantly change the mean results.

An analysis of the results of measles LMC and CF or HI data
showed no correlation between the tests. A comparison of the
two cellular immune tests, the DMI and LMC showed that there was
no correlation between them (Figure 2).

3. Stimulation or Blocking Factors. The results obtained when
testing sera and CSF for stimulation or blocking factors are presented in Figure 3. Treatment of the target cells with MS sera
resulted in a mean percentage blocking of lymphocyte activity of
-19.57 whereas for the "pal" controls the blocking was -22.67.
These differences were not significant. The mean percentage
blocking of CSF from MS patients was -22.6 and -44.7 for controls.
These differences also were not significant at the p = 0.1 level.

4. Rosetting. The mean percentage of measles specific rosette
formation was similar for MS patients (31 ± 16.5) as for matched
controls (33.5 ± 16.9) (Figure 4). In two laboratory personnel

Table 3. The Response of Lymphocytes of MS Patients and Controls
to Various Antigens as Measured by the Direct Migration
Inhibition Assay

Antigen	Patient Pairs	Mean Percent + DMI MS Patient/Control	Standard Error of the Mean MS Patient/Control
Measles			
Flow			
1/10*	53[a]	15.06/17.43	10.95/9.31
	49[b]	16.14/17.41	9.13/9.51
1/100	53	5.53/3.60	12.01/10.72
	49	4.90/3.65	11.23/10.91
Micro			
1/100	41	22.41/21.20	11.19/16.98
	38	22.29/20.18	11.16/16.91
1/1000	34	6.65/1.74**	9.64/10.87
	31	6.94/1.71**	9.53/11.31
Herpes I			
1/100	64	.953/ .953	14.08/11.49
	57	.772/ .246	13.53/11.56
1/1000	70	-2.2 /-1.1	22.86/15.19
	63	-2.94/-.809	23.48/15.88
Herpes II			
1/100	44	2.61/2.59	13.83/18.03
	41	3.33/1.78	13.75/13.99
1/1000	43	.511/2.37	26.6 /14.67
	40	.6 / .57	27.61/12.23
Vaccinia			
1/10	13	-2.15/-9.84	15.13/25.67
	12	-2.66/-9.5	15.69/26.78
1/100	13	-4.31/-1.69	11.34/19.94
	12	-3.5 /-.33	11.45/14.74
CMV			
1/10	22	-1. /-3.45	17.69/15.72
	21	-2.57/-3.24	13.03/16.08
1/100	22	-7.32/-3.32	15.28/25.68
	21	-7.67/-6.48	15.56/21.5

a = Total number of patients studied.
b = Number of patients studied that had not been treated with
    steroids for the past 6 months.
 * = Dilution of antigen used.
** = Significant at the p = <0.05.

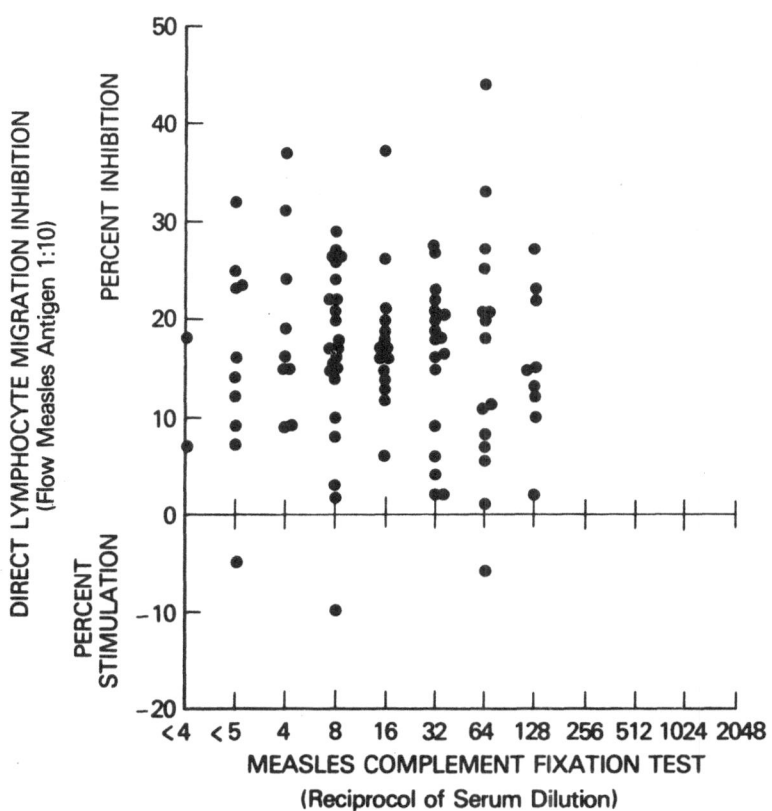

Figure 1. Relationship between humoral immunity (complement-
           fixation) and cellular immunity (direct migration
           inhibition).

tested, the specific rosette formation was 32.7 ± 15.0 for one and
20.9 ± 6.1 for the other. Rosette formation for the MS patients
on the MA-160 control cells was 12.6 ± 10.6 and for the matched
controls 12.3 ± 9.1.

HLA and DW$_2$ Determination

    The HLA antigen frequency for 72 MS patients and matched "pal"
controls are presented in Tables 5 and 6. The HLA-A3 antigen was
increased in MS patient compared to controls (38% vs. 32%). Both
of these values are significantly higher than that for the average

Table 4. The Response of Lymphocytes of MS Patients and Controls
          to Measles and CMV Antigens as Measured by the Lymphocyte
          Cytotoxic Assay

Antigen	Patient Pairs	Mean Specific Release MS Patient/Control	Standard Error of the Mean MS Patient/Control
Measles Virus (SSPE)			
200:1*	20[a]	31.27/30.49	17.86/14.9
	18[b]	32.24/32.26	15.27/14.35
80:1	23	25.64/24.32	19.06/15.64
	21	25.83/25.11	19.72/15.55
40:1	30	27.94/22.84	16.46/11.83
	27	28.18/22.87	16.86/12.25
20:1	45	23.16/23.57	15.70/15.08
	41	23.23/23.71	16.20/15.23
10:1	30	11.63/14.38	12.23/10.66
	27	11.42/14.48	12.26/10.82
5:1	30	9.54/9.40	10.59/10.27
	27	9.90/9.14	11.03/10.24
2.5:1	8	.95/2.89	4.92/3.96
	7	4.85/3.53	5.12/3.80
CMV			
80	28	13.53/16.62	16.73/11.35
	25	13.31/17.21	16.65/11.74
40	34	5.39/9.17	10.51/11.98
	31	5.48/9.69	10.53/12.41
20	36	1.34/2.41	6.22/10.10
	32	1.2 /3.37	6.12/9.89
10	36	-.15/2.1	6.07/6.69
	32	-5.62/2.22	4.82/6.84
5	35	-1.39/-.103	3.83/4.68
	31	-1.29/ .17	3.98/4.63

a = Total number of patients studied.
b = Number of patients studied that had not been treated with
    steroids for the past 6 months.
* = Ratio of lymphocytes to target cell.

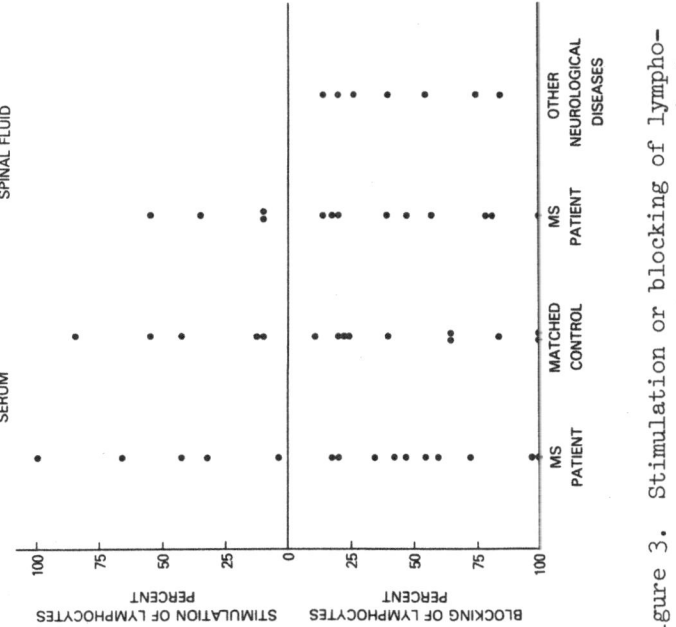

Figure 3. Stimulation or blocking of lymphocyte activity by serum or spinal
fluid from MS patients and controls.

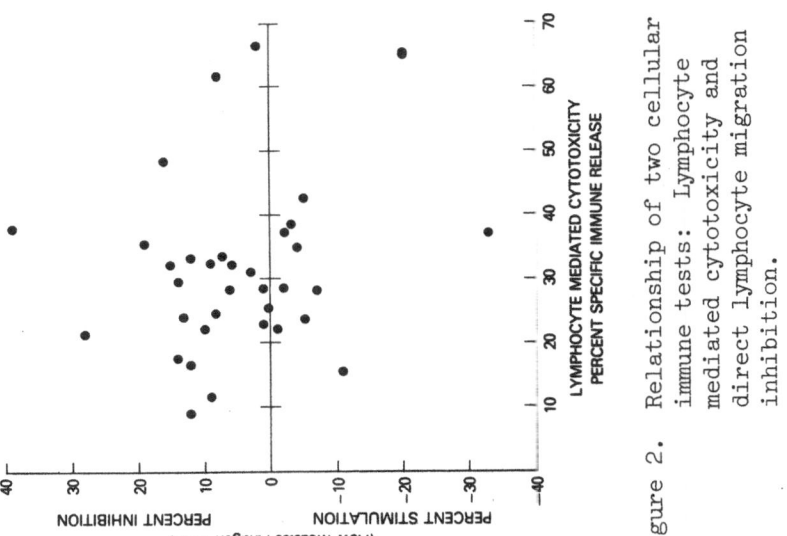

Figure 2. Relationship of two cellular
immune tests: Lymphocyte
mediated cytotoxicity and
direct lymphocyte migration
inhibition.

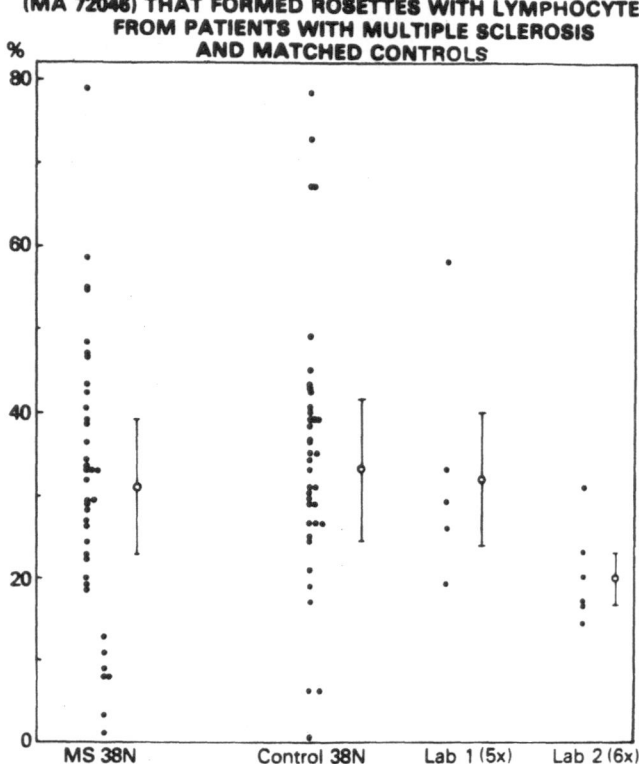

Figure 4. Measles specific rosetting by lymphocytes from MS
           patients, matched controls and laboratory controls.

American population (24%). The frequencies of the HLA-B7 and B8
loci in the MS patients were elevated also, as compared to the
matched controls. The frequency of the HLA-B7 loci was also elevated when compared to the U.S. population; however, the HLA-B8
loci in MS patients was not significantly elevated over the population in general. The frequency of HLA-B12 in MS was decreased
compared to controls; however, compared to the U.S. population,
only a significant decrease in the frequency of the HLA-B12 loci
in the MS patients was identified.

     The frequencies of the measles and HSV-II antibodies in MS
patients and matched controls as associated with HLA antigen type
are presented in Table 7. Although the measles antibody titer was
consistently higher in MS patients compared to controls, none of

Table 5. HLA Antigen Frequency in MS Patients and Matched Controls

HLA A Loci	MS Patients POS**	Frequency	Controls POS	Frequency	U.S. Population* Frequency
A1	23	31.9	20	27.7	30.9
A2	35	48.6	33	45.8	44.1
A3	28	38	22	30.5	23.2
A6	1	1.4	-	-	-
A11	6	8.3	7	9.7	8.7
A23	6	8.3	4	5.5	22.7
A24	14		13	18.5	
A25	4	5.5	1	1.4	11.0
A26	7	9.7	8	11.1	
A28	2	2.8	5	6.9	6.5
A29	3	4.2	5	6.9	8.0
A30	-		3	4.2	
A31	2	2.8	6	8.3	
A32	5	6.9	7	9.7	16.7
A33	-		1	1.4	

*Caucasian - 401 subjects.
**Number of people with this HLA antigen.

the HLA antigen types was significantly elevated from the others to account for this. The frequency of HSV-II antibody in the MS patients and controls was similar. Similar results were also found for HSV-I and CMV.

The distribution of DW_2 antigen in MS patients and matched controls is presented in Table 8. A significant increase in the frequency of DW_2 in the MS patients was found.

DISCUSSION

The possible viral etiology of MS has been based primarily on epidemiological data (1,2,15). The disease is generally most common in the northern latitudes. Population migration studies have shown that the exposure to the primary agent which causes MS almost certainly takes place before 15 years of age (15). These findings were considered important and influenced our selection of an MS population from Milwaukee with stringent criteria in the selection of controls. In this location, patients and controls could be selected who had been born in the same area, resided there and knew each other for the last 10 years.

Table 6.   HLA Antigen Frequency in MS Patients and Matched Controls

| HLA B Loci | MS Patients | | Controls | | U.S. Population* |
	POS**	Frequency	POS	Frequency	Frequency
B5	8	11.1	5	15.3	11.2
B7	28	38.8	18	25	23.7
B8	21	29.1	13	18.5	22.2
B12	11	15.3	15	20.8	26.9
B13	3	4.2	4	5.5	3.5
B14	4	5.5	6	8.3	7.2
B15	7	9.7	9	12.5	7.5
B17	5	6.9	8	11.1	5.7
B18	11	15.3	7	9.6	2
B21	2	2.8	5	6.9	4.6
B22	3	4.2	1	1.4	3.0
B24	1	1.4	-	-	-
B27	9	12.5	13	18.5	9.2
B35	7	9.7	13	18.5	18.5
B37	5	6.9	2	2.8	-
B38	2	2.8	4	5.5	-
B39	3	4.2	2	2.8	-
B40	5	6.9	8	11.1	15.5

*Caucasian - 401 subjects.
**Number of people with this HLA antigen.

    Serum measles antibody levels were found by others to be higher
in MS patients than in controls (1,2) and our results for CF and HI
tests confirm these studies.   However, there was no significant
increase in the level of antibody titers to HSV-I and II and CMV.
This indicated that the humoral immune system of MS patients was
not hyperactive in general.   The CMC antibody test similarly showed
that MS patients had significantly higher titers than "pal" controls.
Inclusion of patients on steroids caused a depression of the measles
antibody titers but not sufficient to eliminate the distinction from
controls.

    Cellular immune responses against several viruses using the
DMI and LMC techniques were used to determine whether MS patients
had sensitized lymphocytes to specific viral antigens.   The results
obtained in the DMI did not conform to the pilot study previously
reported by our laboratory (19) nor with those obtained by Utermohlen and Zabriskie (12).   In our previous study on 15 patients
and controls from the Washington, D.C. area, an impairment of leukocyte migration inhibition by cells from MS patients was found only
with the 1:100 dilution of the Flow measles antigen.   The MS lymphocytes were not affected when a Microbiological Associates measles

Table 7.　Frequency of Antibody in Multiple Sclerosis Patients and Controls as Related to HLA Antigen

| | Measles HI Antibody | | | | Herpes II Antibody | | | |
| | MS Patients | | Pal Controls | | MS Patients | | Pal Controls | |
	No. of Patients	Titers*	No. of Controls	Titers	No. of Patients	Titers	No. of Controls	Titers
HLA-A								
1	23	3.76	20	2.61	23	6.31	20	5.0
2	35	3.29	33	3.0	35	6.70	33	6.71
3	28	3.22	22	3.9	28	6.22	22	5.95
11	6	3.83	7	2.7	6	7.0	7	5.71
23	6	3.0	4	2.75	6	5.8	4	4.25
24	14	3.46	13	3.66	14	4.66	13	3.83
26	7	3.14	8	2.57	7	6.28	8	6.57
32	5	3.8	7	3.71	5	6.2	7	5.71
HLA-B								
5	8	3.75	5	2.5	8	8.37	5	6.25
7	28	3.23	18	3.17	28	4.8	18	6.64
8	21	3.44	13	2.66	21	6.55	13	5.25
12	11	3.55	15	2.8	11	6.22	15	5.0
15	7	2.85	9	2.5	7	6.71	9	7.25
18	11	3.81	7	2.71	11	5.0	7	7.57
27	9	3.4	13	2.9	9	6.81	13	5.38
35	7	4.4	13	3.46	7	5.71	13	5.38

*Mean titer, $\log_2$.

Table 8. Frequency of DW_2 Antigen in MS Patients and Matched
          Controls

	DW_2 Positive	DW_2 Negative	Frequency DW_2
MS	20	10	66.6%
Controls	15	15	50%

antigen or a parinfluenza type 1 antigen were used. In the present
study, we observed a trend towards stimulation instead of depression
of lymphocytes with the Flow measles antigen at a dilution of 1:100
and a significant stimulation with the Microbiological Associates
measles antigen at 1:1000 dilution. The inconsistency of the results
from these two studies using the same measles antigen is difficult
to explain. In our previous study, MS patients were matched with
controls on the basis of age, sex and acquaintanceship for the last
five years. The study group was quite transient and had previously
lived in various parts of the United States. This completely ig-
nored the epidemiological findings that MS infections are more
common in the northern parts of the United States and that acquisi-
tion of infection and/or immunity is thought to occur during the
first 15 years of life. In the present study, the fact that a
larger number of patients and controls were studied and matching
included not only sex, age and association but the same areas of
residence for the first 15 years of life. It is possible that the
larger study and closer matching resulted in the elimination of the
apparent differences in cellular immunity previously reported.

The results obtained using the LMC assay indicated that the
cytotoxic reactivity of lymphocytes from MS patients was similar
to that of matched "pal" controls. The test results of the high
to low ratios of lymphocytes to target cells indicate that the MS
patients' lymphocytotoxic reaction against measles and CMV infected
cells was no more or less active against the antigen than lymphocytes from the "pal" controls.

An additional study using the LMC assay for detection of stimulation or blocking factor was also performed. A substance which
blocks reactivity of lymphocytes in the recognition of measles
infected target cells has been found in the sera and CSF of SSPE
patients (13). In these studies, no evidence of stimulation or
blocking factor was found in the MS sera as compared to control
sera. The difference in effect of MS and control CSF were not
statistically significant and may be related to the heterogenous
nature of the control CSF.

Levy et al. (5) suggested a blood test for MS based upon adherence of lymphocytes to measles infected cells. Offner et al. (24) reported that although they found lymphocytes from MS patients had a considerably higher percentage of rosettes, the values over-lapped with controls, thus, suggesting that a relationship similar to measles antibody in serum may exist. We found no differences between the ability of lymphocytes from MS patients or controls to react with measles infected cells. This is in agreement with our studies using LMC and DMI techniques.

It has been suggested that the genotype particularly HLA and DW_2 determinants of individuals may be associated, at least in part, with responsiveness to disease processes (16,17,18,21). An elevated frequency of HLA-A3 and B7 and a decrease in HLA-A2 and B12 among MS patients has been reported. Our study, except for the A2 loci, showed a similar tendency and depending upon the control used, the statistical significance of these observations may change. Our data also indicated that the DW_2 antigen occurs more often in MS patients; however, its significance is unknown.

The role of specific HLA antigens in antibody production has been suggested (16,22,23). Our study indicates that the elevated measles antibody titers in MS was not associated with a specific genotype, but that a general pattern of increased measles antibody levels for all genotypes exists in MS patients. Using other viruses HSV-I and II and CMV, no one gene seemed to be consistently associated with elevated antibody response in these closely matched individuals. Our data, thus, does not indicate an association of virus antibody production with a specific HLA genotype.

The data presented here from both types of cellular immune studies, DMI and LMC, in contrast to others (12,19) indicated that MS patients have the same capabilities of reacting to measles virus as controls. The very careful matching of "pal" controls in our studies may have eliminated several variables such as differences in exposure to various antigens differences in genotypes and environmental factors. Thus, apparent differences in cellular immunity may have been eliminated.

SUMMARY

Elevated measles antibodies in MS patients was detected using CF or HI tests, and the CMC test. No increase in antibody titers to HSV-I and II or CMV was found. Cellular immune studies using the DMI technique showed no difference between MS and matched control patients with measles virus, CMV, HSV-I and II or Vaccinia virus antigens. Using the LMC tests, no difference between the

MS and matched controls using cultures infected with measles and
CMV was observed. No stimulation or blocking of the LMC by serum
from 15 MS patients and matched controls and cerebrospinal fluid
serum from 13 MS and seven neurological controls was found. No
increase in lymphocyte rosetting of measles infected cells by MS
patients was observed. Thus, in our study, while increased levels
of measles antibody in serum and elevation in frequency of the
HLA-B7 genotype was again demonstrated for the MS patients, there
was no difference in the cellular immunity against measles virus
nor humoral and cellular immunity against the other viruses tested.

REFERENCES

1. Brody, J., Sever, J.L., Edgar, A., and McNew, J., 1972,
    Measles antibody titers of multiple sclerosis patients and
    their siblings, *Neurology* 22:492.

2. Adams, J., and Imagawa, D., 1962, Measles antibodies in
    multiple sclerosis, *Proc. Soc. Exp. Biol. Med.* 111:562.

3. Carp, R.I., Licursi, P.C., Merz, P.A., and Merz, G.S., 1972,
    Decrease percentage of polymorphonucelar neutrophils in mouse
    peripheral blood after inoculation with material from multiple
    sclerosis patients, *J. Exper. Med.* 136:618.

4. Carp, R.I., Licursi, P.C., and Merz, G.S., 1975, Multiple
    sclerosis induced reduction in the yield of a mouse cell
    line, *Infect. Immun.* 11:737.

5. Levy, N.L., Auerbach, P.S., and Hayes, E.C., 1976, A blood
    test for multiple sclerosis based on the adherence of lympho-
    cytes to measles infected cells, *N. Engl. J. Med.* 294:1423.

6. Pertschuk, L.P., Cook, A.W., and Gupta, J., 1976, Measles
    antigen in multiple sclerosis: Identification in the jejunum
    by immunofluorescence, *Life Sci.* 19:1603.

7. Koldovsky, U., Koldovsky, P., Henle, G., Henle, W., Ackermann,
    R., and Haasse, G., 1975, Multiple sclerosis associated agent:
    transmission to animals and some properties of the agent,
    Infect. Immun. 12:1355.

8. Henle, G., Koldovsky, U., Koldovsky, P., Henle, W., Ackerman,
    R., and Haasse, G., 1976, Multiple sclerosis associated agent.
    Neutralization of the agent by human sera, *Infect. Immun.* 12:
    1367.

9. Fuccillo, D.A., Moder, F.L., Catalano, L.W., Vincent, M.M., and Sever, J.L., 1970, Herpesvirus hominis type I and II. A specific micro-indirect hemagglutination test, *Proc. Soc. Biol. Med.* 133:735.

10. Kibler, R., and ter Meulen, V., 1975, Antibody-mediated cyto-toxicity after measles virus infection, *J. Immunol.* 114:93.

11. Steele, R.W., Hensen, S.A., Vincent, M.M., Fuccillo, D.A., and Bellanti, J.H., 1973, A ^{51}Cr microassay technique for cell-mediated immunity to viruses, *J. Immunol.* 110:1502.

12. Utermohlen, V., and Zabriskie, J.B., 1973, A suppression of cell-mediated immunity in patients with multiple sclerosis, *J. Exp. Med.* 138:1591.

13. Steele, R.W., Fuccillo, D.A., Hensen, S.A., Vincent, M.M., and Bellanti, J.A., 1976, Specific inhibitory factors of cellular immunity in children with subacute sclerosing panencephalitis, *J. Pediatr.* 88:56.

14. Prevost, J., Orr, T.W., and Pearson, G.R., 1975, Augmentation of lymphocyte cytotoxicity by antibody to Herpesvirus saimiri associated antigens, *Proc. Nat. Acad. Sci.* 72:1671.

15. Kurtzke, J.F., Kurland, L.T., Goldberg, I.D., and Choi, N.W., 1973, Multiple Sclerosis: Kurland, L.T., Kurtzke, J.F., and Goldberg, I.D. (eds.) Epidemiology of Neurologic and Sense Organ Disorders, Harvard University Press, Cambridge, Mass.

16. Myers, L.W., Ellison, G.W., Feurster, M.E., Teraski, P., and Opetz, G., 1976, HLA and the immune response to measles in multiple sclerosis, *Neurology* 26:54.

17. Winchester, R.J., Ebers, G., Fu, S.M., Espinosa, L., Zabriskie, J., and Kunkel, H.G., 1975, B-cell alloantigens Ag 7a in multi-ple sclerosis, *The Lancet* ii:814.

18. Jersild, C., Fog, T., Hansen, G.S., Thomsen, M., Svejgoard, A., and Dupont, B., 1973, Histocompatibility determinants in multiple sclerosis with special reference to clinical course, *The Lancet* ii:1221.

19. Fuccillo, D.A., Abela, J.E., Traub, R.G., Gillespie, M.M., Beadle, E.L., and Sever, J.L., 1975, Cellular immunity in patients with multiple sclerosis, *The Lancet* i:980.

20. Opelz, G., Terasaki, P., Myers, L., Ellison, G., Ebers, G.,
     Zabriskie, J., Kempe, H., Sibley, W., and Sever, J., 1976,
     HLA-D locus typing in 350 patients with multiple sclerosis,
     In The First International Symposium on the HLA and Disease,
     Paris, June 1976, ISERM, Paris.

21. Alter, M.M., Harshe, M., Anderson, V.E., Emme, L., and Yunis,
     E.J., 1976, Genetic association of multiple sclerosis and HLA-A
     determinants, *Neurology* 26:31.

22. Ilones, J., Herva, E., Reunanen, M., Panelius, M., Meurman, O.,
     Arstila, P., and Tiilikaines, A., 1977, HLA antigens and anti-
     body responses to measles and rubella viruses in multiple
     sclerosis, *Acta. Neurol. Scand.* 55:299.

23. Paty, D., Furesz, J., Boucher, W., Rand, C.G., and Stiller,
     C.R., 1976, Measles antibodies as related to HLA types in
     multiple sclerosis, *Neurology* 26:651.

24. Offner, H., Konat, G., and Clausen, J., 1977, A blood test
     for multiple sclerosis, *N. Eng. J. Med.* 296:451.

CELLULAR IMMUNOLOGY IN MULTIPLE SCLEROSIS

STUDIES ON IMMUNE REGULATORY CELLS

W.C. Wallen, J.L. Sever and D.L. Madden

National Institutes of Health, NINCDS
Bethesda, Maryland, U.S.A.

INTRODUCTION

Multiple sclerosis (MS) is a chronic inflammatory disease of the central nervous system (CNS). Although the etiology of MS remains undefined, many have suggested that immune mechanisms play a central role in the pathogenesis of the disease. Two hypotheses for the pathogenesis of MS have recently received widespread interest: 1) the disease is the result of a chronic viral infection which is not controlled due to a faulty immune response; and 2) the disease is an autoimmune response resulting from an inherent immunological defect. These hypotheses may not be mutually exclusive in that chronic viral infection may result in altered immune function and autoimmunity.

Recently, several studies have shown that the distribution of lymphoid subpopulations is altered in some MS patients compared with normal individuals (1). These fluctuating disturbances may reflect changes in the activity of the immune response during exacerbating or remitting phases of the disease. In some cases, subpopulation changes may be a result of changes in the distribution of the cells which regulate the immune response.

There is increasing evidence for cell-to-cell interactions in the regulation of human immune responses. Two functional activities of immune regulator lymphocytes include "helper" functions for enhancing an immune reaction and a "suppressor" function for inhibiting immune responses. Helper cells have been shown to belong to the T-lymphocyte subpopulation and to enhance the immune response to T-dependent antigens. Suppressor cells, thought to play a central role in immune regulation, have been found to inhibit plasma cell formation, immunoglobulin production and mitogen or allogeneic cell-induced lymphocyte proliferation responses. Several reticulo-endothelial subpopulations have been shown to have suppressor cell activity including T-lymphocytes (2), B-lymphocytes (3) and macro-phages (4).

Human T-lymphocytes with suppressor cell activity may be activated both nonspecifically by general mitogens, such as Concanavalin A (Con A) (5) and specifically in response to various antigens (6). Proper control and function of these cells may have important implications in the pathogenesis of MS. In MS patients, it has been suggested that abnormal suppressor cell activity may be responsible for disease onset as well as periods of disease exacerbations (7).

In this study, we examined the spontaneous and nonspecific Con A induced suppressor cell activity in MS patients and matched normal controls. In some cases, we have also employed measles virus antigen to induce antigen specific lymphocyte stimulation or suppressor cell activity.

MATERIALS AND METHODS

Patients

The study group consisted of 28 MS patients (mean years post diagnosis was 17 years) and matched "pal" controls which were selected from the Milwaukee, Wisconsin area. Patients fulfilled the Schumacher criteria for the diagnosis of MS; however, none were undergoing disease exacerbation at the time of sampling nor were they on steroid therapy. Selection of control individuals for this study was based on the following carefully matched criteria: 1) same sex; 2) age; 3) born and lived in the same general location for first 15 years of life; and 4) acquainted for past 10 years. Sixty milliliters of heparinized (preservative-free) peripheral blood was obtained from patients with MS and matched "pal" controls, at the same time, transported by air to our laboratory and tested within 20 hours.

Preparation of Cells

Lymphocytes were separated from 60 ml of blood by Ficoll-Hypaque (Litton Bionetics, Kensington, Md.) density gradient centrifugation (8). Separated lymphocytes were washed twice in RPMI-

1640 (Grand Island Biological Co., Grand Island, N.Y.) and resuspended in RPMI-1640 supplemented with 5% human AB serum, 1% l-glutamine, 50 units/ml penicillin and 50 µg/ml streptomycin (Microbiological Associates, Walkersville, Md.) and counted to determine the number of viable cells.

Lymphocyte Stimulation Assay

Stimulation of lymphocytes by general mitogen or specific antigens was assessed by microculture technique. The assay assessed the lymphocyte incorporation rate of tritiated thymidine (^{3}H-TdR; New England Nuclear),6.7 Ci(mM) into DNA using 2 X 10^5 cells per microtiter well by scintillation spectroscopy as previously described (9).

Stimulation indices were calculated as follows:

$$SI = \frac{CPM\ Stimulated\ Cultures}{CPM\ Untreated\ Cultures}$$

Differences between mean counts per minutes of treated versus untreated cultures were evaluated for statistical significance using the student's "t" test. Values of SI greater than 2.2 were always highly significant (p<0.05) and were considered positive responses. Replicate counts were always within 10% of the mean for each group tested.

Suppressor Cell Assay

Lymphocytes were resuspended in RPMI-1640 supplemented with 10% fetal calf serum at 5 X 10^6 cells/ml and placed in 12 X 75 mm culture tubes (Falcon Plastics. Oxnard, Calif.) in 1 ml volumes. Concanavalin A (60 µg/ml; Calbiochemicals, Los Angeles, Calif.) or specific antigen (0.1 cc) were added to duplicate cultures which were incubated for four days at 37°C in a humidified 5% CO_2 in air atmosphere. The cells were then treated with mitomycin C (50 µg/ml; Sigma, St. Louis, Mo.) for 45 minutes at 37°C. The suppressor cells were washed three times and resuspended at 2 X 10^6 cells/ml. Responder lymphocytes were obtained from a normal donor peripheral blood and suspended at 2 X 10^6 cells/ml. Responder lymphocytes were added in 0.1 cc volume to microtiter wells with or without 0.1 cc of suppressor cells. Each culture was treated with PHA (5 µg/ml) in 0.05 cc volumes and incubated at 37°C in a humidified 5% CO_2 in air atmosphere for three days. Cells were pulsed and harvested as described above.

Suppressor activity was determined to be positive based on a cut-off level of 10% inhibition of DNA synthesis by the responder

lymphocytes in the presence of suppressor cells. This level was
selected because >90% of the normal individuals had spontaneous
suppressor activity which gave less than 10% inhibition of responder
lymphocyte DNA synthesis.

Antigens

Measles virus was grown in Vero cells in roller bottles with
Eagle's MEM (Microbiological Associates) supplemented with 5% fetal
calf serum. Infection was initiated at a multiplicity of 0.1 and
the virus was allowed to grow for four days at which time the media
was removed and fresh media containing 0.1% fetal calf serum was
added to the cells. After two more days the media was harvested,
centrifuged at 1200 x g for 30 minutes and the virus was concentrated 50-fold by negative pressure membrane dialysis (Millipore
Corp.). Virus was titered at $10^{9.2}$ hemagglutinating units/ml and
UV inactivated for 90 minutes.

RESULTS

Con A Induced Stimulation and Suppression

Twenty-eight patients with MS and matched "pal" controls were
tested simultaneously for their response by lymphocyte stimulation
and suppressor cell activity assays following activation with Concanavalin A. The results are presented in Table 1. Peripheral
blood lymphocytes from both patients and controls were found to
react vigorously to Con A in the stimulation assay. Mean stimulation indexes for MS and controls were 162.1 and 160.9 respectively.
Although there was extensive variation from individual to individual,
all 28 individuals from both patient and control groups had significant DNA synthetic responses to Con A.

Suppressor cell activity was inducible by Con A in 25/28 (89%)
of the control population and slightly fewer of the MS patients
21/28 (75%). The mean percent inhibition for the MS patients,
however, was slightly higher than the control group, 28.8% vs. 32.7%
respectively. Since there was extensive variation in the level of
activity from each individual in both groups this difference in
the mean response was not significant.

Response to Measles Virus Antigen

Lymphocytes from MS patients and controls were tested in both
stimulation and suppressor assays with a measles virus antigen

Table 1. Mitogen (Con A) Induced Lymphocyte Stimulation and Non-
specific (Con A-Induced) Suppressor Cell Activity in
Patients with Multiple Sclerosis and Matched "Pal" Controls

	MS		Matched Controls	
	Lymphocyte Stimulation	Suppressor Activity	Lymphocyte Stimulation	Suppressor Activity
n^a =	28	28	28	28
Mean[b] =	162.1 ± 67	28.8 ± 5.2%	160.9 ± 53	32.7 ± 4.3%
Range =	(19.5-419.4)	(0-81%)	(51.2-378.0)	(5-62%)
No. Pos.[c] (%) =	28/28 (100%)	21/28 (75%)	28/28 (100%)	25/28 (89%)

[a]Number of patients tested.

[b]Lymphocyte stimulation response is presented as stimulation indices
(SI) computed as follows:

$$SI = \frac{CPM\ mitogen\ treated}{CPM\ control}$$

Suppressor activity is presented as the group mean percent inhibition
of normal responder lymphocyte DNA synthesis (±SE).

[c]No. Pos. (%) equals the frequency and percent of positive responses.
Significant lymphocyte stimulation response was an SI = 2.2.
Significant suppressor cell activity was determined as $\geq$10% inhibi-
tion of responder DNA synthesis.

preparation. Results are presented in Table 2. Both MS patients
and matched controls showed the same level of positive cellular
reactivity to measles virus antigen by the stimulation assay. The
MS patients had a mean SI of 3.4 ± 1.4 compared to 2.4 ± 0.9 for
the control group and both groups were similar in percent of individuals with positive cellular responses to measles antigen (25%
vs. 21.4% respectively). However, differences were seen in the
suppressor cell response to measles antigen between the two groups.
MS patients showed a higher frequency of positive suppressor cell
activity 9/28 (32.1%) compared to controls, 2/28 (7.1%) and a higher
mean percent inhibition of normal responder DNA synthesis (9.1% vs.
2.5%, respectively). More significantly, if one considers the combined immune reactivity of both the positive stimulation and negative
suppression, one finds that in MS patients, 13/28 (46.4%) showed
measles virus antigen immune reactivity with three individuals showing both positive and negative reactions while the control group
showed a combined immune response frequency of 7/28 (25%) with one
individual showing both responses. Chi square evaluation of positive

Table 2. Lymphocyte Stimulation and Suppressor Cell Activity of
          Lymphocytes From Patients with Multiple Sclerosis and
          Matched "Pal" Controls in Response to Measles Virus

	MS		Matched Controls	
	Lymphocyte Stimulation	Suppressor Activity	Lymphocyte Stimulation	Suppressor Activity
n^a =	28	28	28	28
Mean^b =	3.4 ± 1.4	9.1 ± 2.4%	2.4 ± 0.9	2.5 ± 1.1%
Range =	(0.8-26.3)	(0-41%)	(0.3-9.1)	(0-18%)
No. Pos.^{c} (%) =	7/28 (25%)	9/28 (32.1%)	6/28 (21.4%)	2/28 (7.1%)

^{a,b,c}Same as Table 1.

or negative immune reaction with measles virus antigen showed that
the groups were different with a high degree of significance (χ^2 =
4.132; p<0.01).

Spontaneous Suppressor Cell Activity

        Finally, the lymphocytes of MS patients and controls were
compared for spontaneous suppressor cell activity. Results are
presented in Table 3. We found only 1 of 28 controls who had spontaneous suppressor activity and the level of inhibition was barely
significant (11%). In the MS patient group 4 of 28 patients had
suppressor activity which occurred spontaneously without antigen or
mitogen activation. In these four cases, the level of inhibition
ranged from 10% to 24%. These results showed that, in some cases,
patients as well as controls have spontaneous active suppressor
cells circulating in their peripheral blood.

DISCUSSION

        This study has demonstrated the presence of nonspecific,
antigen specific and spontaneous suppressor cells in the peripheral
blood of patients with MS. We were unable to demonstrate any difference in the level of mitogen (Con A) induced lymphocyte stimulation between MS patients and carefully matched "pal" controls when
using optimal stimulatory doses of mitogen. This demonstrated that
for this population of stable MS patients, there was no discernible
major defects in the lymphoproliferative response to general mitogens. Simultaneously, we found a slightly lower frequency of Con A

Table 3. Spontaneous Suppressor Lymphocyte Activity in Peripheral
          Blood of Patients with Multiple Sclerosis and Matched
          "Pal" Controls

	Suppressor Activity	
	MS	Matched Controls
n^a =	28	28
Mean Inhibition^b =	4.0 ± 0.8%	2.2 ± 0.7%
Range =	(0-24%)	(0-11%)
No. Pos.^{c} (%) =	4/28 (14.3)	1/28 (3.6%)

a,b,cSame as Table 1.

induced nonspecific suppressor cell activity in MS patients (75%)
when compared with "pal" controls (89%). However, this difference
was not statistically significant and, in fact, the mean percent
inhibition exhibited in the MS group (28.8%) was only slightly lower
than that of the controls (32.7%). These results correspond with
those reported by Antel et al. (7) which previously showed that non-
specific suppressor cell activity could be induced by Con A from
peripheral blood lymphocytes of most patients with MS. However, our
study did not show any significant difference between MS and control
groups.

    One of the most interesting findings was the demonstration of
antigen specific suppressor cells which were induced by measles
virus. Conflicting studies exist over the responsiveness of MS
patients to measles virus antigen. Some have reported positive
cell-mediated response (10) while others have failed to confirm
this finding (11). We found no difference in the level of specific
positive cellular immunity to measles virus antigen using the lymphocyte stimulation assay between MS patients and controls. However,
there was a large group of MS patients (32%) who develop significant
suppressor cell activity following in vitro challenge with measles
virus antigen compared to controls (7%). When frequencies of both
reactivities, stimulation and suppression were combined, it becomes
apparent that a large percentage of these MS patients reacted to
the measles virus antigen with a positive or negative response,
13/28 (46.4%), compared to 7/28 (25%) of controls. This increase
was found to be significant and shows that some MS patients have
enhanced responsiveness to measles virus but that much of this reactivity is from suppressor cells which may prevent the development
of controlling immunity and contribute to a chronic measles virus
infection of these patients.

Although the suppressor cell response to measles virus antigen may be significant, it must be cautioned that measles virus receptors exist on lymphocytes (12) and this may nonspecifically affect the level of reactivity to this particular virus or influence the lymphocyte subpopulations which react to it. However, it is also possible that measles virus can infect brain cells and the subsequent failure to develop controlling immunity to this agent, possibly due to the presence of suppressor cells, may result in a chronic infection and the eventual development of an autoimmune response directed against brain tissue as a result of long-term exposure of small quantities of brain cell-virus antigen complexes from infected cells. Future studies should be directed at this intriguing possibility and a better understanding of the relationship of regulatory cells to immune responses in MS.

SUMMARY

Nonspecific, antigen specific and spontaneous suppressor cell activity was demonstrated in peripheral blood lymphocytes of patients with MS. Positive cell-mediated immune reactivity, as demonstrated by lymphocyte stimulation assay, in response to challenge by measles virus antigen in vitro by MS patients was the same as in the control group. However, most important, was the demonstration of a significantly higher frequency of patients with MS (32%) which had antigen specific suppressor cell activity induced by measles virus antigen than did the matched control group (7%). Although Con A induced nonspecific suppressor activity was demonstrated in both groups, no significant difference in the frequency or level of this activity was demonstrated in patients with multiple sclerosis when compared with carefully matched "pal" controls. In addition, no defect in lymphoproliferative response to the mitogen Con A was demonstrable in these patients either. Finally, spontaneous suppressor cells were found in about 14% of the MS patients and only 3.7% of the controls.

REFERENCES

1.   Symington, G.R., Mackay, I.R., Whittingham, S., White, J., and Buckley, J.D., 1978, A profile of immune responsiveness in multiple sclerosis, *Clin. Exp. Immunol.* 31:141.

2.   Dutton, R.W., 1975, Suppressor T-cells, *Trans. Rev.* 26:39.

3.   Katz, S.J., Parker, D., and Turk, J.L., 1974, B-cell suppression of delayed hypersensitivity, *Nature (London)* 251:550.

4. Kirchner, H., Chused, T.M., Herberman, R.B., Holden, H.T., and Lavrin, D.H., 1974, Evidence of suppressor cell activity in spleens of mice bearing primary tumor induced by Maloney Sarcoma virus, *J. Exp. Med.* 139:1473.

5. Hubert, C., Delespesse, G., and Govaerts, A., 1976, Concanavalin A-activated suppressor cells in normal human peripheral blood lymphocytes, *Clin. Exp. Immunol.* 26:95.

6. Stabo, J.D., Sigrun, P., Van Scoy, R.E., and Hermans, P.E., 1976, Suppressor thymus-derived lymphocytes in fungal infection, *J. Clin. Invest.* 57:319.

7. Antel, J.P., Weinrich, M., and Arnason, B.G.W., (in press), Mitogen responsiveness and suppressor cell function in multiple sclerosis - influence of age and disease activity, *Neurology*.

8. Boyum, A., 1968, Separation of leukocytes from blood and bone marrow, *Scand. J. Clin. Lab. Invest.* 21:S1.

9. Wallen, W.C., Rabin, H., Neubauer, R.H., and Cicmanec, J.L., 1975, Depression in lymphocyte response to general mitogens by owl monkeys infected with herpesvirus saimiri, *J. Nat. Cancer Inst.* 54:679.

10. Utermohlen, U., and Zabriskie, J.B., 1973, A suppression of cell-mediated immunity in patients with multiple sclerosis, *J. Exp. Med.* 138:1591.

11. Fuccillo, D.A., Madden, D.L., Castellano, G.A., Traub, R.G., Mattson, J., Krezlewicz, A., and Sever, J.L., 1978, Multiple sclerosis: cellular and humoral immune responses to several viruses, *Neurology* 28:613.

12. Levy, N.L., Auerbach, P.S., and Hayes, E.C., 1976, A blood test for multiple sclerosis based on the adherance of lymphocytes to measles infected cells, *N. Engl. J. Med.* 294:1423.

HUMORAL IMMUNITY IN DISEASE WITH SPECIAL REFERENCE TO MULTIPLE SCLEROSIS

E.J. Field

M.S. Research Unit, Royal Victoria Infirmary, Newcastle Upon Tyne, U.K.

The varied manifestations of antibody activity (complement fixation, agglutination, opsonization etc.) have been assiduously studied, both in health and disease, for some seventy years or more. The role of circulating antibody in the pathogenesis of diseases remains, however, difficult to assess, for it has to be decided whether antibodies (AB) are the cause or the result of the disease, i.e. whether they are the primary cause of, or merely a consequence of tissue breakdown - an epiphenomenon. Breakdown of tissue in a lesion, from many causes, may liberate antigenic materials with sufficient similarity to intact tissue to react with extracts of the latter so that the disease may appear to be "auto-immune". Indeed it can be said to the assessment of humoral auto-immune disease (AID), on the basis of findings of specific antibodies, that it is just as insecurely founded as AID based on cellular immunity (35). There is no doubt that various AB (with or without complement) can act directly on cells, e.g. lysing erythrocytes or platelets or injuring cells of the thyroid gland, and classifications continue to be put forward (45). Early studies were those by Gajdusek (23, 24) and McKay and Gajdusek (38) who found complement fixing auto-antibodies in hepatic and collagen diseases, as well as paraproteinaemia, using liver and kidney antigens. The number of conditions in which antibodies have been found has expanded greatly since then (Table I) though the significances remain unclear. What is clear, however, is that there are large numbers of cross reactivities in the antigenic determinants involved.

Apart from diseases which may be attributable to the direct action of AB there is a group of Immune Complex diseases—best

TABLE 1

Organ or tissue	Disease	Antigen	Detection of antibody
Thyroid	Hashimoto's thyroiditis (hypothyroidism)	Thyroglobulin	Precipitin; passive hemagglutination; IF on thyroid tissue
		Thyroid cell surface and cytoplasm	IF on thyroid tissue
	Thyrotoxicosis (hyperthyroidism)	Thyroid cell surface	Stimulates mouse thyroid (bioassay)
Gastric mucosa	Pernicious anemia (vitamin B 12 deficiency)	Intrinsic factor (1)	Blocks binding of B 12 or binds to : B 12 complex
		Parietal cells	IF on unfixed gastric mucosa; CF with musocal homogenate
Adrenals	Addison's disease (adrenal insufficiency)	Adrenal cell	IF on unfixed adrenals CF
Skin	Pemphigus vulgaris	Epidermal cells	IF on skin sections
	Pemphigoid	Basement membrane between epidermis - dermis	IF on skin sections
Eye	Sympathetic ophthalmia	Uvea	Delayed-type hypersensitive skin reaction to uveal extract
Kidney glomeruli plus lung	Goodpasture's syndrome	Basement membrane	IF on kidney tissue; linear staining of glomeruli
Red cells	Autoimmune hemolytic anemia	Red cell surface	Coomb's antiglobulin test
Platelets	Idiopathic thrombocytopenic purpura	Platelet surface	Platelet survival

TABLE 1 (cont'd)

Organ or tissue	Disease	Antigen	Detection of antibody
Skeletal and heart muscle	Myasthenia gravis	Muscle cells and thymus "myoid" cells	IF on muscle biopsies
Brain	? Multiple sclerosis	Brain tissue	Cytotoxicity on cultured cerebellar cells
Spermatozoa	Male infertility (rarely)	Sperm	Agglutination of sperm
Liver (biliary tract)	Primary biliary cirrhosis	Mitochondria (mainly)	IF on diverse cells with abundant mitochondria (e.g., distal tubules of kidney)
Salivary and lacrimal glands	Sjögren's disease	Many: secretory ducts, mitochondria, nuclei, IgG	IF on tissue
Synovial membranes, etc.	Rheumatoid arthritis	Fc domain of IgG	Antiglobulin tests: agglutination of latex particles coated with IgGs, etc.
	Systemic lupus erythematosus (SLE)	Many: DNA DNA-protein, cardiolipon, IgG, Microsomes, etc.	Precipitins, IF, CF, LE cells

IF = Immunofluorescence staining, usually with fluorescent anti-human Igs.
CF = complement fixation.
Based on Roitt, I. Essential Immunology. Blackwell, Oxford, 1971.

recognised amongst which is the well recognised disease of the
kidney.

Excellent recent reviews are available in Holborow and
Reeves' book (1977), amongst others, and their tables serve only
to see if what is know of the pathogenesis of MS can readily be
made to fit into any particular category.

The study of circulating antibody (AB) in MS began long ago
and a notable, though much neglected, contribution was made by
Sachs and Steiner (49) who were able to find circulating AB to
MS brain extracts in the serum of MS patients and others - but
not to extracts derived from arteriosclerotic and other brains.
They established "positives" only when CF occurred with MS
brain extract but not with other brain extracts. We may note
this has a curiously modern ring about it when antibodies to
"specific viruses" are being sought for by eager virologists.
Steiner's name later became intimately bound up with the spiro-
chaetal theory of the origin of MS which has received no significant support.

More recently, with the isolation of a relatively pure human
encephalitogenic factor (EF) (12) and the use of the tanned RBC
method of Boyden, circulating AB were found in all destructive
diseases of the nervous system including MS. AB which reacted
with EF also appeared in the serum of young subjects inoculated
with PPD (Table II). Frick (22), indeed, had found that rabbits
immunized with killed tubercle bacilli in lanolin and paraffin
oil developed AB both to tubercle antigen and to aqueous MS
brain extracts. "Sharing of antigens" is important in modern
immunological research.

Granted that with the relatively impure brain antigens then
available circulating AB could be demonstrated, attempts to transfer EAE in animals (accepted almost without demur at the time as
the analogue of human MS) with serum from sick animals were unsuccessful with the exception of the claim by Jancovic et. al.
(30) who thought they could transfer EAE by intraventricular
instillation of acute EAE serum. More recently Lebar et al.
(36) showed that this effect was due to a CF auto-antibody of
the IgG_2 class. Oldstone and Dixon (41) demonstrated CF anti-
basic protein AB in the thoracic duct of rats before the onset
of EAE. However, the general impression remained that EF when
purified and potent was a poor antibody producer but gave rise
readily to lymphocyte sensitization. "The failure to transfer
EAE in vivo with large amounts of serum is a serious objection
to the etiological significance of circulating demyelinating
antibodies" wrote Appel and Bornstein (2) and suggested (as will
be elaborated below) that AB may be only one of several factors
at work.

TABLE II

Subjects	Serum			Significance against normal (x^2 test)
	Positive	Negative	Total	
Normal	9	37	44	..
Acute M.S.	11	7	18	<0.001
Chronic M.S.	27	20	47	<0.001
G.P.I.	62	38	100	<0.001
Neurological disease other than M.S. or G.P.I.	18	14	32	<0.001
Huntington's chorea	6	10	16	0.1
Presenile dementia	9	5	14	< 0.001
Hashimoto's disease	5	14	19	0.8 - 0.9
Rheumatoid arthritis	7	10	17	0.1 - 0.2
B.C.G. subjects	17	14	31	0.02 - 0.01

The most important evidence for AB function in producing EAE
in MS rested for years upon the work instigated by Margaret Murray,
Edith Peterson, M.B. Bornstein and their associates. Bornstein
and Appel (8) demonstrated the presence, in the serum of animals
with EAE, of some factor (complement dependent) which produced
demyelination with sparing of axis cylinders in tissue cultures
of new born rat cerebellum. Much of the work by Bornstein and
his associates was reviewed (by him) in 1973 (7). It is clear
that the effect is not limited to MS but occurs in other destructive diseases, e.g. neurosyphilis, and especially amyotrophic
lateral sclerosis (ALD). Indeed, in a critical review, Hughes
and Field (28) found (like Bornstein) that two-thirds of ALS
sera were highly active in causing demyelination and indeed their
strongest serum was from an ALS patient. It is interesting to
note that demyelinating activity had been shown earlier by
Birkmayer and Neumayer (4) in the serum of MS patients by the
simple process of incubating small pieces of spinal cord at 37°C
over 24 hours. They, too, noted dissolution of myelin with relative preservation of axis cylinders. They concluded that "MS
serum hat die Fähigkeit, in vitro die Markscheiden in fast
elektiver Weise aufzulösen".(In view of the very recent claim

to have isolated an infectious agent from the bone-marrow of
patients with multiple sclerosis (40) it is of further interest to
note that the same Vienna School (5) also reported bone marrow
changes in MS and even attempted prognosis on these grounds).

In addition to AB against myelin there appears in the serum
of MS subjects (as it does in all subjects whose lymphocytes become sensitized to any antigen) a lymphocyte depressing factor
(LDF) - probably that described by Cooperband et. al. (14) and
since clarified - which depresses lymphocyte transformation
(31, 27, 18).

Bornstein and Crain (10) reported that serum from animals
with EAE (10-25 % concentration) caused marked bioelectric changes
in tissue (organ) cultures of rat cerebellum long before morphological changes were visible. Cerf and Carels (13) likewise
found a complement dependent factor in the serum of acute MS
patients capable of producing a reversible alteration in the bioelectric responses of isolated frog cord.

Unfortunately, these results were not well controlled and
the seductive idea that synaptic blockage might account for
transient variation in MS symptoms and signs is without real foundation. Recently Seil et. al. (50) carried out carefully controlled experiments and concluded that "the ability to block evoked
bioelectric responses in tissue cultures is a non-specific
serum property, and that it is not specifically related to the
pathogenesis of demyelinating disease".

The much neglected hypothesis put forward by Tracy Putnam
and his co-workers (42, 43, 44) that MS may be due to temporary
occlusion of small blood vessels, especially veins, by thrombi
(which are commonly known to be short lived only) involves AB.
A really hard fact in the pathology of MS is the relationship
of lesions to small blood vessels (especially veins) (first
observed, naked eye, by Rindfleisch (47) and confirmed by Ribbert
(46)). The lesions are strung out like pearls at intervals over
the course of small branches. Much of Putnam's painstaking
work in reconstructing lesions from serial sections, together
with his own important contribution, is summarized by Fog (21).
Blood platelets are known to be more "sticky" in MS than normal
(12, 53, 39). Ribbert, as long ago as 1882, claimed to have
found small plugs of white blood cells in arterioles in MS brains.
(By strange coincidence, in the paper succeeding that of Ribbert,
Bizzozero (6) describes blood platelets and their function in
clotting). Putnam (42, 43) and Putnam and Adler (44) have suggested that plaques may develop around veins as a result of occlusion by temporary thrombocyte agglutinations. "Sludging" of blood
had indeed been reported by Roizin et. al. (48). Such agglutinates
would stick to the endothelium, pavementing it over some distance

and so altering the resorptive capacity of the venule leading to
a localized perivascular oedema (itself known to lead to demyelination if sustained). Platelet aggregates are, however, unstable and the degree of perivascular change would depend upon the
length of time for which functional occlusion of the venule
occurred and upon its degree. This transitory character of
platelet aggregates (3, 15, 26); as well as the task of finding
them in serial sections, might account for the infrequency with
which they have been reported, though Putnam (42, fig. 6) and
Putnam and Adler (44, fig. 4) have published photographs. Clearly
these ideas are related to the possibilities raised by Wisniewski
and Bloom (52) that primary demyelination might be a non-specific
consequence of a cell-mediated immune reaction. Platelets would
become involved as "innocent bystanders".

Furthermore, once a lesion has been established around a
vein there will be resorption of brain breakdown products into
the lumen and (since AB are more readily formed to broken down
brain than to purified EF) there will be AB developed. Under
certain conditions of blood flow resorbed antigen may meet AB
in optimal proportions (17) and lead to serotonin release from
platelets (29, 11) which might have further effects "downstream".
In view of the recent interest in PUFA as a "treatment" for MS
it is worth recalling that Sim and McCraw (51) have demonstrated
the anti-aggregation properties of γ-linolenate vis à vis
platelets (see below).

Antibodies might thus have a part to play both in the ini-
tiation of plaques and in the mechanism of their expansion.

MORPHOLOGICAL STUDIES

In EAE of guinea pigs (and other animals) the earliest
morphological change in the brain is a reaction of the microglial
elements around small veins - before there is any evidence at
all of lymphocyte infiltration. The endothelium of the vessels
may be swollen and this suggests that some fluid exudate has
came out or that resorption into the vein has been interfered
with (16). In either case there is no visible infiltration
with cells. Electron microscopy has shown the same increased
permeability of small intracerebral veins (20) in EAE of the
rhesus monkey. Indeed, they pointed out that "in addition to
destruction of myelin associated with the presence of a mononuclear cell, myelin lamellae sometimes appeared to have simply
melted away, occasionally all around a nerve fibre but sometimes
only over a part of its circumference." and suggested that at
least some of this melting away might be due to Bornstein's
antibody. Incidentally, in this work the authors issue a strong
note of caution that "variations due to sampling in all electron

microscopic examination of the nervous system can lead to differing
descriptions of a process" and that "seldom is some estimate given
in a description of the frequency with which a given phenomenon
has been encountered and photographic evidence of one good example
may lead to quite misleading estimates of the regularity of a
process". In this study of the rhesus monkey, direct attack upon
myelin sheaths by mononuclear cells was more common than in the
previous study in guinea pigs (19). Incidentally, the special
mononuclear cell attack on the myelin sheath by penetration
along the external mesaxon reported by Lampert (32) and Lampert
and Kies (34) was never observed. On the other hand the earliest
change was an oedema about the small vessels (see above). An
elegant demonstration of the early increased vascular permeability
in EAE in Wistar rats was given by Lampert and Carpenter (33)
using thorotrast as contrast medium and others have followed suit
with peroxidase.

So far as acute MS lesions are concerned they occur without
lymphocyte infiltration.

Turning once again to MS, antimyelin antibodies in neurological diseases in general have been reviewed by Lisak et.al. (37)
who found increases in acute MS, Guillain-Barré syndrome, and
ALS. A lesser degree of binding was found in normals of all ages
and thus corresponds with the non-specific bindings shown by
Allerand and Yahr (1) of the γ-globulin fraction of serum and
spinal fluid from both normal and MS patients. They thus showed
an affinity (by immunofluorescence) of γ-globulin for normal
human nervous tissue.

From the mass of work published on antibodies, both to crude
myelin and to purified EF, the conclusion can only be drawn that
AB are not of themselves a primary cause in the pathogenesis of
MS though they may play an important role in the further development of plaques. Only in the Putnam hypothesis can AB be
assigned a major role. It might be appropriate to conclude, in
view of widespread enlistment of EAE as a "model for MS", (a
mainstay for all those applying for grants to work on EAE) that
this concept has recently been called into question by Gutstein
and Cohen (25) who, working with EAE in sheep, conclude that
serum AB to myelin basic protein are not responsible for induction
of EAE and that "the use of EAE as a model for MS should be
carefully questioned".

REFERENCES

1. Allerand, C.D. and Yahr, M.D. (1964) Science, 144, 1141.
2. Appel, S.H. and Bornstein, M.B. (1964) J. exp. Med. 119, 303.
3. Astrup, T. and Piper, J. (1945) Nord. Med. 28, 2405.

4. Birkmayer, W. and Neumayer, E. (1957) Wien. Klin. Wochenschr. 69, 718.
5. Birkmayer, W., Dittrich, H. and Neumayer, E. (1958) Wien Z. Nervenheilk. 15, 59.
6. Bizzozero, J. (1882) Virch. Arch. 90, 261.
7. Bornstein, M.B. (1973) In "Progress in Neuropathology, vol 2 69. ed. H.M. Zimmerman. Grune & Stratton, New York.
8. Bornstein, M.B. and Appel, S.H. (1961) J. Neuropath. exp. Neurol. 20, 141.
9. Bornstein, M.B. and Appel, S.H. (1965) Ann. N.Y. Acad. Sci. 122, 280.
10. Bornstein, M.B. and Crain, S. (1965) Science 148, 1242.
11. Caspary, E.A. and Field, E.J. (1967) Deutsch. Z. Nervenheilk. 190, 267.
12. Caspary, E.A., Prineas, H., Miller, H. and Field, E.J. (1965) Lancet, 2, 1108.
13. Cerf, J.A. and Carels, G. (1966) Science 152, 1066.
14. Cooperband, S.R., Bondeuik, H., Schmid, K. and Mannick, J.A. (1968) Science, 159, 1243.
15. Copley, A.L. and Houlihan, R.B. (1947) Blood (Spec. Issue N°1) 1, 182.
16. Field, E.J. (1961) Proc. roy. Soc. Med. 54, 15.
17. Field. E.J. and Caspary, E.A. (1964) Lancet, 2, 876.
18. Field, E.J. and Caspary, E.A. (1971) Brit. med. J. 4, 529.
19. Field, E.J. and Raine, C.S. (1966) Amer. J. Path. 49, 537.
20. Field, E.J. and Raine, C.S. (1969) J. Neurol. Sci. 8, 397.
21. Fog, T. (1965) The Topography of Plaques of Multiple Sclerosis Munksgaard, Copenhagen.
22. Frick, E. (1951) Deutsch, Z. Nervenheilk. 166, 54.
23. Gajdusek, C.D. (1957) Nature, 179, 666.
24. Gajdusek, C.D. (1958) A.M.A. Arch. Int. Med., 101, 9.
25. Gutstein, H.S. and Cohen, S.R. (1978) Science, 199, 301.
26. Hirsch, E., Faure-Gilly, J. and Dameshek, W. (1950) Blood 5, 568.
27. Hughes, D., Caspary, E.A. and Field, E.J. (1968) Lancet, 2, 1205.
28. Hughes, D. and Field, E.J. (1967) Clin. exp. Immunol. 2, 295.
29. Humphrey, J.H. and Jacques, R. (1955) J. Physiol. 128, 9.
30. Jancovic, B.D., Draskowski, M. and Janjic, M. (1965) Nature (London) 207, 428.
31. Knowles, M., Hughes, D., Caspary, E.A. and Field, E.J. (1968) Lancet, 2, 1207.
32. Lambert, P.W. (1965) J. Neuropath. exp. Neurol. 24, 371.
33. Lampert, P.W. and Carpenter, S. (1965) J. Neuropath. exp. Neurol. 24, 11.
34. Lampert, P.W. and Kies, M.W. (1967) Exp. Neurol. 18, 210.
35. Lancet, (1971) Leading Article : Immunological aspects of the Guillain-Barré Syndrome.
36. Lebar, R., Boutry, J.M., Vincent, C., Robineaux, R. and Voisin, G.A. (1976) J. Immunol. 116, 1439.

37. Lisak, R.P., Zwiman, B. and Norman, M. (1975) Arch. Neurol. 32, 163.
38. Mackay, I.R. and Gajdusek, C.D. (1958) A.M.A. Arch. Int. Med. 30.
39. Millac, P. (1967) Deutsch. Z. Nervenheilkunde. 191, 74.
40. Mitchell, D.N., Porterfield, J.S., Micheletti, R., Lange, L.S. Goswami, K.K.A., Taylor, P., Jacobs, J.P., Hockley, D.J. and Sailsbury, A.J. (1978) Lancet, 2, 299.
41. Oldstone, M.B.A. and Dixon, F.J. (1968) Amer. J. Path. 52, 251.
42. Putnam, T.J. (1935) Arch. Neurol. 33, 929.
43. Putnam, T.J. (1937) Arch. Neurol. 37, 1298.
44. Putnam, T.J. and Adler, A. (1937) Arch. Neurol. 38, 1.
45. Reeves, W.G. and Holborow, E.J. (1977) In : "Immunology in Medicine" eds. Holborow and Reeves. Academic Press, New York.
46. Ribbert, H. von (1882) Virch. Arch. 90, 243.
47. Rindfleisch, E. von (1863) Virch. Arch. 26, 474.
48. Roizin, L.,Abell, R.C. and Winn, J. (1953) Neurology 3, 250.
49. Sachs, H. and Steiner, G. (1934) Klin. Wochenschr. 13, 1714.
50. Seil, F.J., Leiman, A.L. and Kelly, J.M. (1976) Arch. Neurol. 33, 418.
51. Sim, A.K. and McGraw, A.P. (1977) Thompsons Research. vol 10, p. 385, Perganon Press.
52. Wisniewski, H.M. and Bloom, B.R. (1975) J. exp. Med. 141, 346.
53. Wright, H.P., Thompson, R.H.S., Zilkha, K.J. (1965) Lancet 2, 1109.

CELLULAR IMMUNE FUNCTION TO MEASLES ANTIGEN IN NORMAL SUBJECTS

AND MULTIPLE SCLEROSIS:

SKIN TESTING WITH AUTOLOGOUS CSF AND OTHER ANTIGENS IN MULTIPLE

SCLEROSIS

L. Bannon, J. Dempsey, V. Parameswaran, M. Robinson
and H. Staunton

Department of Neurology, Richmond and Mater Hospitals
Dublin, Ireland

There have been reports of generally depressed cellular immune function in multiple sclerosis (1, 4). Reference has been
made to a selective diminution in the cellular immune response
to measles antigen (3, 2). With a view to testing the latter
hypothesis and, if confirming it, reversing the situation by
administration of transfer factor from unaffected siblings,
we instituted a study of cellular immune function to measles
antigen particularly in normal individuals and in subjects
with multiple sclerosis. In addition, in view of the many criticisms of in vitro tests as an index of cellular immune capacity, an in vivo investigation on the basis of skin testing
with autologous cerebrospinal fluid and a variety of antigens
was also undertaken.

IN VITRO TESTS, MATERIALS AND METHODS

In all, 27 patients at various stages of the disease were
studied. Their mean age was 33.21 years (range 19-52). Patients
were selected based on the criteria of McDonald and Halliday
(1977). Highly probable cases were included on the basis of the
possibility that more active changes might exist. The control
subjects were matched for age as closely as possible. All control subjects had a past history of uneventful measles.

57

Antigens : Measles antigen, Edmonston strain, lot no. M 944055, was obtained from Flow Laboratories. The antigen was diluted to 1:10 for most studies. Tuberculin PPD obtained from Evans Biological was dialysed against physiological saline over 36 hours.

Lymphocyte Transformation Test (LTT)

This test was performed as described by Penhale et al. Various concentrations of phytohaemagglutinin (PHA) and measles antigen were added to the lymphocyte suspensions, and 0.4 μCi/ well of tritiated thymidine added before termination of culture. The transformation index (TI) was calculated as follows :

$$T.I. = \frac{\text{maximum counts per minute in presence of antigen}}{\text{maximum counts per minute in absence of antigen}}$$

Results of LTT

The mean T.I. with PHA for controls and M.S. was not in statistical terms significantly different (p = $<$ .5 $>$ .4), though there was a trend towards a lesser response on the part of the subjects with M.S. (fig. 1). Although repeatable blastogenesis

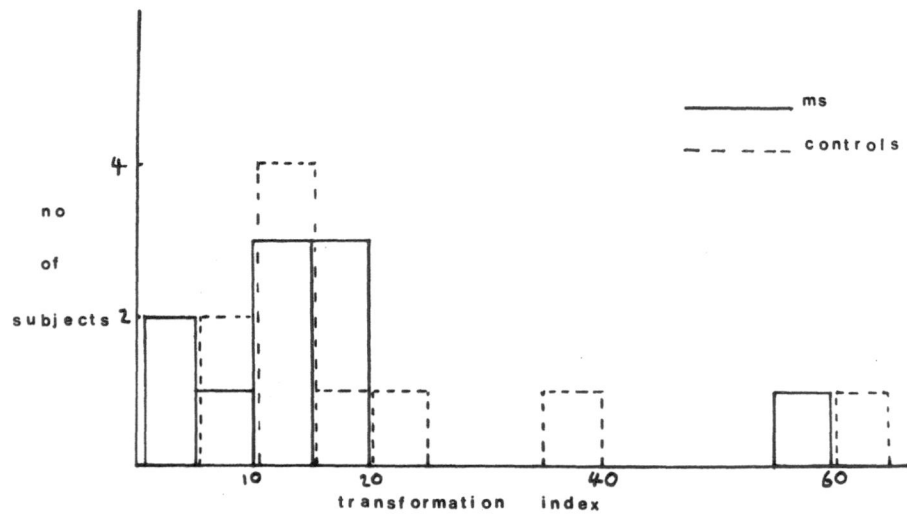

Figure 1

was obtained with PHA in the normal individuals, it proved impossible to show any consistent blastogenic response to measles
antigen in the same group. A few subjects with multiple sclerosis were studied, showing similar responses. However, in the
absence of response in the normal individuals, it would be impossible to demonstrate a depressed response in subjects with
multiple sclerosis.

Leucocyte Migration Inhibition (LMIT)

The LMIT was modified from the method described by Bendixen
and Soborg (1969). The chambers were filled with RPMI containing
the respective antigens. Measles antigen was used at a dilution
of 1:10 of original strength, and PPD at a concentration of 20
µgl/ml. The area of migration was projected on paper and measured
by planimetry. The percentage migration index was calculated as :

$$\% \text{ migration index} = \frac{\text{migration area with antigen}}{\text{migration area without antigen}} \times 100$$

An index of less than 80 % was taken to represent the presence of
cellular immune function.

Results of LMIT

The results of leucocyte migration inhibition with measles
antigen in controls and multiple sclerosis are illustrated in
figure 2. There was no significant difference between the groups
(p = <.2 > .1). Figure 3 illustrates the findings with PPD. There
was a significant difference between the two groups (p = <.01> .001),
the M.S. subjects not showing significant migration inhibition.

Macrophage Migration Inhibition Test (MIT)

This was an indirect test adopted from the procedure described by Rocklin (1976). Lymphocytes were prepared as for the
LTT. Macrophages from guinea pig peritoneal exudate were used
as indicator. The antigens were used in the foregoing concentrations. The migration patterns were measured as in the LMIT.

Results of MIT

It again proved impossible to induce migration inhibition
with measles antigen in control subjects. Using this system,
₤ 4/10 of the normal group showed significant migration inhibition with PPD, whereas one of the M.S. subjects only, showed an
index of less than 80 %.

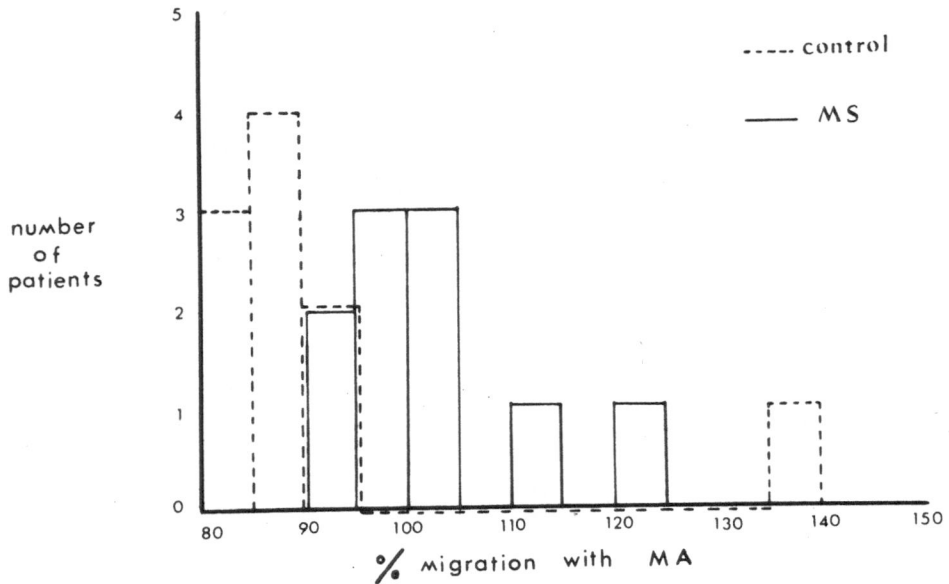

Fig. 2

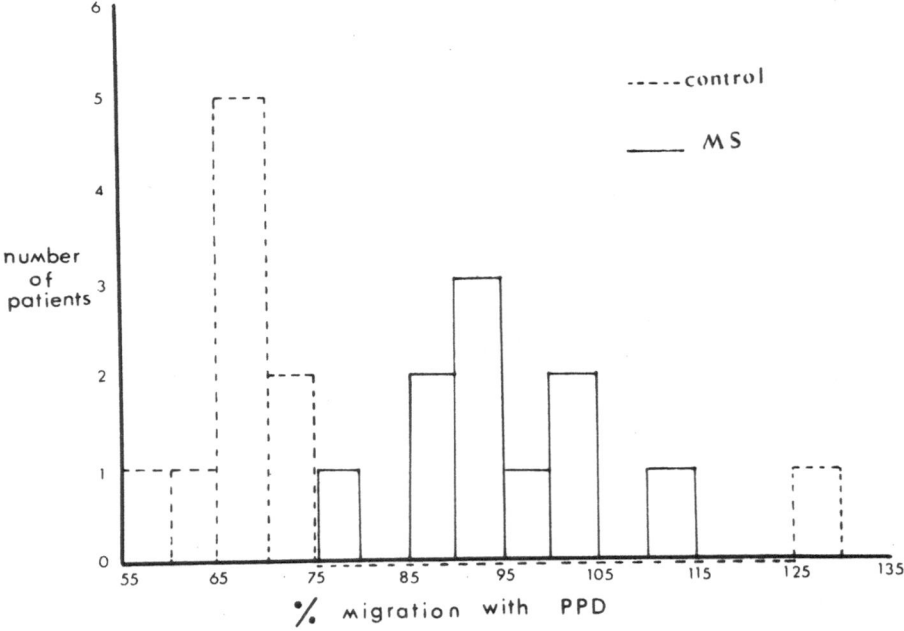

Fig. 3

Comment

It proves impossible to induce signs of cellular immune competence with measles antigen in the foregoing systems, so that
demonstration of depression of function in M.S. would not be
susceptible to demonstration. Furthermore, the vagaries of such
in vitro tests as are described make it unlikely that they will
provide a consistent picture in the abnormal corresponding to a
clinical analogue.

SKIN TESTING

In view of the considerable clinical limitations of the
foregoing in vitro techniques, a parallel in vivo programme was
undertaken. It was also desired to note whether there existed
in patients CSF an antigen to which they had become sensitized,
begging entirely the question of whether it was of endogenous
or exogenous origin.

MATERIALS AND METHODS

Two groups of patients were studied. A variety of skin
antigens were used, including concentrated autologous CSF, measles antigen, measles control fluid, PPD, and streptokinase-
streptodornase (SK-SD).

Antigens

Measles antigen and measles control fluid were obtained
from Evans Biologicals, Liverpool. The antigen was the Schwartz
strain prepared in chick embryo fibroblast cultures and the control fluid prepared from uninfected chick embryo fibroblast
cultures. SK-SD, 'varidase' from Lederle Laboratories and PPD
from Evans Medical Ltd. were used. 0.1 ml. of all antigens was
injected intradermally. Induration in two perpendicular direc-
tions of greater than 0.5 mm. was taken to indicate a positive
response.

Group 1

For this group of 9 patients and four neurological controls
the CSF was concentrated by an Amicon filter membrane (type B15),
filtering all under 15,000 M.W.

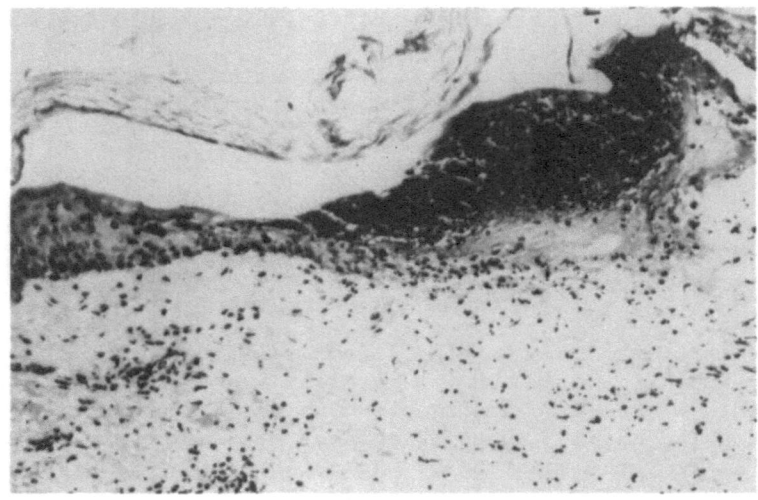

Figure 4

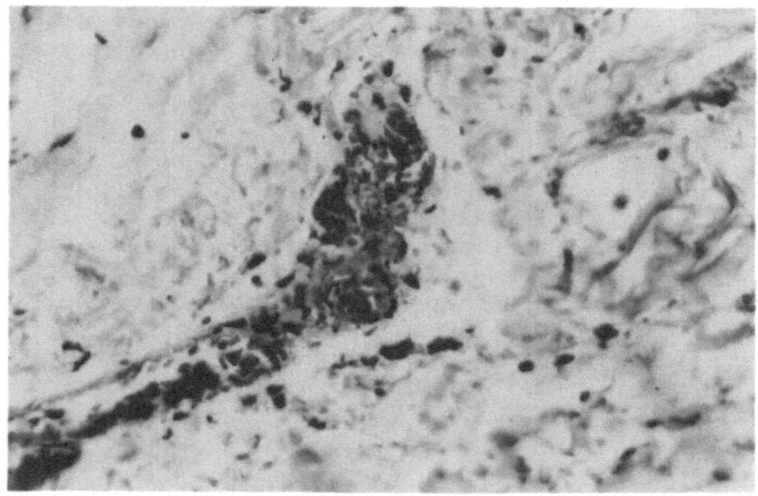

Figure 5

Group 1 Results. There was one positive response to measles antigen (table 1), in the M.S. subjects. All M.S. subjects tested had a positive response to PPD and SK-SD, the expected normal response in an Irish population. There were two positive reactions to CSF in this group. Of the four neurological controls, all had negative responses to CSF, and three reacting positively to PPD and SK-SD.

Group 2

It was felt that the system of concentration in the foregoing study might not be quite satisfactory in view of the very small quantity of protein in the CSF, and the possibility of some getting lost on the membrane. Further, all material under 15,000 M.W. was lost. A further eight patients were therefore studied, on this occasion freeze-drying the CSF, followed by reconstitution with NaCl. The subsequent solution proved to be a very hypertonic salt solution. A 12 grams % solution of NaCl was therefore administered as a control. Three control subjects with spinal disc degeneration were also studied, and one subject with a Guillain-Barré syndrome.

Group 2 Results. 5 of the 8 patients showed a positive response, the response, however, coming up within hours. Two of the non-reactors were on steroids. The concentrated NaCl did not elicit a positive response, and neither the control disc subjects nor the Guillain-Barré subject showed positive responses to either. Skin biopsies were performed on all five subjects. 4 of these showed the changes illustrated in Fig. 4 and 5. There was necrosis of epidermis and underlying collagen, perivascular infiltration by polymorphonuclear cells with swelling of endothelial cells, and exudation of red cells.

Comment

Positive skin reactions to autologous CSF, coming up within hours, have been found in some patients with M.S. The early appearance, coupled with the pathological changes, particularly that of vasculitis, suggest that this may be a specific type of antigen-antibody response of the Arthus type. This requires confirmation by immunofluorescence.

TABLE 1

Testing of M.S. Patients with Specific and

Non Specific Antigens

Patients	Antigens					
	MA	TCF	CSF	WATER	PPD	SK-SD
G.M.	-	-	-	-	+	+
B.M.	+	-	-	-	+	N.D.
A.M.	-	-	+	-	+	+
A.S.	-	-	+	-	+	+
P.K.	-	-	-	-	+	+
G.B.	-	-	-	-	+	+
P.M.	-	-	-	-	+	+
M.C.	-	-	-	-	+	+
M.R.	-	-	-	-	+	+

MA	=	Measles antigen (flow)
TCF	=	Tissue control fluid
CSF	=	Cerebrospinal fluid, concentrated 80 – 100 times.
PPD	=	Purified protein derivates 10 tuberculin units
SK-SD	=	Streptokinase-Streptodornase (20:5)

0.1 ml. of above antigens were injected intradermally.

ACKNOWLEDGEMENTS

    This work was performed with the help of a grant-in-aid from the Irisch Medical Research Council. We also received financial assistance from the Irish Multiple Sclerosis Society.

REFERENCES

1. Salmi, A., Gollmar, Y., Norrby, E. and Panelius, M. Acta Pathol. Microbiol. Scand. Sect. B 81, 627, 1973.
2. Sheremata, W., Sella, G. Triller, H. and Cosgrove, J.B.R. Neurology 26, 377, 1976.
3. Untermohlen, V. and Zabriskie, J.B. J. Exp. Med. 138, 1591, 1973.
4. Vandvik, B. and Degree, M. J. Neurol. Sci. 24, 201, 1975.

CASES OF ACUTE MEASLES INFECTION IN MULTIPLE SCLEROSIS PATIENTS

B. Ryberg [+] and M. Gudnadottir [x]

+ Department of Neurology, University of Lund, Lund, Sweden
x Department of Microbiology, University of Iceland, Reykjavik, Iceland

Immunological findings have suggested an association between measles and multiple sclerosis (MS), and the possibility that MS is an age-dependent response to measles has been discussed. One of the author's patients, a woman of 20 years with firm evidence of early MS including a mononuclear pleocytosis in the CSF and evidence of an intrathecal IgG synthesis, developed a clinically and serologically confirmed acute measles infection after having been in contact with a child with this disease. She had not had measles before and she had never been vaccinated against measles. A follow-up one year later confirmed the MS diagnosis. Thus, if measles can have a causal role in MS, it is probably not the only agent with this ability.

M. Gudnadottir, (Reykjavik) adds the following information :

I might just add to this that in Iceland we have references to 5 rather well documented cases of multiple sclerosis who either contracted clinical measles after the onset of multiple sclerosis or have not yet had measles but were vaccinated against them in an area, where measles had not come for years. These patients were seronegative as well as everybody else, and the fact that they had multiple sclerosis was not known to those who did a study on the effects of the vaccination.

    Case 1. A female born 1921. M.S. began 1937.
            Clinical measles 1946 or nine years after the onset of M.S.

Case 2. Male born 1893.
        Onset of M.S. 1907.
        Clinical measles in 1916 or nine years later.

Case 3. Daughter of case 2 born 1933.
        M.S. began 1948.
        Clinical measles 1951 or 3 years after the onset of
        M.S.

Case 4. Female born 1920.
        Onset of M.S. 1944.
        Vaccinated in 1962.

Case 5. Female born 1921.
        Onset of M.S. 1956.
        Vaccinated in 1962.

PATHOGENETIC CONSIDERATIONS IN MULTIPLE SCLEROSIS : IS MS A

CHRONIC VARIANT OF POSTINFECTIOUS ENCEPHALOMYELITIS ?

J. Simon

Max-Planck-Institute for Psychiatry, München, F.R. Germany

SUMMARY

Experimental data obtained in vaccinia infection are compatible with following hypothesis :
Acute postinfectious and postvaccinal encephalomyelitis and multiple sclerosis (MS) are two variants of demyelination disease which can develop as a neurological complication of an irrelevant systemic infection caused by ubiquitous viruses.

A major factor determining the expression of the disease is the host and its relationship to virus both in the CNS and in the immune system.

INTRODUCTION

Investigation of pathogenetic factors in multiple sclerosis (MS) is hampered by the unavailability of a suitable experimental model. The experimental allergic encephalomyelitis (EAE) employed thus far can explain only some of the mechanisms involved in the complex pathogenesis of MS, i.e. the autoimmune reaction.

However, the primary etiologic agent in MS appears to be a virus, as indirectly evidenced by a variety of data recently reviewed by R.T. Johnson (1) and V. ter Meulen (2). Therefore it was thought that an experimental viral infection which can lead to demyelination disease might provide some additional information regarding the pathogenetic role of viral agent in demyelination.

In our study we used vaccinia virus. This was because of
its well-established role in postvaccinal encephalomyelitis,
which shares common pathomorphological features not only with
the EAE but also with the group of para- and postinfectious encephalomyelitis, with acute MS and, to some extent, with chronic
MS (3).

The resemblance of the pathomorphology as well as of some
virological and immunological parameters provides strong evidence
of a pathogenetic relationship among these conditions.

In order to investigate this possibility, we performed a
series of experiments with the vaccinia virus with variations
in the experimental protocols.

EXPERIMENTAL VACCINIA INFECTION

Two series of experiments were performed:
a) infection of animals with a competent immune system and
b) infection of immunologically compromised animals.

Details of the experiments performed thus far are described
elsewhere (4, 5, 6, 7), and will be summarized only briefly
here.

The results obtained thus far show that vaccinia virus is
capable of producing a broad range of pathological syndromes,
some with an acute and some with a protracted course (the longest observation period was 3 years). After extraneural administration, an irrelevant immunizing infection develops usually.
Infection of the CNS occurs in animals infected intrathecally
or intracerebrally. Two pathogenetically different forms can be
discerned :
a) acute choriomeningitis, ependymitis and vasculitis;
b) postvaccinal encephalomyelitis.

Acute Choriomeningitis, Ependymitis and Vasculitis

This form is limited to the neuronal membranes and vessels.
Pathologically, regressive changes and/or lysis of numerous infected cells of the vessels, choroid plexus, leptomeninges and
ependyma are visible. Simultaneously an acute inflammatory reaction appears, consisting of mononuclear cells: many of these
cells are also damaged.

An adjacent neuroparenchyma shows secondary non specific
lesions, due to damage to the brain-barrier system with leakage
of serum proteins and edema. The glial cells show swelling,

activation and proliferation. In severe cases, hemorrhages
and necrosis are visible.

The virus multiplies rapidly and can be isolated between
the 2nd and 6th day post infection (p.i.). The viral antigens
are detectable by immunofluorescence as a bright fluorescence
limited to the cells of the neuronal membranes and vessels.
Some inflammatory cells are also positive. In severe cases,
a few glial cells can be found which exhibit a weak cytoplasmic
fluorescence. However, these cells display only minimal regressive lesions or none at all, suggesting a noncytocidal (abortive)
infection.

Immunologically, anti-viral humoral and cellular reaction
develop. Less frequently, autoimmunity against brain antigens
is detectable. This form can be regarded as a prototype of an
acute productive viral infection. The direct, cytocidal action
of the virus is the major factor in pathology, with the severity
and extent of the pathology being determined by the biological
properties of the virus on the one hand and by the efficiency
of the defence mechanisms on the other.

The limitation to the neuronal membranes and vessels can
be explained by a restricted permissivity of various cells within
the CNS. Our findings indicate that vaccinia virus (three strains
with different virulance were employed) is almost strictly meso-
dermotrophic; the ependymal cells are the only exception. In
contrast, neuroectodermal glial cells (astrocytes and oligodendroglia) and neurons seem to be nonpermissive. Preferential
infection of the glial cells may be due to the altered permissivity of activated glial cells : the activated cells seem to become
semipermissive. This speculation needs confirmation, however.

Postvaccinal Encephalomyelitis

The pathogenesis of postvaccinal as well as postinfectious
encephalomyelitis is still unclear. Our study of the vaccinia
infection in immunologically compromised animals suggests that
this demyelination disease is not a separate entity but rather
a complication or further progression of the acute choriomeningitis.

Three features characterize the infection in animals which
were x-irradiated (mice) or immunosuppressed with cyclophosphamid
(monkeys, rats, guinea pigs) :
a) non specific changes in neuroparenchyma adjacent to neuronal
membranes and vessels become prominent;
b) the virus spreads into the changed neuroparenchyma and noncytocidal infection of numerous glial cells and some neurons

takes place;
c) pathological autoimmunity frequently appears, with predominantly cellular response. Pathologically,heavy inflammatory
infiltrates and perivascular, periventricular and subpial patches
of demyelination are present, expressed mainly in monkeys. In
fact, the pathological condition is indistinguishable from the
EAE.

    A prerequisite for this pathology seems to be the expression
of efficient effector mechanisms of demyelination. The sequence
of events thought to occur is that first a number of non specific
factors (e.g. edema with water, electrolyte and acid-base imbalance, mediators of inflammation, immune complexes, and direct
enzymatic virus action on membranes), produce non specific, mostly
reversible lesions of adjacent myelin sheaths (bystander effect).
The consequence is an increased release of myelin antigens on
the one hand and an increased vulnerability of damaged myelin
sheaths on the other. The myelin antigens induce an autoimmunity.

    Simultaneously, the noncytocidal infection of glial cells
leads to antigenic membrane changes in these cells, inducing a
"rejection" reaction. Thus, two factors seem to determine the
expression of demyelination :
a) autoimmunity,
b) indirect virus action mediated by immune mechanisms.

        Autoimmunity as Potential Effector of Demyelination

    The pathogenetic role of autoimmunity has been intensively
studied in the EAE. It is now well-documented that a physiological, predominantly humoral, autoimmunity appearing after administration of an encephalitogen in an incomplete Freund's
adjuvant (6) has a homeostatic function. In contrast, the mixture of an encephalitogen with a complete Freund's adjuvant
leads to disregulated proliferation of the autoreactive T-cells
and production of cytotoxic antibodies. Similarly, the infection
of the cells of the immune system may lead to various disorders
of the surveillance function of the immune system, apparent as
a pathogenic autoimmunity.

    Possible mechanisms of virus induced alteration of the
function of the immune system have been reviewed (8).

        Indirect Action of Virus as Inductor of Immune Reaction

    The capacity of viruses associated with postinfectious en-
cephalomyelitis to change the antigenic "make-up" of noncytoci-

dally infected cells is well-known and has been reviewed in several papers (9, 10). By various mechanisms the cells or their
processes are recognized as non-self. The immune system tries
to reject the changed cells, whereby cross-reactivity can lead
to simultaneous injury to normal cells and tissues. The rate
and extent of demyelination due to "rejection" of altered oligodendroglia cells are determined by biological properties of both
virus and host and by the genetically controlled immune reaction.
If our speculation is right, there are two stages of demyelination :
a) non specific, reversible lesions give rise to autoimmunity
and make the myelin sheaths vulnerable to the immunological injury. This non specific stage can be realized in many other
pathological conditions, e.g. trauma, intoxication, hypoxia and
infection;
b) specific interaction of "presensitized" myelin sheaths with
the myelinotoxic antibodies and/or T-effector or with killer-cells
may lead to severe irreversible changes. This specific stage is
realized in postinfectious and postvaccinal encephalomyelitis
and probably in MS.

MULTIPLE SCLEROSIS : A CHRONIC VARIANT OF AN ACUTE POSTINFECTIOUS
                    ENCEPHALOMYELITIS ?

     The main objection to the suggested pathogenetic relation-
ship between postinfectious encephalomyelitis and MS is the difference in their courses. Our experiments with protracted observation period provide evidence that the same virus is capable
of inducing a chronic latent infection. Some of the animals killed at various periods p.i. exhibit localized lesions, consisting
of regressive changes and loss of glial cells and neurons with
or without an inflammatory reaction. Patches of demyelination
are not infrequent. Both acute and chronic foci can be detected
in various regions of the same animal. Occasionally, the immune
complexes are visible in choroid plexus and kidneys, where a
proliferative glomerulonephritis can develop. Clinical signs
are rarely seen. Thus far, no virus has been isolated after
the 12th day. However, viral antigens are detectable by immunofluorescence in the glial cells, neurons and monocytes in 1 %
to 5 % of the animals,if a large number of sections are examined.
Immunologically, antiviral reaction is present in all animals;
autoimmunity is detectable in about 60 % of animals. Two features of MS, i.e. long incubation and a remitting and relapsing
course have been the main reasons so far for arguing that MS is
a separate entity.

Long Incubation Period

A basic feature of MS is the latency period between exposure
to the clausal agent and the clinical manifestations of the disease.

A prerequisite for latency is probably the innocuous persistence of the virus after acute infection, resulting from an incomplete clearance of the virus. Deficient clearance is to be
expected mainly in genetically determined low responders. The
group of factors supporting the persistence in the CNS is beyond
the scope of this paper.

Little is known about the events occurring in the CNS during
the incubation period. In fact, this period may consist of numerous subclinical relapses and remissions in localized areas.
This assumption is supported by findings in some of our animals,
where circumscribed lesions of different ages were found in the
absence of any clinical signs.

The fact that the disease remains subclinical may be due to
the relatively non-essential nature of the infected cells, the
absence of cytolytic response during virus growth or extremely
slow virus growth approaching the condition of total dormancy.

Relapse

Regardless of the mechanism by which the virus remains in
a relatively dormant or clinically unrecognized state, it seems
necessary to postulate some form of induction or reactivation mechanism to explain the deterioration of the clinical picture
during the relapse.

By analogy with RNA tumor viruses, the induction of dormant
viruses may be effected by biochemical changes that temporarily
disrupt cellular protein synthesis. The possibility of hormonal
induction might also be considered. Another mechanism for rescue of a latent or mutant virus from relatively nonpermissive
neural cells may be co-infection of these cells by another virus.
Once activated, the virus may now have access to another cell
type, e.g. to permissive cells of vessels in which normal cytolytic replication is possible, leading to expanded virus synthesis and spread back into the neuroparenchyma. The production
and release of infectious virus particles may result in a situation similar to that occurring in postinfectious encephalomyelitis. This speculation is supported by findings of acute inflammatory lesions in chronic MS. Such "early lesions" are indistinguishable from those found in EAE (3) or in postvaccinal encepha-

lomyelitis. In this situation, the same effector mechanisms of
demyelination may develop as in an acute PPE (postinfectious and
postvaccinal encephalomyelitis).

Remission

Remission necessitates the repression of effector mechanisms
operative during the relapse. A modified or exaggerated autoimmunity might be suppressed by a number of regulatory mechanisms
which are triggered simultaneously with each immune response.
Self-limitation of the pathogenic action is the expected consequence. Only disorders in suppressive mechanisms might lead
to chronic progressive course. Rescue of the dormant viruses
as a cause of a relapse may lead not only to the virus production
but also to activation of defence mechanisms. The outcome of
this situation depends on many host-specific and virus-specific
factors, which provide "fine tuning" of the virus-host relationship. A prerequisite for remission may be an efficient defence
which clears the extracellular particles and rejects the host
cells with antigenic membrane changes. In this case the situation is reestablished in which the virus is in a relatively
dormant or clinically unrecognized state.

ACKNOWLEDGEMENT

This study was supported by grant Si 174/5 from Deutsche
Forschungsgemeinschaft, and performed in collaboration with W.
Mintzel, K. and H. Huber, R. Wenner, Landesimpfanstalt, München.

REFERENCES

1. Johnson, R.T. : Virological data supporting the viral hypothesis in multiple sclerosis; in A.N. Davison, J.H. Humphrey,
A.L. Liversedge, E.I. Mc. Donald, J.S. Porterfield (Eds.) :
Elsevier, Amsterdam, New York 1975, M.S. Research, S. 155.
2. ter Meulen, V. : Multiple sclerosis : a case for viral etiology; in V. ter Meulen, M. Katz (Eds.) : Slow virus infections
of the central nervous system. S. 143. Springer, New York
1977.
3. Adams, C.W.M. : Morphological aspects of myelin and demyelination; in C.W.M. Adams (Eds.) : Research on multiple sclerosis. Thomas, Springfield/III. 1972.
4. Huber, H. Ch., Zinn, K.H., Hochstein-Mintzel, V., Simon, J.,
Stickl, H. : Sensibilisierung gegen Antigene des Zentralner-
vensystems nach experimenteller Infektion mit Vaccinia-Virus.
I. Nachweis einer zellulären Sensibilisierung. Zbl. Bakt.,
I. Alt. Orig. 232, 1 (1975).

5. Simon, J., Huber, H., Hochstein-Mintzel, V., Stickl, H. :
   Vacciniavirusinfektion als Trigger der Autoimmunreaktion.
   Zbl. allg. Path. 119, 119 (1975).
6. Simon, J., Hochstein-Mintzel, V., Huber, H., Gradl, A.,
   Hansert, E. : Die Suppression der experimentellen allergischen
   Encephalomyelitis durch vaccinia-virus-induzierte Hirnantikör-
   per. Z. Immun.-Forsch. 153, 23 (1977).
7. Blinzinger, K., Hochstein-Mintzel, V., Anzil, A.P. : Experimental vaccinia virus meningoencephalitis in adult albino
   mice : Virological, light microscopic and ultrastructural
   studies. Acta neuropath. (Berl.) 40, 193 (1977).
8. Woodruff, J.F., Woodruff, J.J. : The effect of viral infections on the function of the immune system; in : A.L. Notkins
   (Eds.) : Viral immunology and immunopathology. S. 393.
   Academic Press New York, San Francisco, London 1975.
9. Fahey, J.L. : Cell surfaces and immune activity; in : F.
   Wolfgram, G.W. Ellison, J.G. Stevens, J.M. Andrews (Eds.) :
   Multiple sclerosis. S. 417. Academic Press, New York, London
   1972.
10. Harter, D.H., Choppin, P.W. : Possible mechanisms in the
    pathogenesis of "postinfectious" encephalomyelitis; in : L.P.
    Rowland (Eds.) : Immunological disorders of the nervous
    system. S. 342. The Williams and Wilkins Comp., Baltimore
    1971.

HETEROGENEOUS HUMORAL AUTOIMMUNE RESPONSE IN MULTIPLE SCLEROSIS

B. Ryberg

Department of Neurology, University of Lund, Lund,
Sweden

Recent studies (1) have demonstrated that complement-fixing
IgG antibodies against antigens in central nervous tissue frequently occur in CSF from patients with MS but are seldom found in CSF
from patients with other neurological diseases. These antibodies
appeared to be organ-specific and their distribution between CSF
and serum suggested an intrathecal synthesis. Though antibodies to
gangliosides (2), galactosylceramide (3) and myelin basic protein
(4) have been found in serum from MS patients and other patients
with different techniques, the specificity of the complement-
fixing antibrain antibodies has been unknown.

In early attempts to define the specificity of these antibodies, I found antibodies to sulfatide to explain the reactivity
with brain extracts in serum and CSF from one MS patient. Sulfatide is a glycolipid hapten not earlier known as an autoantigen in
man. Continued studies of this hapten with MS samples reactive
with crude brain extracts were, however, negative. It was therefore evident that the antibodies represented different specificities.

In order to get some orientation in this situation I examined
paired serum and CSF samples from 60 MS patients, 15 patients
with chronic myelopathy (CM), and 60 controls (53 with other neurological diseases and 7 patients without neurological disease)
(5). Serum and CSF from these subjects were tested in a complement-fixation test at a standardized IgG concentration of 1000
mg/l against an extract in physiological saline and a lipid
extracts of human brain. The result is shown in Figure 1.

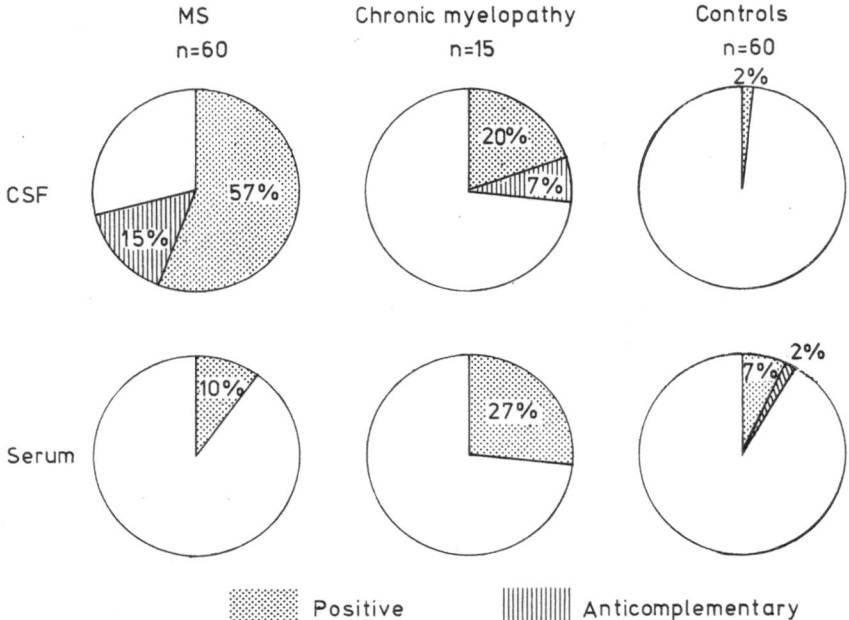

Fig. 1. The result of testing paired serum and CSF samples at 1000 mg IgG/l in the complement-fixation test against saline extract and lipid extract of human brain.

        The proportion of anticomplementary CSF samples was signifi-
cantly higher in the MS group than in the control group. This
property of some samples prevented the evaluation of their ability
to react with the antigens. Though anticomplementary activity
in serum and CSF samples might also be caused by unspecific
aggregates of immunoglobulins, it is not unlikely that it represents circulating immune complexes in these cases.

        Fifty-three per cent of the MS CSF samples had detectable
antibodies against antigens in the saline brain extract, whereas
7 % had antibodies against antigens in the lipid extract. A
number of samples were positive against both the saline extract
and the lipid extract. In total 57 % of the MS CSF samples were
positive against one or the other extract. If the anticomplementary CSF samples are excluded from the calculations, the proportion of positive MS CSF samples rises to 67 %. The CM group which
is likely to contain a number of MS patients not fulfilling the
clinical criteria of a MS diagnosis, also had a considerable
proportion of patients with antibrain antibodies in CSF, whereas
in the control group only a patient with SLE had such antibodies.
The percentual differences between the groups were less pronounced

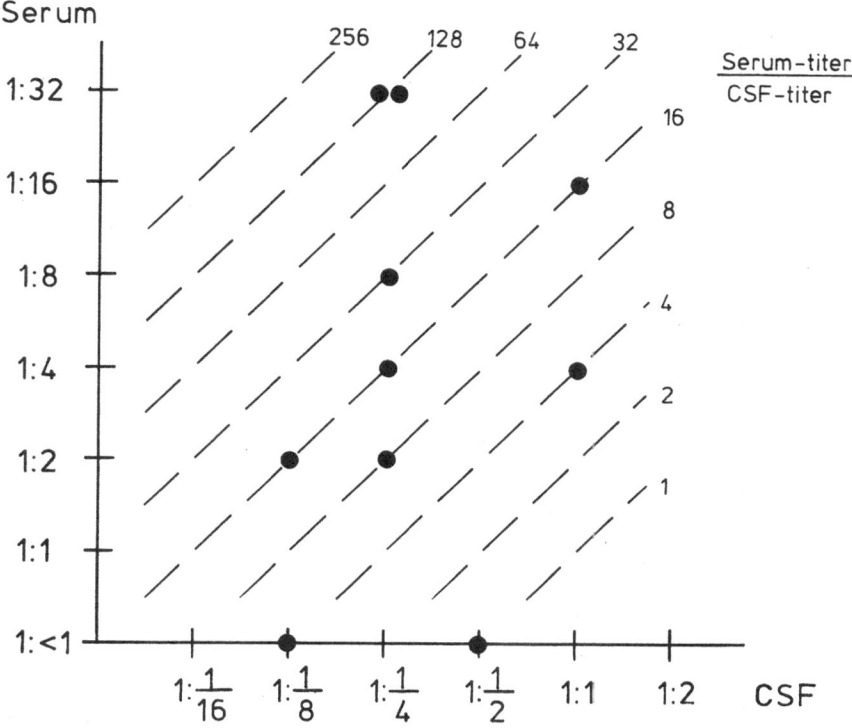

Fig. 2. Correlation between titers in serum and titers in CSF of complement-fixing antibrain antibodies in 10 MS patients.

when sera were compared, but the specificities of the antibodies in the control group differed from those commonly seen in the MS and CM groups.

Gel filtration experiments showed the antibodies to be generally of IgG class. Interestingly, one patient had a transient occurrence of IgM antibrain antibodies in serum in addition to a steady titer of IgG antibodies. This finding suggests that a fresh antigenic stimulation might have taken place. In the majority of the studied cases, the antibody activity was several times higher in CSF than in serum diluted to the same IgG concentration. Comparative titrations of paired serum and CSF samples, irrespective of IgG concentration, gave varying results (Fig. 2). The ratios between the antibody titres in serum and CSF were usually, but not always, much lower than the corresponding ratios of IgG concentrations and usually lower than known ratio values for a number of reference antibodies (6, 7). The most likely explanation for these low ratios is a local antibody synthesis within the CNS.

A large number of MS and CM samples with antibrain antibodies were further studied by testing against extracts of different organs and different tissues from the CNS.· The temperature resistance and the solubility of the antigens were also tested. The reactions caused by non-lipid antigens were extinguished by heating the extract to 80°C for 10 min. The antigens reactive in the saline extract were not solubilized in water or common aqueous buffers. The distribution within the CNS of the antigen that gave most positive reactions (antigen 1, Table 1) suggested an association with myelin. It also turned out that a purified myelin preparation was very rich in this antigen. Preliminary attempts to characterize this antigen indicate that it is an intrinsic membrane protein.

Immunological studies with lipids are complicated by the fact that lipids often get anticomplementary and lose their immunological activity during purification. To counteract this, socalled auxiliary lipids, e.g. lecithin and cholesterol have to be added in specific proportions (8). By purifying brain lipids by thin layer chromatography and by finding out suitable proportions of lecithin and cholesterol, I could demonstrate three specificities among the MS and CM samples positive against brain lipids. Two of these specificities could be identified.

In some CSF samples antibodies to galactosylceramide (galactocerebroside, cerebroside) were found. This is a glycolipid hapten found mainly in myelin. Autoantibodies to this substance have earlier been demonstrated in human sera (3), but not in CSF. Rabbit antisera to galactosylceramide have a demyelinating activity on CNS cultures (9). The antibodies were highly specific as they did not virtually cross react with glucosylceramide, that differs from galactosylceramide in the epimeric configuration at the C-4 position of the hexose. On the other hand substitution with a hydroxyl group on the C-2 position of the fatty acid residue did not seem to change the reactivity.

Antibodies to sulfatide were found in a new patient in the MS group. Sulfatide is a sulfate ester of galactosylceramide (galactosylceramide-3-sulfate) and similar to this substance it has a rich representation in myelin. If the sulfate group is split off by mild acid hydrolysis, the reactivity with the sulfatide antibody is lost and replaced by a reactivity with antibodies to galactosylceramide.

Samples from a few patients with MS, CM, rheumatoid arthritis and SLE gave results compatible with the presence of antibodies to cholesterol. This finding needs, however, further investigation.

Table 1. Properties and distribution of the antigens responsible for the reactions with antibrain antibodies in MS.

| | Antigen | | | | | | |
	I	II	III	IV	V	VI	VII
Lipid	-	-	-	-	Cerebroside	Sulfatide	Cholesterol?
Resistance to 80°C	-	-	-	-	+	+	
Other organs	-	-	-	(+)	(+)	+	+
Activity grey/white matter	1:4 - 1:16	1:4 - 1:8	1:1	4:1	1:4	1:16	
Myelin	+	+	-	-	+	+	
Bovine brain	+	-	+	+			

All the antigens reactive in the saline brain extract are present in all of several human brains tested, including one MS brain. Thus there is no reason to believe that alloantigens are involved in the studied immunological reactions. On the other hand a few samples reactive with human and rodent brain were not reactive with bovine brain.

The results of the investigation of the antigens to which the complement-fixing antibrain antibodies in MS and CM are directed, are summarized in Table 1. Antibodies to antigen 1 can be demonstrated in about half of the MS patients, whereas antibodies to the other six antigens together are found in about 14 % of the MS patients.

The antibrain antibodies of different specificities in MS demonstrate no apparent coupling to each other. Such a coupling would be expected if the MS patients had a generally increased tendency to produce autoantibodies. The selectivity suggested by these findings and the dichotomy of the MS population in patients with and without antibrain antibodies, might reflect a heterogeneity of the MS patients, the disease itself or its causing agent or agents.

A preliminary study of clinical parameters such as duration and severity of the disease and CSF findings did not reveal any impressive correlations with the results in the antibody investigation. Further, long term following of the titers of the antibrain antibodies, that shows interesting fluctuations in some cases, is not easily correlated with other clinical parameters. It will therefore be of interest to see if the autoantibody status is in some way correlated with the histocompatibility antigens of the MS patients. Preliminary results indicate that this is the case.

ACKNOWLEDGEMENT

This work was supported by a grant from the Greta and Johan Kock Foundation.

REFERENCES

1. Ryberg, B., Complement-fixing antibrain antibodies in multiple sclerosis, Acta Neurol. Scand. 12, 1-12 (1976).
2. Yokoyama, M., Trams, E.G. and Brady, R.O., Sphingolipid antibodies in sera of animals and patients with central nervous system lesions, Proc. Soc. exp. Biol. Med. (NY) 111, 350-352 (1962).
3. Dupouey, P., Role of the cerebrosides and galactodiglyceride

in the antigenic cross-reaction between nerve tissue and tre-
ponema, J. Immunol. 109, 146-153 (1972).

4. Sheremata, W., Wood, D.D., Moscarello, A.A. and Cosgrove, J.B.R.,
   Sensitization to myelin basic protein in attacks of multiple
   sclerosis, J. Neurol. Sci. 36, 165-170 (1978).

5. Ryberg, B., Multiple specificities of antibrain antibodies in
   multiple sclerosis and chronic myelopathy, J. neurol. Sci. in
   press.

6. Norrby, E., Link, H. and Olsson, J.E., Measles virus antibodies
   in multiple sclerosis, Arch. Neurol. 30, 285-292 (1974).

7. Fossan, G.O., The transfer of IgG from serum to CSF, evaluated
   by means of a naturally occurring antibody, Eur. Neurol. 15
   231-136 (1977).

8. Rapport, M.M. and Graf, L., Immunochemical reactions of lipids,
   Progr. Allergy 13, 273-331 (1969).

9. Dubois-Dalcq, M., Niedieck, B. and Buyse, M., Action of anti-
   cerebroside sera on myelinated nervous tissue cultures, Path.
   Europ. 5, 331-347 (1970).

SUBACUTE SCLEROSING PANENCEPHALITIS

A. Lowenthal

Born-Bunge Foundation, Department of Neurochemistry
U.I.A., Wilrijk, Belgium

HISTORY

Subacute sclerosing panencephalitis (SSPE) constitutes a
typical example of a neurological disease : first described by
clinicians, later observed by neuropathologists. The disease is
now recognized as a complex basic neurological problem. Although
relatively rare, one case per million children, SSPE has been
mentioned in the last forty years with increasing frequency in
scientific literature pertaining to neurology.

At the turn of the century, genetic and non genetic diseases,
assigned to the group of the so called diffuse sclerosis, were
characterized by a dementia syndrome, epileptic fits and amaurosis,
affecting only children, mainly boys. The pathology was traced
to the white matter of the brain, and the disease presented a
slowly evolutive course, chronical or at the most subacute. Neuropathologists revealed several distinct forms of the affection :
some were hereditary, others non genetic. For the latter three
groups of investigators individualized almost at the same time a
disease described as "panencephalitis", "subacute sclerosing leuco-
encephalitis" or "inclusion encephalitis". Each of the investigators stressed a different morphological aspect of the illness,
yielding only an incomplete picture. It was left to the clinicians
to demonstrate that the three terms designated in fact the same
clinical syndrome.

The first lumbar punctures from SSPE patients indicated that
the cerebrospinal fluid (CSF) total protein was slightly higher
or at the upper limit of the normal levels, and that the colloïdal

reactions, mainly "colloidal benjoin", were abnormal. A cellular reaction was not detected.

Electroencephalography revealed in SSPE anomalies never seen in other diseases. These anomalies appear later after the onset of the disease and less constantly than the changes in CSF. They are also maintained throughout the whole course of the disease.

Bucher, Matzelt and Pette (1) were the first to show the increase of γ -globulin levels in cerebrospinal fluid by paper electrophoresis. Agar gel electrophoresis allowed us to demonstrate that these immunoglobulins migrated in distinct fractions or bands (2). In 1961 (3), for the first time, we could show that SSPE sera often yielded the same anomalies as seen in the CSF.

Around 1967, it was generally accepted that a measles related paramyxovirus could be recovered from biopsies or autopsies of SSPE nervous tissue. The titers in measles antibodies were found to be considerably increased in the biological fluids and tissue from SSPE patients (4).

Beside subacute SSPE cases, chronic forms have been described which may evolve during many years. Recently cases of SSPE correlated with rubeola were reported.

To summarize this clinical description, SSPE is a chronic or subacute encephalitis affecting the grey and white matter, characterized by an immunological reaction which we would describe as an hyperimmune process. Our purpose is to prove this hypothesis.

Clinical Description

It is still not known when the disease really starts. Some authors suggest that it takes about seven years after an acute measles attack to develop SSPE. Seen from a clinical point of view, it causes first, a drop of the scholar achievements and affects mostly boys, who show also apraxia. The disease evolves slowly, affecting children from 2 to 10 years. Surprisingly, it often appears as if transient clusters of SSPE establish themselves in a given region, later to decline and then disappear. After the initial clinical signs, patients present myoclonic jerks and important neurovegetative reactions : hyperthermia, abondant sweating, etc... The evolution of the disease may take a few months or ten or more years (5). One may observe slight remissions or periods of stabilization. Total remissions have been described but appeared unconvincing. In a very few cases, verified anatomically, the electroencephalographic anomalies were never seen.

Various therapies utilising corticoids, immunosuppressors, antibiotics, levamisol, ... have been applied, none of which appeared to be really efficient.

The Immunological Reaction

The immunological manifestations of SSPE should really retain our attention. The increase of the immunoglobulin level, often considerable, was observed in all of the more than 200 samples of cerebrospinal fluid studied in our laboratory. The fractionation of the γ-globulin region can lead to 2 main and 5 minor components, as first demonstrated using agar gel electrophoresis, and later confirmed by agarose and cellulose acetate electrophoresis. A similar fractionation or restricted heterogeneity has been observed in 80 % of the more than 200 SSPE sera analysed in our laboratory. Both immunoelectrophoresis and specific titrations indicate that the increased and fractioned immunoglobulins belong to the IgG class. From the measles antibody titration it is likely that the high titers correspond to the increased IgG. This however has not been demonstrated unequivocally. The altered and increased light chain κ / λ ratio and the aminoterminal sequences of both the light and heavy chain variable regions suggest that the individual IgG are homogeneous proteins (6). It should be mentioned that those IgG's do not contain only one type of light chain. It is interesting to note that free chains have been detected in the cerebrospinal fluid, and also in the serum.

At the end stage of the disease, it means 2 or 3 days before death, the immunological reaction appears to fade away.

Virology

The paramyxovirus recovered from biopsies or autopsies of the SSPE central nervous tissue or lymphnodes is for some authors indistinguishable, for others similar to measles virus. This virus has now been grown in cultures. The fact that this virus is present at all stages of the disease indicates that SSPE should be classified as a slow viral disease or a persistant viral disease. Sigurdsson (9, 10) was first to describe slow virus diseases : these were soon subdivided in 2 types : on the one hand, the"visna" and the other hand the "rida" or "scrapie" type. The first type comprises transmissible diseases which virus is often known, with a typical immunological reaction, it is to say, the fractionation of the γ globulins. We were able to demonstrate the fractionation of the γ globulins in serum and cerebrospinal fluid from sheep affected by visna. Transmission appears to be difficult for the disease affecting humans. However, SSPE could belong to this group. As a virus can be isolated at all stages

of its evolution, SSPE should be considered as a persistant viral
disease.

The rida or scrapie type of disease has hitherto not been
characterized by specific viruses nor has an immunological reaction been reported. This transmissible disease presents a particular anatomo-pathological picture, that of spongiform encephalopathies.

Experimental hyperimmunisation leads to the synthesis of homogeneous antibodies as long as the antigens are injected or
persist but,so far, no neurological reaction has been seen in
animals. Maybe they should be followed for a longer period of
time. If we accept what is said, SSPE could be a slow viral
disease, with a persistant virus, which can be isolated during
the whole course of the disease and stands at par with an hyperimmune process, with synthesis of homogeneous antibodies.

                     Differential Diagnosis

Clinical or anatomopathological syndromes analogous to SSPE
have been described :
a) in treatment with immunosuppressors, of non neurological diseases
   or shortly after a measles infection. The electrophoretic studies we performed in one case gave a pattern identical to that
   of classical SSPE (7);
b) in measles vaccination programs. In these patients no electroencephalographic anomalies were detected. No electrophoretic
   studies were described (8);
c) after rubeola infections;
d) SSPE is representative of a more generalized phenomenon than
   thought initially. It is certain that the classical human measles encephalitis is entirely different clinically, anatomopatho-
   logically and immunochemically from SSPE, although neurological
   anomalies, different from those seen in SSPE, are frequent in
   measles. We performed also electrophoretic studies on material from animals experimentally infected with SSPE virus but
   we could not show any abnormal immunological reaction with the
   exception of one dog.

We conclude these observations concerning the description of
SSPE by stating that it definitely is a neurological viral disease
accompanied by an hyperimmunization process.

Is SSPE due to a specific virus ? Does the disease develop
in a particular environment, immunologically deficient or modified ? These two questions should help define the relationship
between the viral infection and the apparent hyperimmunization
and constitute a point to focus on.

REFERENCES

1. Bucher, Th., Matzlt, D. and Pette, D. Papier Elektrophorese von Liquor cerebrospinalis. Klin. Wschr. 13/14, 1, 325-330, 1952.
2. Karcher, D., van Sande, M. and Lowenthal, A. Microelectrophoresis in agar gel of the proteins of the cerebrospinal fluid and central nervous system. J. Neurochem. 4, 135-140, 1959.
3. Lowenthal, A., Karcher, D. and van Sande, M. Analyse électrophorétique des protéines sériques dans la LESS. Livre Jubilaire du Dr. L. van Bogaert, 506-514, 1962.
4. Measles Virus and Subacute Sclerosing Panencephalitis in "Neurology" 18, n°1, Part 2, 1968.
5. Rappel, M., Dubois-Dalcq, M., Sprecher, S., Thiry, L., Lowenthal A., Pels, S. and Thys, J.P. Diagnosis and treatment of herpes encephalitis. A multidisciplinary approach. J. Neurol. Sci. 12, 443-458, 1971.
6. Strosber, A.D., Karcher, D. and Lowenthal, A. Structure and idiotype of human homogeneous antibodies. Fed. Proc. (abstr.) 969, 1975.
7. Terheggen, H.G. and Lowenthal, A. SSPE in a child with treated acute lymphoblastic leukemia (in Press).
8. Lowenthal, A. and Karcher, D. Diagnosis of SSPE. J. Pediatr. vol. 93, nr 3, 537-538, 1978.
9. Sigurdsson, B., Palsson, P.A. and Grimsson, H. Visna, a demyelinating transmissible disease of sheep. J. Neuropathol. Exp. Neurol., 16, 389-403, 1957.
10. Sigurdsson, B. Observations on three slow infections of sheep. Brit. Vet. J., 110 : 7, 8, 9, 255-270, 307-322, 341-354, 1954.

ACKNOWLEDGEMENT

This study has been supported by grants from the Belgian National Fund for Medical Scientific Research (grant nr 30033), the Belgian Ministry of Education and Culture and the "Universitaire Instelling Antwerpen".

COMPARATIVE NEUROPATHOLOGY OF SUBACUTE SCLEROSING PANENCEPHALITIS

J.J. Martin

Department of Neuropathology, Born-Bunge Foundation,
U.I.A., Wilrijk, Belgium

HUMAN SUBACUTE SCLEROSING PANENCEPHALITIS (SSPE)

The.description of SSPE as a subacute sclerosing leukoencephalitis (1) was initially necessary to isolate this disorder from a heterogeneous group of diseases with a diffuse sclerosis of the white matter such as Schilder's disease, sudanophilic leukodystrophies, metachromatic leukodystrophy and diffuse gliomatosis of the white matter. Since the need for characterizing that disorder by one of its main morphological features has disappeared, it is logical to use the more accurate denomination of subacute sclerosing panencephalitis. Beside the sixty odd cases of the files of the Born-Bunge Foundation, we will especially consider the five cases autopsied during the last three years since they can be considered as representative of the various possible courses of the disease. In four of them, the clinical features and EEGs were highly suggestive of SSPE while confirmatory evidence was brought up by agar gel electrophoresis of CSF and serum or by autopsy or by both. In the fifth case of 14 years duration, the main clinical signs were epilepsy and dementia while typical periodic complexes were never found on EEG. Nevertheless agar gel electrophoresis allowed the diagnosis to be made; postmortem examination revealed still very active SSPE features including Cowdry type A inclusions in neurons and oligodendroglial cells.

Distribution of the Lesions.

Cortical and white matter lesions are the most prominent in SSPE but the involvement of the subcortical white matter and of the centrum ovale are often prevalent as shown by Osetowska (2) in a series of 50 cases from the files of the Born-Bunge Foundation : in 41 cases the white matter was apparently more severely affected than the grey matter. Admittedly these results are based on a qualitative evaluation of the lesions : in fact both grey and white matter are affected in every case but the lesions in the centrum ovale are always more impressive because of the fibrillary gliosis and of the demyelination.

Four major patterns of involvement can be recognized : a parieto-occipital one (28/50), a temporal one (9/50), a frontal motor one (6/50) and a generalized one (7/50). Demyelination is frequent (17/28) and severe in the parieto-occipital group: this reflects probably the initial appearance of the inflammatory foci in the caudal parts of the brain with a forward progression of the disease as suggested by Ohya et al. (3).

Among the deeper located nuclei, the medial part of the thalamus is often severely affected (28/50). Some authors, Petsche et al. (4),have assumed that the thalamic damage occurred very early and have tried to correlate it with the periodic complexes recorded on EEG. It is evident from our own study that the thalamus represents a heavily damaged area in SSPE but considering the ease and rapidity with which retrograde changes can occur in the thalamic association nuclei (5), it is really difficult to date the thalamic lesions with accurateness.

The brain stem involvement is frequent but has more often a nodular character. The inflammatory damage brought to the ventral pontine nuclei leads as in some of our cases to a picture of ponto-cerebellar atrophy. There exists however no direct relationship between the duration of the disorder and a demyelination of the brachia pontis as it was e.g. conspicuously absent in our case of 14 years duration.

In the spinal cord the lesions are essentially of a secondary nature affecting mainly the pyramidal pathways. Spinal ganglia and peripheral nerves have been reported to be affected in one case (6). Retinal involvement with inclusions in the ganglion cells has also been documented (7).

In visceral organs, measles antigen or immune complexes have been demonstrated by immunofluorescence or immuno-ultrastructural methods in liver, lung, renal glomeruli, spleen and lymph nodes (8, 9). Paramyxovirus nucleocapsids have been shown by routine electron microscopy in mononuclear cells present in the lungs (10).

Structure of the Lesions.

Intranuclear inclusions and to a lesser extent intracytoplasmic ones have been found by light- and or by electron microscopy in neurons and oligodendroglial cells in many cases, with some difficulty or not at all in a few other cases. Cowdry type A inclusions are also found in the brain stem (3, our own cases). Immunofluorescent or immuno-ultrastructural studies – see (6) for review – have demonstrated the presence of measles antigen, IgG, complement on the nucleocapsids, the plasma membranes and the external myelin lamellae (9). No autoantibodies were detected which could react with normal brain. It is barely necessary to describe the 16-18 nm wide paramyxovirus nucleocapsids, their electron-lucent core, their smooth outline and the periodic transverse striation distinct at higher magnification. A series of other inclusions have also been described and in some cases their measles antigen nature has been demonstrated by immunoperoxydase staining (11). An interesting electron microscopic feature is the occasional fusion of cell membranes which could suggest that cell to cell transmission is a possible mechanism for the spread of SSPE virus (12).

Neuronophagias, neuronal losses, and, when the course of the disease is of long duration, images of neurofibrillary degeneration have been described.

Among the glial changes, the presence of glial nodules is noteworthy but barely represents a specific feature. A diffuse microglial proliferation under the form of rod cells can be found in the cortex of SSPE patients but also in syphilitic general paresis or in trypanosomiasis. The astrocytosis present in the white matter has a strongly fibrillary character with production of dense bundles of thick filaments. A severe fibrillary gliosis can be found in association with a myelin pallor while a strong demyelination is always associated with a heavy fibrillary gliosis except when there is an edematous necrosis of the white matter (e.g. in the pseudo-tumoral form of SSPE).

The inflammatory reaction is characterized by perivascular cuffs composed of lymphocytes and of numerous plasma cells. Plasma cells with their basophilic cytoplasm can be found everywhere along the capillary walls and also in the adjacent neuropile. They undergo sometimes a transformation into morular cells with hugely distended ergastoplasmic citernae.

Demyelination in SSPE is a complex problem and results from different causes acting mainly in association :
1) a direct viral invasion of the oligodendrocytes with destruction of these myelin-forming cells;

2) as a consequence of immunologic reactions against the virus,
   the virus-infected cells or the plasma membranes having incorporated viral antigens;
3) as a result of permeability changes in the walls of the vessels
   produced by immune complexes deposits, resulting in a brain
   edema, the so-called pseudo-tumoral form of SSPE with secondary anoxia due to circulatory disturbances;
4) as a consequence of neuronal losses with wallerian degeneration;
5) as an autoimmune process of demyelination (?) although no auto-antibodies have been demonstrated by immuno-ultrastructural
   methods (9). The only restriction to the exclusion of autoimmunity is that only very few reports have dealt with that
   problem.

SSPE, Measles-Inclusion Body Encephalitis, Progressive Rubella PE.

    No differences can be noted between the histopathological
features of SSPE and the mononucleosis-associated SSPE reported
by Hochberg et al. (13). In SSPE with agammaglobulinemia (14, 15,
personal data on a Bruton type agammaglobulinemia with SSPE), the
only peculiar and expected feature was the absence of plasma cells.

    Measles-inclusion body encephalitis has been found after
recent measles infection in patients with lymphatic malignancies
and- or treated by immunosuppressants - see (16, 17) for a review.
Although measles nucleocapsids have regularly been found with or
without inflammatory features, there are no typical SSPE lesions
in such cases.

    Progressive rubella panencephalitis (18, 19) is due to another
viral agent. Some of the histopathological features such as the
peri- or paravascular deposits of amorphous material containing
acid mucopolysaccharides can be attributed to congenital rubella.
The panencephalitis lesions closely resemble the ones found in
SSPE.

                        EXPERIMENTAL SSPE

    After many unsuccessful experiments, encephalitides produced
by inoculating various SSPE strains have been described in suckling,
weaned or adult hamsters, ferrets, beagle dogs, calves and lambs
- see (6) for a review. Acute or chronic diseases have been induced by intracerebral infection. Although some histological features remind of SSPE such as the intense astrocytic proliferation
in hamsters (20) or the diffuse microglial proliferation (21),
it is fair to say that no experimentally induced SSPE has adequa-
tely reproduced the features of human SSPE. In their papers,

Raine et al. (22, 23) and Byington and Johnson (24) have described localized ependymal cell infection as a primary event. Multinucleated giant cells are often found and this is a highly unusual
feature in the human disease. The abundance of viral particles
and the ease with which they are shown in experimental SSPE contrast with the difficulty to demonstrate them in human cases.
Finally the dense fibrillary gliosis in the white matter so characteristic of human SSPE is missing in the infected animals.
Clearly other methods of inoculation are needed before satisfactory results can be obtained. However the use of such models enables
to study the different parameters which can influence the pathogenesis of the disease such as the influence of the host immunological competence on the characteristics of the viral agent, the role
of immunosuppression, of a combined administration of viruses,
of potentially therapeutic drugs.

SPONTANEOUS AND EXPERIMENTAL DISTEMPER IN DOGS

Distemper is a naturally occurring infectious disease of dogs
caused by a paramyxovirus closely related to human measles virus.
Neurological signs can appear early or later in the course of the
disease; they reflect an encephalomyelitic process. It is tempting
to try to correlate the different histopathological pictures of
distemper with human disorders. In a retrospective study of 72
cases from the files of the Born-Bunge Foundation, Liégeois et al.
(25) have distinguished four different forms : a hemodynamic form
close to a non-specific postinfectious encephalopathic reaction;
a classical distemper with four main localizations (brain stem,
cerebellum, spinal cord and optic pathways) to be compared with
post-infectious encephalomyelitis; a granulomatous type of distemper with demyelination and a subacute sclerosing panencephalitis
of the dog with features closely similar to human SSPE. A personal review of the same cases has shown that types 2 and 3 were
rather closely similar with numerous intranuclear inclusions in
astrocytes and less often in oligodendroglial cells. The topography of the lesions was very characteristic with a centripetal
progression of the inflammatory lesions starting subpially. Transition pictures were observed between the areas with moderate changes and the granulomatous areas with demyelination. It seems to
us that the histopathology of these two forms is different from
postinfectious encephalomyelitis, rabies postvaccinal encephalomyelitis and experimental allergic encephalomyelitis. Unfortunately it was impossible to tell from the study of the third form
whether the demyelinating lesions were secondary to the thick
perivascular inflammatory infiltrates or whether such cuffs represented relatively late events as suggested by Raine (26) in
an electron microscopic study of acute spontaneous distemper or by
McCullough et al. (27) in experimentally infected dogs. The patho-

genesis of demyelination in distemper is difficult to unravel just like in SSPE since for example Vandevelde and Kristensen (28) using fluorescent antibody techniques have considered it unlikely that demyelination in distemper resulted from a direct destruction of oligodendrocytes by viral activity. Wisniewski et al. (29) have tried to explain the demyelination by a "bystander" effect, as a secondary phenomenon resulting from an immunological conflict in the vicinity of myelin sheaths.

In the SSPE form of canine distemper the lesions can be compared with the ones observed in human SSPE including the diffuse sclerosis of the white matter. However the use of such animal material depends on its discovery which is not an easy task.

CONCLUSION

Although many interesting pathogenetic hypothesis can be derived from experimental or animal studies, human SSPE result from complex events which cannot be satisfactorily reproduced at present.

REFERENCES

1. van Bogaert, L. : J. Neurol. Neurosurg. Psychiat. 8:101-120 (1945).
2. Osetowska, E.: in Encephalitides, pp. 414-469, van Bogaert et al. Elsevier Publ. Co., Amsterdam (1961).
3. Ohya, T., Martinez, A.J., Jabbour, J.T., Lemmi, H., Duenos, D.A. Neurology (Minneap.) 24 : 211-218 (1974).
4. Petsche, H., Schinko, H., Seitelberger, F.: in Encephalitides, pp. 353-385, loco cit.
5. Martin, J.J. : Acta Neurol. Belg. 70 : 5-212 (1970).
6. Martin, J.J. : Riv. Patol. nerv. ment. 95 : 1-25(1974).
7. Font, R.L., Jenis, E.H., Tuck, K.D.: Arch. Pathol. 96 : 168-174 (1973).
8. Dayan, A.D., Stokes, M.I.: Brit. med. J. : 2 : 374-376 (1972).
9. Jenis, E.H., Knieser, M.R., Rothouse, P.A., Jensen, G.E., Scott, R.M. : Arch. Path. 95 : 81-89 (1973).
10. Ishihara, T., Uchino, F., Kamei, T., Yokota, T., Nakamura, H., Etoh, F., Suzuki, E., Konishi, S., Matsumoto, N.: Acta Path. Jap. 28 : 139-155 (1978).
11. Brown, H.R., Thormar, H.: Acta neuropath. (Berl.) 36 : 259-267 (1976).
12. Iwasaki, Y., Koprowski, H.: Lab. Invest. 31 : 187-196 (1974).
13. Hochberg, F.H., Lehrich, J.R., Richardson,Jr., E.P., Feorino, P., Aström, K.E.:Acta Neuropath. (Berl.) 34 : 33-40 (1976).
14. White, H.H., Kepes, J.H., Kirkpatrick, C.H., Schimke, R.N.: Arch. Neurol. 26 : 359-365 (1972).
15. Hanissian, A.S., Jabbour, J.T., Delamerens, S., Garcia, J.H., Horta-Barbosa, L.: Amer. J. Dis. Child. 123 : 151-155 (1972).

16. Drysdale H.C., Jones L.F., Oppenheimer D.R., Tomlinson A.H. : J. clin. Path. 29 : 865-872 (1976).
17. Aicardi J., Goutières F., Arsénio-Nunes M.L., Lebon P. : Pediatrics 59 : 232-239 (1977).
18. Weil M.L., Itabashi H.H., Cremer N.E., Oshiro L.S., Lennette E.H., Carnay L.:N.Engl.J.Med. 292 : 994-998 (1975).
19. Townsend, J.J., Baringer J.R., Wolinsky J.S. , Malamud N., Mednick J.P., Panitch H.S., Scott R.A.T., Oshiro L.S., Cremer N.E. : N. Engl. J. Med. 292 : 990-993 (1975).
20. Zlotnik I., Grant D.P. : British J. exp. Path. 57 : 49-66 (1976).
21. Brown H.R., Jervis G.A., Thormar, H. : J. Neuropath. exp. Neurol. 36 : 653-665 (1977).
22. Raine C.S., Byington D.P., Johnson K.P. : Lab. Invest. 31 : 355-368 (1974).
23. Raine C.S., Byington D.P., Johnson K.P. : Lab. Invest. 33 : 108-116 (1975).
24. Byington D.P., Johnson K.P. : Lab. Invest. 32 : 91-97 (1975).
25. Liégeois F., van Bogaert L., Osetowska E. : Bull. Acad. roy. Med. Belg. 9 : 805-875 (1969).
26. Raine C.S. : J. Neurol. Sci. 30 : 13-28 (1976).
27. McCullough B., Krakowska S., Koestner A. : Lab. invest. 31 : 216-222 (1974).
28. Vandevelde M., Kristensen B. : Acta neuropath. (Berl.) 40 : 233-236 (1977).
29. Wisniewski H., Raine C.S., Kay W.J. : Lab. Invest. 26 : 589-599 (1972).

CROSS-IDIOTYPIC SPECIFICITY AMONG IMMUNOGLOBULINS IN SUBACUTE SCLEROSING PANENCEPHALITIS AND MULTIPLE SCLEROSIS

A.D. Strosberg[*], B. Marescau[*], K. Thielemans[*], B. Vray[+],
D. Karcher[o] and A. Lowenthal[o]

[*] Laboratory of Pathology, V.U.B. Brussels, Belgium
[+] Laboratory of Microbiology and Immunology, U.L.B.,
    Brussels, Belgium
[o] Department of Neurology, Born-Bunge Foundation,
    U.I.A., Wilrijk, Belgium

SUMMARY

The existence of cross-idiotypic determinants among human oligoclonal Subacute Sclerosing Panencephalitis (SSPE) immunoglobulins was shown by the use of monospecific rabbit anti-idiotypic antisera. Sharing of idiotypy was also shown to exist to a lesser extent with sera from patients with Multiple Sclerosis (MS), another disease of the central nervous system. No reaction was observed with sera from other neurological diseases. Appropriate controls excluded artefacts due to a prevalent subclass of immunoglobulins in SSPE or MS. Identity with SSPE cerebrospinal fluid immunoglobulins and SSPE serum proteins was also demonstrated by the anti-idiotypic antibodies.

Our results confirm previous reported patterns of cross-specificity observed for other groups of human monoclonal proteins such as the IgM cold agglutinins or anti-γ globulin (1) antibodies and support the hypothesis of a close involvement of the antigen combining site in the idiotypic specificity.

INTRODUCTION

Previous workers have demonstrated the existence of cross-idiotypic determinants among monoclonal IgM proteins possessing anti-γ globulin activity in the same way that IgM cold agglutinins

97

from different individuals display antigenic specificities which
appear to relate to the combining specificity of these proteins
toward their respective antigens (1, 2, 3, 4). Evidence was obtained both for the cold agglutinins and the anti γ globulins that
the antigen-combining site was involved in these idiotypic specificities. Sequence analyses further confirmed the very marked
similarities of H and L chains of proteins sharing antigenic determinants (1, 5, 6, 7).

More recently idiotypic and cross-idiotypic specificities
were studied for anti-Rh antibodies (8).

The present studies were undertaken in an attempt to demonstrate similar cross-specificity between Subacute Sclerosing Panencephalitis (SSPE) immunoglobulins. In this slow virus disease,
high levels of immunoglobulin of restricted heterogeneity and with
anti-measles antibody activity are found in serum, in cerebrospinal fluid and in brain (9, 10). Idiotypic antisera were raised
by immunizing rabbits with purified immunoglobulin from individual
SSPE and were than used in analyzing cerebrospinal fluid and sera
from other SSPE patients for possible cross-reactions. Since several characteristics of SSPE are found in Multiple Sclerosis (MS),
another and much more prevalent disease of the central nervous system, sera from MS patients were also analyzed.

Our results suggest that patterns of cross-specificity between
SSPE immunoglobulins are similar to those observed for IgM cold
agglutinins or monoclonal IgM proteins with anti- γ globulin activity. A weaker but consistent cross-reaction with immunoglobulin
from MS sera is also observed and supports the idea that the two
central nervous system diseases are related.

                            MATERIALS AND METHODS

The SSPE sera were obtained from patients who clinically and
serologically manifested SSPE. The CSF samples from these patients
were obtained by lumbar puncture. MS sera were obtained from patients who clinically manifested the disease. SSPE immunoglobulins
were purified by ammoniumsulfate precipitation followed by DEAE
cellulose chromatography (9).

Rabbit antisera against SSPE immunoglobulin were produced by
immunization with purified immunoglobulin fractions isolated from
SSPE sera and mixed with equal volumes of complete Freund's adjuvant before injection. Antisera were rendered specific by passing
them through a panel of three human myeloma proteins containing
immunoabsorbent columns.

Agar immunodiffusion tests were performed in 3 % polyethylgly-

col (PEG) to maximize precipitation of soluble complexes. Immunoglobulin concentrations were determined by radial diffusion (11)
and immunoelectrophoresis was performed as described (12).

RESULTS

Three antisera made against different isolated SSPE immunoglobulins were used. After absorption with normal serum all reactivity was lost except for the protein used as antigen. When absorption was performed with immunoabsorbents containing individual or
a mixture of myeloma proteins, reactivity with normal serum was
lost but reactivity with proteins from cerebrospinal fluid from
the donor as well as with immunoglobulins from several other SSPE
patients was retained.

Reaction of Pas anti-Pas proteins from serum and cerebrospinal fluid is illustrated in figure 1. The same two lines of precipitation are visible in both samples.

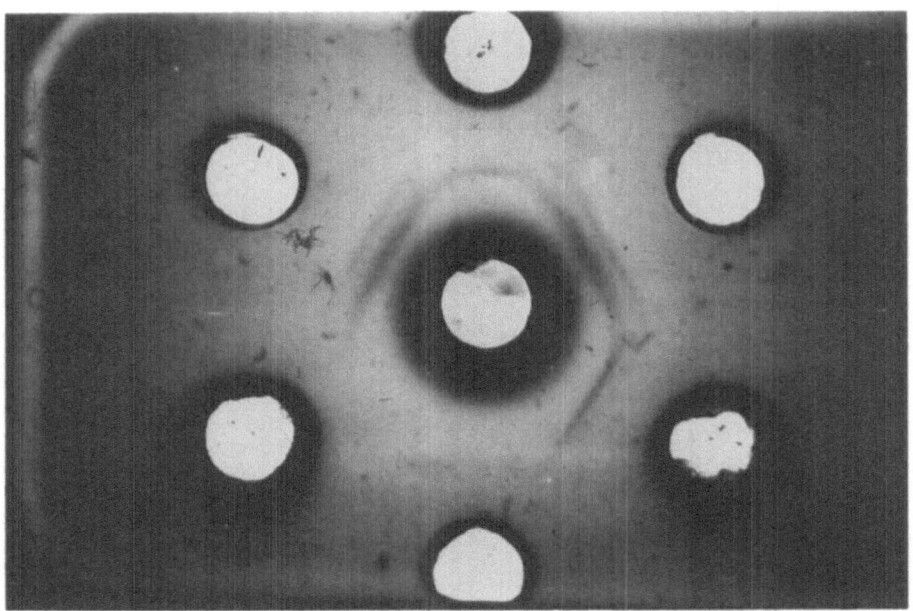

Figure 1 : Agar gel immunodiffusion in 3 % PEG. The central well
contains anti Pas antiserum. Wells 1 and 3 contain Pas purified
immunoglobulins (SSPE), wells 2 and 6 contain concentrated Pas
cerebrospinal fluid (SSPE). Well 5 contains normal pooled immunoglobulin and well 4 contains phosphate buffered saline.

Cross-specificity between SSPE immunoglobulins was also studied by immunodiffusion. Seven out of eighteen patient's sera
react with rabbit antibodies directed against the Sch proteins
and one other serum reacts with anti Pee or anti Pas antibodies.
(Table 1). No correlation of crossreaction with IgG concentration
or anti-measles antibody hemagglutination titers was observed.

No reaction could be detected with control serum samples,
which include a pool of 25 normal sera, twenty five individual
normal sera, twenty myeloma sera belonging to all four IgG subclasses other than SSPE or MS.

Anti Sch antibodies were also tested against MS sera. (Table 2).
Eight out of fifteen sera gave a faint precipitin line in 3 % PEG
agar immunodiffusion : the reaction was definitely weaker than
with SSPE sera but both the IgG content and the measles antibody
titer of MS sera were also generally lower than in SSPE sera.

TABLE 1

Analysis of SSPE sera

Sample	IgG conc. (mg/100ml)	Measles hemag-glutination inhibition titer	Reaction with anti Sch antisera
Dig	1285	4096	−
Ram	1974	4096	−
Gra	1546	8192	−
Zoog	2249	32168	+++
Mar	1778	32168	−
Kle	1862	32168	−
V. Ba	1637	16384	+++
Qui	2024	256	+++
Sch	2094	2048	+++
Pin	2030	64	+++
Dou	1370	256	+++
Car	1875	4096	+
Goe	1244	256	−
Pas	1875	4096	−
Lies	1203	256	−
Cab	1162	1024	−
Jan	1875	8192	−
Pee	1370	256	−

TABLE 2

Analysis of multiple sclerosis sera

Sample	IgG conc. (mg/100ml)	Measles hemag-glutination inhibition titer	Reaction with anti Sch anti-serum
Pee	162	128	-
Beu	1546	16	-
Gou	1875	-	-
Ver	1327	-	-
Deb	1413	-	+
Bas	1413	64	-
De B	1413	-	+
Half	1684	32	-
V. As	1591	-	++
Blo	1162	128	++
Tho	1546	8	++
Bol	892	32	++
Mae	472	-	-
V. Ac	1203	32	++
Ort	1370	512	+

All the SSPE and MS sera studied in this work were examined for the presence of particular immunoglobulin allotype combinations. No correlation was found between sharing of idiotypic determinants and given haplotypes (Van Loghem and Strosberg, unpublished results). These results do not exclude the sharing of a
yet unknown allotype.

The reaction between idiotype and anti-idiotype was analyzed
by immunoelectrophoresis to ascertain that the reaction occurs
between immunoglobulins.

Pepsin digestion of the anti-idiotypic antibodies did not
affect the specific reaction with the idiotype.

DISCUSSION

Subacute sclerosing panencephalitis (SSPE) is a slow virus
disease of the central nervous system characterized by the presence in brain, serum and cerebrospinal fluid of high concentrations
of immunoglobulins of restricted heterogeneity and high titers of
anti-measles antibodies (9). Sequence analysis of the aminoterminal 20 positions of both heavy and light chains from SSPE immunoglobulins from five patients has indicated that the light chains

belong to a subgroup intermediary between II and III subgroups
defined for myeloma and Bence Jones proteins (10). This subgroup
represents only 20 % of the heavy chains in normal serum (13).

In this work anti-idiotypic sera are used first to show that
the SSPE immunoglobulin present in the serum and in the cerebrospinal fluid displays the same antigenic specificities, and second
to detect common determinants on serum proteins from different SSPE
patients. The precise source of SSPE immunoglobulin in cerebrospinal fluid and serum has long been a matter of controversy : our
results would suggest a common origin and thus either a crossing
of the blood brain barrier by the proteins, or the movement of
lymphocytes between these two compartments.

The sharing of idiotypic determinants between immunoglobulins
from various SSPE patients confirms the sequence results which had
suggested common structural characteristics (10). The idiotypic
determinants are generally thought to correspond to the antibody
combining site (7). Since most SSPE immunoglobulins possess anti-
measles virus antibody activity not necessarily correlated with
hemagglutination-inhibition titers, the sharing of idiotypy could
be related to this specificity. This would explain why normal
serum, which contains appreciable amounts of measles antibody,ab-
sorbs out all crossreacting anti-idiotypic antibody. The myeloma
proteins used to prepare immunoabsorbents were devoid of measles
antibody activity.

Alternately, the cross-idiotypic antibodies could detect common features of antiviral antibodies in general, which would explain the reaction with MS sera, or the selection of a rare subclass of immunoglobulins in central nervous system diseases.

Not all anti-idiotypic antisera are equally succesful at detecting crossidiotypic determinants on proteins from different
SSPE patients. Nordal et al. (12) recently described an antiserum
raised against measles virus-specific IgG from a single patient,
which was unable to precipitate with other IgG from this patient
or from 4 other SSPE patients. In our laboratory, anti-Sch
antibodies are considerably more effective than anti-Pee or anti-
Pas idiotypic antisera.

ACKNOWLEDGEMENTS

The authors thank Dr. J.D. Capra for helpful suggestions and
critical review of the manuscript. The constant support of Dr. L.
Kanarek is gratefully recognized.

REFERENCES

1. Kunkel, H.G., M. Mannik and R.C. Williams 1963. Individual antigenic specificity of isolated antibodies. Science 140 : 1218.
2. Kunkel, H.G. 1970. Individual antigenic specificity, cross-specificity and diversity of human antibodies. Fed. Proc. 29: 55.
3. Williams, R.C., H.G. Kunkel and J.D. Capra. 1968. Antigenic specificities related to the cold agglutinin activity of gamma M globulins. Science, 161 : 379.
4. Kunkel, H.G., V. Agnello, F.G., Josling, E.J. Winchester and J.D. Capre 1973. Cross-idiotypic specificity among monoclonal IgM proteins with anti-γ globulin activity. J. Exp. Med. 137 : 331.
5. Capra, J.D., J.M. Kehoe, R.C. Williams, Jr., T. Feizi, and H.G. Kunkel. 1972. Light chain sequences of human IgM cold agglutinins. Proc. Natl. Acad. Sci. 69 : 40.
6. Kunkel, H.G., R.J. Winchester, F.G. Joslin, and J.D. Capra 1974. Similarities in the light chains of anti-γ globulins sharing cross-idiotypic specificities. J. Exp. Med. 139 : 128.
7. Capra, J.D. and J.M. Kehoe. 1975. Hypervariable regions, idiotypy, and the antibody combining site. Adv. Immunol., 20: 1.
8. Natvig, J.B., H.G. Kunkel, R.E. Rosenfield, J.F. Dalton and S. Kochwa 1976. Idiotypic specificities of anti-Rh antibodies. J. Immunol. 116 : 1536.
9. Lowenthal, A. Agar gel electrophoresis in Neurology, Elsevier Publishing C°., Amsterdam, 1964.
10. Strosberg, A.D., D. Karcher, A. Lowenthal. 1975. Structural homogeneity of human subacute sclerosing panencephalitis antibodies. J. Immunol. 115 : 157.
11. Capra, J.D., R.I. Wasserman and J.M. Kehoe. 1973. Phylogenetically associated residues among the V_HIII subgroup of several mammalian species. J. Exp. Med. 138 : 410.
12. Nordal, H.J., Vandvik, B. and Natvig, J.B. 1977. Idiotypy of measles virus nucleocapsid-specific IgG antibody in serum and cerebrospinal fluid in subacute sclerosing panencephalitis. Scand. J. Immunol. 6 : 1351.

THE VIROLOGICAL STATE IN SUBACUTE SCLEROSING PANENCEPHALITIS

J.R. Stephenson and V. ter Meulen

Institute of Virology and Immunobiology, University
of Würzburg, Würzburg, F.R. Germany

Subacute sclerosing panencephalitis (SSPE) is a slow virus
disease of the central nervous system(CNS) associated with a
measles virus infection. This disease has always been linked
to a viral agent after Dawson described in 1933 intracellular
inclusion bodies in SSPE brain tissue. However, only during the
last decade could the etiologic agent be identified (1, 2).
Despite this major discovery the pathogenesis of SSPE is still
not understood (3). Many features of this CNS affection are not
compatible with an ubiquitous measles virus infection. If
measles virus is involved then host or virus derived factors
must play an additional role to account for the rural prevalence,
rarity and the clinical course of SSPE. Moreover, explanations
have to be given for the mechanisms by which measles virus can
persist in the CNS and is activated years after onset of acute
measles. Many studies have been carried out recently to analyze
humoral and cell mediated immune reactions in SSPE and to
characterize the virus agents isolated from SSPE brain (referred
to as SSPE virus) in comparison to standard measles viruses. This
communication gives an account of the virological state in SSPE.

EVIDENCE FOR THE ASSOCIATION OF MEASLES VIRUS WITH SSPE

Presence of Measles-Specific Antibody

Although SSPE patients have normal levels of circulating B
and T lymphocytes, complement and antibodies to antigens other
than measles virus, they possess characteristic high titers of

measles-specific antibodies both in serum and CSF. The proportion
of virus-specific antibody in CSF is much higher than for other
virus-induced encephalitis. The measles-specific Ig is almost
exclusively IgG both in serum and CSF, although some measles-
specific IgM has been reported (4, 5). Evidence is available
that the measles-specific IgG in CSF is produced in the brain
and does not leak through the blood-brain barrier. The IgG in
both serum and CSF is relatively homotypic and has neutralizing
activity against measles virus and reacts with specific antigens
such as haemagglutinin, haemolysin and nucleocapsid (6). In
addition, these antibodies are competent in a complement-dependent
lysis assay using both measles and SSPE infected cells as targets
(7).

Presence of Nucleocapsids in Brain Material

Eosinophilic intranuclear (IN) and intracytoplasmic (ICP)
inclusion bodies are frequently found in neurones, astrocytes
and oligodendrial cells (8, 9). Both IN and ICP inclusions contain RNA by cytochemical staining (10) and consist of paramyxovirus
like nucleocapsid structures of diameter 17-23 nm and of length
up to 500 nm. The nucleocapsids are also found in both nucleus
and cytoplasm of cells persistently or lytically infected with
virus isolated from SSPE patients. The nuclear nucleocapsids
always have a "smooth" appearance and those in the cytoplasm a
rough appearance. This distinction between nuclear and cytoplasmic morphology is constant whether fresh autopsy material is
observed or that from lytically or persistently infected cells
is examined. Only the rough nucleocapsids appear in released
virus, whatever the source (12, 11). Although both IN and ICP
inclusions clearly stain with measles-specific fluorescent antibody, no characteristic cell fusion is noticeable in either brain
or other tissues (2).

Isolation of SSPE Virus

All standard methods for the isolation of SSPE virus from
SSPE brain material failed to recover infectious virus. Only
after cocultivation of SSPE brain tissue culture with cultures
susceptible for measles virus replication were SSPE virus isolated.
However, it is important to emphasize that the isolation of SSPE
virus is an exception rather than a rule (12). Virus has been
recovered not only from biopsy and necropsy material, but also
in one instant from lymph nodes (13). The characteristics of
these virus isolates vary from a virus which produces c.p.e. and
free infectious virus after only a few subcultures to those who
need many subcultures for complete expression. Other isolates
may establish a persistent infection with no free virus produced

and only subgenomic nucleocapsids and viral antigens being detected (14).

COMPARATIVE CHARACTERISTICS OF SSPE AND MEASLES VIRUSES

Morphology

Measles virus is the archetypic member of the genus, morbil-liviruses of the family, paramyxoviruses. It has a single-stranded, negative sense RNA as genome, encapsulated in a characteristic nucleocapsid containing two proteins, usually designated NP and 2, the latter of which is phosphorylated. This nucleocapsid is surrounded by pleomorphic lipid-containing envelope in which are situated the fusion protein and the haemagglutinin. Beneath this layer is the membrane protein, although its precise orientation in respect to the lipid envelope and the nucleocapsid is not known. So far isolates of SSPE virus show no gross morphological differences from that described above for measles virus except that in both persistent and lytic infections with SSPE, the nuclear form of the nucleocapsid predominates, whereas with measles it is the cytoplasmic form which is most common (2).

Biological Characteristics of Measles and SSPE Viruses in Vitro

There are several reports describing differences in host range and growth kinetics between these viruses (2). However, these findings are not consistent and do not rule out that the differences observed are in the range of variability occurring between different measles virus isolates. Similar observations have been made with standard serological assays. It could be shown that minor differences in the immunological reactivity may exist between SSPE and measles viruses in neutralization tests (15) or by a binding inhibition test based on an indirect radio-immunoassay (16). These immunological data suggest minor antigenic differences between SSPE and measles viruses, but they are not sufficient to clearly distinguish these virus strains. Recently, antigenic studies were carried out on isolated membrane (M) proteins from one SSPE and measles virus strain. Antisera against these purified proteins were raised in rabbits and specific antibodies were detected in a solid phase radioimmunoassay. By immunodiffusion and immunoelectrophoresis it could be shown that the M proteins were immunologically distinct, providing a basis for antigenic differentiation of measles and SSPE viruses used in these studies (17).

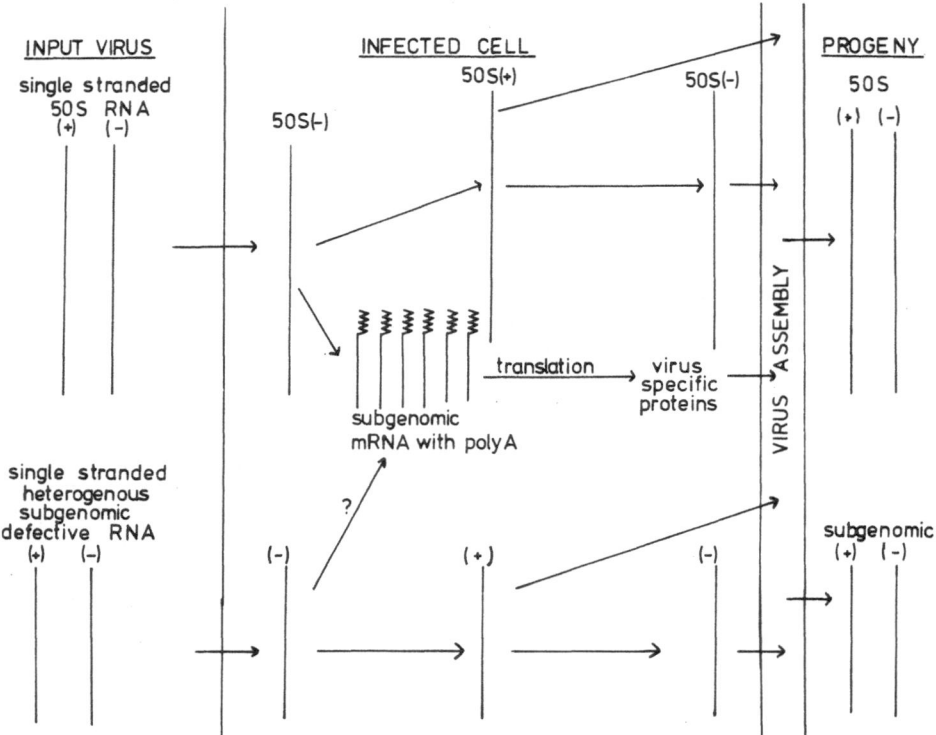

Fig. 1 Replication of Paramyxovirus RNA

Comparative Biochemical Studies

Several recent studies have centered on the biochemistry of
these viruses. Although little is known about the replication of
measles virus, it is assumed to follow the overall replication
pattern of the paramyxoviruses (Fig. 1). The notable features in
this replication scheme is that both positive and negative strands
are incorporated into nucleocapsids and presumably into virions,
and that a significant number of subgenomic defective nucleocapsids
are formed. These defective particles certainly alter the growth
characteristics of the virus in vitro and may lead to the establishment of a persistent infection although their role in the course
of either measles or SSPE has yet to be elucidated.

The RNA's of measles and SSPE viruses have been compared by
hybridization. One study showed that SSPE 50S RNA shared 60 %
homology with measles 18S RNA, although no attempt was made to
determine the role played by negative stranded subgenomic defective

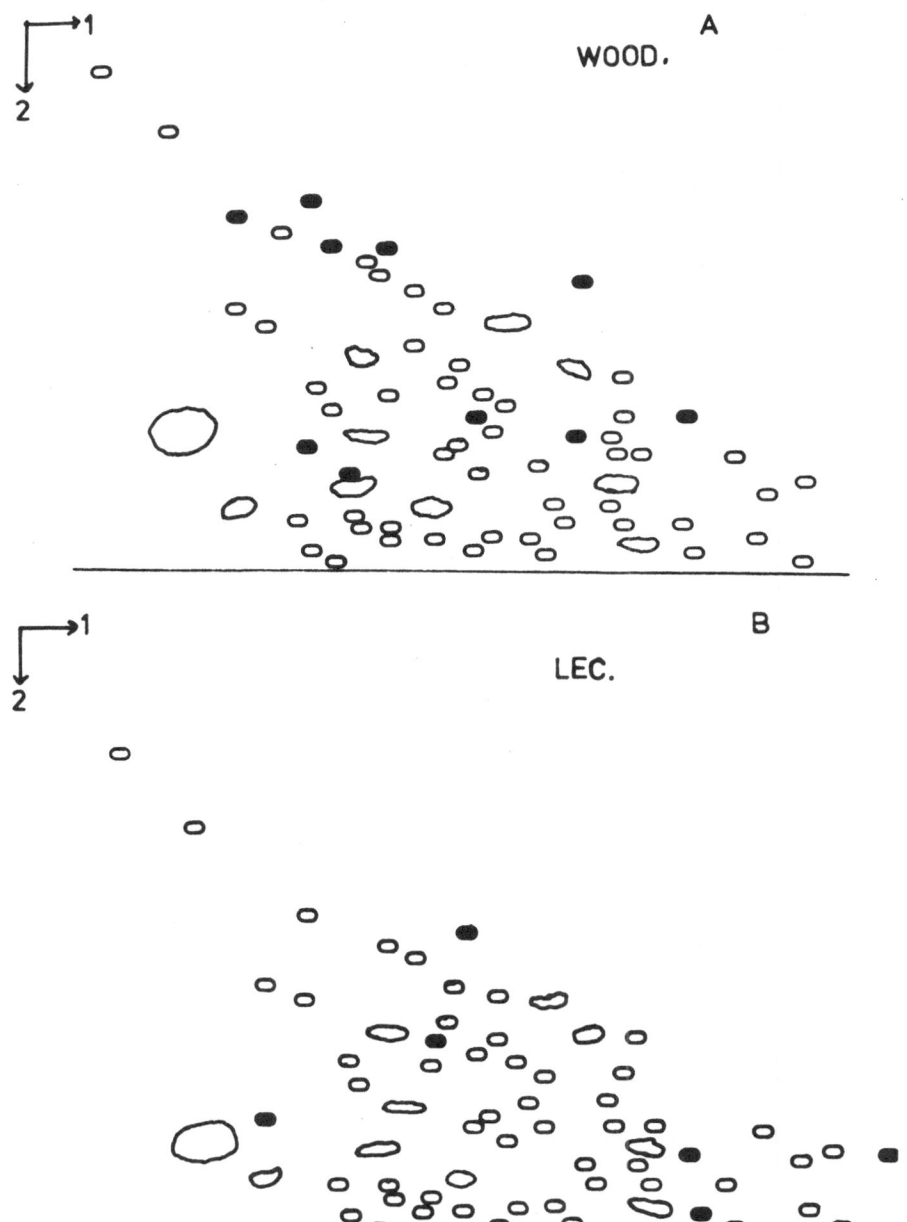

Fig. 2. Two dimensional electrophoresis of T_1 oligonucleotides.
2×10^7 VERO cells were infected with virus at a m.o.i. of O.1.
At the first sign of syncytia, cells were incubated for 1 h with
1 μg/ml of Actinomycin D. Incubation was then continued in the
presence of 10 mCi of ^{32}P orthophosphate until c.p.e. was

complete. Cells were harvested and cytoplasmic RNA extracted as
described previously (22). The final ethanol precipitated RNA
was separated on an aqueous 15-30 % sucrose gradient and the
material sedimenting at 50S was reprecipitated in ethanol and run
on a second sucrose gradient. The 50S material from the second
aqueous gradient was denatured by heating at 37° for 5' in 50%
dimethylformamide, 25 % DMSO, 1 % SDS, 10 mM EDTA and 10 mM Tris
pH 7.4, and run on a 15-30 % sucrose gradient in 50 % formamide.
The material sedimenting between 45 and 50S was taken, digested
with T_1 ribonuclease and analysed by two dimensional electrophoresis as described previously (23). For ease of comparison only
the large oligonucleotides are considered, that is, those migrating slower in the second dimension than an arbitary line drawn
halfway between the cyanol FF and bromophenol blue dyes. The
positions of the oligonucleotides on the X-ray film are transposed
to transparent film and photographed.
A. A two dimensional "map" of Woodfolk 50S RNA. The closed spots
are oligonucleotides present in Woodfolk and absent in LEC.
B. A map of RNA from LEC. The closed spots are oligonucleotides
present in LEC and absent in Woodfolk.

RNAs (18). A more detailed analysis using oligo dT isolated mRNA
and competition hybridization suggested that SSPE mRNA had a
higher genetic complexity than measles mRNA (19). These authors
have also reported differences in migration on SDS P.A.G.E. of
at least one mRNA from SSPE and measles viruses. Similar small
differences in apparent molecular weight have been reported for
the M and P proteins for several strains of SSPE (20) although
these do not appear to be restricted to SSPE viruses (21).

The data so far have only demonstrated differences in the
information contained in mRNA. Recently we have extended these
studies by analyzing the oligonucleotides from a T_1 digest of
single stranded 50S RNA from the cytoplasm of actinomycin D
treated infected cells. If the wild-type measles virus is
compared with an archetypic SSPE virus (LEC) (Fig. 2), it is
seen that although the maps are broadly similar, there is a
significant number of differences, i.e. although the SSPE virus
has lost some oligonucleotides, it also has oligonucleotides
that Woodfolk does not. It has been suggested that such
differences could arise by co-infection and recombination with
an animal paramyxovirus such as that found in isolates from
canine distemper - a known virus-associated CNS disease of
dogs. Fig. 3 shows two oligonucleotide maps of CDV (Onderster-

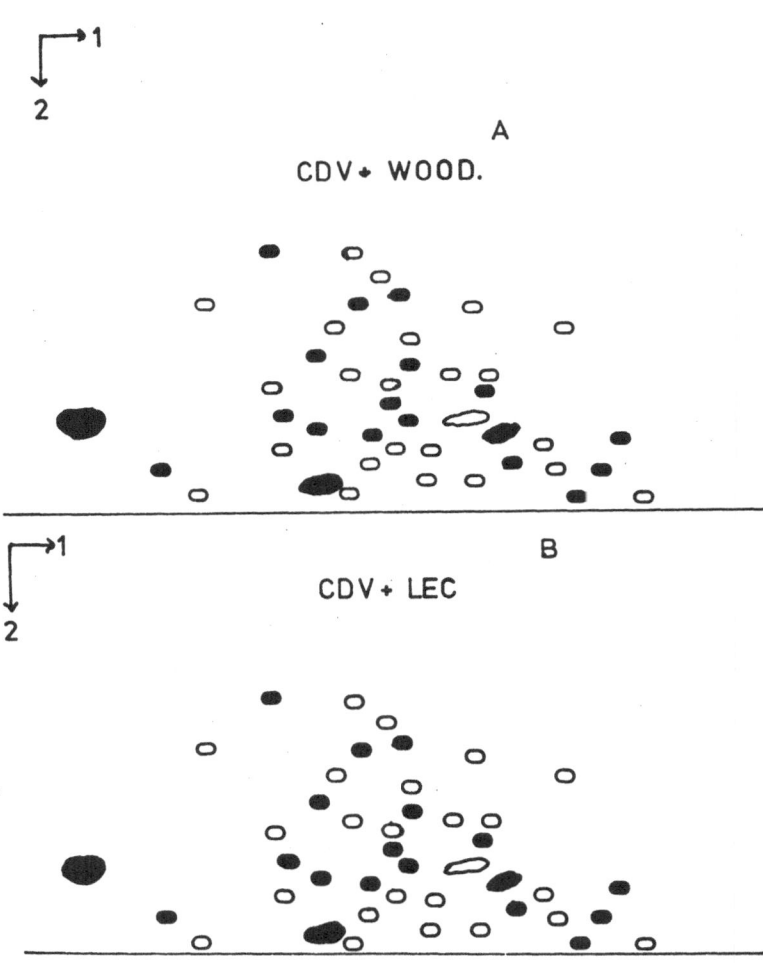

Fig. 3. An oligonucleotide "map" of CDV 50S RNA.
A. The closed spots are oligonucleotides present in CDV and
Woodfolk.
B. The closed spots are oligonucleotides present in CDV and LEC.

poort strain) in which the oligonucleotides found in common
with Woodfolk (3A) and LEC (3B) are shown by the closed spots.
As these diagrams are identical, none of the unique oligonucleotides found can be attributed in Woodfolk or LEC to similar
sequences in CDV.

CONCLUSIONS

The consistent virological findings of virus structure in
SSPE brain material and a humoral hyperimmune reaction against
this virus documents clearly the etiological role of SSPE virus
in this disease. Morover, Koch's first postulate, the occurrence
of the "parasite in every case of the disease in question" seems
to be fulfilled. So far the experimental data on M protein,
mRNA and genomic RNA indicate that SSPE viruses are closely related to measles virus but are not identical.

One of the main virological questions concern the origin
of SSPE viruses. If SSPE viruses primarily represent an independent strain of the measles virus, infecting SSPE patients, one
would expect a clustering of this disease which has not been
observed. Moreover, the three reports of SSPE developing in one
of identical twins only (2) argues against the interpretation
of the occurrence of SSPE viruses as one independent strain
within the group of morbilli viruses. It is more likely, that
SSPE viruses have been derived from measles virus during CNS
persistency. Based on the available biochemical data for SSPE
viruses a mutation has to be postulated, possibly in the region
of the genome, coding for the M protein. This mutation could
be responsible for some of the differences observed between
measles and SSPE viruses. If a non-functional M protein becomes
produced which is incompatible with normal virus assembly, then
the genesis and maintainance of SSPE persistency in the CNS
could be explained. Whether the mutation is host dependent or
not, cannot be identified at present nor the role it may play in
the pathogenesis of the disease.

ACKNOWLEDGEMENT

Supported by the Deutsche Forschungsgemeinschaft grant
Me 270/16.

REFERENCES

1. ter Meulen, V., Katz, M. and Müller, D. (1973) Curr. Top.
   Microbiol. Immunol. 57, 1-38.

2. Agnarsdottir, G. (1977). In "Recent Advances in Clinical Virology" pp. 21-49, ed. A.P. Waterson, Churchill Livingston, London.
3. ter Meulen, V., Hall, W.W. and Kreth, H.W. (1978). In "Persistent Viruses". Academic Press, New York, in press.
4. Kiessling, W.R., Hall, W.W., Yung, L.L.L. and ter Meulen, V. (1977). Lancet 324-325.
5. Salmi, A., Ziola, B. and Halonen, P. (1978) In "International Virology IV" p 223, Pudoc, Wageningen, Holland.
6. Vandvik, B. and Norrby, E. (1973). Proc. Natl. Acad. Sci. USA, 70, 1060-1063.
7. Kibler, R. and ter Meulen, V. (1975). J. Immunol. 114, 93-98.
8. Cowdry, E.V. (1934). Arch. Pathol. 18, 527-542.
9. Herndon, R.M. and Rubinstein, L.J. (1968). Neurology, 18, part 2, 8-18.
10. Müller, D. and ter Meulen, V. (1969) Acta Neuropathol. (Berl.) 12, 227-243.
11. Oyanagi, S., ter Meulen, V., Katz, M. and Koprowski, H. (1971) J. Virol., 7, 176-187.
12. Katz, M. and Koprowski, H. (1973) Arch. ges. Virusforsch. 41, 390.
13. Horta-Barbosa, L., Hamilton, R., Wittig, B., Fuccillo, D.A., Sever, J.L. and Vernon, M.L. (1971). Science, 173, 840-841.
14. Kratzsch, V., Hall, W.W., Nagashima, K. and ter Meulen, V., (1977) J. Med. Virol. 1, 139-154.
15. Payne, F.E. and Baublis, J.V. (1973). J. Infect. Dis. 127, 505.
16. Hall, W.W., Kiessling, W.R. and ter Meulen, V. (1978) in "Negative Strand Viruses and the Host Cell" 143-156, Academic Press, London.
17. Hall, W.W. and ter Meulen, V. (1978) Nature, 272, 460-462.
18. Yeh, J. (1973) J. Virol., 12, 962-968.
19. Hall, W.W. and ter Meulen, V. Nature (1976), 264, 474-477.
20. Wechsler, W. and Fields, B.N. (1978), Nature, 272, 458-459.
21. Hall, W.W. personal communication.
22. Stephenson J.R., Hay, A.J. and Skehel, J.J. (1977) J. Gen. Virol., 36, 237-248.
23. de Wachter, R. and Fiers, W. (1972) Anal. Biochem., 49, 184-193.

CELLULAR IMMUNITY IN SUBACUTE SCLEROSING PANENCEPHALITIS

G. Agnarsdottir [+] and H. Valdimarsson [x]

+ Department of Virology, Hammersmith Hospital, London, U.K.
x Department of Immunology, St. Mary's Hospital, London, U.K.

Subacute sclerosing panencephalitis (SSPE) is a fatal, neurological disease caused by measles or a measles-like virus (1).

THE VIRUS

Measles is an enveloped RNA virus belonging to the paramyxovirus group. When the virus is released from infected cells, it acquires its envelope by budding off the cytoplasmic membrane at a site where virally coded antigens have previously been inserted. The infected cell membrane is capable of fusing readily with an adjacent, uninfected cell membrane, thus allowing continued spread of virus, without exposure to antibodies.

MEASLES VIRUS AND CELLULAR IMMUNITY

We know from experiments in vivo and in vitro that successful control of many enveloped viruses is mainly carried out by cellular immune mechanisms. Furthermore, it is known from clinical experience that intact cellular immune mechanisms are essential for eliminating an infection with measles virus. Individuals suffering from congenital or acquired deficiency of thymus-dependent lymphocytes develop severe, often fatal measles with atypical clinical features. In contrast, hypogammaglobulinaemic children with intact cellular immunity develop normal measles and acquire lasting immunity.

Not only are cellular immune mechanisms critical for the successful elimination of the virus, but lymphocytes are also targets for virus infection. The virus can be isolated from lymphocytes during acute measles and they form giant cells in culture on mitogen stimulation (2). Histopathological changes attributable to measles virus may be seen in lymphoid organs at various times during measles infection from the prodromal stage onwards. These are particularly severe in the thymus of children who die during or shortly after the disease (3).

Impairment of cellular immunity by measles infection has been recognized since von Pirquet described the anergy to tuberculin which occurs during, and for some time after, measles (4). This finding has subsequently been confirmed, and found to apply to other antigens as well. Moreover, activation and spread of tuberculosis has been reported after an attack of measles and the rate of secondary infections following measles is notorious (5, 6).

The susceptibility of lymphoid cells to measles infection may be influenced in vivo by the phenomenon observed in vitro, viz. that 60-70 % of peripheral blood lymphocytes have a receptor for measles virus (7). This immunologically non-specific binding involves predominantly T lymphocytes and it may facilitate infection of these cells by the virus in vivo. Infected lymphocytes may then serve as a vehicle for the spread of virus within the body, even to immunologically privileged sites such as the brain. It is known from in vitro studies that productive, cytolytic infection only takes place in activated lymphocytes (8). However, it has also been reported that non-stimulated lymphocytes may become infected with the virus in vitro, but the infection remains largely non-productive until the lymphocytes are stimulated with mitogen (9).

IMMUNO-EPIDEMIOLOGICAL FEATURES OF SSPE

SSPE is predominantly a disease of childhood, the mean age of onset being 7.2 years, although individuals from two to thirty-two years have been affected. It is very rare and only seen in one child in every two hundred thousand to one million of the childhood population. Boys are affected more frequently than girls, the ratio being 3.3/1[10]. The disease is fatal and the pathological changes involve only one organ, viz. the brain. SSPE patients generally have primary measles which is normal or mild, but a significant observation is that about 50 % of patients have their measles before the age of two. It has been the practice in the U.S.A. for over ten years to give measles immunization to children before the age of two, but there is no evidence of an increased incidence of SSPE following this. On

the contrary it seems to have decreased. So far, no genetic
abnormalities nor HLA associations have been found. Moreover,
SSPE patients have normal resistance to other infections both
before and after the onset of their disease.

CELLULAR IMMUNE RESPONSES IN SSPE PATIENTS

In SSPE we are faced with a persistent measles infection
of the brain in spite of an exaggerated measles antibody
response. Bearing in mind the importance of cellular immune
mechanisms in eliminating measles infections, many investigators
have looked for a defect in cellular immunity in these patients,
especially to measles (1). Unfortunately, most in vitro tests
for cellular immunity to the virus have proved unsatisfactory.
This may be due partly to a suppressive effect mediated by the
virus on specific lymphocyte responses, but specific measles
reactivity is probably also marked by the non-specific
association of the virus with human lymphocytes. Thus, in
lymphocyte transformation assays, very low levels of stimulation
have been obtained with either live or inactivated measles
virus. This suppressive effect has also been noted on
concurrent stimulation with measles virus and non-specific
mitogen (PHA) (11) or specific antigen (PPD) (12). When measles-
infected cells were used to stimulate lymphocytes, a greater
blastogenic response was obtained, but this was already maximal
after three days, a time course which is characteristic of
non-specific mitogens rather than specific antigens. No
significant difference was found between SSPE patients and
normals in this test (13).

Inhibition of leucocyte or macrophage migration has been
described in the presence of measles antigen but is possibly of
a non-specific nature due to receptors for measles virus on T
lymphocytes (14). There are conflicting reports on the ability
of SSPE lymphocytes to respond in these tests. Some describe
intact MIF production, others describe lack of inhibition of
leucocyte migration after exposure to measles virus. The main
in vitro tests which have been used recently to assess cellular
immune responses to measles are cytotoxicity assays. There are
various mechanisms which are known to operate in cell-mediated
cytotoxicity. One is by sensitized T lymphocytes, alone or in
co-operation with macrophages. Another is mediated by K lymphocytes, which possess receptors for the Fc part of cell-bound IgG
antibody molecules, and require the presence of antibody to
become cytotoxic (ADCC). Still another mechanism, not yet
fully investigated, involves the so called "natural killer" cells.
These are non-phagocytic cells with neither T nor B lymphocyte
characteristics which can be non-specifically cytotoxic to
virus-infected as well as to malignant cells. Lastly, it is

possible that, in the case of measles, T lymphocytes can be
non-specifically activated to become cytotoxic because of their
binding to measles-infected cells. The general finding has been
that unfractionated, peripheral blood lymphocytes from SSPE
patients are able to kill measles-infected cells in the presence
of fetal calf serum and in the absence of complement (7). This
killing may be mediated by non-specific T cell activation or by
natural killer cells. Less likely would be local antibody production within the assay system allowing K cell killing. By adding
measles antibodies to the assay system, many workers have found
enhancement of killing by SSPE as well as by normal lymphocytes,
indicating K cell activity. When SSPE serum or cerebrospinal
fluid was added, some workers found inhibition of cytotoxicity,
suggesting the presence of a blocking factor (15, 16). This
blocking effect was more pronounced in some patients than others
and was also found to vary from time to time in the same patient.
The blocking also varies according to the type of target cell
used and it is probably mediated by antigen-antibody complexes.
By using purified lymphocyte populations cytotoxic activity has
been found to be mediated both by K cells and T cells (17, 18,
19). Cytotoxic activity by the latter was found to be somewhat
reduced in SSPE patients compared to controls (19). Histocompatibility restriction of the T cell killing was not observed,
possibly because killing of measles-infected cells by human
lymphocytes may largely be non-specific (7).

Another important parameter of cellular immunity to measles,
and the only one which can be tested in vivo, is delayed
hypersensitivity. Using inactivated measles vaccine as well as
a control antigen we have observed specific anergy to measles
on skin testing 25 SSPE patients at various stages of their
disease. However, in a group of 353 controls, most of whom
were young adults or adolescents, about 50 % were found to
respond to this antigen. It is not clear whether the measles
anergy in SSPE is primary or whether it is secondary to the
infection, or to the high measles antibody levels (immune
deviation). However, positive skin reaction to measles has
been observed in several SSPE patients during intensive Transfer
Factor treatment and this conversion was not associated with
significant reduction in measles antibody levels.

The cellular immune responses to antigens unrelated to
measles, both in vivo and in vitro, have been found to be normal
early in the disease, but in patients with advanced disease
these may become increasingly anergic.

SPECULATIONS ON PATHOGENETIC MECHANISMS IN SSPE

Recent reports (20) suggest that there may be significant
structural differences between measles virus and the viruses

isolated from SSPE brains. However, there is no epidemiological
evidence to support the idea that the SSPE virus as such is
transmitted in the community. If these two viruses turn out
to be different, it is more likely that a wild measles strain
undergoes a change which allows it to persist or to become
reactivated, and if so, it is likely that this occurs within
the host who later develops SSPE. This change may occur due
to pressure from host factors or it may occur spontaneously
as a variant during virus replication.

Infection at an early age with wild measles as opposed
to vaccine virus clearly predisposes a child to develop SSPE.
However, early infection cannot alone be a decisive factor as
there are many children with a similar experience who do not
develop SSPE. Maternal measles antibodies which are present
to a variable degree from one infant to another, may possibly
modify the initial measles infection. This has been observed
in suckling hamsters, which, after intracerebral measles
inoculation, were protected from acute infection by maternal
antibodies but did later develop a persistent neurological
infection (21).

Another possible mechanism could arise if a subpopulation
of lymphocytes became infected with the virus, eg. suppressor
cells involved in controlling antibody production against the
virus. Elimination of measles specific suppressor cells could
lead to an exaggerated measles antibody response. This might
in turn modulate the virus infection further. When measles-
infected cells are grown in vitro in the presence of measles
antibodies, the cells will undergo antigenic modulation and
virally coded antigenic determinants are shed off the cell
membranes in the form of antigen-antibody complexes. In the
continued presence of measles antibodies, the cells do not express
new viral antigens on their surfaces and will thus fail to be
eliminated by relevant, effective immune mechanisms. However,
they still remain infected and may be able to spread virus by
membrane fusion to adjacent cells. If the antibodies are reduced
or removed, the cells will again express viral antigens on their
surfaces (22). It is not known whether these mechanisms apply
in vivo, and the pathogenetic mechanisms of SSPE remain a matter
for speculation.

CONCLUSION

Cellular immune reactions both in vivo and in vitro to
mitogens and measles unrelated antigens are generally normal in
SSPE patients, except in advanced disease when they may become
anergic. Delayed hypersensitivity to measles virus has been
found to be absent in a group of 25 SSPE patients. There are
at present no satisfactory in vitro tests available to assess

specific T lymphocyte reactivity to measles virus. It has therefore not been possible to exclude the presence of a selective defect in cellular immunity to measles virus in patients with SSPE.

REFERENCES

1. Agnarsdottir, G. Recent Advances in Clinical Virology. Churchill Livingstone, 21-49, 1977.
2. Osunkoya, B.O., Cooke, A.R., Ayeni, O. & Adejumo, T.A. Arch. ges. Virusforsch. 44, 313-322, 1974.
3. White, R.G. & Boyd, J.F. Clin. Exp. Immunol. 14, 343-357, 1973.
4. von Pirquet, C. Dtsch. Med. Wochenschr. 34, 1297-1300, 1908.
5. Bech, V. Am. J. Dis. Child. 103, 252-253, 1962.
6. Miller, D.L. Brit. Med. J. 2, 75-79, 1964.
7. Valdimarsson, H., Agnarsdottir, G. & Lachmann, P.J. Nature 255, 554-556, 1975.
8. Sullivan, J.L., Barry, D.W., Lucas, S.J. & Albrecht, P. J. Exp. Med. 142, 773-784, 1975.
9. Lucas, C.J., Ubels-Postma, J.C. & Galama, J.M.D. Abstracts of the Fourth International Congress for Virology, 71, 1978.
10. Jabbour, J.T., Duenas, D.A., Sever, J.L., Krebs, H.M. & Horta-Barbosa, L. J. Am. Med. Ass. 220, 959-962, 1972.
11. Sullivan, J.L., Barry, D.W., Albrecht, P. & Lucas, S.J. J. Immunol. 114, 1458-1461, 1975.
12. Smithwick, E.M. & Berkovich, S. Proc. Soc. Exp. Biol. Med. 123, 276-278, 1966.
13. Thurman, G.B., Ahmed, A., Strong, D.M., Knudsen, R.C., Grace, W.R. & Sell, K.W. J. Exp. Med. 138, 839-846, 1973.
14. Nordal, H.J., Frøland, S.S., Vandvik, B. & Norrby, E. Lancet, 2, 1266-1267, 1975.
15. Valdimarsson, H., Agnarsdottir, G. & Lachmann, P.J. Proc. R. Soc. Med. 67, 1125-1129, 1974.
16. Steele, R.W., Fuccillo, D.A., Hensen, S.A., Vincent, M.M. & Bellanti, J.A. Arch. Neurol. 32, 501, 1975.
17. Kreth, H.W. & Wiegand, G. J. Immunol. 118, 296-301, 1977.
18. Perrin, L., Tishon, A. & Oldstone, M.B.A. J. Immunol. 118, 282-293, 1977.
19. Ewan, P.W. & Lachmann, P.J. Clin. Exp. Immunol. 30, 22-31, 1977.
20. Hall, W.W. & ter Meulen, V. Nature, 264, 424-477, 1976.
21. Wear, D.J. & Rapp, F. J. Immunol. 107, 1593-1598, 1971.
22. Oldstone, M.B.A. & Tishon, A. Clin. Immunol. Immunopathol. 9 55-62, 1978.

PROGRESSIVE RUBELLA PANENCEPHALITIS

M.L. Weil [+], N. Cremer [x], H.H. Itabashi [+], B. Vandvik [o] and E. Norrby [*]

+ Los Angeles County Harbor-UCLA Medical Center, Torrance, U.S.A. x California State Department of Health, Berkeley, U.S.A. o Department of Neurology, Ulleval Hospital, Oslo, Norway. * Department of Virology, Karolinska Institute, Stockholm, Sweden

SUMMARY

Persistent infection with rubella virus can result in slowly progressive degeneration of the central nervous system after an interval of four to twelve years. At least nine cases are known as complications of congenital or acquired rubella. This condition is characterized by progressive dementia, progressive motor dysfunction and seizures. Unusual immune responses characterize this disorder. Endogenous synthesis of oligoclonal rubella-specific IgG antibodies and homogeneous free light chains occur within the central nervous system. Persistence of serum IgM antibodies against rubella virus for at least 12 years has been observed. Circulating immune complexes have been demonstrated using the Clq technique. Persistence of virus has been confirmed by isolation of rubella from brain in one case 12 years after congenital infection and 4 years after onset of symptoms. Inhibition of leukocyte cytotoxicity for rubella infected target cells has been demonstrated for serum but not cerebrospinal fluid in this condition.

Histocompatibility antigens present in one child were HLA-A3, HLA-AW 24, HLA-B7 and HLA-BW 27.

Normal findings include absence of deposits of IgG or complement in brain biopsy specimens and normal serum total and B-1 complement levels.

PROGRESSIVE RUBELLA PANENCEPHALITIS

Rubella virus is now known to cause a chronic progressive
panencephalitis (PRP) after both congenital (16, 20) and acquired
(8, 21) infection. At least nine cases have been recognized during the last few years. In addition to the five reported from
California (20, 16, 21), one has been reported from France (8),
one from the Eastern United States (J. Sever and S. Huff, Bethesda)
one from Israel (O. Abramsky, Jerusalem) and one from Canada
(J.E. Jan, Vancouver).

Clinical manifestations of PRP are those of insidious dementia, progressive pyramidal and extra-pyramidal dysfunction and
multifocal myoclonic seizures. Macular pigmentation may occur.
The group occurring after congenital rubella have the onset of
symptoms at four to twelve years of age. Onset in the acquired
rubella group has been as late as nineteen years of age, twelve
years after the primary infection with rubella (21). All cases
recognized to date have been males. The illness has a duration
of at least seven years in some of the surviving cases, but has
a slow and relentless course characterized by progressive deterioration and death.

Pathological changes have included periventricular enlarge-
ment and cerebellar atrophy. Microscopic evidence of subacute
and chronic inflammatory changes are seen with slight cellular
involvement of the meninges. Perivascular infiltration with
lymphocytes and plasma cells, loss of myelin and later loss of
axons, diffuse astrocytic and microglial proliferation, and microglial modules indicative of cell destruction are present.

Perivascular deposits of iron and acid mucopolysaccharide
are found in the hemispheric white matter, basal ganglia and
cerebellum (17). Such changes have also been described in classical cases of congenital rubella.

PRP patients are of particular interest. They provide the
opportunity to study immune mechanisms in persistent infections
with conventional viral agents. Rubella virus has been isolated
from brain biopsy material(5) and leukocytes (22) from cases of
PRP despite high antibody titers for long periods of time. It
is uncertain if the brain isolate came from infected neural elements or from the mononuclear cells present in the brain specimen. No rubella virus components have been found upon direct
fluorescent antibody or electron microscope examination of the
brain tissue (20, 5).

Humoral immune responses have been striking in the cerebrospinal fluid (CSF) although a pleocytosis of only 0-37 cells/mm^3
and a slight elevation in protein (60-142 mg/dl) has been noted.

The CSF gamma globulin content has ranged from 35 to 52 % of the total protein. In one case endogenous production of IgG in the central nervous system was estimated by the method of Tourtellotte (15) at 532 mg/day (20). The IgG is oligoclonal in character (21, 19).

Serum antibody titers against rubella have been elevated in some cases. Hemagglutination inhibition titers (HAI) of 128 to 2560 and complement fixing titers (CF) of 128 to 8192 have been observed. Initial CSF HAI titers range from 16 to 128 and CF titers from 8 to 256 (22). The ratio of serum to CSF antibody has been markedly lower than that which is found in the usual case of acquired rubella.

The increase in CSF immunoglobulin is selective for IgG; IgA, IgM and IgD have not been increased (19). In one patient, the CSF demonstrated far-cathodic κ IgG bands which were not found in the serum. Free light chains, primarily of the λ class, were present in the anodic region. Only a small amount of κ free light chain was present. The reason for the presence of free light chains is unclear. It may reflect a desynchronisation of heavy and light chain assembly.

After electrophoretic separation of CSF antibody, distribution of IgG and various rubella-specific antibodies were compared (19). The HAI, CF and hemolysis-gel (HIG) (14) antibodies demonstrate a variable distribution in relation to the IgG and to each other. Treatment of serum with rubella infected SIRC or Vero cell pack absorbs microheterogeneous IgG which is not readily apparent in the serum. This can be released from the cell pack by serial elution with pH 4, 3, and 2 buffers. The far cathodic CSF band and possibly the anodic serum band were not represented in the eluates (19). The reason for this is unclear. It may be because the band did not represent rubella antibody, was unstable in acid buffers or was specific for an antigen absent in the rubella infected cell pack.

Prolonged persistence of rubella-specific IgM antibodies is a striking feature of PRP. IgM antibodies to rubella have been identified in serum at titers of 1:2 and 1:4 using sucrose density and HAI techniques. In one patient who had congenital rubella, the IgM antibody titer (HAI) was 1:2 at age 11 and 12, three and four years after onset of PRP. IgM antibodies persist longer in PRP than in congenital infection where first trimester disease results in demonstrable antibody for as long as 16 months following birth (4). In primal postnatal infections, IgM antibodies to rubella virus are present for only two to four months (3, 6, 11). In complicated cases of acute rubella, IgM antibody may persist for seven (7) to 20 (12) months.

Persistence of IgM antibody suggests an active rubella infection of prolonged duration. Prolonged activity is also suggested by the presence of circulating antigen-antibody complexes in the case we have studied. Drs. Luc Perrin and Michael Oldstone, using the method of Nydegger et al. (10) demonstrated a 10 % precipitation of ^{125}I-Clq (normal 3.8 $\pm$ 0.7 %). Elevated levels of circulating immune complexes have also been observed in two other cases (Wolinsky, to be published).

Persistent levels of interferon have been observed in two cases (22) and on one occasion in our case.

The presence of a heat stable inhibitor for cell mediated cytotoxicity has been suggested (23) in studies using PRP patient lymphocytes and BHK-21 cells persistently infected with rubella virus in a ^{51}Cr micro-assay according to the method of Steele (24). These observations are summarized in Table 1. The inhibitory factor was not clearly demonstrable in the CSF. A similar phenomenon has been described for serum and cerebrospinal fluid from parients with SSPE (13).

Genetic factors for immune responsiveness may play a role in PRP. Histocompatibility antigens present in onse case include HLA-A$_3$, HLA-AW$_{24}$, HLA-B$_7$ and HLA-BW$_{27}$. Presence of these antigens in one child suggests that tissue typing should be done for other cases. An association of HLA-A 3 and HLA-B 7 has been suggested for multiple sclerosis, HLA-B 7 with allergy, and HLA-BW 27 with ankylosing spondylitis, Reiters disease and acute anterior uveitis (2, 9).

A number of normal observations have been made in these patients. Brain biopsy specimens have failed to disclose deposits of IgG or complement (Perrin, L. and Oldstone, M.M.B., personal communication). Serum total and beta$_1$ complement have been normal.

The immunological responses of the host in PRP are similar in many ways to those seen in SSPE (18, 1). Humoral responses to persistent infection with these conventional viral agents differ from those characteristic of the conventional acute infection. It is probable that similar humoral immune mechanisms are involved in the pathopoiesis of PRP and SSPE. In both instances, there is evidence of prolonged antigenic stimulation. In addition, there is prolonged persistence of virus with a full complement of genomic material despite the presence of high levels of humoral antibody.

REFERENCES

1. Agnarsdottir, G. : Subacute sclerosing panencephalitis, in Waterson, A.P. (ed.). Recent Advances in Clinical Virology, London, Churchill Livingstone, 1977, p.21.

2. Bach, F.H. and van Rood, J.J. : The major histocompatibility complex-genetics and biology, N. Engl. J. Med. 295 : 806-813, 872-878, 927-936, 1976.

3. Craddock-Watson, J.E., Bourne, M.S. and Vandervelde, E.M. : IgG, IgA and IgM responses in acute rubella determined by the immunofluorescent technique, J. Hyg. (Camb) 70 : 473-485, 1972.

4. Craddock-Watson, J.E., Ridehalgh, M.K.S. and Chantler, S. : Specific immunoglobulins in infants with the congenital rubella syndrome, J. Hyg. (Camb) 76 : 109-123, 1976.

5. Cremer, N.E., Oshiro, L.S., Weil, M.L., et al. : Isolation of rubella virus from brain in chronic progressive panencephalitis. J. Gen. Virol. 29 : 143-153, 1975.

6. Field, P.R. and Murphy, A.M. : The role of specific IgM globulin estimations in the diagnosis of acquired rubella, Med. J. Aust. 2 : 1244-1248, 1972.

7. Haire, M. and Hadden, D.S.M.: Immunoglobulin responses in rubella and its complications, Brit. Med. J. 3 : 13o-132, 1970.

8. Lebon, P. and Lyon, G. : Non-congenital rubella encephalitis, Lancet 2 : 468, 1974.

9. Munro, A. and Bright, S.: Products of the major histocompatibility complex and their relationship to the immune response, Nature 264 : 145-152, 1976.

10. Nydegger, U.E., Lambert, P.H., Gerber, H., et al. : Circulating immune complexes in the serum in systemic lupus erythematosis and in carriers of hepatitis B antigen, J. Clin. Invest. 54 : 297-309, 1974.

11. Ogra, P.L., Kerr-Grant, D., Umana, J.L., et al. : Antibody response in serum and nasopharynx after naturally acquired and vaccine-induced infection with rubella virus, N. Engl. J. Med. 285 : 1333-1339, 1971.

12. Ogra, P.L., Chiba, Y., Ogra, J.L., et al. : Rubella-virus infection in juvenile rheumatoid arthritis, Lancet 1 : 1157-1161, 1975.

13. Steele, R.W., Fuccillo, S.A., Hensen, M.M., et al. : Specific inhibitory factors of cellular immunity in children with subacute sclerosing panencephalitis, J. Pediatr. 88 : 56-62, 1976.

14. Strennegård, Ø., Grillner, L. and Lindberg, I.-M. : Hemolysis in gel test for the demonstration of antibodies to rubella virus, J. Clin. Microbiol. 1 : 491-494, 1975.

15. Tourtellotte, W.W. : What is multiple sclerosis : laboratory criteria for diagnosis : in Multiple Sclerosis Research. Edited by A.N. Davison, J.H. Humphrey, A.L. Leiversedge, et

al. : N.Y., Elsevier Scientific Publishing Co., pp. 9-26, 1975.

16. Townsend, J.J., Baringer, J.R., Wolinsky, J.S., et al. : Progressive rubella panencephalitis : late onset after congenital rubella, N. Engl. J. Med. 292 : 990-993, 1975.

17. Townsend, J.J., Wolinsky, J.S. and Baringer, J.R. : The neuropathology of progressive rubella panencephalitis of late onset, Brain 99 : 81-90, 1976.

18. Vandvik, B., Norrby, E., Nordal, H.J., et al. : Oligoclonal measles virus-specific IgG antibodies isolated from cerebrospinal fluids, brain extracts and sera of patients with subacute sclerosing panencephalitis and multiple sclerosis, Scand. J. Immunol. 5 : 979-992, 1976.

19. Vandvik, B., Weil, M.L., Grandien, M., et al. : Progressive rubella panencephalitis : synthesis of oligoclonal virus-specific IgG antibodies and homogeneous free light chains in the central nervous system. Acta. Neurol. Scand. 57 : 53-64, 1978.

20. Weil, M.L., Itabashi, H.H., Cremer, N.E., et al. : Chronic progressive panencephalitis due to rubella virus simulating subacute progressive panencephalitis, N. Engl. J. Med. 292 : 994-998, 1975a.
    Weil, M.L., Itabashi, H.H., Rola-Pleszczynski, M., et al. : Chronic progressive panencephalitis due to rubella virus, Arch. Neurol. 32 : 501-502A, 1975b.

21. Wolinsky, J.S., Berg, B.O. and Mailand, C.J. : Progressive rubella encephalitis, Arch. Neurol. 33 : 722-723, 1976.

22. Wolinsky, J.S., 1978, Handbook of Neurology, Vol. 34 in press.

23. Weil, M.L., Perrin, L., Buimovici-Klein, E., Oldstone, M., Cooper, L.Z. : Immunological abnormalities associated with chronic progressive panencephalitis due to congenital infection with rubella virus. Clin. Res. 24, 185A, 1976.

24. Steele, R.W., S.A. Hensen, M.M. Vincent, D.A. Fuccillo and J.A. Bellanti : A 51 Cr micro-assay tecjnique for cell-mediated immunity to viruses. J. Immunol. 110 : 1502-1510, 1973.

MULTIPLE SCLEROSIS AND THE HLA DETERMINANTS

M. Alter

Department of Neurology, Temple University School of
Medicine, Philadelphia, U.S.A.

HLA AND DISEASE

There is a region on chromosome six in man which contains
genes which are major determinants of histocompatibility. These
are the genes which confer uniqueness upon the cellular characteristics of every individual. These uniqueness markers enable the
immune system to recognize tissue which is self from foreign, non-
self tissue. The region, called HLA, contains four loci labelled
respectively HLA-A, B, C, and D. Each of these loci has many
allelic forms. In addition, there are loci believed to contain
immune response genes, complement genes and a closely related
region which is labelled Dr. A gene which determines B cell
antigens is located in or near the HLA locus.

Our knowledge of this genetic system received a major impetus
when its importance for tissue transplantation became evident but
the value of the HLA genes to general medicine was appreciated only after association between the HLA genes and particular diseases was shown. The most impressive association exists with ankylosing spondylitis; 95 % of patients with ankylosing spondylitis
have the B27 HLA determinant. The association apparently involves
a heightened susceptibility or a genetic predisposition among individuals with B27 who, after an appropriate triggering illness
such as a bacterial infection, have an increased risk of developing
ankylosing spondylitis. Thus, not every carrier of the B27 gene
develops the disease and there are some patients who fit rigid
criteria for ankylosing spondylitis who do not have the B27 determinant.

MULTIPLE SCLEROSIS AND HLA GENES

In the last several years, during which the relationship
between HLA genes and disease was being explored, a weak association between HLA genes and multiple sclerosis (MS) was found. In
most populations studied, the HLA A3 and B7 genes were increased.
Later, an even stronger association was found between a D locus
gene, Dw2, and MS (Table 1). While the statistical significance
of the association of these genes with MS seems firmly established,
the biological significance remains obscure. Many patients otherwise "typical" examples of MS do not have A3 or B7 or Dw2 genes
and many individuals who possess these genes do not have MS. Moreover, the association with these particular genes and MS has not
been found in all populations : Israeli patients and Japanese
patients with MS do not show an excess of HLA A3 or B7
Clearly, the relationship between MS and the HLA genes is more
complex than the relationship between ankylosing spondylitis and
B27.

POSSIBLE SIGNIFICANCE OF HLA-A3, B7 AND Dw2 IN MS

There is some evidence that individuals with MS who have the
HLA A3, B7 genotype, may have a more malignant course. However,
not all investigators have been able to confirm that the clinical
course in MS is affected by the HLA system. Another line of investigation suggests that individuals with A3 or B7 may be better
humoral antibody formers when challenged with certain common viruses such as rubeola, a fact which would help explain the higher
humoral antibody level to measles (rubeola) in MS patients than
in controls. If a viral response is, in fact, involved in MS,
the population-specific associations between MS and particular
HLA genes might mean that different viruses trigger MS in different populations - a condition which would make the search for a
single "virus of MS" more difficult. However, it is not known
whether the HLA genes really render individuals susceptible to
MS by virtue of inducing a special response to viral infection,
as is believed to occur with ankylosing spondylitis, or whether
the mechanism explaining the weak association in MS is due to
some entirely different mechanism. One idea which has been put
forth is that the HLA genes are actually markers for another
closely linked hypothetical gene called "MSS" for multiple sclerosis susceptibility. If there is such an MSS gene, then one
should be able to trace its inheritance in families with more
than one member who has MS.

HLA HAPLOTYPES IN MULTIPLEX MS FAMILIES

     The HLA haplotype consists of the HLA gene-set inherited from
a parent. Thus, each person has two HLA haplotypes. Multiplex
families are those with two or more members affected with MS.
Such constellations of cases should, theoretically, provide information on presence of an MSS gene. The reasoning is as follows :
if MS is due to a dominant gene which is closely linked to an
HLA gene, the affected members in a family should share an HLA
haplotype significantly more often than non-affected members. Reduced penetrance of MS and the possible need for an exogenous event
to trigger clinical expression of MS are two factors which might
complicate analysis of multiplex families. More important, however, is the high inherent likelihood that members of a family
will share a given haplotype. Indeed, if a parent and child have
MS, the likelihood that they will share one haplotype is a certain-
ty. Among siblings, the probabilities are as follows : the chance of inheriting one haplotype is 50 per cent. That given type
will be shared by 25 per cent of siblings (1/2 x 1/2 = .25).
Because the shared haplotype is determined after inspection of
the pedigree, a statistical test of significant association must
be applied to the unaffected sibs. This test assumes that unaffected sibs will inherit the shared haplotype significantly less
often than affected sibs. Thus, if there is no association, then
50 per cent of the unaffected sibs will inherit the same haplotype as was shared by the affected sibs; if there is an association,
then the unaffected will inherit the shared haplotype significantly less often than 50 per cent of the time. An alternative method
utilizes Norton's lod score method for demonstrating linkage
rather than merely association between an HL-A linked susceptibility gene and MS.

     A sizeable number of multiplex families with MS have now
been collected and the inheritance of HLA haplotypes has been analyzed. On balance, these studies have failed to demonstrate that
MS is inherited with a particular HLA haplotype in simple mendelian fashion. Thus, there is no evidence, as yet, to support the
notion of an MSS gene.

     It is still possible that the HLA genes studied are not clo-
sely enough linked to the MSS gene. Therefore, some investigators recommend studying inheritance of B cell antigens in multiplex MS families. They assume that the B cell antigen determinant is more closely linked to MSS than HLA-A, B, C or Dw. However, it seems unlikely, at this juncture, that this approach
will be fruitful. An alternative is that there are different
types of MS and only some are influenced by HLA genes. This possibility also seems rather unattractive at present. Whatever the
correct explanation, it seems definite now that the association

between the HLA genes and MS represents more than a fortuitous
connection. It is true that the connection is not so simple as
was once hoped, when the association between HLA gene and MS was
first discovered. However, the solution to the cause and pathogenesis of MS has an elusiveness of which these new data of HLA
genes are but another example. On the other hand, investigators
who have chosen MS as a research area have for their part consistently demonstrated an ingenuity and a tenaciousness which one
day will certainly prove a match for this enigmatic disease.

TABLE 1

Distribution of HL-A Antigens

In Multiple Sclerosis

(Sachs, 1947)

Source	A 3		BM		DW 2		BT 101		B 4	
	MS	CT	MS	CT	MS	CT	MS	CT	MS	CT
Compston 1976	33	20	57	33	–	–	83	32	–	–
Terasaki 1976	50	32	39	33	50	20	–	–	83	33
Jersild 1973	48	25	49	26	70	16	–	–	–	–

HLA AND MULTIPLE SCLEROSIS

GENETIC CONSIDERATIONS

P. Platz, L.P. Ryder, M. Thomsen, A. Svejgaard, T. Fog[*]

Tissue-Typing Laboratory, University Hospital (Rigshos-
pitalet) Copenhagen, Denmark
[*] Neurological Department, Municipal Hospital, Copenhagen, Denmark

INTRODUCTION

Familial occurrence of multiple sclerosis (MS) is rare and
was originally considered exceptional. Studies since the 1950'es
have, however, confirmed that the familial prevalence of MS is
approximately 20 times more than that of the general population.
The prevalence is higher the closer the relationship and highest
in siblings and twins (for review see 39, 25).

Familial clustering of a condition is an indication but no
proof of genetic influence. It may equally well imply common exposure to environmental factors. The family studies and especially
studies in twins (25,50) were in fact unable to convincingly establish the importance of genetic factors, but they strongly supported
the importance of environmental factors. This situation has changed
since 1972, when three groups (4, 21, 29) reported increased frequencies of the histocompatibility antigens, HLA-A3 and -B7 in
Northern European and North American Caucasians. This association
was later shown to be due to a primary association with another
HLA marker, HLA-Dw2 (22). Thus, it has finally been proven that
at least one genetic factor predisposes to MS.

In this chapter we will present an extract of earlier reported
family data, give a short survey of the HLA system, present own HLA
data as well as combined HLA data from the literature on MS, and
finally try to reevaluate the earlier family data in the view of
the recently obtained HLA data.

FAMILY DATA

     Since the first systematic family study by Curtius and Speer
in 1937 (9), several family studies have confirmed an increase of
MS especially in siblings of MS patients, but also in other family
members. Various methods of ascertainment have been employed in
different studies and the figures of the prevalence in siblings
differ but all agree that siblings of MS patients have the highest
risk of developing MS.

     Mackay and Myrianthopoulos (25) studied both twins and other
relatives. Table 1 gives their data on the relative frequency of
MS in various groups of relatives of MS propositi. Accepting only
definite MS, this gives a prevalence of MS in siblings 76 times
higher than in the general population compared to 35 and 28 times
higher frequencies in parents and children, respectively.

     The classical method of determining the degree of genetic in-
volvement is the twin method. It is a very cumbersome method,
and as discussed by Hauge (16) it has many possibilities of biased
ascertainments. It has repeatedly been shown that most case reports
and smaller series contain too many monozygotic (MZ) pairs. In
most populations, (in western Europe) MZ twins represent about
1/3 of all twins, but in some series of twins with MS the proportion of MZ twins is as high as 80 %. The extensive twin study of
Mackay and Myrianthopoulos has an overrepresentation of MZ twins
and dizygotic (DZ) twins of same sex. This overrepresentation is
probably due to the ascertainment procedure : the twins volunteered

TABLE 1

Category	Percentage	
	only definite MS	including possible MS
General population	0.05	
Parents	1.7	
Children	1.4	
Siblings	4.1	6.4
Dizygotic twins (DZ)	10.3	20.7
Monozygotic twins (MZ)	15.4	23.1
First cousins and other relatives	0.3	0.4

(From ref. 25.)

in a nationwide appeal for twins with MS. By this method, concordant twins are more likely to be ascertained than are disconcordant. Thus, the figures for MZ and DZ given in table I are probably an overestimate. Thums (50) found only 1 of 13 MZ twins to be concordant. With these reservations in mind two important points can be made, (i) the genetically identical MZ twins have only a slightly higher concordance rate than the genetically non-identical DZ twins which suggests that genetic factors are only of minor importance, (ii) perhaps more impressive is the higher frequency of MS in DZ twins compared with other siblings. The major difference between DZ twins and other pairs of sibs is a higher degree of simultaneous exposure to environmental factors in early life, and thus, the figures in table I argue for the influence of environmental factors.

                            THE HLA SYSTEM

     The term HLA refers to : Human Leucocyte System A, i.e. the first leucocyte group system discovered in man (reviews : Snell et al. (1976), Svejgaard et al. (1975), Histocompatibility Testing 1977 (1978)). HLA is the major histocompatibility complex (MHC) in man, and like MHCs in other species it controls three different sets of characters : 1. alloantigens, 2. some components of the complement cascade, C2 and C4 and factor Bf of the alternative complement pathway, and 3. some immune responses.

     The HLA system is a genetic system of closely linked genes on the short arm of the sixth chromosome. Two categories of antigen-controlling genes are known :
1. the HLA-A, B and C genes on three different loci controls antigens present on the surfaces of all nucleated cells. These antigens are detected by serological techniques and have been shown to consist of a glycopeptide of molecular weight of 44,000. On the cell surface these antigens are linked to β2 microglobulin - a non-polymorphic peptide coded for by chromosome fifteen,
2. the HLA-D and DR genes which control antigens present on some cells only (macrophages and B-lymphocytes among others). These antigens are not associated with β2 microglobulin.

     The HLA-D antigens are defined by cell culture techniques, i.e. by mixed lymphocyte culture typing (MLC) or by primed lymphocyte typing (PLT) (47), while the HLA-DR antigens are recognized by serological methods (Histocompatibility Testing 1977 (1978)). It is still a matter of controversy whether these techniques are detecting products of genes from the same locus (HLA-D/DR) or closely linked loci (HLA-D and HLA-DR). The recent histocompatibility workshop did not produce a definite answer, but seemed to favour the "unitarian" hypothesis.

Locus:	←centromere	PGM$_3$	HLA-D	Bf	HLA-B	HLA-C	HLA-A

No. alleles:		3	>8	3	>20	>5	>17

Determinants:

HLA-D	HLA-B	HLA-C	HLA-A
HLA-Dw1	HLA-B5	HLA-Cw1	HLA-A1
-Dw2	-B7	-Cw2	-A2
-Dw3	-B8	-Cw3	-A3
-Dw4	-B12	-Cw4	-Aw23 } A9
-Dw5	-B13	-Cw5	-Aw24
-Dw6	-B14	-T7	-Aw25 } A10
-LD107	-B18		-Aw26
-LD108	-B27		-A11
	-Bw15		-A28
	-Bw17		-A29
	-Bw21		-Aw30
	-Bw22		-Aw31 } Aw19
	-Bw35		-Aw32
	-Bw37		-Aw33
	-Bw38 } Bw16		-Aw34
	-Bw39		-Aw36
	-Bw40		-Aw43
	-Bw41		
	-Bw42		

Figure 1. The HLA system.

The immune response (Ir) genes are not yet very well defined in man, but in other species, these genes are known to be closely related to the homologues of the HLA-D/DR genes and it is possible that Ir and HLA-D/DR genes may be identical. In animals, Ir genes are involved in the specific cell-mediated immune response and in the formation of IgG antibody production to thymus-dependent antigens (20).

The HLA system is extremely polymorphic at each locus (except those controlling complement components) : between seven and 30 alleles are known at each of the loci, HLA-A, B, C, and D. There is pronounced linkage disequilibrium between these various loci, i.e. some HLA genes and antigens occur much more frequently together in the same individual than would be expected from their individual frequencies. This phenomenon is of crucial importance for the understanding of the associations between HLA and disease. For example, the antigens, HLA-B7 and Dw2, are positively associated in Caucasians and when one of these antigens occurs with increased frequency in a disease, there is a secondary increase of the other. Occasionally, it is difficult to decide which antigens show the strongest association. Moreover, still unknown HLA factors are likely to show linkage disequilibrium too and thus we do not know whether it is the action of such hypothetical HLA factors which are truly responsible for the HLA disease associations now known.

The strength of the association between a given HLA antigen and the disease is usually expressed as the relative risk (RR)

which indicates how many times more frequently the disease occurs
in individuals with the HLA antigen than in those lacking it.
Even if the relative risk deviates from one, the statistical significance has to be taken into consideration. Chance deviations
are to be expected as a large number of antigens is usually tested
for. Often it is necessary to investigate a large number of
patients or to pool the results from different studies to confirm
an association.

HLA DATA ON MS

In 1972 three groups (7, 4, 21) reported increased frequencies of HLA-A3 and -B17 in MS, and these findings have now been
confirmed by many other investigators. Table 2 shows the data
accumulated at the HLA and Disease Registry of Copenhagen until
May 1978.

TABLE 2

Multiple Sclerosis

Combined HLA-A, B, C data (Caucasians) from the HLA and
Disease Registry in Copenhagen, Denmark.

	No. of studies	No. of patients investigated	Relative risk	% $\longrightarrow$ %
Increased				
HLA-A3	15	2,592	1.4	27 $\longrightarrow$ 34
HLA-B7	16	2,638	1.7	27 $\longrightarrow$ 39
Decreased				
HLA-A2	14	2,262	0.7	54 $\longrightarrow$ 45
HLA-B12	14	2,262	0.7	25 $\longrightarrow$ 19
HLA-B15	13	2,188	0.7	18 $\longrightarrow$ 13

Only deviations significant below 10^{-4} are recorded.
"% $\longrightarrow$ %" indicates frequency in control group $\longrightarrow$ frequency in patient groups.

More than 2,500 patients with MS have now been studied. The increase of B7 as well as the decrease of B12 are now confirmed
beyond any doubt, although the relative risk for HLA-B7 positive
is only 1.74. In addition, the finding of Jersild et al. (22)
that the DLA-D locus antigen, Dw2, showed a stronger association
with MS than HLA-B7 has now been extended and confirmed by ourselves and others.

The frequencies of the HLA-D antigens, Dw1 to HLA-Dw8 in
the Copenhagen series of MS patients are shown in table 3, and
the combined data from the literature on HLA-Dw2 in Caucasians
MS patients are given in table IV.

The frequency of HLA-Dw2 in the MS patient groups varies
from 47% to 68% compared with 18%-33% in the control group.
The combined relative estimate of the relative risk for Dw2 is
4.05 compared to the 1.74 for B7, a difference which is significant. This indicates that the primary association is with Dw2
and that the increase of B7 (and A3) is most probably due to
the known linkage disequilibrium between these factors.

Not only does Dw2 increase the risk for MS, but it also influences the clinical course. In figure II the progression coefficient of the disease is compared in the two groups of Dw2 positive and negative patients, and the disease progresses significantly faster in the Dw2 positive patients (p < .01 by rank
sum test). These results have been confirmed by Ilonen et al.
(19), and Bertrams et al. (6) who found that B7 positive MS patients have a more severe clinical course than B7 negative.

Only few studies on HLA-DR have been reported to date (17),
but the data have shown nearly identical results for HLA-D and -DR
typing. Table 5 shows the results in 27 MS patients typed with the
1977 workshop DR sera and both homozygous typing cells and PLT
as previously described (46). Only one discrepant result was
obtained. Thus we do not anticipate that HLA-DR typing will reveal
a closer association between HLA and MS as originally suggested
by Winchester (51).

Studies in other ethnic groups have shown somewhat conflicting results. In American Blacks, Dupont et al. (12) found MS
strongly associated with Dw2, whereas this antigen does not
seem to be associated with MS in Japanese or Jews (8, 29). Recently, Kurdi et al. (24) found that in Arab MS patients from
Lebanon,MS was not associated with DRw2, but with another DR
antigen, and there are indications that MS in Italy is associated
with the same DR antigen (17). If confirmed these results may
suggest that different environmental factors are involved in
different parts of the world.

TABLE 3

HLA-D frequencies in Danish patients with multiple sclerosis and in controls.

	CONTROLS		MULTIPLE SCLEROSIS			
	No. investigated	Per cent positive	No. investigated	Per cent positive	Relative risk	p
Dw1	272	19.9	48	10.4	0.5	n.s.
Dw2	345	25.8	97	59.7	4.3	$<10^{-9}$
Dw3	334	26.3	69	27.5	1.1	n.s.
Dw4	345	19.4	69	20.3	1.1	n.s.
Dw5	191	5.8	27	3.7	0.6	n.s.
Dw6	281	16.0	48	20.8	1.3	n.s.
Dw7	345	18.0	69	21.7	1.3	n.s.
Dw8	335	7.5	69	2.9	0.4	n.s.

TABLE 4

HLA-D frequencies in multiple sclerosis.
Combined data from the HLA and Disease Registry, May 1978.

HLA	No. of studies	No. of patients	No. of controls	Relative risk	p
Dw1	3	280	759	0.86	> .05
Dw2	9	932	1387	4.05	$<$IE-10
Dw3	3	301	814	1.31	> .05
Dw4	2	190	443	0.96	> .05
Dw5	1	27	191	0.89	> .05
Dw6	2	169	379	1.60	> .05
Dw7	1	69	345	1.29	> .05
Dw8	1	69	335	0.45	> .05
Dw11	1	111	394	1.67	> .05

Data from ref. 3, 15, 19, 28, 32, 33, 43, 48 and Table 3.

P. PLATZ ET AL.

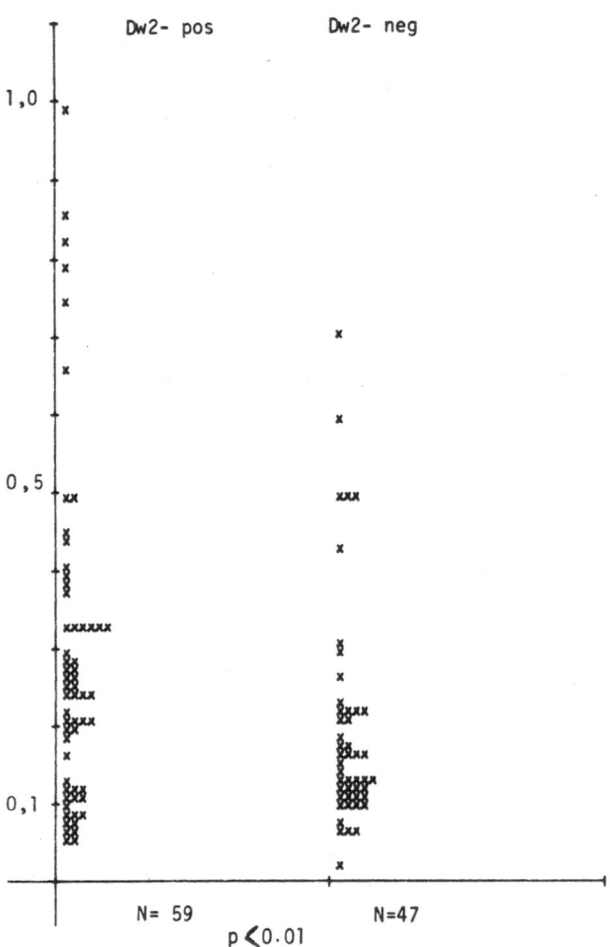

Fig. 2. Progression coefficient in 106 patients with MS

TABLE 5

DRw2 assignment compared with the Dw2 assignment by means of
homozygous typing cells (HTC) and primed lymphocyte typing (PLT).

	++	+-	-+	--	Total
DRw2 versus HTC	19	0	1	7	27
DRw2 versus PLT	19	0	1	7	27
HTC versus PLT	20	0	0	7	27

Only a few families with more than one member suffering from
MS have so far been HLA typed. Table 6 shows the data from the
literature on pairs of siblings both of whom suffering from MS.

OPTIC NEURITIS

Acute monosymptomatic optic neuritis (ON) often precedes MS,
although there are conflicting reports as to the frequency with
which patients with ON later develop MS. Figures from 11 to 76
per cent have been mentioned (37). Following the discovery
of an association between HLA and MS, it was therefore of obvious
interest to investigate the HLA profile in ON patients, in particular to see whether HLA typing could be used to predict a
later development of MS.

HLA-A, B, C typing in ON has been reported by 3 groups (2,
28, 28) but only a slight and insignificant increase in HLA-B7
was found in the combined data. We have performed HLA-D typing
on 73 patients with ON from a prospectively ascertained series
selected by Dr. Sandberg-Wollheim in Lund, Sweden. The results
from 54 of the patients have previously been published (38).
Thirty five (48%) of the 73 patients carried the HLA-Dw2 antigen
compared to 25.8 per cent of 345 normal controls, a difference
which is highly significant (p = 2.2×10^{-4}, Fisher's exact test).
13 patients have developed MS during the observation period
(mean 6.2 year), and 7 of these were HLA-Dw2 and 6 were not.
Thus, HLA-Dw2 is increased in primary ON nearly to the same extent
as in MS, but the presence of HLA-Dw2 does not seem to predict
the later development of MS. The observation period is, however,
still short and Stendahl-Brodin and coworkers (42) found in a
retrospective study an increased frequency of HLA-Dw2 in MS
patients where ON was the first symptom, but only a slight increase of Dw2 in patients with ON who did not develop MS.

DISCUSSION

The pathogenesis of MS is probably complex, and considerable
evidence has now been accumulated indicating that both environmental and genetic factors are involved (34). Familial MS is rare
and constitutes less than 10% of all MS cases (26). Nevertheless,
HLA-linked genetic factors are strongly associated with MS in
unrelated patients. How can this apparent paradox be explained?
Firstly, familial cases of MS may not be representative of all
MS cases, but could represent a "biased sample". Secondly, the
twin data show that the majority (75-80%) of genetically identical
twins of an MS propositus will not develop MS, and furthermore
fraternal twins have a higher risk than other sibs of developing

P. PLATZ ET AL.

TABLE 6

Nr. of HLA haplotypes shared by siblings both suffering from MS.

	No. of families	No. of haplotypes shared		
		0	1	2
combined data from ref. 1, 7, 11, 13* 17, 22, 31, 43	45	8 (17.0%)	20 (42.6%)	19 (40.3%)
Expected (1) no linkage		25.0%	50.0%	25.0%
(2) one gene dose gene frequency .15		11.1%	48.8%	40.1%
(3) two gene doses gene frequency .15		1.7%	22.7%	75.6%

* 2 sibships with 3 affected sibs.

The observed frequency of siblings sharing 0, 1, and 2 HLA haplotypes deviated only significantly from the third expectation, p   0.001.

MS, although they are not more genetically alike than other sibs. The most straightforward interpretation of these observations is that environmental factors are of major importance for the development of overt MS. Thus, we have to accept that genetic factors play a minor role, but the question still remains : what is the nature of these genetic factors?

The prevalence of MS in relatives of MS patients (table 1) is higher in siblings to the propositi than in both parents and children. This would immediately suggest that a double dose of an "MS susceptibility" (MSS) gene was necessary, and Mackay and Myrianthopoulos (25) concluded from their data that MS was inherited as an autosomal recessive trait with a penetrance of 43 %. Against this hypothesis can be argued as did Schapira et al. (39) that "such an explanation can be manipulated to explain any disease with familial occurrence". A stronger argument against this recessive hypothesis is the HLA-data on sibpairs with MS. If the MSS gene closely linked to the HLA region as suggested from the HLA data in unrelated MS patients then nearly all the sibpairs according to the double dose theory should be HLA identical (independently of the penetrance, because both sibs have manifested MS), unless the MS gene exists in the normal population in a very high frequency (49).

Recently, Terasaki and Mickey (45) have forwarded a single mutation hypothesis according to which the MSS gene originated in a single prehistoric individual by mutation. This MS suscep- tibility gene should thus have been transmitted from generation to generation, and all present MS patients are descendants of the original MS homoid. The original MS haplotype should then have been A3, B7, Dw2 and MSS. The observed association with HLA-Dw2 could be explained on the assumption that the original MSS-Dw2 coupling has not yet been broken by crossing-overs. If the MSS gene was due to a single mutation one would expect it to be a rare gene with a low frequency in the population, and accordingly the sibpairs should either be HLA identical (if a double dose was needed), or one half should be HLA identical and the other half haplo-identical (if only one dose was suffi- cient) (49). Although the HLA data from the literature on sib- pairs with MS (table 6) have to be considered with some caution (familial cases are rare and may not be representative of MS, and the diagnosis of MS is always difficult) they argue against both the recessive theory and the mutation hypothesis because in case of a rare gene no HLA unidentical sibpairs should be expected.

Thus, it seems that we have to reject the theory of a rare MSS gene in close linkage with the HLA region. The association between HLA-Dw2 and MS in the population studies (table 4) is, however, very consistent and new explanations must be considered.

Both the recessive hypothesis with reduced penetrance and especially the mutation theory implies that a rare MSS gene fairly commonly (influenced by environmental factors) leads to overt MS. In fact, both theories suggest genetic factors to be of major importance, but if we accept that environmental factors are the most important, an alternative explanation would be that the genetic contribution to MS comes from a gene(s) commonly found in the normal population. This gene might in most environ- mental situations confer advantage to the normal population on the expense that,in rare and special environmental conditions, it increases susceptibility to MS.

Such an hypothesis of a common gene which only in rare conditions leads to MS is fully compatible with the HLA-Dw2 data from population studies, HLA-Dw2 is found in approx. 1/4 of the normal Caucasian population, and the gene frequency of HLA-Dw2 has been found to be 0.145 in the normal Copenhagen population (Thomsen et al. unpublished). Curiously, if we use a gene fre- quency of .15 (as for Dw2) the observed frequency of haplotype distribution shows a remarkable good fit to the distribution (from ref. 49) which would be expected from a dominant hypothesis (expectation 2 in table 6). In fact, with our present knowledge it may be accepted as a working hypothesis that it is the HLA-Dw2

determinant itself which confers susceptibility to MS. We also
wish to emphasize that it has not been ruled out that MS in
some cases may arise without HLA factors being involved.

If we accept that it is a common gene which only in rare
and special environmental conditions gives rise to MS, the family
cases would reflect heavy and common environmental pressure within
the family, rather than a common genetic predisposition.

Thus, both the HLA data from population studies and the
family data are in agreement with the hypothesis : MS is not
inherited in the classical sense, but HLA linked genes confer
a hereditary predisposition which produces overt disease only
in the presence of appropriate environmental stimuli. This is
in agreement with a conclusion reached in 1963 by Schapira et
al. (39) based on family data alone.

There are in fact data which could indicate that HLA-Dw2
or HLA-Dw2 linked genes may confer advantage in the general
population. Insulin-dependent diabetes (IDD) is associated
with both HLA-Dw3 and -Dw4 (46), but perhaps more remarkably
Dw2 was not found in any of 124 HLA-D typed IDD patients in
Copenhagen. This indicates that HLA-Dw2 may have a protective
effect against IDD, a disease which is much more common than
MS and was invariable fatal in young age prior to the discovery
of insulin.

The mere associations between a genetic marker and a disease
does not in itself contribute very much to the understanding
of the etiology and pathogenesis of the disease, unless it is
the biological activity of the marker itself, which is responsible for the association. In the case of MS with the well
established association to Dw2, it must be recalled from the
section in the HLA system that it is possible, that the HLA-D/DR
genes in man are identical with or very closely linked to the
human Ir genes It is therefore possible that the different
HLA-Dw2 associations with MS and IDD reflect the existence
of a common Ir gene(s) closely linked to Dw2 which in some circumstances give an advantage, but in others increases the susceptibility to MS. This would also be in agreement with the
numerous reports of immunological abnormalities in MS which
all point towards some involvement of the immunological system
(primary or secondary) in the development of MS.

One of the consequences of this hypothesis is that it is
not only of interest to investigate MS patients but that it is
equally important to investigate normal individuals to discover
HLA-D dependent variations in their immunological reactivity
to a variety of environmental stimuli e.g. viruses, bacteria
and other antigens. Such differences might give clues to further

investigations on the etiology of MS. The possibility that
MS is not a single disease but may be heterogeneous is also
possible within the framework of this hypothesis, e.g. is MS
in Dw2-positive subjects a different disease from MS in Dw2-
negative individuals ? The observation that MS in Dw2-positive
patients progresses faster than in Dw2-negative patients would
support this assumption, but could also be explained by a secondary effect of Dw2 (or Dw2 associated genes) when MS is first
established. Studies comparing different parameters such as
age at onset, sex, immunological parameters in Dw2-positive
and Dw2-negative patients would help to clarify this problem
and are certainly warranted.

In the above discussion we have only considered hypotheses
involving one gene, or a set of closely linked genes. We are
well aware, however, that the genetic predisposition to MS could
be polygenic and involve many genes in addition to the HLA gene.
Nevertheless, we will however, leave speculations along these
lines until there are data which force us to do otherwise.

ACKNOWLEDGEMENTS

This work has been supported by a grant from the Danish Multiple Sclerosis Society, the Danish Medical Research Council
and the EEC. The excellent assistance of Elly Andersen, the
HLA and Disease Registry, was invaluable.

REFERENCES

1. Alter, M., Harshe, M., Anderson, N., Elving, V., Emme, L.
   and Yunis, E.J.: Neurology, 26 : 31-36, 1976.
2. Arnason, B.G.W., Fuller, T.C., Lehrich, J.R. and Wraym, S.H.
   J. Neurol. Sci. 22 : 419-428, 1974.
3. Berg-Loonen, E.V. van and Lucas, K.J. : Histocompatibility
   Testing, 1975, pp. 773-777 (Munksgaard, Copenhagen).
4. Bertrams, J., Kuwert, E. and Liedtke, U. : Tissue Antigens
   2 : 405-408, 1972.
5. Bertrams, J. and Kuwert, E. : Thesis 1974.
6. Bertrams, J., Höher, P.G. and Kuwert, E. : Lancet i : 1287,
   1974.
7. Bertrams, J. and Kuwert, E. : Z. Immun-forsch. 152 : 200-208,
   1976.
8. Brautbar, C., Cohen, I., Kahana, E., Alter, M., Jørgensen, F.
   and Lamm, L. : Tissue Antigens 10 : 291-302, 1977.
9. Curtius, F. and Speer, H. : Z. Ges. Neurol. Psychiat. 160 :
   226, 1937.
10. Dausset, J. and Hors, J. : Transplant. Rev. 22: 44-74, 1975.

11. Drachman, D.A., Davison, W.C. and Mittal, K.K. : Arch. Neurol. 33 : 406-413, 1976.
12. Dupont, B., Lisak, R.P., Jersild, C., Hansen, J.A., Silberberg, D.H., Whitsett, C., Zwieman, B. and Ciongoli, K. : Transplant. Proc. 1978 (in press).
13. Eldridge, R., McFarland, H. and Sever, J. : Ann. Neurol. 3 : 72-80, 1978.
14. Fewster, M.E., Myers, L.W., Ellison, G.W. and Walford, R.L. : J. Neurol. Sci. 34 : 287-296, 1977.
15. Grosse-Wilde, H., Bertrams, J., Schuppien, W., Netzel, B., Ruppelt, W. and Kuvert, E.K. : Immunogenetics 4:481-488, 1977.
16. Hauge, M. : Acta Neurol. Scand. 55, Supple. 63 : 49-53, 1977.
17. Hens, L. & Carton H., : Tissue Antigens 11 : 75-80, 1978.
18. Histocompatibility Testing 1977. (Bodmer, W.F., Batchelor, J.R., Bodmer, J.G., Festenstein, H., and Morris, P.J., eds.), Munksgaard, Copenhagen.
19. Ilonen, J., Herva, E., Reunanen, M., Panelius, M., Meurman, O., Arstila, P. and Tiilikainen, A. : Acta Neurol. Scand. 55 : 299-209, 1977.
20. Immunological Reviews 38, 1978. (Möller, G. ed.), Munksgaard, Copenhagen.
21. Jersild, C., Svejgaard, A. and Fog, T. : Lancet i : 1240-1241, 1972.
22. Jersild, C., Fog, T., Hansen, G.S., Thomsen, M., Svejgaard, A. and Dupont, B. : Lancet ii : 1221-1225, 1973.
23. Jersild, C., Dupont, B., Fog, T., Platz, P. and Svejgaard, A. : Transplant. Rev. 22 : 148-163, 1975.
24. Kurdi, A., Ayesh, I., Abdallat, A., Maayta, U., McDonald, W.I., Compston, D.A.S. and Batchelor, J.R. : Lancet i : 1123-1125, 1977.
25. Mackay, R.P. and Myrianthopoulos, N.C. : Arch. Neurol. 15 : 449-462, 1966.
26. McAlpine, D., Compston, N.D. and Lumsden, C.E. : Multiple Sclerosis, Edinburgh, 1955.
27. Morris, P.J., Vaughan, H., Tait, B.D. and Mackay, I.R. : Aust. N. Z. J. 7 : 616-624, 1977.
28. Möller, E., Link, H., Matell, G., Olhagen, B. and Stendahl, L. : Histocompatibility Testing 1975 p. 778-781 (Munksgaard, Copenhagen).
29. Naito, S., Namerow, N., Mickey, M.R. and Terasaki, P.I. : Tissue Antigens 2 : 1-4, 1972.
30. Naito, S., Kuroiwa, Y., Itoyama, T., Tsubaki, T., Horikawa, A., Sasazuki, T., Noguchi, S., Ohtsuki, S., Tokuomi, H., Miyatake, T., Takahata, N., Kawanami, S. and McMichael, A.J. : Tissue Antigens 12 : 19-24, 1978.
31. Olsson, J.-E., Möller, E. and Link, H. : Arch. Neurol. 33 : 808-812, 1976.
32. Opelz, G., Terasaki, P., Myers, L., Ellison, G., Ebers, G., Zabrieskie, J., Weiner, H., Kempe, H. and Sibley, W. : Tissue Antigens 9 : 54-58, 1977.

33. Paty, D.W., Cousin, H.K., Stiller, C.R., Boucher, D.W., Furesz, J., Warren, K.G., Marchuk, L. and Dosseter, J.B. : Transplant. Proc. IX : 1845-1848, 1977.

34. Platz, P., Jersild, C., Thomsen, M. Svejgaard, A., Fog, T., Midholm, S., Raun, N., Hansen, S.K. and Grob, P. : In : Transfer Factor (Ascher, M.S., Gotlieb, A.A. and Kirkpatrick, eds.), Academic Press, Inc., New York, San Francisco, London, pp. 649-662, 1976.

35. Reekers, P., Hommes, O.R., Creemers-Molenaar, J., Wijnings, J., Kunst, V.A.J.M. and van Rood, J.J. : J. Neurol. Sci. 33 : 143-153, 1977.

36. Sabourad, O., Fauchet, R., Genetet, B. and Genetet, N. : data submitted to the Registry, 1976.

37. Sandberg, M. and Bynke, H. : Acta Neurol. Scand. 49 : 443-452, 1973.

38. Sandberg-Wollheim, M., Platz, P., Ryder, L.P., Nielsen, L. Staub & Thomsen, M. : Acta Neurol. Scand. 52 : 161 - 166, 1975.

39. Schapira, K.,Postkanzer,D.C. and Miller, H. : Brain 86 : 315-332, 1963.

40. Smeraldi, E. : Boll 1st Sieroter Milan 51 : 220-223, 1972.

41. Snell, G.D., Dausset, J. and Nathenson, S. : Histocompatibility, Academic Press, New York, San Francisco, London, pp. 1-401, 1976.

42. Stendahl-Brodin, L., Link, H., Möller, E. and Norrby, E. : Acta Neurol. Scand. 57 : 418-431, 1978.

43. Stewart, G.J., Basten, A., Guinan, J., Bashir, H.V., Cameron, J. and McLeod, J.G. J. Neurol. Sci. 32 : 153-167, 1977.

44. Svejgaard, A., Hauge, M., Jersild, C., Platz, P., Ryder, L.P., Nielsen, L., Stab and Thomsen, M. : Monographs in Human Genetics 7 : 1975. (Beckman, L. and Hauge, M., eds.) S. Karger, Basel.

45. Terasaki, P.I. and Mickey, M.R. : Neurology, June 1976, part 2, 56-58.

46. Thomsen, M., Platz, P. Andersen, O., Ortved, Christy, M., Lyngsøe, J., Nerup, J., Rasmussen, K., Ryder, L.P., Nielsen, L., Staub and Svejgaard, A. :   Transpl. Rev. 22 : 125-147, 1975.

47. Thomsen, M., Ryder, L.P. and Svejgaard, A. : Scand. J. Immunol. 5, supple. 5 : 157-174, 1976.

48. Thorsby, E., Helgesen, A., Solheim, B.G. and Vandvik, B. : J. Neurol. Sci. 32 : 187-193, 1977.

49. Thomson, G. and Bodmer, W. : In : HLA and Disease (Dausset, J. and Svejgaard, A., eds.) Munksgaard, Copenhagen, p. 84-93, 1977.

50. Thums, K.: Wien. Z. für Nervenheilkunde und deren Grenzgebiete IV : 173-203, 1952.

51. Winchester, R.J., Ebers, G., Fu, S.M., Espinosa, L., Zabrieskie, J. and Kunkel, H.G. : Lancet ii : 814, 1975.

FAMILIAL ASPECTS OF MULTIPLE SCLEROSIS : A RATIONAL PROPHYLACTIC
THERAPY

E.J. Field

M.S. Research Unit, Royal Victoria Infirmary
Newcastle Upon Tyne, U.K.

   Multiple Sclerosis, in the present state of our understanding,
is not an hereditary disease, though like so many other diseases
in medicine (e.g. diabetes, coronary disease, etc.) it does tend
to cluster in families. It is estimated that the disease is 5
to 20 times more common in the first degree relatives of a propositus than in the general population (18). The problem is
enormously complicated by the existence of "benign" cases - those
whose symptomatology may be so slight that they visit the doctor
once only with a minor undiagnosed complaint which never recurs;
and "latent" cases whose lesions are found only at postmortem
but who had no neurological complaint during their lifetime (14,
23, 15). Indeed Myrianthopoulos (18) points out that, because
of uncertainty of diagnosis and extension of the time of attack,
even if MS were completely genetic in origin monozygotic twins
could not be expected to show more than 50 % concordance at any
one time. "Latent" and "benign" cases are lost to epidemiological and genetic studies and so may well distort results.

   With the MEM-LAD or E-UFA tests (11, 8) it is possible to
verify that the surface of lymphocytes and RBC are different in
MS from other neurological diseases (OND) and normals. For
lymphocytes this is borne out by the finding that unrelated MS
patients' lymphocytes mount a poor MLR as compared with unrelated OND (other neurological disease) or normal subjects (16, 13).
It would thus appear that the surface of quite unrelated
lymphocytes have something in common in all cases of MS.

   In 1966 R.H.S. Thompson (21) propounded a most significant and
fruitful hypothesis, elaborated with further evidence in 1973,
that MS occurred against an inborn background of mishandling of

147

unsaturated fatty acids of the linoleic (LA) and arachidonic (AA)
type. Such acids (as phospholipid components) play an important
part in the make up of the surface membranes of all cells. The
MEM-LAD test shows the difference between MS and other lymphocytes
in respect of reactivity with LA and AA. In the E-UFA test the
RBC, too, are found to be different in MS from OND and normals.
There must be some altered biochemical - biophysical make up of
the lymphocyte and RBC surface membrane in MS. If this difference
extends to all cells of the body (a testable hypothesis) then
oligodendrocytes, which produce myelin from an extrusion of their
surface in extended layering around the axon, would be expected
to lay down abnormal myelin even in areas away from lesions.
Such areas away from naked eye plaques might well appear normal
and yet show microscopic demyelinative or other lesions. Thompson
has reviewed the relative literature and Dr. Ingrid Allen has
shown, in an extensive series of brain examinations, that white
matter apparently normal is indeed very largely so, there being
only mild astrocytic hypertrophy and minor perivascular cuffings
with lymphocytes in about 7 % of cases. The chemical anomalies
(deficiency in UFA) reported by many workers in the apparently
normal areas of white matter away from lesions in MS would thus
appear to be genuine and not secondary. This is precisely what
would be expected if Thompson's anomaly extended to the surface
of the oligodendrocytes. The MS brain is thus an abnormally chemically constituted brain ab initio, abnormal myelin being laid
down right from the beginning, on account of the anomalous
unsaturated fatty acid make up of the oligodendroglial surface.

The study of many families in which an MS propositus occurs,
has shown (by the MEM-LAD and E-UFA tests) that anomalies are much
more frequent in the female near-relatives than amongst the males.
Apart from the propositus who shows a full MS type result (with
MEM-LAD about 90 % reduction with LA; with E-UFA, slow with both
LA and AA at 0.08 mgm/ml concentration) "half-way houses" appear
in both tests. In the former there are relatives who give about
77 % reduction of lymphocyte - thyroid (antigen) interaction (i.
e. midway between the normal of 57 % and the MS of 90+ %) and
with the E-UFA test possess RBC which travel slowly with LA yet
fast with AA. Early Tables (1 a, b) are shown for both, but since
these publications (11, 8) very many more subjects have been
examined, especially with the simpler E-UFA test, with the same
sort of distribution of "anomalous" results. Thus all of over
100 mothers have shown this result, a very few fathers and the
preponderance amongst sisters and daughters holds good. Full
figures will be published elsewhere (6). Typical family trees (10)
are shown in Table II (see also 5). The distribution of "anomalous" results appears to follow no clear Mendelian pattern but
probably represent some minor membrane modification which is not
bound up with the development of MS for such subjects never develop
MS, even though mothers have been followed into their nineties.

TABLE Ia

	Control	LA	AA	FUR LA .00167 μg/ml	FUR AA .00167 μg/ml	FUR LA .0000167 μg/ml	FUR AA .0000167 μg/ml	FUR LA .00000167 μg/ml	FUR AA .00000167 μg/ml
A.M. (MS) M 38	.991 ± .020	.863 ± .014	.871 ± .018	1.087 ± .032	1.037 ± .029				
Fur .00167 μg/ml	.992 ± .021								
K.V. (N) M 22	.991 ± .012	1.052 ± .027		.943 ± .027					
Prof M.S. (MS) M 40	.992 ± .015	.865 ± .019	.879 ± .018	1.043 ± .026					
L.M. (MS) F 22	.986 ± .024	.876 ± .017	.871 ± .015	1.034 ± .020	1.028 ± .020	.949 ± .015	.919 ± .020	.873 ± .021	.875 ± .019
K.H. (N) M 27	.989 ± .021	1.052 ± .022	1.051 ± .017	.913 ± .013	.921 ± .021				
Fur .00167 μg/ml	.991 ± .020					.965 ± .021			
Fur .0000167 μg/ml	.987 ± .018						.935 ± .021		
Fur .00000167 μg/ml								1.052 ± .020	1.052 ± .017
J.M. (N) F 22 Sister of MS A.M. above	.990 ± .018	.937 ± .026	1.045 ± .019	1.054 ± .018	.928 ± .031				

CONCLUSION

Furadantin reverses results at concentrations down to $\frac{1.67 \text{ ng/ml}}{.00167 \text{ μg/ml}}$ in MS

Furadantin gives abnormal results down to $\frac{16.74 \text{ pg/ml}}{.00001674 \text{ μg/ml}}$ in Normals but at $\frac{.167 \text{ pg/ml}}{.00000167 \text{ μg/ml}}$ gives normal result again

i.e. MS less sensitive to Furadantin than is Normal.   Red circle is reversed at .00167 μg/ml - not timed below

TABLE Ib

	Control	LA	AA	5.57pg/ml	3.34 pg/ml	1.67 pg/ml
D.P. (N) F 50	.989 ± .016	1.050 ± .017	1.054 ± .020	LA .973 ± .020 AA .938 ± .019 CON .996 ± .021	LA 1.047 ± .020	LA 1.055 ± .019 CON .990 ± .023

Amongst whole families young children, apparently in perfect health, were discovered who nevertheless showed a full MS type result in the E-UFA test (i.e. slowing of RBC with LA and AA). When examined for lymphocyte sensitization to EF (encephalitogenic factor) they showed positive results (a sign of organic brain destruction of some sort - here presumably, though not certainly, MS (2)) suggesting that MS lesion(s) were already present though of course symptomatology could hardly be expected from immature brains. Altogether 5 such children have so far been picked up ranging from 1.5 to 13 years of age.

In addition 15 "silent" adult MS cases have been found who presented as relatives of a propositus. Only one has (for obvious psychological reasons) been examined and found to have unequal reflexes and occasional right ankle clonus. None complains at all save one other who is "depressed". These 15 are out of a total of 600 making approximately 1 in 40 near relatives, "MS". This figure seemed very high until it was learned (personal communication from Professor Roberts, Newcastle) that in the Shetland Isles 1 in 50 amongst the same degree of relatives displays clinical MS. This raises many theoretical questions of environment, especially the high saturated fat intake in the Shetlands.

Prolonged treatment of an MS patient with γ-linolenate (Naudicelle Capsules, Bio-Oil Research Limited, England) leads to the conversion of a positive into a negative MS result. This has been followed in 53 patients (8) and generally takes (in English patients) about 3 to 4 months to begin (first with AA and later with LA) (Table III). In countries (e.g. West Germany) where saturated fat intake is very heavy the E-UFA test must be modified, i.e. using 0.16 mgm/ml of LA or AA instead of 0.08 mgm/ml. Moreover, ingestion of large quantities of heavily unsaturated margarines (or even the consumption of especially highly saturated oils) may give rise to difficulties since even small γ-linolenate treatment will then lead to conversion. A further complication is the heavily drug-treated case encountered more on the Continent than in England where most cases tested have had little more than valium, ACTH or prednisolone or perhaps a gluten free diet. It is now known that certain drugs interfere with the E-UFA test (the MEM-LAD has not been tested). Furadantin (Eaton Laboratories, England) enjoys some popularity in the BRD and treatment for bladder infection will completely reverse a positive MS E-UFA test. Indeed in England we have carried out experiments to test this drug and found that amounts as small as 6 pg/ml will reverse the test in a normal subject (Table I a/b) (9). Hence the observer must beware of applying the test where several drugs have been used. ACTH, prednisolone and valium are

TABLE II

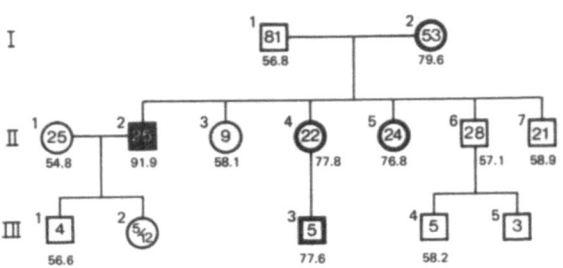

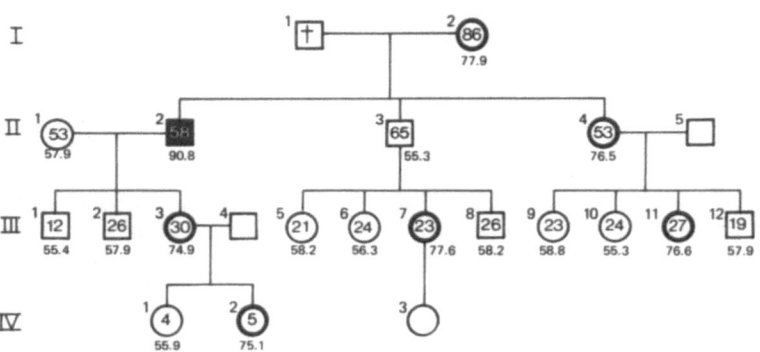

Typical MS family trees (□ = male
with age inserted, o = female with
age inserted; MEM-LAD test percentage given beneath each subject;
propositus : solid shading; anomalous (77% type) outlined in thick
line; normal children with full
MS result : stippled)

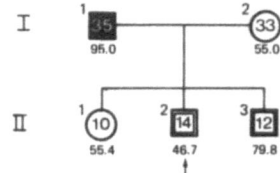

Difficult
  Birth
? Residual
Epilepsy
brain damage

TABLE III
Patients with M.S. Beginning Treatment at Date Shown on First Line

Date	CON	SD	LA	SD	AA	SD	% change	
							LA	AA
G.H. (female) age 29								
24.4.76	1.113	± 0.037	1.073	± 0.036	1.073	± 0.034	− 3.64	− 3.63
4.5.76	1.101	± 0.034	1.058	± 0.035	1.068	± 0.032	− 3.86	− 3.02
18.5.76	1.108	± 0.036	1.074	± 0.040	1.075	± 0.035	− 3.04	−2.95
8.6.76	1.172	± 0.035	1.117	± 0.037	1.166	± 0.030	− 4.65	− 0.52
28.6.76	1.144	± 0.030	1.091	± 0.029	1.162	± 0.029	− 4.64	+ 1.59
26.7.76	0.902	± 0.024	0.879	± 0.030	0.970	± 0.041	− 2.65	+ 7.45
6.9.76	0.980	± 0.031	0.994	± 0.034	1.024	± 0.032	+ 1.41	+ 4.50
4.10.76	0.970	± 0.041	1.036	± 0.043	1.043	± 0.037	+ 6.78	+ 7.49
8.12.76	1.002	± 0.024	1.042	± 0.035	1.047	± 0.035	+ 4.03	+ 4.47
5.1.77[1]	1.018	± 0.026	1.072	± 0.027	1.120	± 0.043	+ 5.33	+ 10.03
5.5.77	0.998	± 0.027	1.063	± 0.022	1.062	± 0.021	+ 6.52	+ 6.39
P.P. (female) age 24								
24.6.76	1.174	± 0.034	1.124	± 0.030	1.128	± 0.027	− 4.28	− 3.88
28.7.76	0.935	± 0.024	0.900	± 0.025	0.909	± 0.025	−3.80	− 2.77
15.9.76	0.983	± 0.023	0.951	± 0.023	1.004	± 0.034	− 3.31	+ 2.15
25.10.76	0.978	± 0.030	0.951	± 0.040	0.991	± 0.037	− 2.76	+ 1.31
29.11.76	1.004	± 0.031	1.031	± 0.034	1.025	± 0.028	+ 2.65	+ 2.12
10.1.77	1.025	± 0.023	1.079	± 0.037	1.095	± 0.030	+ 5.27	+ 6.83
10.2.77	1.071	± 0.032	1.117	± 0.028	1.130	± 0.020	+ 4.33	+ 5.49
30.2.77	0.987	± 0.031	1.085	± 0.029	1.111	± 0.030	+ 10.00	+ 12.64
M.D. (female) age 29								
27.9.76	0.987	± 0.035	0.950	± 0.035	0.942	± 0.030	− 3.7	−4.56
15.11.76	0.996	± 0.035	0.944	± 0.038	0.919	± 0.033	−5.22	−7.7
20.12.76	1.168	± 0.044	1.125	± 0.041	1.176	± 0.045	− 3.68	+ 0.6
7.2.77	1.019	± 0.027	0.979	± 0.027	1.079	± 0.030	− 3.9	+ 5.88
29.3.77	0.976	± 0.030	1.043	± 0.031	1.050	± 0.028	+ 6.86	+ 7.58
20.5.77	1.020	± 0.017	1.072	± 0.016	1.083	± 0.019	+ 5.09	+ 6.18
J.G. (female) age 30								
7.7.76	1.201	± 0.043	1.161	± 0.036	1.163	± 0.032	−3.29	−3.16
19.8.76	0.976	± 0.031	0.922	± 0.023	0.952	± 0.026	−5.46	−2.37
27.9.76	0.982	± 0.024	0.965	± 0.026	0.988	± 0.029	−1.77	+ 0.66
14.11.76	0.998	± 0.025	0.936	± 0.031	0.994	± 0.030	− 6.20	− 0.37
20.12.76	1.144	± 0.029	1.195	± 0.029	1.228	± 0.027	+ 4.47	+ 7.31
7.2.77	1.026	± 0.022	1.074	± 0.024	1.101	± 0.025	+ 4.65	+ 7.27
28.3.77	0.977	± 0.030	1.056	± 0.034	1.079	± 0.027	+ 8.04	+ 10.40
20.5.77	1.023	± 0.021	1.075	± 0.020	1.079	± 0.020	+ 5.13	+ 5.52

Note the retardation produced by 0.08 mg/ml LA and AA. After some months' treatment with γ-linolenate all begin to show a reversion to the normal type of response (i.e. increased speed with these acids) beginning first with AA and followed a month or two later by LA so that ultimately they give full normal response. All figures are significant at p <0.001, except around about the transition stage, for example, the AA reading for G.H. on 8.6.76 or the AA reading for M.D. on 20.12.76.

[1] On 5.1.77 capsules reduced to 1 tds.

without effect but there is no doubt a whole field of iatrogenic
false results are awaiting discovery and publication.

USES OF γ -LINOLENATE

The double blind trial of Bates et.al. (1) was announced at
the Göttingen Symposium "Progress in MS Research" (September 14th
to 16th, 1978) by Dr. J. Mertin as having been successful in the
acute episodic cases of MS, i.e. cases similar to those employed
by Millar et.al. (17) in the sun flower seed oil (LA) double
blind trial, as predicted by Field and Shenton (12). The "chronic
case" part of the Bates trial has long been made public and was, as
expected, negative (1). Thus in the early MS (and diagnosis can
now be made within days of the first episode) it is possible to
reduce the number, severity and duration of MS attacks and so
delay (if indeed it will ever come on) any ultimate downward
progress. The diagnosis of MS rests nowadays on "dissemination
in space and (wasted) time". There is no need to wait for a second attack. Such may very well come, even with γ-linolenate
therapy, though it is likely to be short-lived and mild, avoiding
ACTH or prednisolone therapy so unpleasant (and indeed dangerous)
to many patients. But there is no cure for MS. This must be
clearly emphasized at the present time. Of much greater importance as a practical way forward - and by no means costly when
measured by the millions of dollars spent on EAE, virological
and "basic" lymphocyte research - is the establishment of testing
stations throughout the country where children born as near relatives into MS families, and hence especially liable to develop
MS (see above), can be tested as early as possible after birth.
Myelin is laid down very actively in the brain from about mid-foe-
tal life until at least five years of age and thereafter actively,
but with diminishing tempo, until 16 years of age. The turnover
of some constituents appears to go on much longer, but human data
are difficult, if indeed possible, to come by. It is essential
to ensure that the child who inherits Thompson's anomaly of his
or her membranes (i.e. an abnormal biochemical -biophysical make
up rendered manifest in the E-UFA test) should at once have this
anomaly corrected by treatment with γ -linolenate. If this
correction extends to the oligodendrocytes then they will, from
this time forward, lay down normal myelin not susceptible to the
MS process whatever its aetiology may ultimately turn out to be.
Clearly the important time for such prophylactic treatment is
before myelin is laid down and one should not depend upon
replacement turnover, of which we know so little, in adult life.
It is the early childhood period that is important. It is perhaps
of secondary importance that saturated fat depletion in later
life with substitution of unsaturated fats leads to slowing of
deterioration, as Swank (20) maintains, depending upon the slow
and unascertained turnover in the adult. It is almost certainly

significant that human milk contains about 7 times as much linoleic acid (a real "essential" fatty acid) than does cow's milk.
In tropical countries children are undoubtedly breast fed much
longer than children in the 40°-60° latitude high incidence belt
of MS. It is probably of less importance what happens after the
crucial myelination period, so that the absence of MS in primitive South African peoples, who as adults consume large amounts
of saturated fats (as argued by Dean against the importance of
UFA), is not significant. Their children are kept at the breast
much longer over the major myelin formative years.

THEORETICAL CONSIDERATIONS

It is very largely from the surface of the oligodendrocyte
that myelin is laid down and the surface appears as the intraperiod line in the electron microscope. Slippage along this line
has often been observed when myelin breaks down - it is clearly
a weak place in the holding of myelin together. The forces which
"bind" opposed oligodendrocyte surfaces together at the intraperiod line are clearly important. Abramsky (this meeting) has
shown, in his beautiful scanning electron microscope preparations
of apparently living (though unfortunately non-human) oligodendrocytes, that their surface is much smoother than that of
astrocytes. It is tempting to suppose that in the surface anomaly
of oligodendrocytes, which goes with MS, residual electric change
and H-bonding might be so reduced so that disintegration of con-
structed (chemically abnormal) myelin might be facilitated. Particular HLA antigens known to protrude from the surface of the
cell membrane commonly associated with MS, such as W40, might
indeed add to the weakness of binding of adjacent lamellae so
that in their presence (i.e. with this particular haplotype) MS
is especially liable to develop. It is possible that slippage
(disintegration of myelin) might occur "spontaneously" i.e.
without recognizable cause. For some reason, however, lesions
are nearly always (though not absolutely invariably) associated
with small blood vessels. Here all sorts of mischief might be
set afoot - e.g. antigen - antibody reactivity, mechanical disturbances, temporary damming back of tissue fluid absorption with
oedema of transient nature, virus invasion with subsequent immunological interactions, and so on. For any of these reasons a
congenitally "weak" myelin might "slip" and breakdown. Indeed
Clausen and Møller (3) have shown that poor PUFA feeding of rats
in the myelin formative (postnatal) period leads to especial
susceptibility to EAE. Any antigen - antibody reaction might
set off the avalanche of myelin disintegration (24). All phenomena which follow might then be secondary - lymphocyte sensitization, antibody formation, etc. etc.

These ideas (which will be elaborated elsewhere (6) are susceptible of disproof or verification and thus fulfil Popper's criteria of "scientific"though many years might be required.(19) It involves setting up two groups of children, picked out as MS "candidates" at an early age, and a blind trial - one "candidate" group being given γ -linolenate and the other placebo. If by the age of (say) 21 years, none of the γ -linolenate treated children has developed clinical signs of MS whilst some of the placebo group have already done so, it would be very encouraging and of course as the years go by more data would unfold. Although a long experiment, whose outcome the writer is hardly likely to live to see, it nevertheless seems a good sound rational approach opposed to the current Research Zeitgeist (SPQR - small profits quick return) in a field where 100 years have gone by without real understanding of the disease.

Finally, the writer has observed again and again that early patients commonly feel better long before there has been time for "conversion" to occur. It might be that linoleic acid (every bit as much a Vitamin as Vitamin C) is of value per se in some as yet ill understood manner in the subclinically deficient patient.

In addition, brief reference may be made to those childhood cases of MS in which there is a failure to mount an adequate lymphocyte sensitization response against measles after clinical infection. Here it is conceivable that the virus may fail to be eliminated from the brain, as almost always happens, and persists as a "slow" infection. There may well be a small group of MS cases which begin in this way and to which measles, as a "slow" infection, is related (4, 5).

ACKNOWLEDGEMENTS

The author is indebted to Messrs. Karger, Basel for permission to reproduce Table III, from European Neurology, 17 : 67-76 (1978) - Field and Joyce, Effect of Prolonged Ingestion of γ -linolenate by MS Patients. The author is also indebted to the Journal of Neurology for permission to reproduce Table II from : J. Neurol. 216, 135-146 (1977).

REFERENCES

1. Bates, D., Fawcett, P.R.W., Shaw, D.A., Weightman, D. (1977) Brit. Med. J. 2, 932.
2. Caspary, E.A. and Field, E.J. (1970) Europ. Neurol. 4, 256.
3. Clausen, J. and Møller, J. (1967) Acta. Neurol. Scand. 43, 375.
4. Field, E.J. (1975) Acta. Neurol. Scand. 51, 285.

5. Field, E.J. (1976) Akt. Neurologie, 3, 23.
6. Field, E.J. "Multiple Sclerosis in Childhood : its diagnosis and prophylaxis". C.C. Thomas (to appear).
7. Field, E.J., Joyce, G. and Smith, B.M. (1977) J. Neurol. 214, 113.
8. Field, E.J. and Joyce, G. (1978) Europ. Neurol. 17, 67.
9. Field, E.J. and Joyce, G. - unpublished.
10. Field, E.J., Meyer-Rienecker, H.J., Shenton, B.K., Jenssen, H.L. and Kohler, H. (1977) J. Neurol. 216, 135.
11. Field, E.J., Shenton, B.K. and Joyce, G. (1974) Brit. Med.J. 1, 412.
12. Field, E.J. and Shenton, B.K. (1975) Acta. Neurol. Scand. 52, 121.
13. Field, E.J., Shenton, B.K. and Meyer-Rienecker, H.J. (1976) Acta. Neurol. Scand. 54, 181.
14. Georgi, W. (1961) Schweiz. med. Wschr. 91, 605.
15. Ghatak, N.R., Hirano, A., Littmaer, H., and Zimmerman, H. (1974) Arch. Neurol. 30, 484.
16. Källen, B. and Nilsson, O. (1971) Nature (New Biol.)229, 91.
17. Millar, J.H.D., Zilkha, K.H., Langman, M.J.S., Payling-Wright, H., Smith, A.D., Belin, J. and Thompson, R.H.S. (1973) Brit. Med. J. 1, 765.
18. Myrianthopoulos, N.C. (1970) Genetics of Multiple Sclerosis. In "Handbook of Clinical Neurology" vol. 9, Ed. P.J. Vinken and G.W. Bruyn. North Holland Publishing Co.
19. Popper, K.R. (1965) Conjectures and Refutations; the growth of scientific knowledge. Second Edition. Routledge and Kegan Paul, London.
20. Swank, R.L. (1970) Arch. Neurol. 23, 460.
21. Thompson, R.H.S. (1966) Proc. roy. Soc. Med. 59, 269.
22. Thompson, R.H.S. (1973) Biochem. Soc. Symp. 35, 103.
23. Vost, A., Wolochon, D.A., and Howell, D.A. (1964) J. Path. Bact. 88, 463.
24. Wisniewski, H.M. and Bloom, B.R. (1975) J. exp. Med. 141, 346.

DISTRIBUTION OF SCRAPIE INFECTIVITY IN VARIOUS MOUSE TISSUES AT
EARLY TIMES AFTER INFECTION

G.C. Millson, R.H. Kimberlin, E.J. Manning and S.C.Collis

Agricultural Research Council, Institute for Research
on Animal Diseases, Compton, Newbury, Berkshire, U.K.

SUMMARY

Pilot studies with 99m-technetium labelled liposomes showed
that radioactivity was widely distributed in mouse tissues 30
minutes after injection by the intracerebral (i.c.), intraperito-
neal (i.p.), intravenous (i.v.) or subcutaneous (s.c.) route.
However, most radioactivity was taken up by liver, lung and spleen.
A similar pattern was seen when scrapie infectivity (Chandler
strain of agent) was assayed in tissues 30 minutes after the injection of high doses of agent (in brain homogenates) using the
same four routes. Although there was a significant infectivity in
blood 5 minutes after the injection of scrapie agent (particularly with the i.c. and i.v. routes), infectivity was barely detectable after 16 hours and only accounted for a small proportion of
the infectivity found in tissues.

The infectivity in liver decreased steadily during the 16
hours after injection, with very low levels persisting for the
next 135 days. In contrast to lung and liver, the amount of infectivity in spleen and salivary was initially low but increased
rapidly during the first 11 days after infection and reached
maximum levels well before the onset of clinical disease.

It is concluded that agent is rapidly distributed very early
after infection by the four routes tested, but the large amount
of agent taken up by the liver may not contribute to the pathogenesis of disease.

159

IMMUNOGLOBULIN G LEVELS IN THE SERA OF HERDWICK SHEEP WITH

NATURAL SCRAPIE

S.C. Collis, R.H. Kimberlin and G.C. Millson

Agricultural Research Council, Institute for Research
on Animal Diseases, Compton, Newbury, Berkshire, U.K.

SUMMARY

Studies have been made of a flock of Herdwick sheep, genetically selected for susceptibility to experimental infection
with scrapie, in which an extensive outbreak of the natural disease has occurred. One hundred and fifteen sheep in 3 lamb crops
(1974, 1975 and 1976) were bled at approximately 6 months intervals and measurements made of the concentration of IgG in serum.
Sixty-seven of these sheep developed natural scrapie at 21 to 28
months of age. Between 41 and 88 per cent of the scrapie cases
(depending on the lamb crop) had greatly increased levels of IgG
in the clinical stage of the disease. On average, the increases
were about 70 to 90 per cent above the levels of IgG found in
normal and scrapie sheep of 2-18 months of age. The significance
of these changes is not known but it is suggested that they may
be associated with the deposition of cerebral amyloid which is
known to a feature of some experimental models of scrapie in
mice.

VISNA IN SHEEP

M. Gudnadottir

Department of Microbiology, University of Iceland, Reykjavik, Iceland

HISTORICAL REVIEW

Natural History

In 1935 the first cases of a previously unknown paralytic
disease were seen in older age-groups of sheep in a south-western
region of Iceland (Fig 1). From 1935-1952 cases were increasing
causing considerable loss of sheep in the affected flocks (1, 2,
3). For a period of about 50 years prior to the occurrence of
these cases a paralytic disease of sheep, "rida", similar or
identical to scrapie, had been found on a few farms in a north-
western region. (Fig 1) (19-20). There, rida had remained localized
and not spread further (19). When a paralytic disease was found
in the south-western region the first thought was, that now rida
had spread south of the inland mountains separating these two
areas. Clinical and pathological studies soon revealed, that
these cases were not rida, but a new disease, not described
elsewhere before (2, 3). This new disease acquired the Icelandic
name "visna" a word which means "wasting", referring to the
clinical appearance of the paralytic sheep.

A few months earlier, pulmonary adenomatosis or "jaagziekte"
was found in the same area (1, 14, 15). Its origin could be
traced to the importation of sheep from Germany in 1933 (15). In
1939, another new lung disease of sheep, progressive pneumonia,
was found in a remote north-eastern region (12). Its origin could
be traced to the same importation of German sheep (15). The
progressive pneumonia acquired the Icelandic name "maedi", a word
meaning dyspnoea, referring to the cardinal clinical sign of this
disease. When progressive pneumonia had been recognized it became

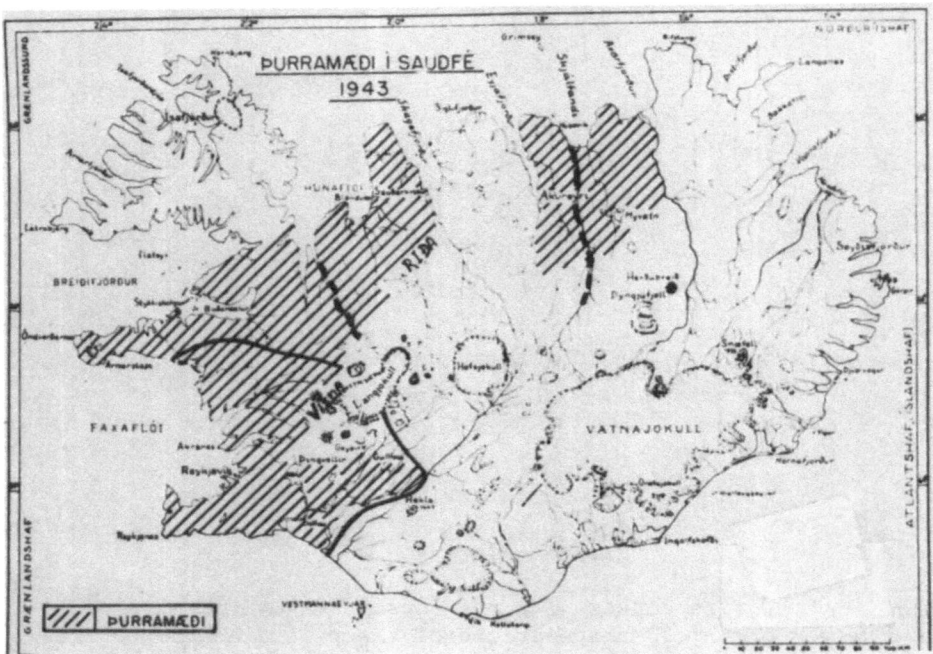

Fig. 1. A map of Iceland, showing maedi in 1943. The visna and
rida areas are marked on the map. In the large western maedi
area it was mixed with adenomatosis, but clean maedi without a
single case of visna was in the remote smaller eastern area,
where maedi was first found.

evident, that in the western and southern districts, where adenomatosis had caused great losses of affected flocks and masked all
other pathological conditions of the lungs, many lungs did not
only have adenomatosis, they also had maedi (12).

      The fourth serious sheep disease that could be traced to the
same importation of sheep was paratuberculosis (1).

                          Epidemiology

      Origin. The origin of visna, maedi, pulmonary adenomatosis
and paratuberculosis could be traced to the unfortunate importation
of 20 apparently healthy sheep of the Karakul breed from Halle,
Germany in 1933 (15). This importation was no accident. It was
decided upon by the Icelandic Ministry of Agriculture, supervised

by their experts and carried out after careful selection of place
and sheep flock from which these sheep were purchased. They underwent thorough veterinary examination both in Germany and Iceland
and were kept in isolation for 2 months on an island near Reykjavik
before they were released to 14 good farms in the best sheep
farming areas of the country (15).

    Soil. Sheep-farming has always been the main way of Icelandic
farming. The Icelandic sheep is a breed of hill sheep originally
brought there by the first settlers from Norway about 1100 years
ago. Since then, it has lived in Iceland isolated and undisturbed
and is well adapted to the hard survival so far north. The few
attempts to breed it with foreign sheep have all ended in difficulties with infectious diseases. Thus sheep scab was introduced and
caused great economical losses in the 18th and 19th centuries. Rida
was imported from Scotland late in the 19th century, and the great
disasters, jaagziekte, maedi, visna and paratuberculosis all at
the same time with the Karakul sheep in 1933. These diseases all
landed in a virgin soil living on the limits of survival, probably
also genetically different from most other sheep and more suceptible
than average at least to jaagziekte, maedi and visna. None of these
3 diseases were recognized in the German sheep flock from which the
20 Karakul sheep came, and none was at that time a veterinary
problem in Germany.

    Spread. Most likely 2 of the 20 imported Karakul sheep
were originally affected. The close contact they had during importation by sea and 2 months of quarantine created beautiful means
of infecting all of them before they were released to the farmers.
Such close contact seemed to be needed in order to transmit these
infections from one sheep-farm to another. During short, bright
and cold Icelandic summers, sheep **graze** freely in the mountainous
inland. This was harmless. During autumns sheep are chased from
the inland to large outdoors fences where sheep from large areas
mix for a night or two before they are brought to their home farms.
Only very rarely was this a suspected source of infection in a
new flock. During long and dark winters all sheep are housed in
huts for 4-6 months and fed hay indoors. In almost all cases could
a new infection be traced to the sheep huts, where neighbouring
sheep from infected flocks came in bad weather and stayed a few
days, and nights, often prior to the discovery of the infection in
the flock they came from (13).

    The mode of transmission of visna-maedi infection is not yet
clear. Respiratory infection is suspected, but it has been difficult
to prove. Most attempts at growing virus from throat swabs and saliva
in experimental infections have been negative (16, 21, 22, 23). The
milk is infective (16). Intra-uterine transmission is not proven,
and all attempts to prove it are negative so far (16, 27).

Geographical distribution of natural visna infection. The visna area shown in Fig. 1 is only a part of a larger area where mixed infection of jaagziekte and maedi occurred. In remote places each of the 2 lung diseases was found in a clean form. In none of these foci did visna occur. Therefore, there was no clear epidemiological evidence pointing at a common cause of any two of these three diseases. From 1949-1952, all infected flocks were slaughtered and the farms repopulated with sheep from the western peninsula, where these diseases never came (30). Thus visna and adenomatosis disappeared but maedi reappeared and caused localized outbreaks in an area where eradication was probably not thoroughly carried out. No cases of visna were seen in these herds, but the animals were all killed as soon as possible after confirmation of the first maedi case.

Incubation period. Almost 2 years elapsed from the importation of the Karakul sheep until the first cases of pulmonary adenomatosis appeared (15). Two years elapsed until visna was recognized and four year until maedi was found. The same or even a longer lapse of time between the infection of a flock and the clinical appearance of the first case was noted. From epidemiological experience it was very clear, that no acute type illness was ever seen in these cases. Insidious onset of a progressive clinical illness leading to death after exceptionally long incubation period was the general rule.

Age and sex distribution. Visna and maedi were diseases of older sheep, never found under the age of 2 years, but often much later (1, 2, 3). Life span of a sheep on a farm is 6-8 years. Adenomatosis could be found in sheep in their second year (13). None of these diseases affected small lambs. Both sexes seemed to be equally vulnerable.

Transmissions Experiments

Dr Björn Sigurdsson and his coworkers at the Institute for Experimental Pathology in Reykjavik successfully transmitted visna and rida to healthy sheep by inoculating brain material and cerebrospinal fluid (CSF) intracerebrally into them (1, 2, 3, 19). Adenomatosis and maedi were also successfully transmitted by intrapulmonary inoculation of material from infected lungs (6, 7, 8). Results of filtrations experiments indicated that these were viral infections.

Origin of the Concept: "Slow Viral Infection"

Studies on these four diseases, maedi, visna, rida and adenomatosis, their epidemiological pattern in virgin soil, and observations on their experimental transmission in sheep, besides a tremendous

amount of work on paratuberculosis at the same time, lead Dr. Björn
Sigurdsson to a recognition and description of a new previously
unknown group of viral infections, which he named "Slow Viral
Infections". In 1954 he described this group of infections (1).

His criteria for a slow viral infection were as follows :
1) A very long initial period of latency, lasting from several
months to several years.
2) A rather regular protracted course after clinical signs have
appeared, usually ending in a serious disease or death.
3) Limitation of the infection to a single host species and
anatomical lesions in only a single organ or tissue system.
The statements in the last paragraph were put forward with the
remarks, that they might have to be modified as knowledge increased.

In 1954, when Dr. Björn Sigurdsson published his criteria
for a slow viral infection, these criteria were solely based on
clinicopathological and epidemiological observations of diseases,
and on experimental work when the afore mentioned diseases were
transmitted into their healthy natural host, the sheep. While these
criteria were founded tissue culture work on viruses was still in
its infancy. Very few growth curves of viruses at cellular level
were available, except for polioviruses, and measles and rubella
viruses had not been isolated from clinical specimens for the first
time. Therefore, Sigurdsson's criteria for a slow viral infection
refer to the course of events in the disease itself in its natural
host, but are no guesswork on growth or replication in tissue culture
of viruses that had not even been isolated for the first time.

Isolation in Tissue Culture of the First Viruses Causing a Slow

Infection

In 1957 Sigurdsson and his coworkers succeeded in isolating
a virus in tissue culture from choroid plexuses and central nervous
system of experimental visna sheep. This virus produced visna when
inoculated into sheep (4). In 1958 Sigurdsson isolated a similar
virus from lungs of sheep in a localized outbreak of maedi (9).
His successors later isolated identical viruses from other outbreaks
of maedi and produced maedi by inoculating these viruses intrapulmonarily into sheep (10, 11). Some of these sheep also contracted visna (11).

The Visna-Maedi Virus

This new virus turned out to be a middle sized enveloped
lipid containing virus with many properties in common with the
Friend's leucemia virus and viruses causing chicken leucoses, but
not serologically related to them. Many more common properties

have since then be found, f.ex. reverse transcriptase. Therefore
the visna-maedi virus is preliminarily classified as a retrovirus.
Recently its properties were thoroughly reviewed (28, 29, 30).

The Visna Disease

Clinical signs of visna were clearly described in the original
work of Sigurdsson, who also studied clinicopathological changes
in the cerebrospinal fluid and blood of naturally and experimentally infected cases (1, 2, 3, 5). Histopathological lesions in
the central nervous system were described by Sigurdsson, van Bogaert
and Palsson (2, 3, 12). Further work on the histopathology and ultrastructure of the visna lesions has recently been done (18, 30).
Immunosuppression was recently found to diminish the inflammatory
reaction in experimentally infected sheep (31, 32).

COURSE OF EVENTS IN VISNA INFECTION OF ICELANDIC SHEEP

This review is based on studies carried out in collaboration
with Dr. Pall A Palsson, Institute for Experimental Pathology,
Reykjavik, during the period from 1960-1971, with references to
more recent data from Palsson and his present coworkers.

In October 1960, 34 female sheep 5 months of age were infected
with a visna strain called K796 (see fig. 3). Of these sheep
24 were infected intracerebrally (i.c.) with 300.000 $TCID_{50}$ and
10 were infected intrapulmonarily (i.p.) with 5 million $TCID_{50}$.
It was decided not to terminate these experiments until all sheep
had died of natural causes.

Incubation Period and Clinical Course

During almost 11 years 30 cases of clinical visna occurred in
these sheep. Maedi lesions in lungs were frequently found and
clinical cases of maedi were seen (22, 23, 27). The lapse of time
from the inoculation to the beginning of clinical visna disease
varied considerably as shown in Table 1.

No acute illness was detectable during the first weeks of these
experiments, neither were any prodromal symptoms or signs detectable
at the beginning of the clinical phase. Paralysis began insidiously.
Sometimes the clinical course lead to death rapidly. In other cases
paralytic disease progressed slowly and the clinical phase lasted
for years, in one case 6 years. There were no remissions.

Table 1

Clinical signs of visna begin :

	Years after inoculation :						
	1st	2nd	3rd	4th	5th-6th	7th-9th	No ill-ness.
inoc. i.c.	2/24	5/24	4/24	5/24	1/24	5/24	2/24
inoc. i.pulm.			1/10	4/10	1/10	2/10	2/10

number of sheep with first signs/number inoculated.

The Cerebrospinal Fluid

Cell counts and inoculations into tissue culture were carried out on samples of cerebrospinal fluid (CSF) from all these sheep at regular intervals throughout the observation period. Examples of the results are given in Table 2.

Subclinical meningitis could in all cases be detected during the first months .after inoculation, and at 6 months all sheep had elevated cell counts regardless of the mode of inoculation. Cellular reaction in the cerebrospinal fluid is considerably less in the intrapulmonarily inoculated group. Yet 8 cases of visna occurred in this group. Inoculation of 0,3-0,5 ml of CSF into each of 2 choroid plexus tissue culture tubes, directly, gave positive results at any time in some cases (Fig 2 A)but less frequently in others (Fig 4). Both samples with high and low or normal counts could give positive results. (Fig 2). Low titer of neutralizing antibodies was irregularly found in CSF when looked for in the later years but early CSF samples were not tested. Neutralizing antibodies have now been found at a high titer in CSF early in the visna infection (32).

Viremia

In the second week after inoculation viremia was detected. In the i.p. inoculated group it began on the 11th day and lasted a few days in all cases. It was more irregular in the i.c. inoculated group. Viremia became persistent in some cases and lasted for years in the presence of high neutralizing antibodies. Although the virus was readily isolated from whole blood in such cases, few experiments indicated that infectivity was connected with the white cells. This has been confirmed (16).

Table II : Examples of cell counts and results of virus isolations from CSF during a 10 year period of observations. Each example is plotted as number sheep with the stated amount of cells or number positive visna virus isolations at the given time/number sheep counted or cultivated from.

Time	Group I					Group II				Control.
	Number of cells				Virus	Number of cells			Virus	cell count
	< 10	10-50	50-500	>500	+	< 10	10-50	50-500	+	< 10
Day 0	24/24				0/24	10/10			0/10	5/5
" 13	18/21	3/21			0/21	8/10	2/10		0/10	"
2 months		8/24	9/24	7/24	20/24	2/10	7/10	1/10	1/10	"
3 "	1/24	8/24	14/24	1/24	9/24	2/10	6/10	2/10	1/10	"
6 "		5/23	18/23		4/23		9/10	1/10	1/10	"
1 year	1/23	14/23	7/23	1/23	7/23	5/10	5/10		0/10	"
2 "	6/17	4/17	7/17		3/17	6/10	4/10		1/10	"
3 "	7/11	2/11	2/11		3/11	5/10	5/10		1/10	"
4 "	5/11	3/11	3/11*		3/11	7/9	2/9		0/9	"
5 "	4/11	1/11	5/11	1/11	2/11	2/6	4/6		1/6	"
6 "	5/10	1/10	2/10	2/10	1/10	4/5	1/5		0/5	"
7 "	4/7	1/7	2/7		1/7	5/5			0/5	"
8 "	2/4		2/4		0/4	3/5	2/5		1/5	"
9 "	2/3	1/3			0/3	1/1			0/1	"
10 "	1/3	1/3	1/3		0/3					"

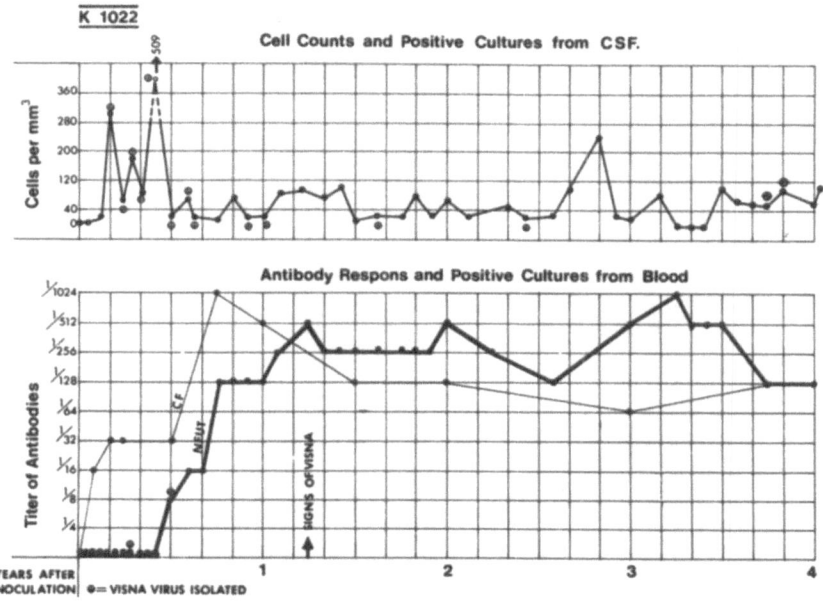

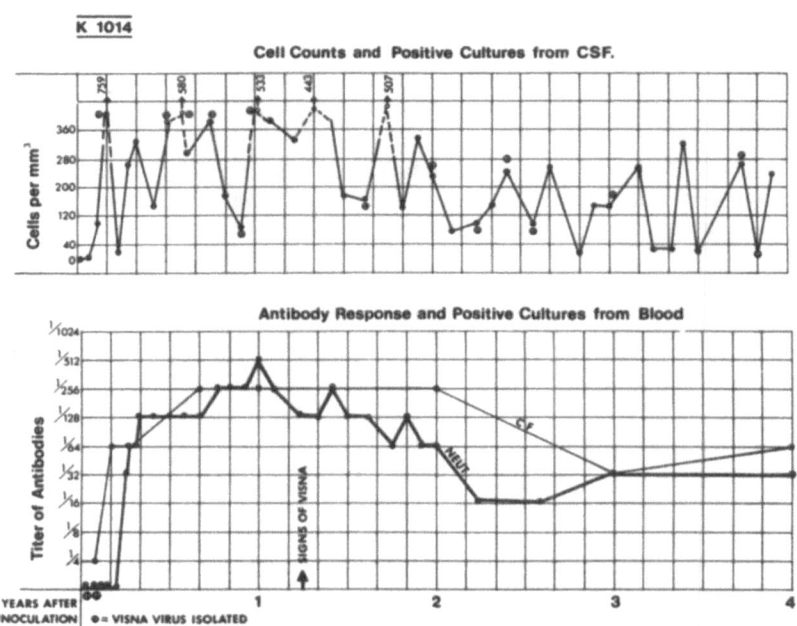

Fig. 2 A and B.   Course of events in 2 cases of visna with early onset.

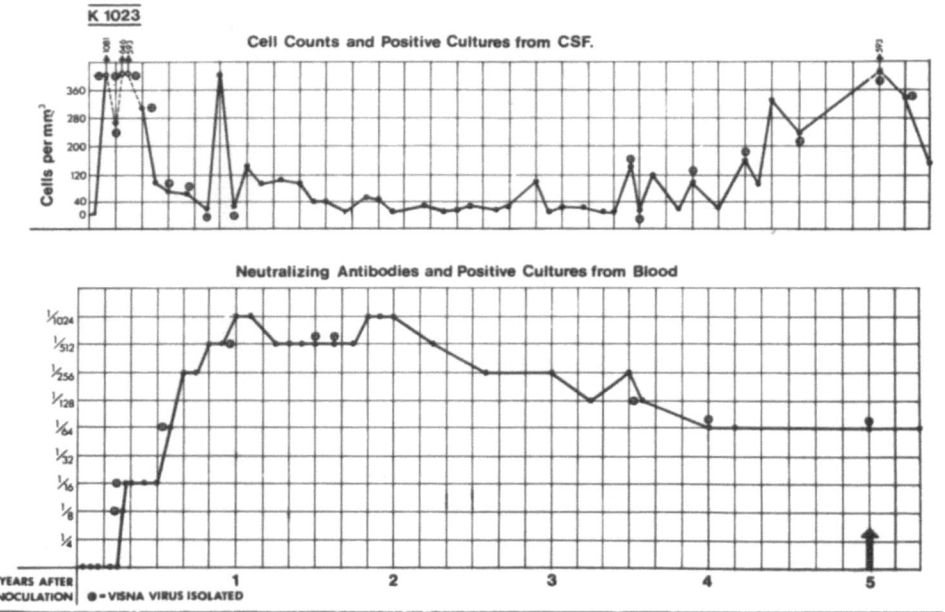

Fig. 2 C. A late case of visna with diphasic subclinical
meningitis and viremia for 6 years.

Virus in other Body Fluids, Excreta and Tissues

Search for virus in throat swabs and saliva during the first
years were mostly unsuccessful, and so were a few attempts to
isolate virus from faecal samples in early years. Virus was
easily isolated from many tissues by explanting them in plasma
clots and passing both fluid and cells into fresh choroid plexus
tissue cultures 3-4 weeks later. From 32 of the 34 sheep could
virus be isolated from both spleen and mediastinal lymph node.
In two very slow clinical cases no virus was detectable in any
organ. Isolations of virus from lungs were frequent but not quite
as frequent as from the lymphoid tissues. Viruses were found
in every other salivary gland tested, but rarely in kidney
tissue. Virus was isolated from all but one choroid plexus
of the i.c. inoculated group. Only 3 of 10 choroid plexuses of
the i.p. inoculated sheep were positive by using the same
methods. A similar proportion of positive virus isolations from
choroid plexuses was found in natural cases of maedi (24). This,
and the considerably diminished cellular reaction in the CSF of
the i.p. inoculated group might mean, that i.c. inoculation of
virus creates more artificial and less reliable surroundings in
the CNS than will be created there if the virus gets there by
a more natural route.

Antibody Response

Neutralisation tests were regularly carried out on serial
2-fold dilutions of sera from these sheep against 100 $TCID_{50}$
of the inoculated strain K796. Examples of the results of these
tests are shown in Table 3; which shows titers of neutralizing
antibodies in 16 of the i.c. inoculated sheep. In these animals
a period of 2.5 months elapsed until the first neutralizing antibodies were detected but 1.5 months in the i.p. injected group.
The course of the infection could not be predicted by looking
at the level of neutralizing antibodies in individual sheep.
Sheep K1013 and K1019, the lowest and the highest, were the
two sheep, that had the longest lifespan.

The methods used in neutralization of visna virus deserve
a comment : most consistant results are obtained by using the
old method of Sigurdsson, "incubating" the serum-virus mixture
in ice-water (0°C) in a refrigerator for 48 hrs. Visna virus is
easily heat-inactivated and does not survive long in protein-free
buffers at any temperature. Shorter fixation at 37°C gives less
consistent results than the 48 hrs fixation in the cold. Conventional neutralization for 1-3 hrs. at room temperature is useless.
Neutralizing antibodies seem to have a very low avidity. Complement fixing antibodies behave conventionally and were detectable in less than a month after inoculation. A hemagglutination-
inhibition test is not yet available.

Fig 2 illustrates the course of events in 3 cases of visna,
2 early cases and one late case with persistent viremia.

CHANGES IN VISNA VIRUS AND INDIVIDUAL VARIATIONS IN ANTIBODY
RESPONSE OF SHEEP DURING VISNA INFECTION

The afore mentioned long-term experiments were carried out
by using a visna strain called K796. Its origin is shown in
Fig. 3. In 1958 strain K 796 was isolated in tissue culture from
explants of choroid plexus of sheep K796 in the 5th brain to
brain passage of visna. Four natural cases of visna from two
parts of the visna district contributed to the brain material
that was passed 5 times in sheep in 9 years (Fig 3). The inoculated strain K796 in this work was also in the 5th passage in
sheep choroid plexus tissue culture. In further passages used
in neutralizations tests during 18 years of laboratory work it
has remained stable and given most consistant results from one
passage level to another.

In 1957 when visna virus was first isolated all natural
cases had disappeared, no new cases have been found since before

Table III. Neutralizing antibodies against visna strain K796 in 16 sheep infected i.c. with 300.000 TCID$_{50}$ and observed for 10 years

Time	\ Sheep no. 1010	1011	1012	1013	1014	1015	1016	1017	1018	1019	1020	1021	1022	1023	1024	1025
Prae inoc.	<4	<4	<4	<4	<4	<4	<4	<4	<4	<4	<4	<4	<4	<4	<4	<4
0-2 1/2 mnt	<4	<4	<4	<4	<4	<4	<4	<4	<4	<4	<4	<4	<4	<4	<4	<4
3 months	4	4	4	4	32	4	32	<4	4	<4	4	<4	<4	<4	<4	<4
4 "	8	4	8	4	128	8	128	<4	4	8	4	<4	<4	<4	<4	<4
6 "	16	16	16	4	128	32	128	8	8	8	32	8	8	16	4	4[x]
9 "	32	32	32	4	256	64	256	32	16	4	64	8	128	16	16	
1 year	64	64	128	8	512	256	256	256	128	512	128	32	128	256	64	
16 months	32	32	64	4	128	128[x]	128	512	256	512	256	16	128	1024	512	
21 "	32	128	32	4	64		128	512	128	512	256	16	256	512	512	
2 years	32	128	128	4	64		128	512	512	2048	256	16	512	512	512	
27 months	8	32	64	4	16		32	1024	512	2048	256	16	256	1024	512	
31 "	8	32[x]	64	4	16		64	512	256	1024	128	16	128	512	128	
3 years	16		64	4	32		128	256	256	512	128	16	512	256	128	
3 1/2 yrs	8		64	16	64		128	256	256	512	16	8	512	256	128	
4 years	8		16[x]	16	32[x]		64	256	128	1024	16	32	128[x]	128	128	
5 "	8			16			64	128	64[x]	1024	32	32		64	512	
6 "	8[x]			16			32[x]	128[x]		1024	32	16		64	512	
7 "				32						1024	16[x]	16		64[x]	1024	
8 "				8						128		16			512[x]	
9 "				8[x]						256		16				
10 "										128		16[x]				

x Last serum specimen before death of visna

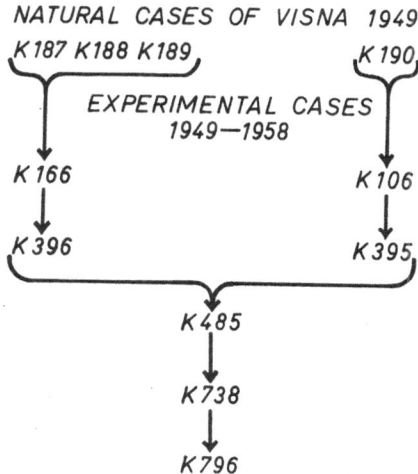

Fig. 3. Origin of visna strain K796. 5 brain to brain passages
in 9 years of brain material from 4 natural cases occurring in 2
different parts of the visna area.

the eradications programme, which ended in 1952. Therefore all
available Icelandic visna strains have a background similar to
strain K796. They are all isolated from experimental visna cases
in which mixed brain material from more than 2 natural visna
cases was used to begin with. These old transmission experiments
were designed in order to find out that visna was an infectious
disease. Therefore mixed brain material was considered more suitable than individual brains, probably with very low infectivity.
The Icelandic visna strains may all be genetic recombinants of 2 or
more natural visna strains from old brain material. If so, this
does not disturb everydays work with them in tissue culture in which
they are very stable.

    The last sheep to die in these long experiments was killed
without signs of visna 10.5 years after inoculation. Visna lesions
corresponding to late preclinical phase were found in its central
nervous system and virus isolated its choroid plexus, mediastinal
lymph node and spleen. When the reisolated virus from spleen was
neutralized against a few sera from this sheep, it was observed,
that early sera did not neutralize this virus, although they
had high titer against strain K796, when retested. Less neutralization of the reisolated strain than that of K796 was found in
later samples (Fig. 4).

These findings were confirmed when testing reisolated viruses from other sheep against their own sera. Sometimes there was no neutralization for years (Fig. 5) (26, 27).

Table 4 shows results of neutralization tests on sera from one of the intrapulmonarily inoculated sheep against its own virus from choroid plexus, the spleen strain from sheep K1019 and 3 strains isolated from CSF at 3 and 5 years after inoculation of K796, which also was neutralized for comparison. A marked difference was found.

Strain K1010 isolated from a CSF sample taken at the beginning of a second meningeal phase of preclinical visna, just before onset of clinical illness seemed to differ a great deal from the originally inoculated strain K796. This strain was inoculated intra-cerebrally into 4 sheep (300000 TCID$_{50}$ per sheep). Fig. 6 shows results of cell counts in CSF and neutralizing antibody response of these sheep during the first 7 months after inoculation.

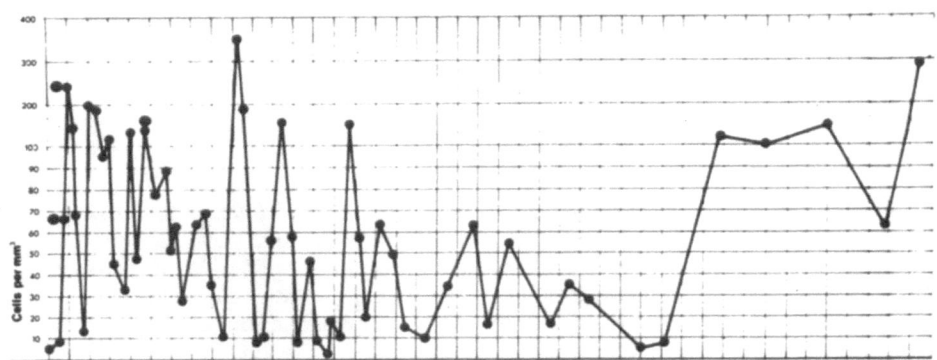

K 1019   Cell counts and positive cultures from CSF

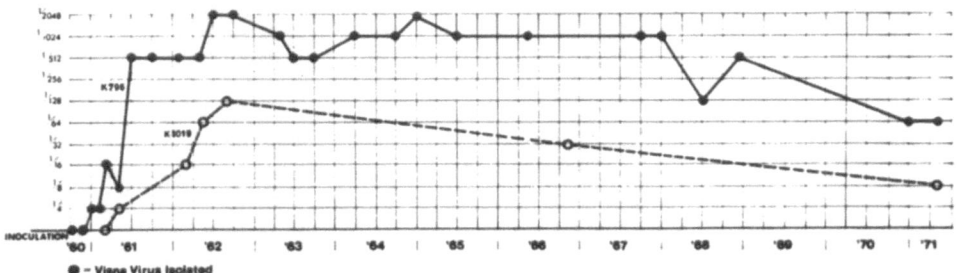

● - Visna Virus Isolated

Fig. 4. Comparison of originally inoculated visna strain K796 and reisolated strain K1019, from spleen 10 1/2 years after inoculation, by neutralization tests on sera from sheep K1019 at different times.

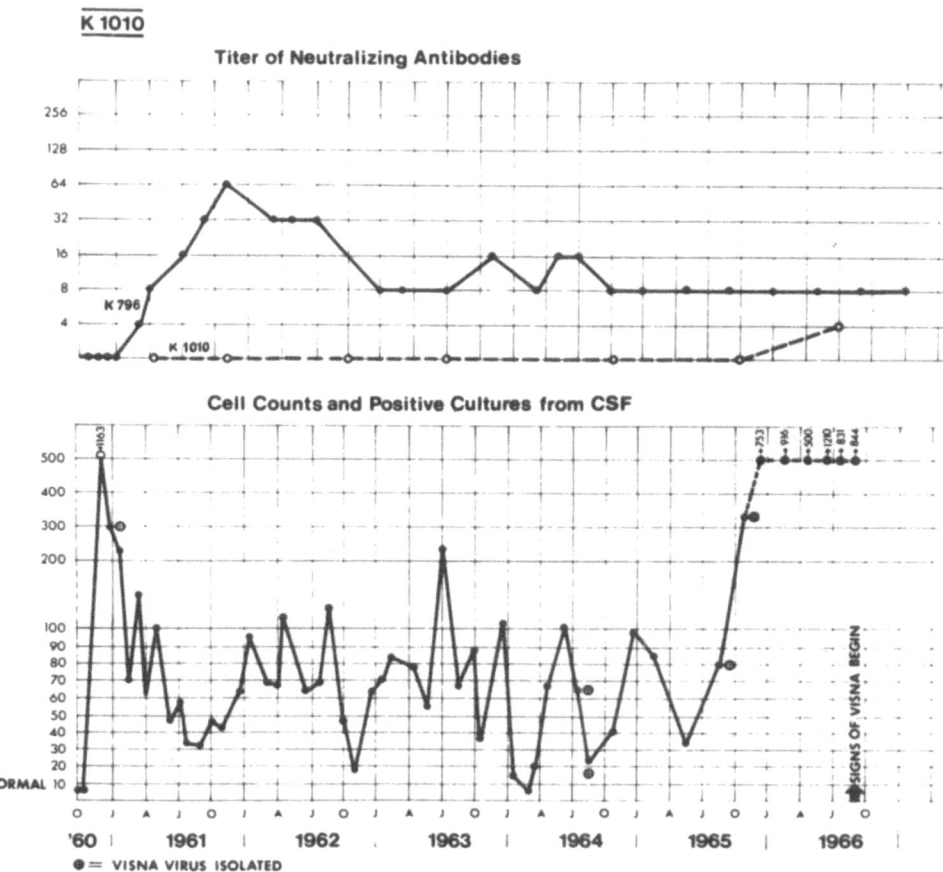

Fig. 5. Late visna case with diphasic meningitis, at the beginning of which strain K1010 was isolated from CSF. No neutralization of this strain for 4 years in sera from sheep K1010, and a titer of 4 at time of death from visna.

They all developed good neutralizing antibodies at the same time to strain K1010. They also developed antibodies against the mother strain K796, three of them during the first 7 months. Two reisolated viruses from early CSF samples were tested. Differences were found in sera from 3 sheep but one sheep neutralized all four strains almost equally well (Fig. 6), and did not recognize differences in antigenic structure of strains K1010 and K796 (Fig. 7). The other sheep showed variable amount of neutralization of strain K796, in two of them only a low late response was found, less than one would expect if both strains were

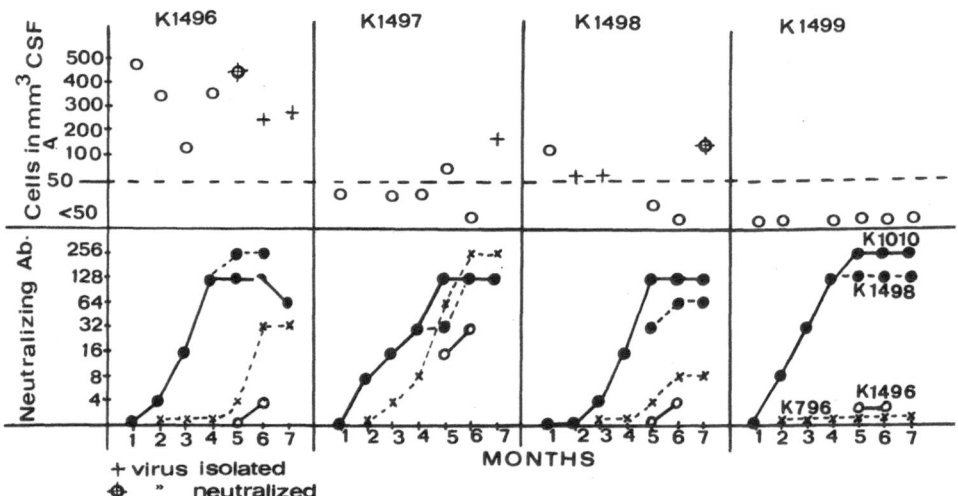

Fig. 6. Cell counts, positive cultures from CSF and neutralizing antibodies to 4 visna strains during the first 7 months, in 4 sheep inoculated i.c. with strain K 1010. The sheep were tested against strains K1010, K796, and two reisolated strains K 1496 from CSF of one of them at 4 months, and K1498 from another of them at 7 months after inoculation.

Table IV

Reisolated strains vary, when they are compared in neutralization tests on same sera. Only slight variations are observed in CF tests.

Séra from Sheep K1029	Neutralizing antibodies to original K796 and 5 reisolated strains.				
taken at	Original K796	K 1029 · choroid plexus 9 years	K1019 Spleen 10 1/2 year	K1017 CSF 3 years	K1023 CSF 5 years	K1010 CSF 5 years
6 months	8	< 4	4	< 4	< 4	< 4
1 year	16	< 4	4	< 4	< 4	< 4
2 years	128	32	16	< 4	8	< 4
3-4 years	256	128	64	4	32	4
6 years	512	128	64	8	32	16
9 years	256	256	32	8	8	8

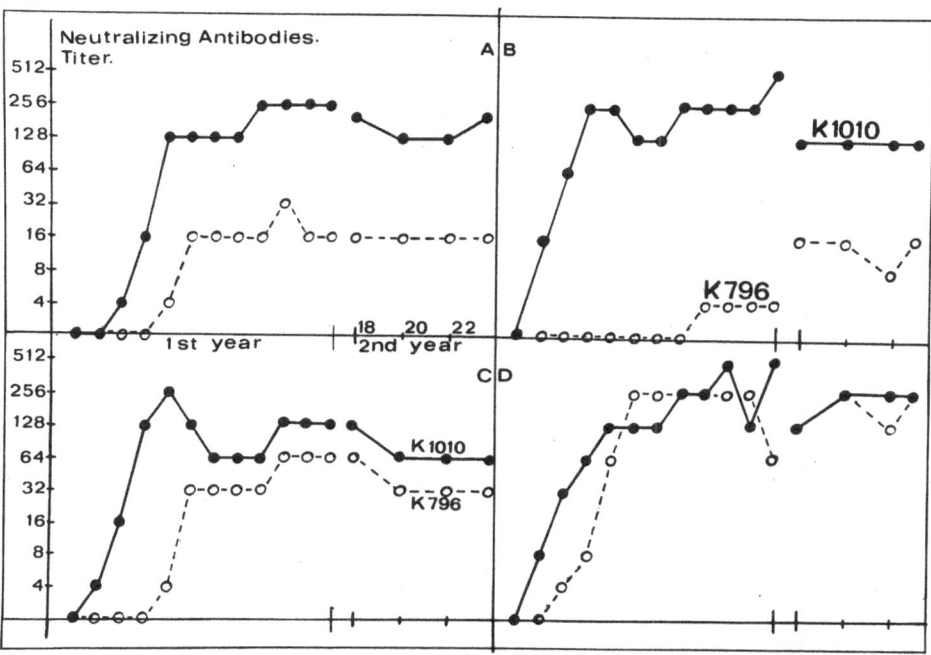

Fig. 7. Neutralizing antibodies against strains K1010 and K796 in sera of the 4 sheep inoculated with strain K1010 during the first 2 years after inoculation.

actively infecting the sheep tested, as could be the case as judged by the neutralization tests on the early reisolates from CSF of two of them. Similar heterogeneity of neutralizing antibodies was observed when a few sheep from the older experiments were used to compare these and other reisolated visna viruses.

These findings may mean that the visna virus, persisting in one host for years as a low grade productive infection in the presence of antibodies, undergoes changes comparable with influenza virus in the whole human population. These differences could also be due to impaired antibody production of an infected lymphoid tissue, where in some cases only a narrow range of antigenic determinants can be detected because only a few stem cells are well enough to carry out their normal function, the others are impaired or dead. The sheep, that do not detect these differences in surface structure, would then be individuals with healthy lymphoid cells. Both factors could operate in the visna infection.

CONCLUSIONS

Visna and maedi are two forms of the same infection, which both progressively lead to death. These are systemic diseases and the third target organ is in all cases the lymphoid tissue, probably functionally very much disturbed because of the persistent virus infection, which in the experiments here reported appeared productive. In most of the cases, the virus was easily detectable during the whole course of the visna infection and easily reisolated at any time from many tissues, CSF and sometimes from whole blood for years in spite of good humoral antibody response. Direct inoculations of specimens gave positive virus isolations and special procedures had to be applied. This indicates a low grade productive infection in various tissues of the infected animal. The visna infection appears to be a classical slow infection fulfilling the two first criteria of Sigurdsson's original concepts of this type of disease. Changes in surface antigens of the virus may occur during persistence. Marked individual heterogeneity in neutralizing antibody response was observed.

Accumulating evidence of the behavior of the agents so far involved in slow infections shows, that they all multiply and persist in lymphoid tissues probably impairing the immune response of the host by causing infectious immunological diseases, a concept, that has not yet attracted any attention. Production of CF antibodies goes on for years at a high titer in contrast to most of the acute infections, with the possibilities of a slow damage of altered cells through the complement system. Nothing is known of the composition of the complement system in visna, its production or fitness for function. Further work on the immunopathology of the slow infections might be fruitful. Workers of the future should probably pay more attention to the features that these diseases have in common than to the differences in structure at the molecule level of the agents causing them.

REFERENCES

1. Sigurdsson B.: Observations on three slow infections of sheep. Maedi. Paratuberculosis. Rida, a chronic encephalitis of sheep with general remarks on infections, which develop slowly, and some of their special characteristics. Brit. Vet. J. 110: 255-270, 307-322, 341-354 (1954).
2. Sigurdsson B.; Palsson P.A. and Grimsson H.: Visna, a demyelinating transmissable disease of sheep. J. Neuropath. exp. Neurol. 16: 389-403 (1957).
3. Sigurdsson, B. and Palsson, P.A.: Visna of sheep. A slow demyelinating infection. Brit. J. exp. Path. 39:519-528 (1958).

4. Sigurdsson, B.; Thormar, H. and Palsson, P.A.: Cultivation of visna virus in tissue culture. Arch. ges Virusforsch. 10 : 368-381 (1960).

5. Sigurdsson, B.; Karcher, D.; van Sande, M. and Lowenthal, A.: Electrophoresis of serum and CSF proteins in sheep neurological diseases. In : Proc. 8th Coll. Protides of the Biological Fluids, Bruges 1960, pp. 110-111. (Elsevier, Amsterdam 1960).

6. Sigurdsson, B.: Adenomatosis of sheep's lungs. Experimental transmission. Arch. ges Virusforsch. 8:51-58 (1958).

7. Sigurdsson, B.; Grimsson, H. and Palsson, P.A. : Maedi. A chronic progressive infection of sheep's lungs. J. Infect. Dis. 90: 233-241 (1952).

8. Sigurdsson, B.; Palsson, P.A.; and Tryggvadottir, A.: Transmission experiments with maedi. J. Infect. Dis. 93: 166-175 (1953).

9. Sigurdsson, B.: Unpublished work.

10. Sigurdardottir, B. and Thormar, H.: Isolation of a viral agent from the lungs of sheep affected with maedi. J. Infect. Dis. 114, 55-60 (1964).

11. Gudnadottir, M., and Palsson, P.A.: Transmission of maedi by inoculation of a virus grown in tissue culture from maedi affected lungs. J. Infect. Dis. 117: 1-6 (1967).

12. Gislason, G.: Maedi. In International encyclopedia of veterinary medicine, vol 3, pp 1780-1784 (Green, Edinburgh, 1966).

13. Gislason, G.: Unpublished work 1935-1965.

14. Dungal, N.; Gislason, G. and Taylor, E.L.: Epizootic adenomatosis in the lungs of sheep. Comparison with Jaagziekte, verminous pneumonia and progressive pneumonia. J. Comp. Path. 51: 46-68 (1938).

15. Gislason, G.: Yhaettir um innflutning bufjar og karakylsjukdoma. Icelandic Ministry of Agric. Publ. pp 235-254 (1947).

16. De Boer, G.F.: Zwogerziekte een persisterende virusinfektie bij schapen. Proefschrift, Drukkerij Elinkwijk Utrecht (1970).

17. Sigurdsson, B.; Palsson, P.A. and van Bogaert, L. : Pathology of visna. Acta Neuropath. 1: 343-362, (1962).

18. Georgsson, G.; Palsson, P.A., Panitch, H.; Nathanson, N.; and Pétursson, G.: The ultrastructure of early visna lesions. Acta Neuropath. (Berl.)37, 137-135 (1977).

19. Palsson, P.A. and Sigurdsson, B.: Rida, En langsom, progredierende infektios nervesygdom hos far. Proceedings of the 8th scandinavian veterinary congress in Finland. Publ. Vammalan kirjanpaino Oy (1958).

20. van Bogaert, L.; Dewulf, A. and Palsson, P.A. : Rida in Sheep. Pathological and clinical aspects. Acta Neuropath. (Berl.) 41, 201-206 (1978).

21. Gudnadottir, M. and Palsson, P.A.: Transmission of Maedi by inoculation of a virus grown in tissue culture from maedi affected lungs. J. Infect. Dis. 117: 1-6 (1967).

22. Gudnadottir, M. and Palsson, P.A.: Host-virus interaction in Visna infected sheep. J. Immunol. 95: 116-1120 (1966).

23. Gudnadottir, M. and Palsson, P.A.: Successful transmission of visna by intrapulmonary inoculation. J. Infect. Dis. 115 217–225 (1965).

24. Gudnadottir, M.; Gislason, G. and Palsson, P.A.: Studies on natural cases of maedi in search for diagnostic laboratory methods. Res. Vet. Sci. 9: 65–67 (1968).

25. Gudnadottir, M. and Kristinsdottir, K.: Complement fixing antibodies in sera of sheep affected with visna and maedi. J. Immunol. 98: 663–667 (1967).

26. Gudnadottir, M. : Preliminary reports on strain differences in visna. 4th meeting of the Noth-West European Microbiology Group, Bristol (1972).

27. Gudnadottir, M.: Visna-Maedi in sheep. In: Progress in Medical Virology 18: 336–349 (1974).

28. Thormar, H.: Lin, F.H. and Throwbridge, R.S.: Visna and Maedi viruses in tissue culture. Progress in Medical Virology 18: 323–335 (1974).

29. Haase, A.T.: The slow infection caused by visna virus. In : Current topics in Microbiology and Immunology. 72: 101–156 (1975).

30. Kimberlin, R.H. ed: Visna-Maedi. In:Slow virus diseases of animals and man. North-Holland Research Monographs Frontiers of Biology 44 (1976).

31. Petursson, G.; Georgsson, G.; Nathanson, N.; Palsson, P.A and Panitch, H. : Pathogenesis of Visna, I, II, III. Lab. Invest.

32. Pétursson, G.; Nathansen, N.; Palsson, P.A.; Martin, J. and Georgsson, G.: Immunopathogenesis of visna. A slow virus disease of the central nervous system. Acta Neurol. Scand 58 Suppl. 67 (1978).

OLD DOG ENCEPHALITIS

A CLINICAL AND SEROLOGICAL STUDY

J.M. ADAMS [+], M.J. Appel [x], E. Norrby [o] and S.H. Snow [*]

+ Department of Pediatrics, University of California
Medical Center, Los Angeles; x The James A. Baker Insti-
tute for Animal Health, Cornell University, Ithaca, New
York; ° Karolinska Institute, Stockholm, Sweden; * The
Leo Rigler Center for Radiological Sciences, Los Angeles,
California, U.S.A.

ABSTRACT

Antibody tests for measles (rubeola) and canine distemper on
sera and cerebrospinal fluid of 36 dogs with probable Old Dog
Encephalitis (ODE) have revealed positive titers in sera or spinal
fluid in 18 of the suspect animals. Antibody tests performed on
similar samples were normal or absent in 18 control animals of
similar breeds, ages and sex. The following tests were performed :
measles virus hemolysis-inhibition (HLI), measles hemagglutination-
inhibition (HI), measles nucleo-capsid C.F., distemper complement-
fixation (C.F.) and a microneutralization test for canine distemper
virus. All dogs had canine distemper antibody in sera. Measles
titers in C.S.F. were found in 3 dogs and distemper titers were
positive in C.S.F. in 5 dogs. All serological tests were performed
in two different laboratories on identical samples. Results of
tests are compared. Clinical features are cited, and pathological
findings are illustrated by photomicrographs from cases of ODE.

INTRODUCTION

The need for an animal model of human demyelinating diseases
was emphasized by J.R.M. Innes (1) in a discussion of demyelinating diseases in animals. He asked the question : "Could encephalitis 'in dog' occupy exactly the same peculiar position to
distemper as the so-called postinfectious encephalitides in man
due to smallpox, measles, chickenpox and influenza?" Several
authors (2, 3, 4) likewise called attention to similar patholo-

gical findings in disseminated encephalomyelitis of the dog and
acute and subacute disseminated sclerosis in man.

Cordy, D.R. (5) called attention to encephalitis in mature
dogs characterized by perivascular accumulations of mononuclear
cells in the central nervous system and by intranuclear inclusion
bodies. This rare disease of middle aged dogs, now known as
old dog encephalitis (ODE), is characterized by an insidious
onset of dyspraxia, periods of depression and circling. Convulsions are rarely seen early in the illness which is one of progressive impairment in mental and motor abilities leading to
death in a few months.

Lincoln, S.D. and associates (6) described brain lesions
characterized by disseminated encephalitis with perivascular and
diffuse lymphoplasmocytic infiltrations. Lincoln, S.D. (7) demonstrated immune gamma globulin (IgG) in brain sections employing direct fluorescent antibody tests. Cutler, R.W.P. and
Averill, D.R. Jr. (8) presented supporting evidence that immunoglobulin-G (IgG) is produced locally within the nervous system
in canine distemper encephalitis.

The objective of this study was to increase our understanding of the pathogenesis of slow virus infections with emphasis
directed to measles (rubeola) and canine distemper - RNA viruses
in the paramyxoviridae family (9).

Human sera and human gamma globulin were reported by one of
us (JMA) to neutralize canine distemper virus (10). Subsequently, the immunologic relationship between measles, distemper and
rinderpest was reported from our laboratory (11).

MATERIALS AND METHODS

The animals, dogs of various breeds, varied in age from 2
to 15 years with no particular sex predominance. Although a
rare disease among dogs, symptoms and signs indicating a probable diagnosis of ODE were studied. Thirty-six animals have
been observed clinically and a few pathologically confirming
the diagnosis of ODE. The canine patients were anesthetized
intravenously, at which time a 10 ml sample of blood was drawn
for serologic study. The animal was placed on his side, a tra-
cheal respiratory tube was placed, and a small area on the back
of the head in the cisternal area was shaved in preparation for
a spinal tap. A 20 gauge spinal needle was used. Following
preparation of the area, the needle was inserted in the midline
approximately 2.5 cm below the occipital tubercle. Five to 6 ml
of clear spinal fluid was obtained for serologic study.

The results of the microneutralization tests for canine distemper virus were recorded initially to Log 10 (12). Figures have been converted to compare with results of measles and distemper antibodies reported from Karolinska Institutet (13). It should be pointed out that clinical criteria for making a diagnosis of ODE are difficult to obtain from owners and are usually only suspect, such as lameness, weakness, abnormal gait and convulsions. All of these symptons and signs may be related to various causes and not ODE as recently emphasized by Sullivan, C.B. and Haile, R.W. (14).

RESULTS

Published reports (15, 16) from this laboratory implicated ODE as a possible animal model for further study of the pathogenesis of severe demyelinating diseases related to slow virus infections.

Data from two different laboratories (12, 13) using different methods have been recorded in the accompanying Tables I and II for comparison. Dogs with positive findings have been listed by name, breed, age and sex. Table III sumarizes Clinical and Serological data from Tables I and II. Control animals were selected with no history suggesting the classic clinical features

TABLE I

DOGS WITH PROBABLE ODE

				MEASLES				DISTEMPER		
Name	Breed	Age	Sex	HI	HLI	NC-CF (CSF)		CD-CF	CD-SN	
SASHA	GOLDEN	7	M	40	40	10	4	80	100	
TOSH	GR.SH.	11	M	4	32	20		40	4000	CSF 32
GIMSLEY	GR.SH.	8	F	40	16	10		8o	32	CSF 6
MAJOR	GR.DA.	5	M	32	256	2			4400	CSF 6
CHICO	TERR.	3	M	2	32	32	4		320	CSF 32
BATDORF	GR.SH.	8,5	F	16	32	64			500	CSF 6
MAUI	X LAB.	8	M	2	32	128			500	CSF 6
BUDDY	X SH.	10	M	2	64	2			160	CSF 6
MIDNIGHT	GR.SH.	13	M	2	2	4	4		320	CSF 6
BRUTUS	GR.SH.	9	M	2	64	4			790	CSF 6

186 J. M. ADAMS ET AL.

of old dog encephalitis. A few of the dogs had a history of
convulsions and a diagnosis of epilepsy. Most of the control
dogs had some distemper antibody titer in their serum varying
from low to high, depending on recent immunization. None of
the control dogs had any measurable titer in spinal fluid as
recorded by the two laboratories.

The photomicrographs (fig. 1 to 5) from two dogs illustrate the pathological changes.

TABLE II

DOGS WITH PROBABLE ODE

NAME	BREED	AGE	SEX	MEASLES				DISTEMPER		
				HI	HIL	NC-CF	CD-CF	CD-SN		
JOE	POINTER	7	M					1600	CSF	160
MELISSA	LABR.	9	F					13.000	CSF	10
REX	GR.SH.	11	M	2	4	4		790	CSF	6
SHAWN	GR.SH.	10	M	2	4	4		160	CSF	6
TORO	GR.SH.	8	M	2	4	8		6	CSF	6
TY	GR.SH.	11	M	2	4	4		31	CSF	6
CLEO	GR.SH.	6	M	4	4	5	20	160	CSF	6
ZANKY	GR.SH.	9	M	4	4	5	10	100	CSF	6

DISCUSSION

The earliest serologic study revealed high titers against
distemper virus by the fluorescent antibody (FA) technique, titers of 1:512 to 1:2048 were found. A technique for obtaining
cerebrospinal fluid (CSF) was learned and found to be acceptable
to owners.

Measles antibodies were reported in CSF in Sasha whose recovery without therapy was uneventful. Sasha is alive and well to-
day, having had what appears to be a complete remission. No
good method of control is apparent at this time, apart from critical evaluation of the disease and further research into possible effective approaches to diagnosis and treatment. The best
treatment may be widespread prevention by reliable methods of immunization against canine distemper. Drugs that directly stimulate cell-mediated immunity are being investigated for their
use in increasing host resistance to viral infections. Levami-

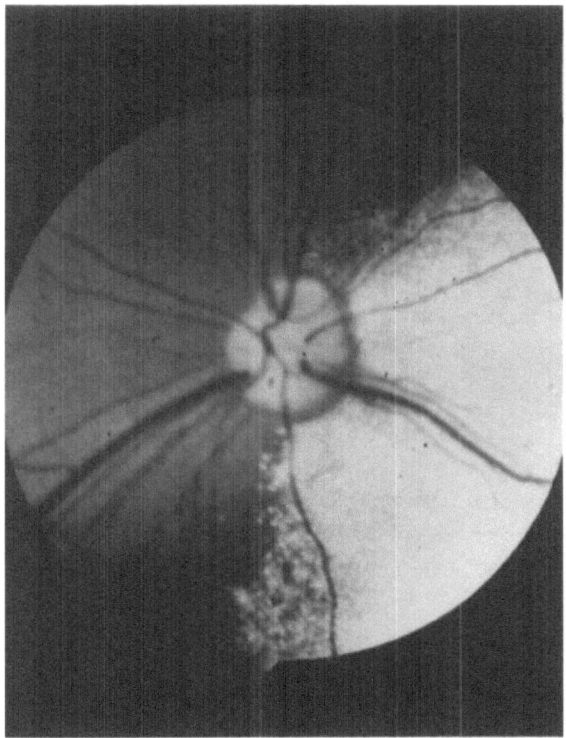

Figure 1: picture of fundus of eye, dog Joe, showing palor of
           disc.

sole is one of these drugs under study in our laboratory.

     The conventional antibody techniques employed in this pa-
per as compared with the highly sensitive radioimmunoassay (RIA)
method have merit for detecting elevated levels of antibody in
specimens such as cerebrospinal fluid (CSF). Elevated levels
of 'IgG', for example, higher than normal, indicate the production of antibody in the nervous system; pointing to the presence of antigen or virus, consequently implicating the cause of
abnormal pathological findings such as areas of demyelination,
referred to as plaques.

     Antibodies may enter the spinal fluid by passive diffusion
(17), especially when high in the serum of the host; and consequently may account for their presence in CSF detected in minute
amounts by the exquisite sensitivity of the RIA method (18).

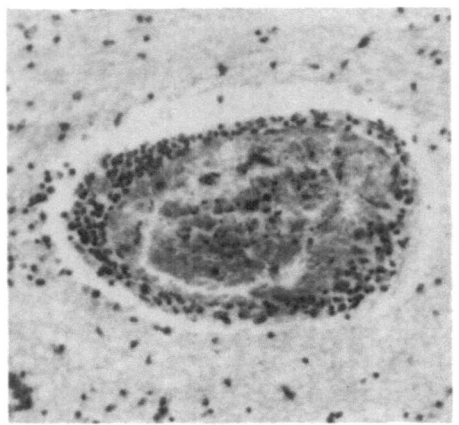 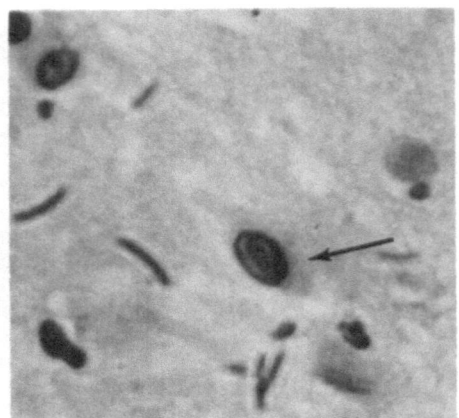

Fig. 2   Fig. 3

Figure 2 : photomicrograph showing perivascular lymphoplasmocytic infiltration in demyelinated plaque in brain of dog Joe.

Figure 3 : Intranuclear inclusion body (arrow) from dog brain of
animal shown in Fig. 1 x 500.

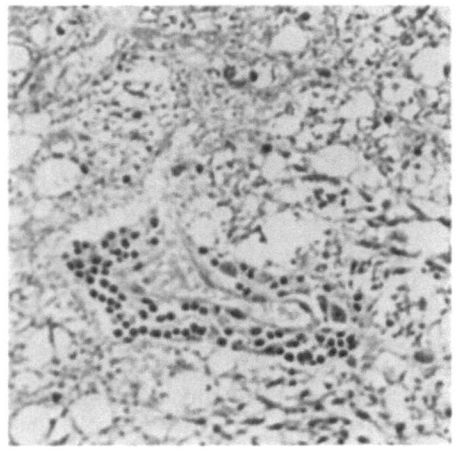 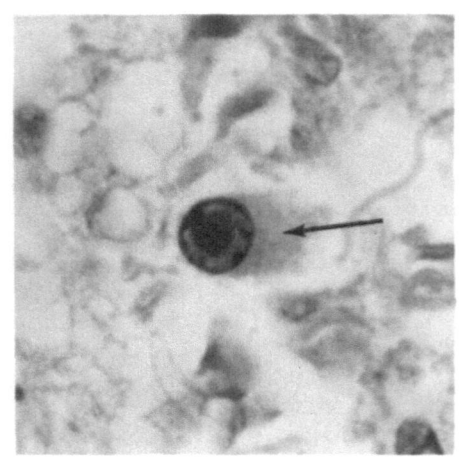

Fig. 4   Fig. 5

Figure 4 : perivascular reaction from brain of dog Chico.

Figure 5 : intranuclear inclusion body from brain of dog Chico
in oligodendroglial cell. x 500.

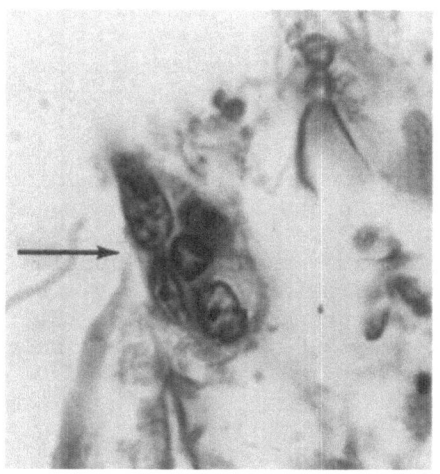

Fig. 6

Figure 6 : multinucleated giant cell from brain of dog Chico
x 500.

TABLE III

SUMMARY OF CLINICAL AND LABORATORY DATA

36 dogs, ages 3 - 13 years, males 20 females 16
ANTIBODY TESTS, KAROLINSKA INSTITUTET

    MEASLES HI : 16 - 40 (4 dogs)

    MEASLES HLI : 4 - 256 (12 dogs)

    MEASLES NUC CAPSID C.F. : 4 - 128 (14 dogs)

    MEASLES NUC CAPSID C.S.F. : 4 (3 dogs)

    DISTEMPER - CF : 10 - 80 (5 dogs)

ANTIBODY TESTS, JAMES A. BAKER INSTITUTE, CORNELL

    CANINE DISTEMPER - SN SERA 32 - 13,000 (17 dogs)

    CANINE DISTEMPER - SN C.S.F. 10 - 160 (4 dogs)

TITERS IN C.S.F. MEASLES 3 DOGS, DISTEMPER 4 DOGS

    CONTROLS : 18 DOGS, AGES 2 - 10, MALES 8, FEMALES 10

Such small amounts do not disturb or upset the normal serum/spinal ratio. The conventional methods employed in this report are reliable indicators of abnormal findings.

Success on antiviral or chemotherapy depends in knowledge of the specific cause of an infection, understanding pathogenesis and virus replication.

Clinical, pathological and serological findings on dogs with probable old dog encephalitis (ODE) are recorded. ODE is a severe demyelinating disease of dogs. Canine distemper virus (CDV) shares antigenic components with measles virus (MV). Immunohistologic findings implicate CDV, providing an animal model for further study of neuromyelitis optica (NO), subacute sclerosing panencephalitis (SSPE) and multiple sclerosis (MS) in man.

REFERENCES

1. Innes, J.R.M. : The relation of distemper infection to the aetiology of canine encephalopathies. Assoc. for Research and Mental Dis. Research Publ. Williams & Wilkins Co., Baltimore, 1950.
2. Perdrau, J.R., and Pugh, L.P. : The pathology of disseminated encephalomyelitis of the dog ("The nervous form of distemper"). J. Path. Bact. 33 : 79, 1930.
3. Scherer, H.J. and Collet, L. : Contribution à la neuropathologie du chien avec remarques sur la pathologie de la maladie de Carré. J. Belge. Neurol. 39 : 132, 1939.
4. Scherer, H.J. : "Vergleichende Pathologie des Nervensystems des Saugtiere". Thieme. Leipzig., 1944.
5. Cordy, D.R.: Canine encephalitis. Cornell Vet. 32: 11, 1942.
6. Lincoln, S.D., Gorham, J.R., Ott, R.T., and Hegreberg, G.A. : Etiologic studies of old dog encephalitis. Vet. Pathol. 8 : 1, 1971.
7. Lincoln, S.D., Gorham, J.R., Davis, W.C., and Ott, R.T. : Studies of old dog encephalitis. II. Electron microscopic and immunohistologic findings. Vet. Pathol. 10 : 124, 1973.
8. Cutler, R.W.P., and Averill, D.R., Jr. : Cerebrospinal fluid gamma globulins in canine distemper encephalitis. An immunoelectrophoretic study. Neurology. 19 : 1111, 1969.
9. Melnick, J.L. : The classification of viruses. Human Diseases caused by Viruses. Oxford University Press, New York, 1978.
10. Adams, J.M. : Comparative study of canine distemper and a respiratory disease of man. Pediatr. 11 : 15, 1953.
11. Imagawa, D.T., Goret, P. and Adams, J.M. : Immunological re-

lationships of measles, distemper and rinderpest viruses.
Proc. Natl. Acad. Sci., USA. 46 : 1119,1960.

12. Appel, M. and Robson, D.S. : A microneutralization test for
    canine distemper virus. Am. J. Vet. Res., 34 : 1459,
    1973.

13. Orvell, C., and Norrby, E. : Further studies on the immunolo-
    gic relationship among measles, distemper and rinderpest vi-
    ruses. J. Immunol. 113 : 1850, 1974.

14. Sullivan, C.B., and Haile, R.W. : Multiple sclerosis, canine
    distemper, and measles immunisation. Lancet, i, 1204,
    1978.

15. Adams, J.M. : A possible animal model for severe demyelinating
    diseases of man. N. Engl. J. Med. 290 : 973, 1974.

16. Adams, J.M., et al. : Old dog encephalitis and demyelinating
    diseases in man. Vet Pathol. 12 : 220, 1975.

17. Gutstein, H.S., and Cohen, S.R. : Spinal fluid differences in
    experimental encephalomyelitis and multiple sclerosis.
    Science 199 : 301, 1978.

18. Forghani, B., Cremer, N.E., Johnson, K.P., Ginsberg, A.H.,
    and Likosky, W.H. : Viral antibodies in cerebrospinal fluid
    of multiple sclerosis and control patients : Comparison be-
    tween radioimmunoassay and conventional techniques. J.
    Clin. Microbiol., 7 : 63, 1978.

EXPERIMENTAL MURINE AUTOIMMUNE ENCEPHALOMYELITIS

D.S. Linthicum, I.R. Mackay and P.R. Carnegie

The Clinical Research Unit of The Walter and Eliza
Hall Institute of Medical Research, Royal Melbourne
Hospital and the Russel Grimwade School of Biochemis-
try, University of Melbourne, Australia.

INTRODUCTION

Experimental autoimmune (allergic) encephalomyelitis is
an inflammatory and demyelinating disease of the central nervous
system (CNS) mediated by the cellular component of the immune
response. EAE is induced in laboratory animals when CNS tissue
homogenates or myelin are injected together with oil adjuvants
containing mycobacteria (Freund's complete adjuvant). The sole
encephalitogenic moiety of myelin has been identified as myelin
basic protein (MBP) (1), and peptides of MBP (2) or even syn-
thetically prepared peptides of MBP (3, 4) can induce EAE. EAE
can be transferred with sensitized lymphoid cells, and requires
T lymphocytes (thymus derived) for the induction, (5, 6) and
effector (7) phases of the disease. Transfer of EAE by immune
serum containing anti-MBP antibody has not been successful (8),
and the level of serum antibody to MBP does not correlate with
the intensity or time of onset of disease (9). The autoimmune
response to MBP exemplifies cell-mediated immune damage in that
the delayed-type hypersensitivity (DTH) response to MBP can be
correlated with the severity and time of onset of EAE.

At present, methods for detecting and measuring DTH and
DTH-like inflammatory responses in mice have been greatly improved by the radioisotopic labelling technique known as the
"ear assay" (10), as follows. Since the mononuclear cells responsible for DTH inflammatory reactions are derived from a rapidly dividing progenitor pool (11), they can be labelled with
radio-active analogues of precursors of DNA. Radiometric assay

of an antigen depot site, as in a cutaneous DTH test, or an
organ site of DTH inflammation, can provide a measurable index
of the response. Moreover autoradiographic analysis of tissues
affected by DTH reactions has revealed that the infiltrating
radiolabelled mononuclear cells are hematogenous in origin,
and proliferate actively at the inflammation site (12). We
have exploited the radiometric technique to assess the onset
and severity of the cell-mediated inflammation in EAE by direct
isotope counting of brains and spinal cords from mice immunized
for induction of EAE, and have used the radiometric "ear assay"
for serial detection and quantitation of the DTH response to
MBP during the 14 day induction period.

MATERIALS AND METHODS

Immunization for EAE

(SJL/J x Balb/c)F_1 hybrid female mice were immunized with
mouse spinal cord homogenate (MSCH), 10 mg dry weight, suspended in saline and emulsified in an equal volume of Freund's complete adjuvant (FCA) supplemented with 5 mg/ml M. tuberculosis
(Difco, H37RA). All four foot pads were injected, the total
inoculum volume being 0.1 ml. Immediately thereafter and 48 hrs
later Bordetella pertussis vaccine, 15×10^9 organisms, was
given iv. This immunization procedure produces 95-100 % incidence of EAE. Immunization with 200 µg of purified mouse MBP
and 200 µg of keyhole limpet haemocyanin (KLH), as a control
antigen, was performed in an identical manner.

Radioisotopic Ear Assay for DTH

On various days after immunization for EAE, groups of mice
were injected i.p. with 0.1 ml of 10^{-3} M FUdR in saline and 20-30
min later, 1 µCi (0.1 ml) of ^{125}I-UdR (specific activity 5 µCi/
mg, Radiochemical Center Amersham) was injected i.p. Immediately
thereafter, the pinna of the left ear was injected intradermally
with 10 µg purified mouse MBP in 10 µl saline, the right ear
being uninjected. The next day the mice were killed, the ears
were excised at the hairline, the uptake of ^{125}I-UdR was measured by gammaspectrometry, and the results were expressed as
the left/right cpm ratio. Typical counts obtained were 530
and 476 cpm, giving a L/R ratio of 1.1 for a normal test. Cytochrome C (lo µg) was used as a control antigen for the ear assay
to determine the specificity of the DTH reaction.

Radioisotopic whole Organ Assay for Inflammation

At various times after immunization for EAE with MSCH, or immunization with MBP or KLH, groups of six mice were given FUdR and ^{125}I-UdR as described for the ear assay. 18-24 hr later, mice were anaesthetized with ether and killed by exsanguination. Brain, spinal cord, spleen and popliteal lymph node were removed and placed in separate plastic tubes containing 10 % neutral buffered formalin for gamma-counting. In addition, 25 μl of whole blood drawn into a calibrated disposable pipette was placed in a plastic tube for gammacounting. The "whole organ" assay results are expressed as a ratio of ^{125}I-radioactivity (cpm) in the tissue to that of 25 μl of whole blood. Typical counts obtained from normal brain and blood were 122 and 101, giving a brain-blood index of 1.2.

RESULTS

The radiometric ear assay was used to measure the DTH response to MBP after immunization for EAE with MSCH. The requirement for adjuvants (FCA and pertussis) and the specificity of the DTH reaction elicited were examined. Mice were tested 7 days after injection of MSCH with adjuvants, or adjuvants alone. Naive mice receiving neither antigen nor adjuvant gave a mean L/R ear assay of 1.06 and 1.09 to MBP and cytochrome C, respectively, and mice injected only with adjuvants gave comparable indices, 1.35 and 1.27. Mice immunized with MSCH in FCA with or without pertussis vaccine gave significantly higher indices of 1.93 and 1.81 (p < 0.05) when tested with MBP. Cytochrome C was used as a control antigen and a normal response elicited in all cases indicated that the DTH response was specific for MBP.

The time kinetics of the onset and magnitude of the DTH response to MBP is presented in Fig. 1. Some groups of mice given cyclophosphamide, 200 mg/kg, 2 days before the initial immunization for EAE with MSCH gave positive DTH reactions by day 5, whereas those not receiving cyclophosphamide did not develop DTH reactions until day 7, and the L/R ratios obtained from mice pre-treated with cyclophosphamide were consistently higher (Fig. 1). On day 12-14 post-immunization, surviving mice developed signs and characteristic histological lesions of EAE.

Mice were immunized with either MSCH, MBP or KLH for the radioisotopic assessment of immune mediated inflammation in the brain and spinal cord during the induction of EAE.

^{125}I-radiometry of the brain and spinal cords from variously immunized mice is presented in Figures 2 and 3. Throughout

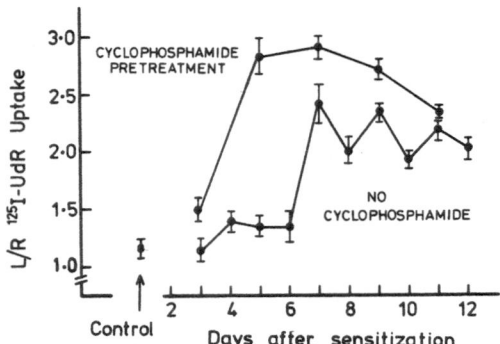

Figure 1 : Kinetics of the DTH response to MBP as measured by
the radiometric ear assay. Mice were immunized with an encephalitogenic dose of MSCH in FCA. Antigen challenge (MBP) for DTH
was given in the left ear pinna and ^{125}I-UdR is given immediately thereafter. Ears were excised 24 hr later and the mean
left : right (L/R) cpm ratio ± SEM is shown. Mice receiving pretreatment of cyclophosphamide (200 mg/kg) 2 days before immunization with MSCH showed a DTH response as early as 5 days post-
sensitization, whereas other mice gave a DTH response on day 7.
The control value is obtained from non-immunized mice.

the entire course of the experiment the radiometric brain-blood
and spinal cord-blood indices of mice immunized with KLH remained stable, the mean brain indices ranging from 0.9 - 1.2, and
the mean spinal cord indices ranging from 0.9 - 1.1. Mice immunized with MBP showed little or no significant changes in
the radiometric indices except that on day 8 there was a significant increase in the brain-blood index (p<0.001). In sharp
contrast, the brain-blood and spinal cord-blood indices from
mice immunized with MSCH increased to significant levels on day
8 and 10, respectively.

DISCUSSION

The inflammation of the CNS tissues in EAE is a classical
manifestation of DTH and cell-mediated immunity, and cell-mediated immune reactions to nervous tissue antigens might determine
immunopathic diseases of the CNS in man, claimed examples being
multiple sclerosis (14) and possibly Huntington's chorea (15).

We have exploited the radioisotopic assay to measure both
DTH responses to intradermal inoculation of MBP and cell-media-

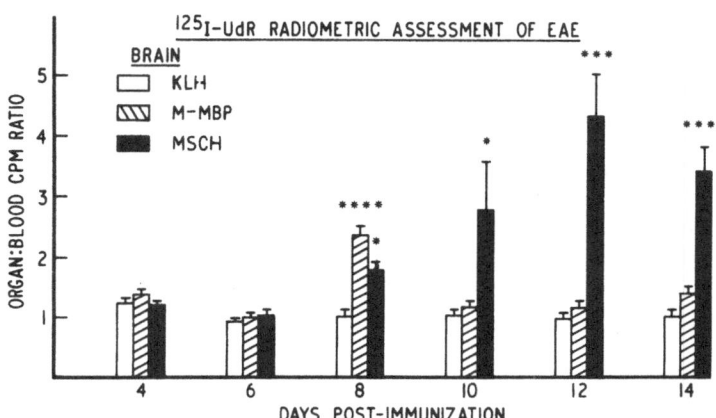

Figure 2 : ^{125}I-UdR uptake in brains from mice immunized with KLH (200 ug) MBP (200 µg) or MSCH (10 mg). ^{125}I-UdR was given 24 hr before excising tissues for radiometry. Results are expressed as mean brain:blood cpm ratios ± SEM. Four to five-fold increases in brain:blood indices were observed in mice immunized with MSCH. Signs of EAE appeared at day 11-12. * Significant difference from the control (KLH), $p < 0.05$; *** $p < 0.01$; **** $p < 0.001$ (n = 6).

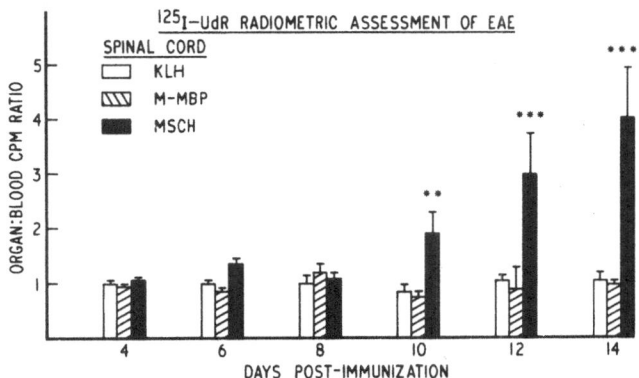

Figure 3 : ^{125}I-UdR uptake in spinal cords from mice immunized with KLH, MBP or MSCH (doses as in Fig. 2). Results are expressed as organ:blood cpm ratios ± SEM. Significant increases in the spinal cord-blood ratios were observed from day 10-14 in mice receiving MSCH. Signs of EAE appeared on day 11. ** Significant difference from control (KLH) $p < 0.02$; *** $p < 0.01$; **** $p < 0.001$ (n = 6).

ted inflammatory reactions in the CNS during the onset of EAE
in mice. Cells participating in DTH reactions to MBP could be
detected in the peripheral circulation as early as 5-7 days after
initial immunization with MSCH. Notably, the adjuvant effect
of B. pertussis was not required for DTH, but was necessary for
EAE, suggesting it may play a role in altering the blood-brain
barrier. Pretreatment with cyclophosphamide, before immunization
with MSCH, advanced the onset (day 5) and increased the magnitude
(L/R ratios above 2.5) of the DTH responses to MBP. Cyclophosphamide has been reported to eliminate B cells, referred to by some
authors (16) as "suppressor" B cells with respect to DTH responses, since specific antibody produced by B cells can depress DTH
responses. In addition to B cell elimination, cyclophosphamide
may diminish those suppressor T cells that may act to regulate
other T cell functions such as cytotoxicity and DTH reactivity.
Suppressor T cells have been reported to be sensitive to cortisone, cyclophosphamide and x-irradiation (17).

     Cell-mediated inflammation of the brain was detectable by
radioisotopic assay 3-4 days before onset of signs of EAE. Although high brain ^{125}I-UdR uptake indices were usually in agreement with the degree of histological lesions, several mice on
day 8 had high brain uptake indices but were assessed microsco-
pically as "negative" for histological lesions. Increased 125
I-radioactivity was detected in the spinal cord on or about the
same day that signs of EAE developed.

     Mice immunized with mouse MBP were relatively resistant to
EAE induction, in that only a few animals developed histopathological lesions (day 14) and none developed signs of EAE. Previous work (13) has demonstrated that high doses of MBP are required for induction of EAE in SJL mice, and the hybrid used in
this study (SJL x Balb/c) could be more resistant than the susceptible SJL parental strain.

     We can conclude by emphasizing that various experimentally
induced autoimmune diseases have a cell-mediated component which
is essential to the pathogenesis of the disease, e.g. orchitis,
thyroiditis, adrenalitis, and that inflammatory reactions which
are cell-mediated or DTH like, and are organ-specific could be
readily studied by the radiometric assay to measure the onset
and magnitude of the inflammatory reaction. In these diseases
as in EAE, effector T cells which immigrate from rapidly dividing
precursor pools, as well as non-specific inflammatory cells (monocytes) which are attracted to the site of inflammation by che-
motactic agents, could be radiolabelled with DNA precursor analogues, and the tissue site of inflammation assessed by radiometry. In particular this technique should prove useful in experimental disease models in which the histopathological changes

are not readily discerned, and the signs of the disease are not self-evident.

ACKNOWLEDGEMENTS

This work was supported by grants 887-C-4 and 10022-A-7 from the National Multiple Sclerosis Society (USA) and grants from the National Health and Medical Research Council of Australia. D.S. Linthicum is a post-doctoral Research Fellow of the National Multiple Sclerosis Society (USA).

REFERENCES

1. Kies, M.W., Alvord, E.C. Jr., (eds). In : Allergic Encephalomyelitis, p 293-299 (1959) Thomas Co. Springfield, III.
2. Eylar, E.H., Caccam, J., Jackson, J., Westall, F., Robinson, A.P., Science 168, 1220-1223 (1970).
3. Nagai, Y. et al, Cell. Immunol. 35 : 158-167 (1978).
4. Hashim, G.A., Sharpe, R.D., Immunochemistry 11: 633-640 (1974).
5. Paterson, P.Y., J. Exp. Med. 111 : 119-136 (1960).
6. Gonatas, N.K., Howard, J.C., Science 186 : 839-841 (1974).
7. Ortiz-Ortiz, L., Nakamura, R.M., Weigle, W.O., J. Immunol. 117 : 576-579 (1976).
8. Bernard, C.C.A., Leydon, J., Mackay, I., Eur. J. Immunol. 6 : 655-660 (1976).
9. Bernard, C.C.A., J. Immunogenet. 3: 263-274 (1976).
10. Vadas, M.A., Miller, J.F.A.P., Gamble, J., Whitelaw, A., Int. Archs. Allergy appl. Immunology 49: 670-692 (1975).
11. Volkman, A., Collins, F.M., J. Immunol. 101 : 846-859 (1968).
12. Kosuner, T.U., Waksman, B.H., Samuelsson, I.K., J. Neuropath. exp. Neurol. 22 : 367-380 (1963).
13. Bernard, C.C.A., Carnegie, P.R., J. Immunol. 114 : 1537-1540 (1975).
14. Colby, S.P., Sheremata, W., Bain, B., Eylar, E., Neurology 27, 132-139 (1977).
15. Barkley, D.S., Hardiwidjaja, S., Menkes, J.H., Science 195 : 314-316 (1977).
16. Lagrange, P.H., Mackaness, G.B., Miller, T.E., J.Exp. Med. 139 : 1529-1539 (1974).
17. Nachtigal, D., Zan-Bar, I., Feldman, M., Transplant. Rev. 26 : 87-105 (1975).

ISOELECTRIC FOCUSING AND CROSSED IMMUNOELECTRO-FOCUSING OF CSF

PROTEINS — ESPECIALLY IMMUNOGLOBULINS

A. Sidén

Department of Neurology, Karolinska Hospital, Stockholm,
Sweden

SUMMARY

Thin-layer IEF and CIEF has been found to be of great value
for the separation and qualitative evaluation of CSF proteins.
In 350 patients with MS, infections of the nervous system or
Guillain-Barré syndromes non-immunoglobulin aberrations (including
transferrin, the tau-fraction and gamma-trace protein) were observed in frequencies varying from about 5 to 55 %. Oligoclonal
bands and/or regional increases of immunoglobulins were found in
the following approximate frequencies : respectively 95 and 80 %
in clinically verified and probable MS, 70 % in (meningo)-encepha-
litis, 50 % in (meningo-) myelitis/radiculitis, respectively 15
and 20 % in meningitis and Guillain-Barré syndromes. In MS these
immunoglobulin abnormalities were entirely or almost entirely of
IgG kappa identity.

INTRODUCTION

On IEF the protein molecules are separated and focused on
the basis of their isoelectric points (pI). Such small differences in pI-values of between 0.01 - 0.02 pH-units allow separation
and this high degree of resolution has been made possible by the
development of synthetic ampholytes (17, 20). Evidence has accumulated favouring the performance of IEF in thin layers of polyacrylamide gel (1, 18, 19). Many samples can be run in parallel, which is helpful for comparative purposes, and µg quantities
of proteins can be examined.

    After the potentialities of isoelectric focusing (IEF) for
the separation of cerebrospinal fluid (CSF) proteins had been pointed out by Fossard, Dale and Latner (5), thin-layer IEF techniques
used for such examinations were reported by Delmotte (2, 3) and
Kjellin and Vesterberg (8). The protein fractions found by IEF
can be further studied by different identification methods, crossed immunoelectrofocusing (CIEF) has been developed into a reproducible and relatively simple method (15, 16) and CIEF techniques
have been shown to be promising tools for CSF-protein examinations
(11, 13, 14).

    This report present some data from studies of the CSF protein
with IEF and immunoglobulin (Ig) examination with CIEF in patients
with MS or infections of the nervous system (including Guillain-
Barré syndromes).

                            MATERIAL AND METHODS

    The CSF-protein findings on IEF were studied in 350 consecu-
tive patients with the following diagnoses : clinically verified
or probable multiple sclerosis (MS) according to the diagnostic
criteria of Schumacher and Kurtzke (10), known or probable infections of the nervous system and Guillain-Barré syndromes. Table 3
gives the number of patients for each diagnostic subgroup.

    IEF was performed in thin layers of polyacrylamide gel as
described by Kjellin and Vesterberg (9). The gels had the dimen-
sions 10 x 20 x 0.1 cm, the gel concentrations were T = 6 % and
C = 3 % and the Ampholine (LKB-produkter, Bromma, Sweden) composition was : pH 3.5 - 10.0 (1.4 ml), pH 4 - 6 (0.1 ml), pH 5 - 7
(0.1 ml) and pH 9 - 11 (0.4 ml). The approximate protein contents
of the CSF and serum samples applied to the gel were 200 - 250 µg.
The separation was carried out with a distance of 8 cm between
the electrodes and a maximal voltage and wattage of 1000 V and
40 W. The gels were stained with Coomassie Brilliant Blue R 250
(ICI) (18). The CSF-protein fractions were divided into 10 num-
bered regions (Figure 1 a, Table 1) and the abnormal findings in
the gammaglobulin range were classified in mean patterns (Table 1)
indicating ("a - e modified" patterns) or uniform ("f" pattern)
increases of protein.

    The CIEF techniques previously described (11, 13, 14) were
used. The immunoelectrophoretic procedure was either performed
in veronal buffer (pH 8.6) using native antibodies or in acetate
buffer (pH 5.0) using carbamylated antibodies, isoelectric at this
pH. The following monospecific rabbit anti-human antibodies (Da-
kopatts, Copenhagen, Denmark) were used : anti-IgG specific for
γ -chains, anti-IgA specific for α -chains, anti-IgM specific
for μ -chains, anti-kappa light chains and anti-lambda light chains.

The electrophoresis was carried out at 5 V/cm overnight. The immunoprecipitates were stained with Coomassie Brilliant Blue R 250 (ICI).

RESULTS

It was found that 345 of the 350 patients (98.6 per cent) exhibited one or more of the CSF-protein findings listed in Table 2 and exemplified in Figure 1 b and 2. The individual occurrence of these findings is summarized in Table 3.

The four types of non-immunoglobulin fractions occurred in frequencies varying from about 5 to 55 per cent. A highly alkaline fraction was found in about half of the patients, while a single fraction in region "7" as well as a double fraction in region "5" and prominent fraction(s) in region "4" were observed in up to one fourth of the subjects.

The gammaglobulin range exhibited an abnormal mean pattern in 90 to 100 per cent of the patients. Patterns with regional increases of gammaglobulins were predominant in MS and (meningo-) encephalitis and occurred in about half of the subjects with (meningo-)myelitis/radiculitis, while an "f" pattern was found in the majority of patients with meningitis or Guillain-Barré syndromes. Oligoclonal Ig bands were exhibited by about 40 to nearly 90 per cent of patients with (meningo-)myelitis/radiculitis, (meningo-)encephalitis and MS; such changes were found in 10 per cent of subjects with meningitis or Guillain-Barré syndromes. These Ig bands were of slight to very marked intensity and had the following positions : region "8", region "9(-10)", region "8 - 9(10)" or region "7 - 9(10)". The band spectra were most frequently situated in region "8-9" or "9".

At present about 60 CSF samples from MS patients have been examined with CIEF (Sidén, to be published); examples of the findings on such examinations are shown in Figure 3. IgG was the only of the three main Ig classes that was detected in region "7 - 10". The immunoprecipitates of IgG in all cases had profiles differing from those of normal CSF or serum and exhibited peaks corresponding to the abnormalities (regional increases of proteins and spectra of oligoclonal bands) found on IEF. Examinations of the light-chain determinants indicated that the abnormal IgG fractions were entirely or almost entirely of IgG kappa identity. The maximal anodal extension observed from IgG was to region "4". IgA was detected in region "2 - 6", however, the main components of the immunoprecipitates had positions corresponding to region "2 - 4". CIEF examinations with anti-IgM have so far been negative.

DISCUSSION

Thin-layer IEF, due to its excellent separation capacity,
has been found to be of great value for CSF-protein examinations;
one important advantage of the method being its very high ability
to detect oligoclonal Ig fractions. Delmotte and Gonsette (4),
in a study in 262 MS patients reported that oligoclonal fractions
in the gammaglobulin range were detected in 91 per cent of the
patients with thin-layer IEF, while the corresponding figure for
agar-gel electrophoresis was 65 per cent.

In our laboratory, a thin-layer IEF technique has been used
for several years and over 3000 CSF- and serum-protein examinations in about 2500 patients have been performed. Data from these examinations have emphasized the great value of the method for
the analysis of normal and abnormal proteins. Descriptive studies
in demyelinating and infectious neurological disorders have shown
different types of CSF-protein aberrations (6, Sidén and Kjellin,
to be published). These changes can be grouped into two main categories. Findings also observed in other neurological disorders
are the following : prominent fraction(s) in the cathodal part
of region "4" (including transferrin), double tau-fractions in
region "5", a single fraction in region "7" (at present unidentified), a highly alkaline fraction in region "10" (including gamma-
trace protein) and an "f" pattern. The "f" pattern generally indicates damage to the blood-CSF barrier, although in some cases
it might refer to a polyclonal intrathecal Ig synthesis. The
second, and from a diagnostic point of view more significant group
of aberrations, are spectra of oligoclonal Ig bands and mean patterns with regional increases of gammaglobulins - the latter being
caused by clusters of more homogeneous Ig fractions within a wider
pI-range. These abnormalities are compatible with intrathecal
Ig synthesis and with few exceptions are found only in demyelinating and infectious/inflammatory neurological diseases. In spite
of the very high sensitivity of this technique according to our
experience there is no significant risk of "false positive" results. A sample from the same patient is always examined in parallel in order to eliminate the risk, that bands reflecting serum abnormalities caused by e.g. a plasma cell dyscrasia (12)
are misinterpreted. CIEF techniques, making use of the excellent
separation capacity of IEF and the specificity of immunoelectrophoresis, have been shown to be very valuable for qualitative evaluation of CSF proteins and identification of CSF-protein abnormalities. The major aberrant Ig fractions found on IEF, in MS,
evidently are of IgG kappa identity.

CSF-protein examinations are of great importance in routine
as well as research work in neurology. High-separation techniques such as IEF and CIEF are obviously very valuable for studies
of the CSF proteins in different neurological disorders.

TABLE 1

The pH-intervals corresponding to regions "1 - 10" (7) and the mean patterns of the CSF gammaglobulin range. Sample application = s.a.

Region	pH-interval	Pattern	Relative increase of proteins in regions "7 - 10"
1	2.5 - 4.6	a	8 - 10, especially 9 - 10
2	4.6 - 5.0	b	8 - 10, rather uniformly
3	5.0 - 5.4	c	7 - 10, especially 8 - 10
4	5.4 - 5.8	d	8 - 9, rather uniformly
5	5.8 - 6.0	e	7 - 9, especially 9
6	6.0 - 6.2	e modified	7 - 9, especially 8 - 9
s.a.	6.2 - 6.4	f	7 - 9, rather uniformly and usually very similar to a "fingerprint" of the corresponding serum γ-globulin range
7	6.4 - 7.4		
8	7.4 - 8.2		
9	8.2 - 8.9		
10	8.9 - 11.0		

TABLE 2

CSF-protein findings on IEF

Number	CSF-protein findings
1	Prominent fraction(s) in the cathodal part of region "4"
2	Double fraction in region "5"
3	Single fraction in the middle of region "7"
4	Highly alkaline fraction (HAF)
5 a	Regional increases of γ-globulins ("a - e modified" patterns)
5 b	Uniform increases of γ-globulins ("f" pattern)
6	Oligoclonal Ig bands

TABLE 3

Occurrence (per cent) of the CSF-protein findings listed in Table 2.

Diagnosis, number of cases in brackets		CSF-protein findings (numbered as in Table 2)						
		1	2	3	4	5 a	5b	6
Clinically verified MS	(125)	4	20	13	40	95	3	88
Probable MS	(105)	12	23	13	56	80	10	63
(Meningo-)encephalitis	(51)	25	22	14	41	69	29	65
(Meningo-)myelitis/radiculitis	(21)	14	24	5	43	48	43	43
Meningitis	(21)	19	10	24	43	14	86	10
Guillain-Barré syndromes	(27)	7	15	4	48	19	81	11

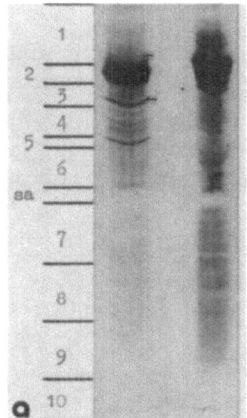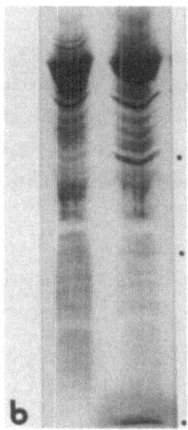

Figure 1 a : normal CSF; serum sample from the same patient to the right. The anode was at the top. The division of the CSF-protein fractions is given to the left (sa = sample application).

Figure 1 b : CSF sample exhibiting a double fraction in region "5", a single fraction in region "7" and a HAF. These fractions are indicated by dots. Serum sample from the same patient to the left.

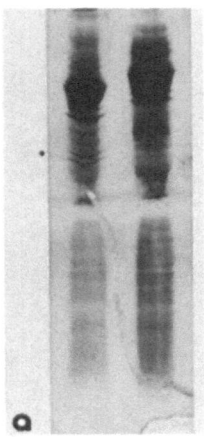 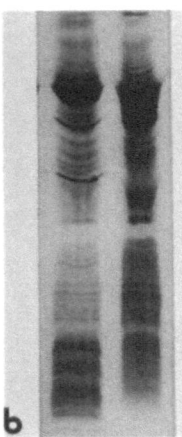

Figure 2 a : CSF sample exhibiting an "f" pattern and a prominent fraction in region "4" (indicated by a dot). Serum sample from the same patient to the right.

Figure 2 b : CSF sample exhibiting a regional increase of gamma-globulins and oligoclonal bands. Serum sample from the same patient to the right.

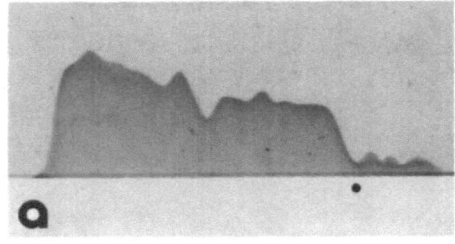 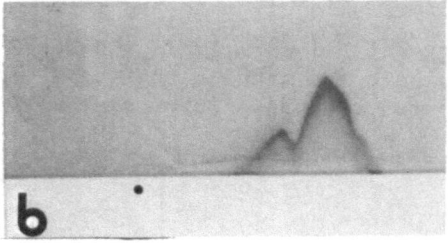

Figure 3 a : CIEF performed at pH 5.0 with carbamylated anti-IgG. The cathodal end of the polyacrylamide gel strip was to the left and the sample application was at the dot.

Figure 3 b : CIEF performed at pH 8.6 with native anti-IgA. The anodal end of the polyacrylamide gel strip was to the right and the sample application was at the dot.

REFERENCES

1. Davies, H. (1975).Thin-layer gel isoelectric focusing. In :
   Arbuthnott, J.P. and J.A. Beeley (eds.), Isoelectric Focusing,
   Butterworths, London, 1975, pp. 97-113.
2. Delmotte, P. (1971). Gel isoelectric focusing of cerebrospinal
   fluid proteins : a potential diagnostic tool, Z. klin. Chem. u.
   klin. Biochem., 9 : 334 - 336.
3. Delmotte, P. (1972) .Comparative results of agar gel electrophoresis and isoelectric focusing examination of the gammaglobulins of the cerebrospinal fluid, Acta neurol. belg. 72 :
   226-234.
4. Delmotte, P. and R. Gonsette (1977). Biochemical findings in
   multiple sclerosis, Part 4 (Isoelectric focusing of the CSF
   gammaglobulins in multiple sclerosis (262 cases) and other
   neurological diseases (272 cases)), J. Neurol., 215 : 27-37.
5. Fossard, C., G. Dale and A. Latner (1970).Separation of proteins
   of cerebrospinal fluid using gel electrofocusing followed by
   electrophoresis, J. clin. Path. 23 : 586-589.
6. Kjellin, K.G. and A. Sidén (1978).Isoelectric focusing and
   isotachophoresis for investigation of CSF and serum proteins
   in demyelinating and infectious neurological diseases. In :
   J. Palo (ed.), Myelination and Demyelination, Plenum Press,
   New York and London, 1978, pp. 545-559.
7. Kjellin, K.G. and H. Stibler (1976).Isoelectric focusing and
   electrophoresis of cerebrospinal fluid proteins in muscular
   dystrophies and spinal muscular atrophies, J. neurol. Sci.,
   27 : 45-57.
8. Kjellin, K.G. O. Vesterberg (1972). Thin-layer isoelectric focusing of cerebrospinal fluid proteins - A preliminary report
   with special reference to the diagnostic significance in multiple sclerosis. In : Proceedings of the 20th Congress of
   Scandinavian Neurologists, Universitetsforlaget, Oslo, 1972,
   pp. 379-380.
9. Kjellin, K.G. and O. Vesterberg (1974). Isoelectric focusing
   of CSF-proteins in neurological diseases, J. neurol. Sci.,
   23 : 199-213.
10. Kurtzke, J.F. (1970). Diagnosis and differential diagnosis of
    multiple sclerosis, Acta neurol. scand., 46 : 484-492.
11. Sidén, A. (1977) .Crossed immunoelectrofocusing of cerebrospi-
    nal fluid immunoglobulins, J. Neurol., 217 : 103-109.
12. Sidén, A. and K.G. Kjellin (1977). Isoelectric focusing of CSF
    and serum proteins in neurological disorders combined with
    benign and malignant proliferations of reticulocytes, lympho-
    cytes and plasmocytes, J. Neurol., 216, 251-264.
13. Stibler, H. (1977) .Crossed immunoelectrofocusing for the
    identification of normal and abnormal cerebrospinal fluid pro-
    teins, J. neurol. Sci., 32 : 331-336.

14. Stibler, H. (1978). The normal cerebrospinal fluid proteins
    identified by means of thin-layer isoelectric focusing and cros-
    sed immunoelectrofocusing, J. neurol. Sci, 36 : 273-288.
15. Söderholm, J. and C.J. Smyth (1975). Crossed immunoelectrofo-
    cusing for studies on protein microheterogeneity. In : P.G.
    Righetti (ed.), Progress in Isoelectric Focusing and Isotacho-
    phoresis, North-Holland Publishing Company, Amsterdam, 1975,
    pp. 99-114.
16. Söderholm, J., C.J. Smyth and T. Wadström (1975). A simple
    and reproducible method for crossed immunoelectrofocusing,
    Scand. J. Immunol., 4 (suppl. no. 2): 107-113.
17. Vesterberg, O. (1969). Synthesis and isoelectric focusing
    of carrier ampholytes, Acta Chem. Scand., 23 : 2653-2666.
18. Vesterberg, O. (1972).Isoelectric focusing of proteins in po-
    lyacrylamide gels, Biochim. Biophys. Acta, 257 : 11-19.
19. Vesterberg, O. (1975). Some aspects of isoelectric focusing
    in polyacrylamide gel. In : Arbuthnott, J.P. and J.A. Beeley
    (eds.), Isoelectric Focusing, Butterworths, London, 1975, pp.
    78-96.
20. Vesterberg, O. and H. Svensson (1966).Isoelectric fractiona-
    tion, analysis and characterization of ampholytes in natural
    pH gradients, Part 4 (Further studies of the resolving power
    in connection with separation of myoglobins), Acta chem. Scand.,
    20 : 820-834.

ACKNOWLEDGEMENT

    Supported by grants from the Swedish Multiple Sclerosis So-
ciety. The invaluable support from ass. prof. K.G. Kjellin as
well as the skilful technical assistance of Mrs. Ann-Marie Olsson
and Mrs. Vera Snikvalds is gratefully acknowledged.

STUDY OF OLIGOCLONAL C.S.F. BY NEW IMMUNOFIXATION TECHNIQUES

FOLLOWING ELECTROPHORESIS ON CELLULOSE ACETATE GEL

J.M. Perini, J. Lebas, P. Roussel and G. Biserte

Département de Biochimie des UER Médicales, Lille,
France

Oligoclonal bands are usually revealed by electrophoresis on
agar gel (1) or on cellulose acetate strip (2). We have used a
particular cellogel, the Cellogel RS (Sebia Lab.) to explore the
CSF of patients with multiple sclerosis (MS) (3). The oligoclonal
patterns show several fine and close bands in the cathodic part of
the electropherogram. We report here an electroimmunofixation
technique to study the antigenic determinants of the gammaglobulinic
bands. We describe briefly the method and more details will be
published further.

METHODS

1) Standard electrophoresis is performed on a Cellogel RS
strip n° 1 using concentrated CSF, and stained by Amidoschwarz.

2) Direct immunofixation procedure : a Cellogel RS strip
(n° 2) is used for immunofixation of the oligoclonal gammaglobulins heavy chains determinants. Another strip (n°3) for immunofixation of the light chains determinants. Upon the completion
of electrophoresis, the cathodic part of the strip n° 2 is cut
off and immediately transferred into a thin plastic cell containing the solution of rabbit antiserum against human gamma chains.
The cell fits the shape of the "wedge" strip. The strip n° 3 is
cut along the length in two equal parts. Each cathodic half is
transferred into a half-cell containing a solution of rabbit antiserum against human κ(or λ) light chains. After incubation, the
strips are washed and finally stained with Amidoschwarz.

3) Indirect immunofixation procedure : unconcentrated CSF

may be used in this second technique fivefold more sensible than the first one. At the completion of electrophoresis, the cathodic part of the strip n° 2 is transferred for a first immunofixation into a cell containing a solution of rabbit anti-human gamma chains serum. In the same way, each cathodic half of strip n° 2 is transferred into a half-cell containing a solution of rabbit anti- κ (or λ) serum. After incubation and wash, the strips are transferred for a second immunofixation into their respective cell containing a solution of pig anti-rabbit (H + L) IgG peroxidase conjugated serum. A second wash is performed. The peroxidase activity of the pig antibodies let reveal the oligoclonal bands after staining by diaminobenzidine and hydrogen peroxide.

RESULTS

The findings obtained comparing the standard electrophoresis patterns and the direct or indirect immunofixation procedures in 10 C.S.F. are summarized in table 1.

The following conclusions can be drawn :
1) It is possible to distinguish discrete oligoclonal bands not visible on standard electropherogram (CSF 6).
2) We observe that oligoclonal bands do not migrate only in the broad γ_4 zone, but may have also the same mobility as the β trace proteins ($\gamma_1 \gamma_2 \gamma_3$) (CSF 1, 3 or 7) or as the slow gamma-globulins (CSF 1, 3, 6, 7 and 8).
3) Some oligoclonal bands possess the two antigenic determinants of light chains : κ and λ . They are heterogeneous and not monoclonal (CSF 1, 2, 3 and 8). Other bands are homogeneous. We have found 17 homogeneous bands of λ type and 13 homogeneous bands of κ type. In CSF 5, 6, 7 all oligoclonal bands appear homogeneous. In CSF 1, 2, 3 and 8 homogeneous and heterogeneous bands are mixed. Generally, the heterogeneous bands migrate in the cathodic part of γ_4 (CSF 1, 2, 3, 8 and 10).
4) Incomplete immunoglobulins may occur in some CSF : the two oligoclonal bands in CSF 5 are revealed by immunofixation with an antiserum against light chains and not with an anti-neavy chain serum. CSF 5 may possess free light chains. On the other hand, the occurrence of free heavy chains may be suspected in CSF 4 because of a band revealed by an anti-heavy chain serum and not by an anti-light chain serum. CSF 3 and 9 possess both free light chains and free heavy chains.

The λ type free light chains in CSF 3 have a more anodic electrophoretic mobility than those of the κ type free light chains in CSF 5 and 9.

	slow γ	broad γ$_4$	γ$_3$	γ$_2$	γ$_1$	Anode →
	1	2	1	1		St *
CSF 1	1(γ)	1(γ,λ) 1(γ,κ,λ)	1(γ,λ)	1(γ,λ)		** D.Im.F.
		3	1			St
CSF 2		2(γ,λ) 1(γ,κ,λ)	1(γ,κ,λ)			D.Im.F.
	1	2	1			St
CSF 3	1(γ,λ)	1(γ) 1(γ,λ) 1(γ,κ,λ)	1(γ,λ)	1(λ)	1(λ)	D.Im.F.
		4	1	1	1	St
CSF 4		2(γ,κ) 2(γ,λ)	1(γ)			D.Im.F.
		2				St
CSF 5		2(κ)				D.Im.F.
		2				St
CSF 6	1(γ,κ)	4(γ,λ)				I.Im.F. ***
		3				St
CSF 7	1(γ,λ)	1(γ,λ) 2(γ,κ)	1(γ,κ)			I.Im.F.
		2				St
CSF 8	1(γ,κ)	1(γ,κ) 1(γ,κ,λ)				I.Im.F.
		4	1	1		St
CSF 9		1(γ,κ) 1(γ,λ) 2(γ)	1(κ)			I.Im.F.
		3	1	1	1	St
CSF 10		1(γ,κ,λ) 1(γ,κ)				I.Im.F.

* St : Standard electrophoresis of concentrated CSF stained by Amidoschwarz

** D.Im.F. Direct immunofixation procedure

*** I.Im.F. Indirect immunofixation procedure

DISCUSSION

Our results are in relative good agreement with the literature. Vandvik (4, 5) has already reported the homogeneous or
heterogeneous character of the gammaglobulins bands. This author
(5) has also published that the homogeneous oligoclonal bands are
the most often κ type. We have found them to be generally λ
type (17 cases/13 cases). We did not think that an antigen excess
level of some oligoclonal bands may explain this contradictory
results. We believe our 10 CSF represent a poor sample of MS population where a synthesis of κ type gammaglobulins is usually
predominant. Bollengier (6) has observed a major λ type gammaglobulins synthesis in some MS cases.

The occurence of free light chains in oligoclonal CSF is
well accepted to-day and has been particularly demonstrated by
Vandvik (7, 8). The presence of free heavy chains in CSF has
never yet been reported to our knowledge.

REFERENCES

1. Link, H. (1967) Acta Neurol. Scand. (suppl.) 28, 45-58.
2. Vandvik, B. and Skrede, S. (1973) Europ. Neurol., 9, 224-241.
3. Doutriaux, C., Clerc, M. and Giordano, C. (1975) Clin. Chim.
   Acta, 37, 15-23.
4. Vandvik, B. and Norrby, F. (1973) Proc. Nat. Acad. Sci. US,
   70, 1060-1063.
5. Vandvik, B. (1977) Scand. J. Immunol., 6, 914-922.
6. Bollengier, F., Delmotte, P. and Lowenthal, A. (1976) J. Neurol.
   212, 151-158.
7. Vandvik, B. (1977) Acta Path. Microbiol. Scand. Sect. C, 85,
   324-332.
8. Vandvik, B., Norrby, E., Nordal, H.J. and Degre, M. (1976)
   Scand. J. Immunol., 5, 979-992.

RADIOIMMUNOASSAY OF IMMUNOGLOBULINS IN CEREBROSPINAL FLUID

T.A.Out,[+] H.K. van Walbeek,[x] E.E. Reerink-Brongers[+]
and H.J. van der Helm[x]

[+]   Central Laboratory of the Netherlands Red Cross,
       Blood Transfusion Service, Amsterdam, The Netherlands
[x]   Neurological Department of the Academic Hospital,
       University of Amsterdam, The Netherlands

In several neurological diseases abnormalities of immunoglobulin G in cerebrospinal fluid (CSF) are observed. These abnormalities can be qualitative (1) (restricted heterogeneity of IgG)
and quantitative (2) (increased concentration of IgG in CSF).
There are four other classes of immunoglobulins : IgA, IgM, IgD
and IgE, some of which have particular functions. It will be of
interest to obtain information on these immunoglobulins in CSF
in order to arrive at a better understanding of immune-processes
in neurological disease. Since the normal concentrations of IgM,
IgA, IgD and IgE in CSF are much lower than that of IgG these
immunoglobulins can only be measured by very sensitive assay
methods, unless CSF is concentrated first.

We have developed radioimmunoassays for measuring IgA, IgM
and IgD (for IgE an assay was already available) and used these
to determine immunoglobulins in CSF. In this paper some aspects
of the radioimmunoassays are described and some results of the
measurements are shown.

Many proteins in CSF are derived from the blood. The concentration of these proteins in CSF depends on the following
factors : the permeability of the blood-CSF barrier, the concentration of that protein in the blood, and the hydrodynamic radius of the protein (3). It has been shown that for IgG these
parameters can be taken into account by measuring the concentration of IgG and albumin both in serum and in CSF (4) : under
normal conditions a linear relationship was found between the

CSF/serum ratio of IgG (i.e. the concentration of IgG in CSF divided
by that in serum) on the one hand and the CSF/serum ratio of albumin
on the other hand (4). Deviations from such a relationship were
found in several groups of patients with neurological diseases.

Method of Radioimmunoassay

The radioimmunoassays (RIA) were performed as shown schematically in Fig. 1. Antisera, prepared in our laboratory, were
coupled to the solid phase (sepharose 4B, activated with CNBr).
The following batches were used : aIgH, KH 15-19-01; aIgA, SH 14-04-04;
aIgD, KH 20-06-01; aIgE. SH 25-02-08; aIgG, KH 16-103-03. The
antibodies used in the second incubation step were isolated from
the same sources, except for the aIgM-antibodies. These were
isolated from batch KH 15-18-02. The procedure for preparing the
reagents and performing the incubations were similar to those described for the RIA of IgE (5).

The lower detection limit in the RIAs used for the measurements described here was about 0,5 ng Ig; thus, when 50 µl of CSF

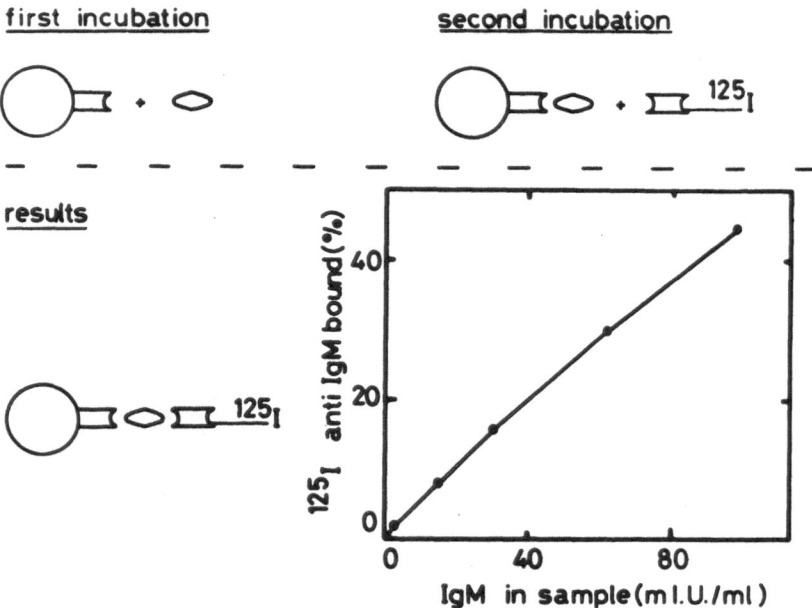

Fig. 1. Procedure of the radioimmunoassays.

was used, levels down to 14 ng/ml could be analyzed. Lower concentrations were measured by addition of larger volumes of CSF
(controls for changes in the final incubation volumes were done).
The coefficients of variation of the RIAs were: within assay, 5
to 7%; inter-assay 7 to 10%.

Specificity Test of the Radioimmunoassay

To establish the specificity of the antisera and ^{125}I-labelled
antibodies in this particular system, we tested the ^{125}I-labelled
antibodies by immunoelectrophoresis. Fig. 2 shows an example of
immunoelectrophoretic analysis. After electrophoresis of normal
human serum a rabbit antiserum, raised against human serum proteins, and ^{125}I-anti IgM were applied in the antiserum-trough.
Many serum proteins were precipitated (upper part, staining for
protein). The ^{125}I-antibodies bound to the precipitated IgM
(lower part,radioautography). A very faint binding to the precipitate containing IgG was also observed. Similarly the other
^{125}I-antibodies bound to their corresponding antigen and showed
a very faint binding to the precipitated IgG. Anti-IgD did not
show any binding to the precipitated IgG.

Next, possible cross-reactions in the actual RIA were investigated. The following results were obtained :

1) In the RIA for IgM, less than 0.002% of IgM was observed in a
   preparation of polyclonal IgG (purified by precipitation, gel
   filtration and ion exchange chromatography; purified monoclonal
   IgG3 and IgG4 were added to this preparation).
2) In the RIA for IgA, less than 1 ng of IgA per ml was found in
   sera of several patients having a selective IgA deficiency.
   In those sera the concentrations of IgM and IgG were normal.
3) The RIA of IgD showed less than 7 ng of IgD per ml, in several
   sera that contained normal amounts of other immunoglobulins.

anti human serum
proteins   +
(^{125}I) anti IgM

radioautography

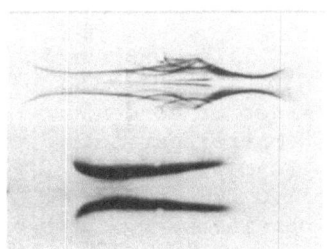

Fig. 2. Immunoelectrophoretic analysis of ^{125}I-labelled anti IgM.

From those values and from the concentrations of immunoglobulins
measured in CSF (see later in this paper), we conclude that the
specificity of the RIAs is sufficient for measurements of Igs in
CSF.

Comparison of the Radioimmunoassay with other Assay Methods

The assay method used for measurements in CSF should yield the
same values for Ig concentrations as the methods used for measurements in serum. In this aspect it is essential to use a proper
standard preparation of immunoglobulins.

In table 1 results of measurements of IgD and IgM in pooled
human serum are summarized. IgD was measured by RIA and radial
immunodiffusion (RID). IgM was measured by RIA, RID and automated
nephelometric immunoassay (ANIA) (our methods for RID and ANIA
have been described elsewhere (6)). The measurements were performed as follows. Five or six different dilutions of the standard preparations and at least four different dilutions of the
pooled human serum were prepared. Each dilution was measured in
triplicate. The mean value of the concentrations measured in the
different dilutions of the serum is given. The IgD concentrations
determined by RIA were the same as those measured by RID, if the
measurements were made relative to standard preparation 67/37
(WHO standard, freeze preparation of pooled human serum). With
the other standard preparation, however, the concentration of IgD
measured by RIA was different from that measured by RID: 60 and
43 I.U./ml, respectively. The IgM concentration measured by the
different methods were the same when the measurements were made
relative to H-00-01 (laboratory standard, prepared in the same
way as WHO standards). However, when the concentration of IgM was
measured relative to K1001, the different methods yielded various
results. Thus, only if a proper standard preparation is used is
it possible to obtain the same quantitative results by different
methods.

Ig-Concentrations determined in CSF

The ranges of concentrations of immunoglobulins measured in
CSF of 33 "control patients" were : IgA, 0.03 to 0.27 I.U./ml;
IgM, 0.004 to 0.069 I.U./ml; IgD, $\leq$ 0.002 to 0.085 I.U./ml; IgE,
$\leq$ 0.15 to 1.0 I.U./ml. More information on the meaning of these
values is obtained by plotting the CSF/serum ratios of the particular immunoglobulin against those of albumin. Fig. 3 shows the
results for IgD and IgM. It can be seen that the CSF/serum ratios
of the immunoglobulins increase as the CSF/serum ratios of albumin
increase. These data will probably prove to be a useful tool in

Table 1

IgM and IgD in pooled serum

	IgM		IgD	
	1*	2	1**	2
RIA	200 ± 13+	135 ± 8	60 ± 6	42 ± 3
RID	153 ± 2	128 ± 2	43 ± 1.6	43 ± 1.6
ANIA	115 ± 8	137 ± 9	n.d.	n.d.

*   standard preparation : 1, K 1001; 2, H-00-01
** standard preparation : 1, 6401 F; 2, 67/37
+   I.U./ml, mean ± standard deviation.

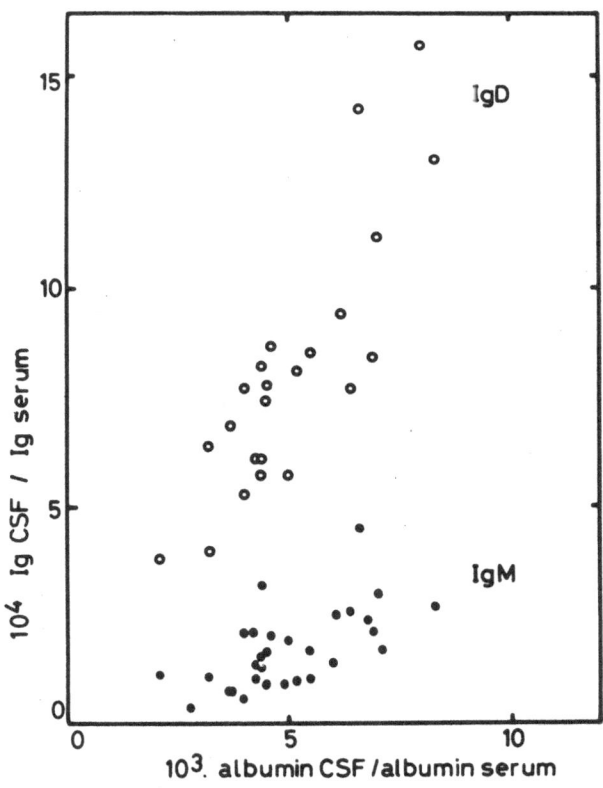

Fig. 3. The relation between the CSF/serum ratios of IgM and IgD, and the CSF/serum ratio of albumin. O——O, IgD; •——•, IgM.

establishing increases of IgD and IgM concentrations in CSF due to production of IgD and IgM within the central nervous system. Our results for IgG were similar to those reported by others (4).

We have observed deviations from the results shown in Fig. 3 in several groups of patients having neurological diseases.

Concluding Remarks

Our data show that IgM, IgA, IgD and IgE can be measured in cerebrospinal fluid by radioimmunoassays. Since CSF/serum ratios are to be used to analyze the concentrations of these proteins in CSF, results of assay methods for CSF should be comparable to results of assay methods for serum. This is possible by using a proper standard preparation. Analysis of neuro-immunological processes can be made now with the use of data on all known classes of immunoglobulins.

REFERENCES

1. Lowenthal, A., Agar gel electrophoresis in neurology. Elsevier, Amsterdam, 1964.
2. Tourtelotte, W. (1970), J. Neurol. Sci. 10, 279-304.
3. Felgenhauer, K. (1974), Klin. Wschr. 52, 1158-1164.
4. Ganrot, K. and Laurell, C.B. (1974), Clin. Chem. 20, 571-573.
5. Stallman, P.J. and Aalberse, R.C. (1977). Int. Arch. Allergy 54, 9-18.
6. Out, T.A., Duimel, W.J., Aalberse, R.C. and Reerinck-Brongers E.E. (1978), La Ricerca Clin. Lab. 8 (Suppl. no. 1) 133-144.

MEASUREMENT OF BLOOD/CSF PERMEABILITY COEFFICIENTS AND OF INTRATHECAL SYNTHESIS OF IgG BY CAPILLARY ISOTACHOPHORESIS

P. Delmotte

National Center for Multiple Sclerosis, Melsbroek,
Belgium

Although a considerable amount of time and effort has been spent to study the immunological response on the cellular level in multiple sclerosis, no clear-cut pattern has emerged until now. The difficulties to standardize the cellular tests and the overlapping of results between multiple sclerosis and other neurological diseases, have hampered their use for diagnostic purposes.

On the contrary, it is a well established fact, that the qualitative and quantitative study of the humoral immunological response within the central nervous system, remains, until now, one of the most important parameters for the diagnosis of inflammatory diseases of the central nervous system, and this is especially true for multiple sclerosis, (1).

For this purpose, several techniques have been proposed and used : zone electrophoresis, immunoelectrophoresis, rocket electrophoresis, isoelectric focusing, to only name some of them.

During the last two years, we have been experimenting with capillary isotachophoresis of the serum and cerebrospinal fluid proteins. We have been able to show that this new electrophoretic technique offers some interesting advantages :
1) exactly controlled working conditions lead to very reproducible results and sample solutions can be quantitatively injected.
2) protein fractions are detected by their UV absorbance under dynamic equilibrium conditions.

    3) peak areas of separated protein fractions are a direct
       measure of the absolute amount of protein present.

    A detailed description of the entire experimental set-up is
beyond the scope of this presentation. For technical details
see Delmotte (2).

    The lower limit of detection lies around 10 nanograms of
protein.

    Unconcentrated cerebrospinal fluid can be used, but the
high salt content adversely influences the separation results.

    We concentrate the cerebrospinal fluid about 10 times and
4 microliter of this concentrate are injected. For serum only
0,6 microliter are used.

    Figure 1 shows the isotachophoretic separation patterns of
the serum and cerebrospinal fluid of the same normal individual.
By manipulation of the composition of the spacer mobility gradient, one can get a clear cut separation of albumin and at the
same time a mobility subfractionation of the immunoglobulin G
fraction. The non-UV absorbing zones are due to amino-acids injected together with the sample.

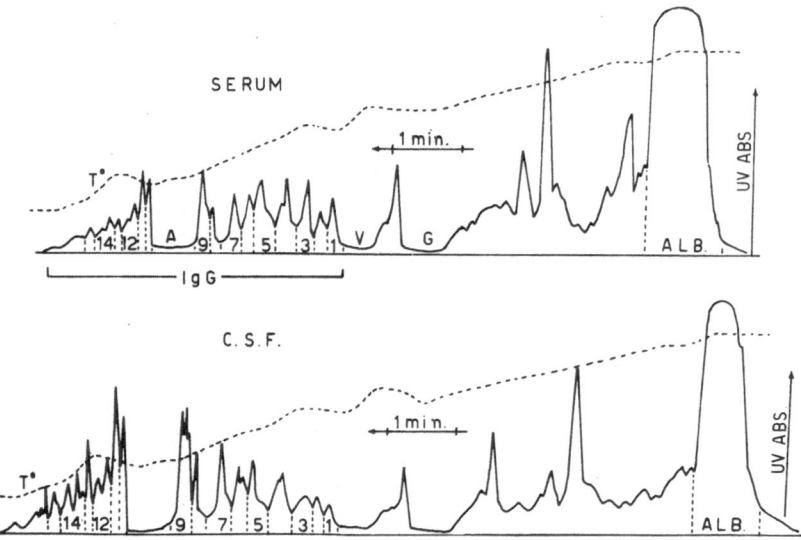

Figure 1 : a-(upper fig.) Capillary isotachophoresis of serum.
            b-(lower fig.) Idem for cerebrospinal fluid from same
                           individual.
Marker amino-acids: A=beta-alanine; V=valine; G=glycine.

As already mentioned, the integrated peak areas are a direct measure of the absolute amount of protein present in a zone.

By taking into account the injected volumes of serum and cerebrospinal fluid, and also the concentration factor of the latter, the blood/cerebrospinal fluid permeability coefficients can be calculated by using the integrated peak surfaces.

The results obtained for a group of 20 normal individuals are presented in Figure 2. The mean and range of the permeability coefficients for albumin and for total IgG correlate well with results obtained by immunological determination of the same fractions. (3, 4).

The most important feature of capillary isotachophoresis lies in the fact that the heterogeneous population of immunoglobulin G molecules, with isoelectric points ranging from around pH 6,8 to 8,6 can be reproducibly subfractionated in about 15 fractions. This subfractionation is solely based on differences in electrophoretic mobility and the delimitation of the fractions depends exclusively on the composition of the spacer mobility gradient used.

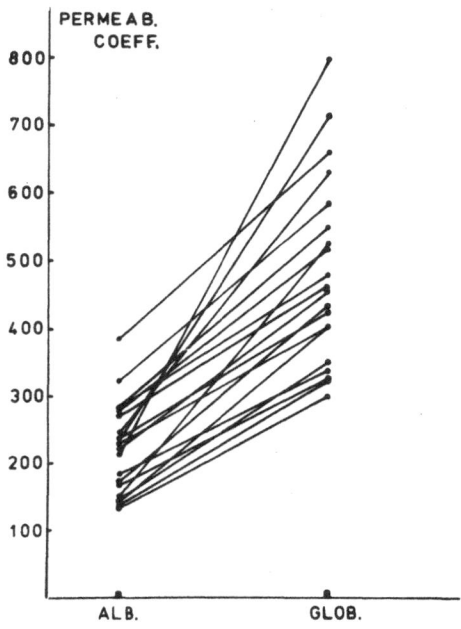

Figure 2 : Blood/CSF barrier permeability for albumin and IgG from 20 normal individuals as obtained by capillary isotachophoresis.

The integration of the peak surfaces of the individual immunoglobulin subfractions in serum and cerebrospinal fluid permits
to calculate the barrier permeability for all of these subfractions. Considering the fact that all immunoglobulin G molecules
have the same molecular size, it is evident that these permeability coefficients must be nearly the same and of the same value
as calculated for the total IgG's. All capillary isotachophore-
tic determinations carried out on serum and cerebrospinal fluid
of normal individuals have confirmed this observation.

The situation is entirely different when serum and cerebrospinal fluid of patients suffering from certain neurological disorders are submitted to the same experiments. Figure 3 shows
the separation patterns of serum and cerebrospinal fluid from a
typical multiple sclerosis patient. As can be expected from the
overall composition of the two fluids and from the fact that the
same mobility spacer gradient is used, the qualitative aspect
of the two patterns is quite similar.

However, the integration of the individual immunoglobulin
subfractions, brings to light some striking differences. The
permeability coefficients for the fastest moving IgG subfractions
were exactly as could be expected from the permeability coefficient calculated for albumin. But, as can be seen on Figure 4,
most, but not all of the slower moving fractions show dramati-

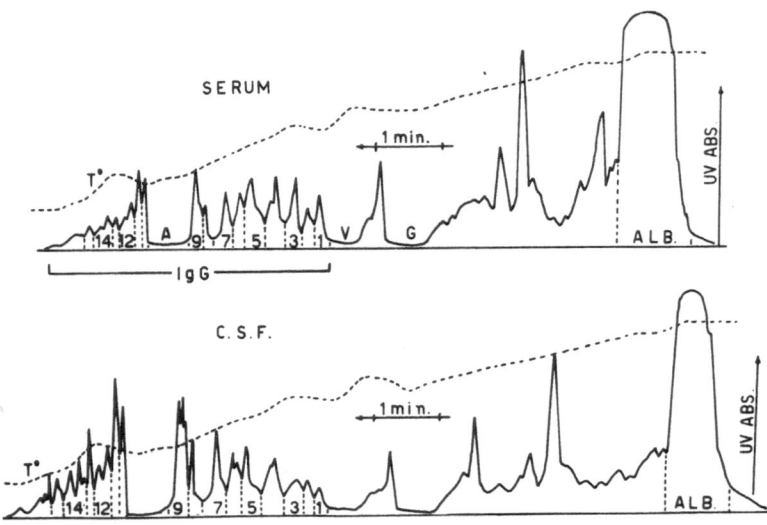

Figure 3 : a-(upper fig.) Capillary isotachophoresis of serum
from a multiple sclerosis patient.
b-(lower fig.) idem for cerebrospinal fluid from same patient.
Marker amino acids : A=beta-alanine; V=valine; G=glycine.

cally lower values for the permeability coefficients. The open
square is the value for albumin and the open circles are the
values for the IgG subfractions. The permeability coefficient
for total IgG is indicated by the line.

In this case, the value for total IgG left no doubt about
the presence of intracerebrally synthetized IgG. However, it
is well to draw attention to the striking differences in values
for the permeability coefficients for the different IgG subfractions.

An entirely different picture is shown in Figure 5. Here,
the permeability coefficient calculated for total IgG was about
twice the value calculated for the albumin fraction : as this
result fell within the range of values found for normal individuals, there was absolutely no evidence for intrathecal synthesis of IgG.

However, the permeability values of the IgG subfractions
leave no doubt about this case. The fastest moving fractions
have values in accordance with the results found for albumin,
and also well above the value calculated for total IgG. But,

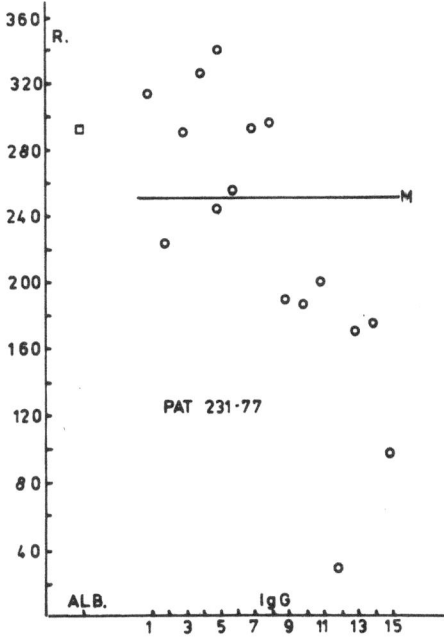

Figure 4 : Blood/CSF barrier permeability for albumin and IgG
subfractions from a multiple sclerosis patient.

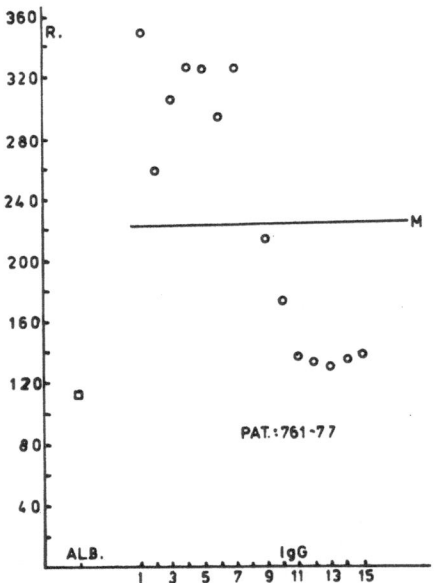

Figure 5 : Blood/CSF barrier permeability for albumin and IgG
subfractions from a multiple sclerosis patient.

for the slower moving fractions, the values are dramatically different and leave not the slightest doubt about the intrathecal
synthesis of IgG.

The same quantitative approach can be used to estimate the
amount of intrathecally synthetized IgG. Instead of using a
base line value the permeability coefficient of albumin, we can
now use as base line value the mean permeability coefficient of
the IgG subfractions which show the highest permeability coefficients (5).

For a group of about 70 clinically confirmed cases of multiple sclerosis, we found for most of them a percentage of intrathecally synthetized IgG of between 20 and 40 % of total IgG,
with cases reaching values as high as 65 %.

Even in cases with very low total CSF protein and having
at the same time a low percentage of IgG, capillary isotachophoresis can detect local synthesis of IgG.

Isoelectric focusing in thin layers of acrylamide of the
CSF IgG's has proven itself to be the most sensitive method to

detect the presence of oligoclonal IgG fractions in the CSF.
Parallel studies between isoelectric focusing and capillary
isotachophoresis has shown a 100 % correlaticn between these two
methods for the detection of local IgG synthesis. Capillary
isotachophoresis has the added advantage of speed and quantitation.

In conclusion we can state the following :
-- capillary isotachophoresis gives not only an overall qualitative picture of the protein composition of serum and CSF, but
   the separation pattern can be quantitatively interpreted.
-- total analysis time for one individual takes only 1 hour
-- the reproducible subfractionation of the IgG's gives not only
   very interesting information for diagnostic purpose, but at
   the same time has brought additional strong evidence for the
   intracerebral synthesis of IgC's in some neurological diseases, especially multiple sclerosis.

REFERENCES

1. Link H., Möller E., Muller R., Norrby E., Olsson J.E., Stend-
   hal L., Tibbling G. : Immunoglobulin Abnormalities in Spinal
   Fluid in Multiple Sclerosis. Acta Neurol. Scand. 55, suppl.
   63, 172-188, 1977.
2. Delmotte P. : Analysis of complex Protein Mixtures by capillary Isotachophoresis - Some qualitative and quantitative
   Aspects. Science Tools 24, 33-41, 1977.
3. Link H., Zettervall O., Blennow G.: Individual Cerebrospinal
   Fluid Proteins in the Evaluation of increased CSF total protein. J. Neurol. 203, 119-132, 1972.
4. Felgenhauer K., Schliep G., Rapic N. : Evaluation of the Blood-
   CSF Barrier by Protein Gradients and the humoral Response
   within the central nervous system. J. of the Neurol. Sciences
   30, 113-128, 1976.
5. Link H., Tibbling G.: Principles of Albumin and IgG Analysis
   in neurological Disorders. III. Evaluation of IgG Synthesis
   within the central nervous system in Multiple Sclerosis.
   Scand. J. clin. Lab. Invest. 37, 387-401, 1977.

STUDY OF THE IMMUNOGLOBULINS (IgG, IgA and IgM) IN THE CEREBRO-

SPINAL FLUID AND SERUM IN CASES OF SUPPURATIVE MENINGITIS AND

VIRAL ENCEPHALITIS

M.R. Kandil, M. Elrehawi

Faculty of Medicine, University of Assiut, Assiut,
Egypt

SUMMARY

Quantitative estimation of the immunoglobulins IgG, IgA and
IgM in serum and CSF of 42 patients (25 had viral encephalitis
and 17 had suppurative meningitis) and 20 controls were done using
the single diffusion precipitation method.

In the control group, the immunoglobulin level in CSF was
very low and IgM could not be detected. In the diseased group
however, the immunoglobulin level was significantly higher, particularly in S. meningitis, the values were several-fold those
found in V. encephalitis, and especially so with IgM. A significant difference was observed between the levels of the 3 immunoglobulins in severe when compared to the mild cases in both
encephalitis and meningitis. This change was not affected by
previous treatment in the meningitis cases.

There was no correlation between immunoglobulin levels in
serum and CSF, and the changes in serum immunoglobulins had no
specific pattern characteristic of either diseases.

The material of this study consisted of 42 patients who
were examined during the first two weeks of their disease. 17
of these patients had purulent meningitis, including 9 with
meningococcal meningitis, 5 with pneumococcal meningitis, 2
with streptococcal meningitis, and one patient with haemophilus
influenza meningitis diagnosed by culture from cerebrospinal
fluid and blood and direct smear from the samples. The remaining

25 patients had aseptic meningo-encephalitis presumed to be viral in origin.

All patients were adults and adolescents except for 2 children with viral encephalitis, with a mean of age 24 ± 11.2 comprising 18 females and 24 males.

The control group consisted of 20 adult patients admitted to the hospital for minor surgical operations, and had no medical illness.

In all these controls, anaesthesia was carried out by the spinal pool, when samples of CSF were collected. CSF samples from all patients were immediately obtained after admission for routine analysis. Two ml of each sample were stored at − 20 degree centigrad for immunoglobulin estimation (IgG, IgA and IgM) at the same time 5 ml of blood were drawn and the serum was separated for estimation of total proteins and immunoglobulins. Immunoglobulin level was estimated by the radial immunodiffusion method of Mancini using the single diffusion precipitation technique (1).

In the control group the immunoglobulin concentration in CSF was very low and its major part was formed of IgG, while IgA was detected in 9 samples only, IgM was not detected in any of the samples. The values of immunoglobulins in serum were within normal. In the diseased group, although a significant difference in the level of the total proteins in CSF was noticed between the two diseases, both were elevated, there was no specific value characteristic of any of the two diseases nor of the severity of the disease.

The elevation of the level of immunoglobulins in CSF was highly significant, even cases with normal total CSF proteins could show an abnormal CSF immunoglobulins (such as IgM). The increase in immunoglobulin levels in S. meningitis exceeds that in V. encephalitis several fold, and especially so with IgM (4:1) all cases of viral encephalitis had IgM level lower than 2.5 mg/100 ml, while 82 % of meningitis cases had levels above this value, this increase was most marked in the early stage of the disease.

Similar values were obtained by Smith et al (2). It was also found that the level of the 3 immunoglobulins in cases of encephalitis was below 15 mg/100 ml, while in 82 % of meningitis cases it was higher. Of the 17 cases with S. meningitis, 13 received some treatment for a few days prior to being investigated. The other 4 cases were investigated afresh (before treatment) and no significant difference was noticed between the mean of immunoglobulins in the two groups. A second CSF sample could be taken 4 weeks later in only 8 patients, 3 with S. meningitis and 5 with V. encephalitis. Out of those 8 cases, 3 patients recovered completely, and their immunoglobulins returned back to normal except for one patient, where there was a trace of IgM. The remaining 5 cases had a protracted course of the disease with changing pattern of their immunoglobulins in the form of either an increase in the level of one or more of the 3 immunoglobulins or a persistant high level especially IgG and IgM. This change may be taken as an index for chronicity of the disease and a bad prognostic pointer to the patient. The increasing level of IgG and IgM may suggest the presence of an allergic or altered immune reaction within the central nervous system, or a persistant damage to the blood brain barrier. Nevertheless the number of such cases was too small to establish such a conclusion and more elaborate work is needed.

REFERENCES

1. Soothill, J.F. et al. (1955) International Symposium on Immunological Methods of Biological Standardisation 4 : 37.
2. Smith, H., Bannister, B. et al; (1973) CSF immunoglobulins in meningitis. Lancet 2: 59 1-3.

VIRAL ANTIBODY AND PROTEIN STUDIES OF CEREBROSPINAL FLUID:

DIAGNOSTIC USEFULNESS IN MULTIPLE SCLEROSIS

K.P. Johnson [+], N.E. Cremer [x] and B. Forghani [x]

+Department of Neurology, Veterans Administration Hos-
pital and University of California, San Francisco,
U.S.S.; x Viral and Rickettsial Disease Laboratory,
California State Department of Health, Berkeley,
CA, U.S.A.

The most consistently useful laboratory aids to the diagnosis of
multiple sclerosis (MS) have come from the study of cerebrospinal
fluid (CSF) (1). In addition, interesting and possibly significant
clues to the etiology of the disease have come from such studies
(2). The determination of the CSF immunoglobulin G (IgG) content
expressed as a percent of total protein was first found by Kabat
(3) and remains, in many hospitals, the most useful diagnostic
test for MS. Lowenthal and coworkers (4) early noted that MS-CSF
when concentrated and separated by agar electrophoresis, showed
oligoclonal IgG bands in the cathodic, immunoglobulin zone. Using
such methods, several workers have found that between 80 and 95%
of clinically definite MS patients display such bands whereas few
patients with other noninflammatory neurologic diseases do (5,6).
Of interest, patients with a variety of chronic neurologic infections
such as neurosyphilis, subacute sclerosing panencephalitis and
progressive rubella panencephalitis invariably show such CSF bands
thus contributing to the idea that MS may be related to a chronic
CNS infection. IgG bands may occur transiently in acute CNS
infections as well (7).

The first evidence implicating a specific virus in MS was the
finding by Adams (8) of increased levels of measles virus antibody
in the serum of MS patients. This finding was extended to CSF and
repeatedly confirmed (2). Norrby, et al. (9) noted that amounts
of measles antibody were increased in CSF out of proportion to
serum, indicating that they were produced somewhere within the

CNS. The relationship between a previous or containing virus infection and MS was complicated with the finding that antibodies to several viruses might be increased in amount in the CSF of a single patient (2). During the past several years, radioimmuno-assays (RIA) for antibodies to many viral antigens have been described and found to be much more sensitive than standard sero-logic techniques (10). We therefore planned a study employing multiple viral serologic techniques including RIA to obtain infor-mation of viral antibodies in CSF of MS patients and patients with other noninflammatory neurologic diseases (OND). The most useful of these techniques in discriminating the MS patients from controls were then compared with electrophoresis of concentrated CSF in an attempt to find a combination of CSF assays which would most surely identify the MS patients.

Serum and CSF specimens were obtained from 87 patients with clinically definite MS using the criteria of McDonald (11) and from 129 patients with OND. Care was taken to exclude patients with evidence of an inflammatory process in the CNS. The viral serologic assays to which CSF was subjected are listed in Table 1. The standard assays were performed according to the methods des-cribed by Lennette and Schmidt (12) the RIA procedures by the method of Forghani (10) and the vaccinia complement dependent plaque reduction assay, (CPR) by the method of Takabayashi and McIntosh (13). The CSF cell count and IgG% amount were determined by standard methods while the IgG/albumin ratio employed the method described by Laurel (14). CSF oligoclonal IgG bands were detected by the method described by Johnson, et al. (15) in com-mercially available, performed agarose gels.

Viral Antibody Tests of Cerebrospinal Fluid

Virus Tests	RIA	HI	CF	CPR
Measles	+	+	+	
Rubella	+	+	+	
Vaccinia	+			+
Herpes Simplex I	+		+	
Mumps	+	+	+	
ParaFlu-6/94	+	+	+	
Varicella Zoster	+		+	
Cytomegalovirus			+	

* RIA, radioimmunoassay; HI, hemagglutination inhibition; CF, complement fixation; CPR, complement dependent plaque reduction.

When complement fixing antibody methods were used, only
measles antibodies were significantly different, appearing in 7%
of MS CSF's but less than 2% of controls. By hemagglutination
inhibition, CSF antibody to both measles and rubella appeared
significantly more often in MS patients however the positive
group was still only about 25% of the MS patients. Similar numbers
of MS patients displayed CSF vaccinia antibodies using the CPR
method. The RIA method used in this study measured antibodies to
all the various antigens of the viruses tested. Comparative
studies on several CSF specimens showed that it was at least 500
times more sensitive than the HI method for measles. Measles
antibody was again the most commonly noted, appearing in 53% of
MS-CSF but only 13% of controls (p >.0001). Rubella, varicella
and vaccinia antibodies appeared significantly more often in MS-
CSF but at lower rates than measles. Of interest, antibodies to
herpes simplex I were noted significantly more often in control
CSF.

To determine other laboratory tests of greatest sensivity in
MS, a number of nonviral methods were also employed. Increased
numbers of cells appeared in 33% of MS CSF's but in only 5% of
controls while the IgG% of total protein was increased in 61% of
MS patients. The reported increase in sensitivy found when IgG
was compared to CSF albumin to give an IgG/albumin ratio (14) was
confirmed for 73% of MS vs 20% of controls had an elevated ratio.
Using a simple, yet sensitive method to determine oligoclonal IgG
bands in prepoured agarose gels the greatest difference between MS
and control CSF's was noted: over 80% in MS and less than 10% in
controls.

A computer study of the CSF viral serologic changes employing
a stepwise discriminant function analysis showed that the tests
which best described the MS-CSF profile were: (a) positive measles
RIA, (b) negative herpes RIA, (c) high vaccinia CPR titer and (d)
high measles titer. When all of these were used in combination,
they discriminated the MS population correctly 70% of the time. A
comparison of CSF viral serologic changes with the presences of
oligoclonal IgG bands indicated that both types of change occurred
most commonly in the same patient population thus no diagnostic
advantage was gained by using both multiple serologic studies and
agarose electrophoresis of concentrated CSF.

One purpose of this study was to find the most sensitive test
or combination of tests available for the laboratory confirmation
of multiple sclerosis. Even when multiple, relatively expensive
viral serologic tests were used (which are available in only a few
research laboratories) no diagnostic advantage was gained over a
simplified agarose electrophoresis method employing commercially
available reagents. The continued study of immunological changes
in MS patients including their response to past or possible

persistent viral infection is probably critical in understanding
the nature of the disease. Nevertheless, such studies presently
confer no advantage in the diagnostic analysis of the individual
MS patients over simple CSF assay for oligoclonal IgG bands.

Supported by grants RG 1010-A-1 and RG 1008-A-2 from the
National Multiple Sclerosis Society, by Public Health Service
grants AI-01475 from the National Institute of Allergy and Infectious Diseases and NS-12064 from the National Institute of Neurological Diseases and Stroke.

REFERENCES

1. Johnson, K.P., Nelson, B.J. : Multiple sclerosis: Diagnostic
   usefulness of cerebrospinal fluid. Ann. Neurol. 2:425-431,
   1977.
2. Norrby, E.: Viral antibodies in multiple sclerosis in Melnick,
   J.L. (ed.): Progress in Medical Virology. Switzerland, 1978.
3. Kabat, E.A., Moore, D.H., Landow, H.: An electrophoretic study
   of the protein components in cerebrospinal fluid and their
   relationships to the serum proteins. J. Clin. Invest. 21:571-
   577, 1942.
4. Lowenthal, A., van Sande, M., Karcher, D.: The differential
   diagnosis of neurological diseases by fractionating electrophoretically the CSF γ -globulins. J. Neurochem. 6:51-56, 1960.
5. Link, H., Muller, R.: Immunoglobulins in multiple sclerosis
   and infections of the nervous system. Arch. Neurol. 25:326-
   344, 1971.
6. Vandvik, B., Skrede, S.: Electrophoretic examination of cerebrospinal fluid proteins in multiple sclerosis and other neurological diseases. Eur. Neurol. 9:224-241, 1973.
7. Vandvik, B., Norrby, E., Steen-Johnsen, J., Stensvold, K.: Mumps
   meningitis: Prolonged pleocytosis and occurrence of mumps
   virus-specific oligoclonal IgG in the cerebrospinal fluid.
   Eur. Neurol. 17:13-22, 1978.
8. Adams, J.M.: Measles antibodies in patients with multiple
   sclerosis. Neurology (Minneap) 17:707-710, 1967.
9. Norrby, E., Link, H., Olsson, J.E., et al.: Comparison of antibodies against different viruses in cerebrospinal fluid and
   serum samples from patients with multiple sclerosis. Infect.
   Immun. 10:688-694, 1974.
10. Forghani, B., Schmidt, N.J., Lennette, H.: Sensitivity of radio-
    immunoassay method for detection of certain viral antibodies in
    sera and cerebrospinal fluids. J. Clin. Microbiol. 4:470-478,
    1976.
11. McDonald, W.I., Halliday, A.M.: Diagnosis and classification of
    multiple sclerosis. Br. Med. Bull. 33:4-8, 1977.

12. Lennette, E.H., Schmidt, N.J. (ed). Diagnostic procedures for viral and rickettsial infections, 4th ed., p. 52-58, 524. American Public Health Association, Inc., New York, 1969.
13. Takabayashi, K., McIntosh, K.: Effect of heat-labile factors on the neutralization of vaccinia virus by human sera. Infect. Immun. 8:582-589, 1973.
14. Laurell, C.B.: Electroimmunoassay, Scand. J. Clin. Lab. Invest 29: Suppl. 124:21, 1972.
15. Johnson, K.P., Arrigo, S.C., Nelson, B.J., et al.: Agarose electrophoresis of cerebrospinal fluid in multiple sclerosis. Neurology (Minneap) 27:273-277, 1977.

THE CLINICAL SIGNIFICANCE OF IMMUNOGLOBULIN G (IgG)

DETERMINATIONS IN THE CSF OF MULTIPLE SCLEROSIS PATIENTS

H.K. van Walbeek, H.J. van der Helm

Neurological Department of the Academic Hospital,
University of Amsterdam, Amsterdam, The Netherlands

The IgG concentration in the cerebrospinal fluid (CSF) is commonly expressed as a percentage of the protein concentration, because the condition of the blood–CSF barrier must be taken into account. Another method of expressing IgG–CSF results is the calculation of albumin and IgG ratio's (CSF concentration/ serum concentration), in which not only the permeability of the blood–CSF barrier but also the IgG concentration in the serum is taken into consideration (1). In a disease in which IgG–CSF elevations are found frequently (multiple sclerosis), it is important to establish the clinical value of this increase.

It is not only necessary to obtain normal reference values of a test, but also to determine at various levels the sensitivity (i.e. percentage of MS patients with a positive outcome) and specificity (i.e. percentage of patients with other diseases and a negative outcome). The diagnostic power is determined by these two properties.

The relative IgG content of the CSF and the IgG index (IgG ratio / albumin ratio) were calculated from 753 patients with various neurological diseases at random selected in our hospital, and from 70 MS patients. In 35 control patients the $\bar{x} \pm 2s$ values were for the relative IgG content of the CSF : 3.0–10.6, and for the IgG index : 0.30–0.62.

At any comparable specificity value of both methods the IgG index shows a higher sensitivity than the relative IgG content of the CSF (Table I and II). For instance, at the arbitrarily chosen value of the IgG index = 0.70, the specificity is 89.5 and the sensitivity 75.7. When the relative IgG content of the CSF

TABLE 1

relative IgG–CSF content	sensitivity	specificity
8	91.4	51.1
9	82.9	63.1
10	75.8	72.6
11	72.9	81.4
12	64.3	86.3
13	61.5	89.5
14	57.1	92.6
15	47.1	94.4
16	37.1	95.8
17	34.3	96.5
18	27.2	97.6
19	24.3	98.4

TABLE II

IgG index	sensitivity	specificity
0.40	95.7	15.9
0.50	92.9	47.4
0.60	84.3	80.9
0.70	75.7	89.5
0.80	67.1	93.2
0.90	55.7	94.8
1.00	47.1	95.2

is 13 %, the specificity is also 89.5, but the sensitivity is 61.5.

From this we can conclude that the IgG index is more advantageous than the relative IgG content of the CSF if used in the diagnostic process to detect MS.

REFERENCES

1. Ganrot, K., Laurell, C.B. : Measurement of IgG and albumin content of cerebrospinal fluid, and its interpretation. Clin. Chem. 20 : 571-573, 1974.

DETERMINATION OF IgM IN THE CEREBROSPINAL FLUID BY PARTICLE COUNTING IMMUNOASSAY (PACIA)

C. Sindic [*], C. Cambiaso, P.L. Masson and E.C. Laterre

Unit of Experimental Medicine, International Institute
of Cellular and Molecular Pathology, Laboratory of
Neurochemistry, University of Louvain, Brussels, Belgium.

INTRODUCTION

The determination of plasma proteins in cerebrospinal fluid
(CSF) enables us to assess the filtration process through the
blood-brain barrier. Their increase generally indicates the existence of an inflammatory reaction in neurological tissues. Particular attention has been paid to IgG because of its possible local
origin and its determination is now fairly common. On a theoretical basis, the determination of IgM in CSF should be more useful
than that of IgG. Because IgM is less liable to gain access to
CSF by mere transsudation on account of its large molecular size,
an increase in IgM concentration should be a better index of the
local immune response. Moreover, IgM should become detectable at
earlier stages of the immune process as it is generally the first
antibody to be produced. However, in practice, the determination
of IgM in CSF is not easy as it requires very sensitive methods.

We will report here the preliminary results of a study of
the clinical relevance of IgM determination in CSF of patients
with various neurological disorders. IgM was determined by a novel method called Particle Counting ImmunoAssay (PACIA). Its
principle is based on the agglutination of antibody-coated particles (latex) by the antigen to be determined. The agglutination is measured by counting the residual, non-agglutinated particles, with a device designed for counting blood cells.

---

[*] Aspirant at the "Fonds National de la Recherche Scientifique",
Brussels.

MATERIALS AND METHODS

The PACIA system has been automated using a Technicon Auto-Analyzer with a special sampler and an AutoCounter (Technicon Instruments Corporation, Tarrytown, N.Y.). The height of the recorded peaks is directly proportional to the number of free particles.

Calibrated polystyrene particles of 0.8 μ diameter, a gift from Rhône-Poulenc (Courbevoie, France), were coated with antibody as described by Cambiaso et al. (1). Briefly, IgG purified from goat anti-IgM antiserum, was absorbed on particles by simple mixing of the reagents.

Standard curves were obtained by making serial dilutions of a standard serum from Technicon. Samples of CSF had been stored frozen in the presence of sodium azide (0.I %). For the immunoassay, it was generally necessary to dilute the samples by a factor of at least four with 0.1 M glycine-HCl buffer, pH 9.2, containing 0.17 M sodium chloride, 0.1 % bovine serum albumin and 50 mM EDTA. To increase sensitivity, a solution of polyethylene glycol was added into the incubating tube to reach a final concentration of 1.33 %.

PATIENTS

We have considered four groups of patients :
- 10 with non-neurological disorders (minor neurosis, or uveitis without neurological signs)
- 73 with various neurological disorders but normal CSF, i.e. level of proteins below 40 mg/ %, number of cells below or equal to 5 per mm^3, and normal appearance in agar gel elctrophoresis
- 42 with clinically definite multiple sclerosis (MS)
- 18 with viral or bacterial (including tuberculous) meningo-encephalitis.

RESULTS AND DISCUSSION

In the group of 10 patients with non-neurological disorders (Fig. 1), the level of IgM in the CSF ranged from 30 to 400 ng/ml with a logarithmico-normal distribution and a median value of 117 ng/ml. Adding two standard deviations, the upper normal limit was set at 540 ng/ml. Of the 73 patients with neurological disorders and normal CSF, 12 had abnormally high levels of CSF IgM. The level of IgM in the 42 patients with clinically definite MS exceeded the normal upper limit in 28 cases (66 %), whereas in

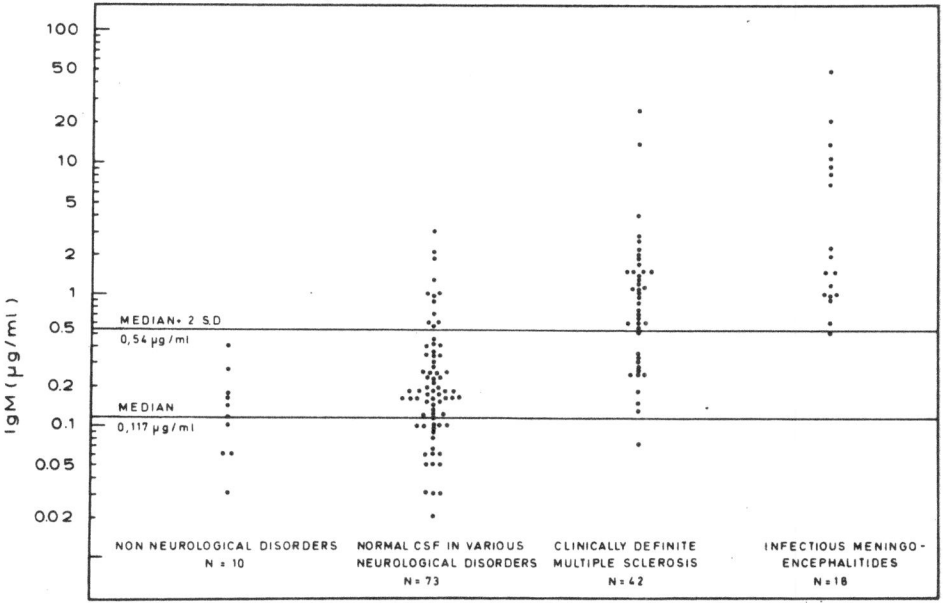

Fig. 1. Levels of CSF IgM in the four groups of patients.

meningo-encephalitis, all patients, but 1, gave abnormal IgM
values.

To distinguish between passive transfer of IgM or local biosynthesis, we have studied the ratio between the levels of IgM
and albumin $\frac{\text{IgM} \quad (\mu g/ml)}{\text{Alb} \quad (\mu g/ml)} \cdot 10^3$, the latter being determined by
immunonephelometry (Fig. 2). In the group of non-neurological
disorders, the ratio ranged from 0.16 to 2.86 (median : 0.73;
median + 2 S.D. : 3.9). In the group with neurological disorders
and normal CSF, 9 patients had a ratio exceeding 3.9 : 2 with
peripheric neuropathies of unknown aetiology, 1 with possible
MS and normal agar gel electrophoresis, 1 with arteritis of the
central nervous system of unknown aetiology, 1 with idiopathic
megaencephaly and mental deficit, 1 with sciatica, and 3 without
definite diagnosis.

In the group of clinically definite MS, 50 % had an abnormally high ratio compatible with local production of IgM, whereas
16 % had a normal ratio despite an abnormally high concentration
of IgM. In the group of meningoencephalitis, high ratios were
observed in most cases (14/18).

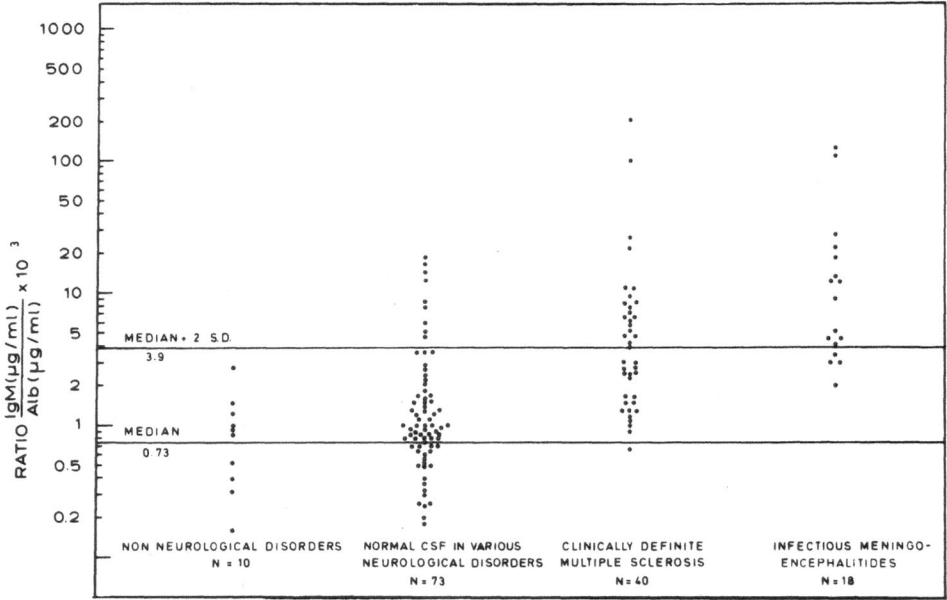

Fig. 2.   Ratio IgM. 10^3/Alb in the four groups of patients.

        No correlation was found between the levels of IgM and IgG
(determined by immunonephelometry) in the CSF of clinically definite MS (r = 0.006). However, highly significant correlation
was found between the presence of oligoclonal bands and a high
concentration of IgM (Table 1).

        The association of oligoclonal bands with high levels of IgM
is reminiscent of what is seen in reconstitution experiments (2).
The immunoglobulin pattern in the sera of children with severe
combined immunodeficiency is characterized, in the days following

Table 1. Correlation between the occurence of oligoclonal bands
and IgM concentration in the CSF of patients with MS

Concentration of IgM in CSF (µg/ml)	Oligoclonal bands in CSF		
	Present	Absent	Total
More than 0.54 µg/ml	28	1	29
Less than 0.54 µg/ml	14	10	24
Total	42	11	53

x^2 = 9.37; 0.005   P   0.001

transplantation with bone marrow, by the appearance of homogeneous immunoglobulins and predominant IgM concentration (3).

Finally, when the number of cells in CSF of patients with definite MS was above $10/mm^3$, the level of IgM always exceeded the upper normal limit. However, abnormally high values of IgM were also detected in patients with normal cell counts.

Our results, by confirming and extending those of Schuller et al. (4) and Williams et al. (5), suggest that the IgM concentration in CSF could be a useful index of immunological disorders affecting the central nervous system.

REFERENCES

1. Cambiaso, C.L., Leek, A.E., De Steenwinkel, F., Billen, J. and Masson, P.L. : Particle Counting ImmunoAssay (PACIA).
   1. - A general method for the determination of antibodies, antigens and haptens. J. Immunol. Methods 18, 33-44 (1978).
2. Radl, J., Van Den Berg, P., Voormolen, M., Hendriks, W.D.H. and Schaefer, U.W. : Homogeneous immunoglobulins in sera of Rhesus monkeys after lethal irradiation and bone-marrow transplantation. Clin. Exp. Immunol. 16, 259-266 (1974).
3. Radl, J., Dooren, L.J., Eijsvoogel, V.P., Van Went, J.J. and Hijmans, W. : An immunological study during posttransplantation follow-up of a case of severe combined immunodeficiency. Clin. Exp. Immunol. 10, 367-382 (1972).
4. Schuller, E., Delasnerie, N., Hélary, M. and Lefevre, M. : Serum and cerebrospinal fluid IgM in 203 neurological patients. Eur. Neurol. 17: 77-82 (1978).
5. Williams, A.C., Mingioli, E.S., McFarland, H., Tourtellotte, W.W. and Mc Farlin, D.E. : Elevated CSF IgM in multiple sclerosis. Neurology 28, 393 (1978).

LOCAL AND GENERAL IMMUNITY IN CNS DISEASES

E. Schuller

Laboratoire de Neuro-immunologie, Hôpital de la Salpêtrière, Paris, France

The most important problem, in the study of CSF-immunoglo-
bulins, is not their specific and precise determination, now
solved by various methods at the level of nanogram, but rather
search for their origin.

Obviously 3 processes may explain presence of immunoglobulins in a CSF :
- a selective filtration (the only physiological one)
- a transudation, if blood-CSF and/or blood-brain barriers are
  altered, as in many diseases
- and a local synthesis by mononuclear cells (cell-mediated immunity) in certain CNS diseases, especially demyelinating diseases.
These 3 processes are well-known today for IgG and 5 different
immunological patterns (table 1) can be proposed with the use
of albumin as the marker of blood-CSF exchanges and the percentage of IgG as the sign of a possible inflammatory reaction
(table 2).

Normal CSF shows neither alteration of blood-CSF exchanges
nor local inflammatory reaction. Inflammatory CSF is a pure local (intrathecal) synthesis of IgG without alteration of blood-
CSF barriers : the level of CSF albumin remains within normal
limits. Two types of transudate can be described :
1) Non inflammatory : transudation of a serum with normal IgG
   level (i.e. :≤15 g/l) in a normal CSF.
2) Inflammatory transudate : transudation of increased IgG serum in a normal CSF, expressing only a general immunity
   reaction, without any local process.

TABLE 1

Classification of CSF in five immunological patterns

C.S.F. patterns	C.S.F. albumin (mg/l)	C.S.F. IgG percentage	IgG origin
1. Normal	normal	normal	filtration (physiological)
2. Inflammatory	normal	increased	local (intrathecal) synthesis
3. Non-inflammatory transudate	increased	normal	transudation from a serum with normal IgG
4. Inflammatory transudate	increased	increased	transudation from a serum with increased IgG
5. Meningitic	increased	increased	association of transudation and local synthesis of IgG

TABLE 2

The 5 immunological CSF patterns

	Meningitis	
	Non Inflammatory Transudate	Inflammatory Transudate
	Normal	Inflammatory

C.S.F. Albumin : 334 mg/l (increased)   (normal)

(normal)   14.5 %   (elevated)

C.S.F. IgG percentage

The fifth pattern, association of a transudation and a local synthesis of IgG is called "Meningitis". The distinction between transudate and meningitis is important, as demonstrated by many samples. In practice : the percentage of albumin increase is evaluated from the serum albumin (40 mg/ml) and the mean CSF albumin (240 mg/l), and called "transudation index". Thus a transudation of 0.1 % (table 3) corresponds to an increase of 40 mg/l in the CSF. Transudations of 0.1 % (280 mg/l) and 0.2 % (320 mg/l) are still physiological considering 334 mg/l as our above usual limit for CSF albumin. Transudation of IgG can be estimated by using this transudation index according to serum IgG. Adjunction of the maximum IgG physiological filtration (40 mg/l) gives the total of "blood IgG" (IgG of plasmatic origin). This total is compared with CSF IgG :
- if "blood IgG" $\geqslant$ CSF IgG $\longrightarrow$ transudation
- if "blood IgG" $<$ CSF IgG : a local synthesis is associated
to the transudation $\longrightarrow$ meningitis

TABLE 3

Calcul of the transudation index

Percentage	C.S.F. Albumin (mg/l)	Total Protein (g/l)
0.3 %	360	0.61
0.5 %	440	0.75
1 %	640	1.10
2 %	1.040	1.80

TABLE 4

Influence of serum IgG in a transudate

Transudation	C.S.F. protein (g/l)	C.S.F. albumin (mg/l)	C.S.F. IgG	
			if serum IgG (10 g/l)	if serum IgG (20 g/l)
0.3 %	0.61	360	70 (11.5 %)	100 (16 %)
0.5 %	0.75	440	90 (12 %)	140 (19 %)
1 %	1.10	640	140 (13 %)	240 (22 %)

Conclusion : if serum IgG $>$ 16 g/l, any transudate is of inflammatory type (IgG percentage $\geqslant$ 15 %).

Influence of serum IgG on a transudate is obvious, as demonstrated in table 4 : all transudates in the left column are non inflammatory and in opposite an inflammatory transudate is observed following the smallest transudation in the presence of a light serum IgG increase (20 g/l in this case).

A meningitis pattern can be detected by this easy calculation in some CSF without increased IgG percentage (table 5).

An inflammatory CSF and an inflammatory transudate are given as example in table 6.

TABLE 5

A fallacious "non inflammatory transudate"

		Total protein	:	0.68 g/l	
C.S.F.	{	Albumin	:	360 mg/l	(53 %)
		IgG	.:	95 mg/l	(14 %)

Transudation index   :   0.3 %

Serum IgG: 10 g/l

IgG Transudation   : 30 mg/l

                          +

                        40 mg/l   (CSF, normal IgG)
                        ─────────
                        70 mg/l

Conclusion : Local synthesis of 25 mg/l (26 %)
             Meningitis (confirmed by oligoclonal aspect)
             (association of transudation and local synthesis).

TABLE 6

Inflammatory CSF and Inflammatory transudate (examples)

CSF Protein	0.68 g/l	0.68 g/l
CSF Albumin	300 mg/l (44 %) no transudation	400 mg/l (59 % transudation 0.4 %
CSF IgG	204 mg/l (30 %)	140 mg/l (21 %)
Serum IgG	normal	25 g/l

$$
\begin{array}{rl}
\text{Transudation} & : \quad 100 \\
+ \quad \text{normal IgG} & : \quad \underline{40} \\
& \quad \ 140
\end{array}
$$

Conclusion   Inflammatory CSF   Inflammatory transudate

TABLE 7

The differen IgG ratios

Ratios	Normal values	Normal ratio	Pathological example with normal ratios	
$\dfrac{\text{IgG}}{\text{Total protein}}$	$\dfrac{40}{400}$	10 %	$\dfrac{80}{800}$ =	$\dfrac{160}{160}$
$\dfrac{\text{IgG}}{\text{Albumin}}$	$\dfrac{30}{200}$	15 %	$\dfrac{60}{400}$ =	$\dfrac{120}{800}$
$\dfrac{\text{CSF IgG}}{\text{CSF Albumin}}$	$\dfrac{40}{200}$	80 %	$\dfrac{80^{+}}{200}$	$\dfrac{300^{++}}{900}$
$\dfrac{\text{serum IgG}}{\text{Serum Albumin}}$	$\dfrac{10.000}{40.000}$		$\dfrac{20.000}{40.000}$	$\dfrac{12.500}{30.000}$
$\dfrac{\text{CSF IgG}}{\text{Serum IgG}}$.	$\dfrac{40}{10.000}$	80 %	$\dfrac{200^{++}}{20.000}$	$\dfrac{80^{+}}{15.000}$
	$\dfrac{200}{40.000}$		$\dfrac{500}{40.000}$	$\dfrac{295}{45.000}$

+   inflammatory CSF
++   meningitis

TABLE 8

CSF Immunological patterns in 203 neurological patients

DIAGNOSES	Normal (56)	Inflam- matory (73)	Non inflamma- tory transudate (36)	Inflam- matory transudate (19)	Me- ningitis (19)
M.S. (63)	14	35	5	1	8
S.S.P.E. (12)	0	11	1	0	0
Infectious di- seases (34)	12	9	7	2	4
Inflammatory diseases (26)	12	5	4	4	1
Malignant diseases (18)	1	3	8	4	2
Peripheral neu- ropathies (24)	5	5	5	7	2
Degenerative diseases (13)	5	4	3	1	0
Miscellaneous (13)	7	1	3	0	2

DISCUSSION

This very easy classification, now used in France, offers some advantages in comparison with the different ratios previously proposed. Any ratio may be "normal" in obvious pathological situations (table 7) and this fact is difficult to conciliate with clinical data.

The immunological status of the patient is more precisely defined by the 5 patterns proposed, and not only the origin of IgG. A recent survey of 203 neurological patients (table 8) shows the frequency of inflammatory pattern in demyelinating (50 à 60 % in M.S. patients) and infectious or inflammatory CNS diseases, contrasting with the prevalence of non inflammatory transudate in malignant diseases and in polyradiculoneuritis. A typical meningitis pattern is observed in 15 % of M.S. patients : as presented elsewhere (3) there is a strong link between this pattern and a special type of immunological reactivity including simultaneous local synthesis of nucleic and viral antibodies. The origin of CSF IgA and CSF IgM may be analysed using these 5 patterns : as demonstrated in two precedent papers (1 and 2) they are not correlated with IgG variations. This line of argument may be used for any antibody present in the CSF. But overall this classification is an attempt to define a common language between laboratories working with different methods (i.e. : different normal limits) and between clinicians and biologists, which is perhaps the most important.

ACKNOWLEDGEMENTS

    This research was supported by Institut national pour la santé et la recherche médicale (I.N.S.E.R.M. - grant n° 77-5-181-6) and Association pour la Recherche sur la Sclérose en Plaques. I thank Pr. W.W. Tourtellotte for stimulating discussions, and Miss L. Tömpe for expert technical assistance.

REFERENCES

1. Schuller, E., Delasnerie, N., Reboul, J., Lefevre, M. Serum and C.S.F. IgA (25th Colloquium "Protides of the biological fluids") edited by H. Peeters. Pergamon Press Oxford and New York, 881-885, 1978.
2. Schuller, E., Delasnerie, N., Helary, M., Lefevre, M. Serum and CSF IgM in 203 neurological patients. Europ. Neurol. 17-77, 1978.
3. Schuller, E., Lebon, P., Allinquant, B., Moreau, N., Reboul, J., and Deloche, G. Nucleic and viral antibodies in serum and CSF of Multiple Sclerosis patients. Nato Advanced Institute on Humoral Immunity in Neurological Diseases (Antwerp-September 10-22, 1978).

NUCLEIC AND VIRAL ANTIBODIES IN SERUM AND CSF OF MS PATIENTS

E. Schuller, P. Lebon [*], B. Allinquant, N. Moreau[*],
J. Reboul and G. Deloche

Laboratoire de Neuro-immunologie (INSERM U-134) Hôpital de la Salpêtrière, Paris, France and Unité de Recherche sur les Infections Virales (INSERM U-43) Hôpital
Saint Vincent de Paul, Paris, France

Two years ago, we described (6) a new method of counter
immunoelectrophoresis which allows the determination of DNA and
RNA (7) antibodies in serum and unconcentrated CSF. This type
of IgG antibody is found in normal serum but in pathological
CSF only.

A precedent work (8) showed a very probable correlation between oligoclonal aspect, local synthesis of viral (measles and
rubella) antibodies (VAB) and local synthesis of nucleic antibodies (NAB) in some MS-CSF.

MATERIAL AND METHODS

We present here the results obtained in 101 MS, 12 SSPE and
30 control cases (other neurological diseases).

For each patient, serum and CSF were investigated :
1) by electrophoresis on cellulose acetate after standardised
concentration (2).
2) by electroimmunodiffusion for IgA, IgM, IgG, C3, C4 and CRP,
as previously described (3, 4, 5).
3) DNA and RNA antibodies were determined by counterimmunoelectrophoresis and expressed in absolute value (serological dilution) and percentage (6). CSF patterns were analysed following our classification in 5 types (8).
4) Measles and rubella antibodies were determined by hemagluti-
nation inhibition.

Clinical data (sex, age of the patient, duration of the disease, clinical stage, type of course, disability grade using Kurtzke's scale) were collected for each patient after careful analysis of the criteria for MS diagnosis.

RESULTS

Table 1 shows the increase of NAB in 58 serum and their abnormal presence in 31 CSF of MS patients without apparent correlation.

In SSPE, NAB were increased in serum and present in CSF in all but one patient, in contrast with their rare variations in controls. Presence of NAB and VAB were analysed according to CSF patterns (tables 2 and 3).

They are clearly linked to a local synthesis of IgG (inflammatory and meningitis patterns only for NAB and even "normal" pattern for VAB) in MS and SSPE patients. On the contrary, a transudation is generally present in controls with NAB and/or VAB in their CSF. In order to analyse the eventual relations between NAB and VAB in CSF of MS patients, we divided our MS population into 3 groups : the first without NAB and VAB (n = 42), the second with VAB only (n = 28) and the third with both (n = 31). Significant differences appear between the frequencies of CSF patterns in the 3 groups (table 4).

Table 1 : NAB IN SERUM AND CSF

NAB percentage in serum	NAB IN CSF					
	MS (101)		SSPE (12)		CONTROLS (30)	
	absence (70)	presence (31)	absence (1)	presence (11)	absence (21)	presence (9)
Normal	31	12	0	2	16	5
Increased	39	19	1	9	5	4

Table 2 : NAB AND CSF IMMUNOLOGICAL PATTERNS

CSF Patterns (143)	MS (101) absence (70)	presence (31)	SSPE (12) absence (1)	presence (11)	CONTROLS (30) absence (21)	presence (9)
Normal (34)	26	--	-	--	8	-
Inflammatory (69)	34	21	1	8	4	1
Non inflammatory transudate (19)	6	--	-	1	9	3
Inflammatory transudate (3)	--	--	-	1	-	2
Meningitis (18)	4	10	-	1	-	3

Table 3 : VAB AND CSF IMMUNOLOGICAL PATTERNS

CSF Patterns (143)	MS (101) absence (49)	presence (52)	SSPE (12) absence (0)	presence (12)	CONTROLS (30) absence (19)	presence (11)
Normal (34)	19	7	-	--	8	--
Inflammatory (69)	24	31	-	9	2	3
Non inflammatory transudate (19)	3	3	-	1	6	6
Inflammatory transudate (3)	--	--	-	1	1	1
Meningitis (18)	3	11	-	1	2	1

A clear predominance of normal pattern is seen in the first
(contrasting with its absence in the third) and, in opposite,
obvious prevalence of meningitis pattern in the third. Some
other significant correlations may be observed in CSF :
- a lymphocytic pleiocytosis in the third group, contrasting with
  normal mean in the first (table 5).

E. SCHULLER ET AL.

Table 4 : CSF IMMUNOLOGICAL PATTERNS IN THE 3 MS GROUPS (n = 101)

CSF PATTERNS	Group 1 absence of AB in CSF (n = 42)	Group II VAB only in CSF (n = 28)	Group III VAB and NAB in CSF (n = 31)
Normal (26)	19 **	7 *	-- **
Inflammatory (55)	19	15	21
Non Inflammatory transudate (6)	3	3	--
Meningitis (14)	1 **	3	10 **

*   p < 0.05
**   p < 0.01

Table 5 : CSF LYMPHOCYTES IN THE 3 MS GROUPS (n = 90)

	Group 1 absence of AB in CSF (n = 38)	Group II VAB only in CSF (n = 24)	Group III VAB and NAB in CSF (n = 28)
Lymphocyte Mean (by mm^3)	2.7 ± 2.6 *	4.3 ± 4.9	6.9 ± 7.0 *

*   p < 0.05

- highest frequency of oligoclonal aspect in the third (73 %) which is relatively rare in the first (table 6).
- important increase of IgG in the third, with significant differences between the second and the first : IgG mean is only slightly elevated in this last (table 7).
- frequent presence of IgM in the third (42 %) significantly higher than in the two others (17 %) (table 8).

    As previously proposed, an obvious correlation is found between simultaneous presence or absence of NAB and VAB (table 9).

Table 6 : OLIGOCLONAL ASPECT IN THE 3 MS GROUPS (n = 99)

O.A.	Group I absence of AB in CSF (n = 41)	Group II VAB only in CSF (n = 28)	Group III VAB and NAB in CSF (n = 30)
Absent (42)	23	11	8
Present (57)	18 *	17	22 *

$* \chi^2 = 6.30$ $(p < 0.05)$

Table 7 : CSF IMMUNOGLOBULINS IN THE 3 MS GROUPS

CSF Immunoglobulins	Group I absence of AB in CSF (n = 42)	Group II VAB only in CSF (n = 28)	Group III VAB and NAB in CSF (n = 31)
IgA (mg/l)	2.8 ± 2.0	3.2 ± 2.0	5.8 ± 9.0
IgG (mg/l)	58 ± 28 *	90 ± 101 *	151 ± 75 *
IgM (mg/l)	0.4 ± 1.0 *	0.6 ± 1.5 *	2.0 ± 3.4 *

* $p < 0.05$ between III and I
                        III and II

Table 8 : CSF IgM IN THE 3 MS GROUPS (n = 101)

CSF IgM	Group I absence of AB in CSF (n = 42)	Group II VAB only in CSF (n = 28)	Group III VAB and NAB in CSF (n = 31)
Absence (76)	35	23	18
Presence (25)	7	5	13

$p < 0.02$: between I and III ($\chi^2 = 5.73$)
$p < 0.05$: between II and III ($\chi^2 = 4.02$)

Table 9 : <u>CSF NAB AND VAB IN 101 MS PATIENTS</u>

<u>VIRAL</u> <u>ANTIBODIES</u>	<u>NUCLEIC ANTIBODIES</u>	
	Absence (70)	Presence (31)
Absence (49)	42	7
Presence (52)	28	24

$\chi^2 = 12.04$ ($p < 0.001$)

Table 10 : <u>SERUM IMMUNOGLOBULINS AND CRP IN THE 3 MS GROUPS</u>

Proteins	Group I absence of AB in CSF (n = 42)	Group II VAB only in CSF (n = 28)	Group III VAB and NAB in CSF (n = 31)
IgA (mg/l)	1974 ± 835 *	2069 ± 816	2346 ± 643 *
IgG (mg/l)	13228 ± 2754 *	13374 ± 3196 *	15348 ± 2995 *
IgM (mg/l)	883 ± 333	836 ± 247	1036 ± 289
CRP (59) Absence (44)	17	15	12
Presence (15)	10 *	2 *	3

* significant for $p < 0.05$

Other interesting facts may be observed in the serum :
- IgA and IgG means are significantly elevated in the third group (table 10) in comparison with the first.

Another unexpected fact is the frequent (and abnormal) presence of CRP in blood of patients of the first group, contrary to others.

Table 11 : <u>SERUM NAB AND VAB IN THE 3 GROUPS</u>
(serological dilution and percentage)

Antibodies	Group I absence of AB in CSF (n = 42)	Group II VAB only in CSF (n = 28)	Group III VAB and NAB in CSF (n = 31)
NAB			
DNA	109 ± 26 **	112 ± 21 *	148 ± 44 **
	(4.1 ± 0.8) *	(4.4 ± 0.9)	(4.8 ± 0.8) *
RNA	204 ± 46 *	220 ± 43	248 ± 80 *
	(7.9 ± 1.9)	(8.8 ± 2.3)	(8.1 ± 2.2)
VAB			
Measles	46 ± 31 *	180 ± 142	135 ± 100 *
	(0.4 ± 0.3)	(1.5 ± 1.3)	(0.9 ± 0.7)
Rubella	88 ± 114 *	179 ± 131 *	125 ± 87
	(0.8 ± 1.3)	(1.4 ± 1.1)	(0.8 ± 0.6)

* $p < 0.05$ ** $p < 0.01$

(for each antibody, the first line gives the reciprocal of the serological dilution : the percentage is indicated in parenthesis).

Table 12 : <u>SEX DIFFERENCES IN THE 3 MS GROUPS</u>

SEX	Group I absence of AB in CSF (n = 42)	Group II VAB only in CSF (n = 28)	Group III VAB and NAB in CSF (n = 31)
Men	22	11	8
Women	20	17	23

$p < 0.05$ between   I and III   (χ^2 : 5.20)

I and II + III (χ^2 : 4.14)

I + II and III (χ^2 : 4.05)

- a significant increase of DNA antibodies (in absolute value
  and percentage) is found in the third group, contrasting
  with rather normal values in others (table 11). Measles and
  rubella antibodies were increased in groups II and II compara-
  tively with normal values in group 1.

Clinical data show no differences between the 3 groups (especially no differences between age of the patients, duration of the
disease, clinical stage, and type of course) with an interesting
exception concerning sex repartition (table 12). A clear prevalence of women exists in the third, contrasting with the slight
dominance of men in the first, and a classical repartition (60 %
of women and 40 % of men) in the second. The mean disability grade
is clearly the same in the 3 groups, not influenced by sex, age of
the patient or duration of the disease, but only by the type of
course (table 13) as demonstrated preciously by Fog and al. (1).

CONCLUSION

Different hypotheses may be discussed, from the clinical,
immunological and virological data (table 14).

Table 13 : DISABILITY GRADE AND COURSE ACCORDING TO THE 3 MS GROUPS

Course	Group I absence of AB in CSF (n = 42)	Group II VAB only in CSF (n = 28)	Group III VAB and NAB in CSF (n = 31)
Intermittent (50)	2.6 ± 1.6 **	2.7 ± 1.8 *	2.2 ± 1.4 **
Progressive (51)	4.4 ± 1.8 **	5.0 ± 2.0 *	5.3 ± 2.2 **

* $p < 0.05$

** $p < 0.01$

(S.D. in each group between intermittent and progressive course)

Table 14 : <u>CSF NAB AND VAB IN 101 MS PATIENTS : SUMMARY OF THE DATA</u>

	Group I absence of AB in CSF (n = 42)	Group II VAB only in CSF (n = 28)	Group III VAB and NAB in CSF (n = 31)
SEX	men : 52 % women : 48 %	men : 40 % women : 60 %	men : 26 % women : 74 %
Viral immunity reaction	normal	increased in serum and present in CSF	increased in serum and present in CSF
Nucleic immunity reaction	normal	normal	increased in serum and present in CSF
Blood-CRP	frequent	rare	rare

These 3 MS populations may represent 3 successive steps in the same disease. However, this hypothesis seems very improbable in regards to the same duration of the disease, and the same disability grade in the 3 groups. Another hypothesis suggests 3 events during the same disease, with alternance of silent phase (type I) and viral (type II) or viral and autoimmune reactions (type III). Two other hypotheses may also be proposed :
1) the possibility of a unique agent involved in 3 different immunogenetically determined processes, in connection with sex differences observed. Type I may be supported by an immunological defect, type II correlated with a pure viral processus, and type III conditionned by an immunological hyperreactivity (auto-immunity after viral persistance) as observed in SLE and in female NZB-mice, which develop much more IgG anti DNA than do males (9).
2) the eventuality of different agents for a same disease , with immunosuppressing action in the first type and immunostimulating effect in the third. Obviously the choice of an efficient therapy depend on a confirmed hypothesis.

ACKNOWLEDGEMENTS

This work was supported by INSERM (grant N° 77-5-181-6), DRET (grant n° 78/209) and Association pour le Recherche sur la Sclérose en Plaques. We thank M. Helary and L. Tömpe for technical assistance, and M. Meshaka for the presentation of this manuscript.

REFERENCES

1. Fog, T., Linnemann, F. The course of multiple sclerosis. Acta Neur. Scand. supp. 47, 46 (1970).
2. Schuller, E., Rouques, C., Loridan, M. Das Eiweisspektrum des Liquors im Verlauf der Multiplen Sklerose. Wien Z. Nervenheilk. (Supplt II) 104 (1966).
3. Schuller, E., Lefevre, M., Tompe, L. Electroimmunodiffusion of Alpha-2 M, IgA and IgM in nanogram quantities with a hydroxy-éthylcellulose-agarose gel : application to the un-concentrated CSF. Clin. Chim. Acta, 42-5 (1972).
4. Schuller, E., Allinquant, B. Determination of C-Reactive protein by electroimmunodiffusion in blood and CSF of neuro-logical patients. Europ. Neurol. 9-216 (1973).
5. Schuller, E., Tömpe, L. Electroimmunodiffusion of IgG heavy chains in nanogram quantities with a carboxymethyl-cellulose agarose gel. Clin. Chim. Acta. 54-131 (1974).
6. Schuller, E., Fournier, C., Reboul, J., Cosson, A., Dry, J., Bach, J.F. Determination of DNA antibodies in normal and pathological sera by a new counterimmunoelectrophoresis method. J. Immunol. Methods. II-355 (1976).
7. Schuller, E., Allinquant, B., Delasnerie, N., Reboul, J. De-termination of RNA antibodies in serum and CSF by counter-immunoelectrophoresis. J. Immunol. Methods 14-177 (1977).
8. Schuller, E., Delasnerie, N., Lebon, P. DNA and RNA antibo-dies in serum and CSF of multiple sclerosis and subacute sclerosing panencephalitis patients. J. Neurol. Sci. 37-31-36 (1978).
9. Talal, N. Autoimmunity and lymphoïd malignancy : manifesta-tions of immunoregulatory disequilibrium : in Talal "Auto-immunity genetic, immunologic, virologic and clinical aspects" Academic Press, 184-206 (1977).

PROBLEMS WITH QUALITATIVE CSF ANTIBODY TESTS

L.E. Davis

Department of Neurology, University of New Mexico School
of Medicine and Veterans Administration Hospital, Albu-
querque, NM, U.S.A.

For a cerebrospinal fluid antibody test to be helpful in the
diagnosis of CNS infectious disease, it must be sensitive and
specific enough to detect antibody against the infectious agent
that is produced by plasma cells within the brain or meninges, but
not so sensitive as to detect the minute amounts of antibody entering the CSF following production by plasma cells elsewhere in the
body. The immunoglobulins in normal CSF are believed to originate
from plasma and to enter the CSF primarily via the choroid plexus
(1, 2). These immunoglobulins are chiefly of the IgG class and
are believed to reflect a proportion of the IgG antibodies in the
blood. Therefore, using CSF to diagnose central nervous system
(CNS) infections differs from using blood to diagnose systemic
infections. If a diagnostic test were very sensitive, it could
detect the presence of antibodies in normal CSF that originated
only from plasma and were, therefore, not indicative of a CNS infection. The newer antibody tests (immunofluorescence, radio-
immuno-assay (RIA), and enzyme-linked immunoabsorbent assay (ELISA))
are achieving the sensitivity that allows detection of viral, bacterial, and protozoan antibodies in normal CSF. As these tests
come into wider usage, the interpretation of their results will
be, at best, difficult. In fact, the meaningful use of sensitive
qualitative tests to detect antibodies in the CSF may be impossible because of the uncertainties in interpretation. One such qualitative test that already has these difficulties is the fluores-
cent-treponemal antibody (FTA) test.

The FTA test and the fluorescent-treponemal-antibody-absorp-
tion (FTA-ABS) test on serum have been well studied. Both are
sensitive. The FTA-ABS test is highly specific for an infection

with T. Pallidum and is widely used in the diagnosis of systemic syphilis (3). In 1960 the cerebrospinal fluid-fluorescent treponemal-antibody (CSF-FTA) test was described as an aid in the diagnosis of neurosyphilis (4) and several subsequent studies have repeated this opinion (4, 6, 7, 8, 9). One study even recommended its use as a screening test (10). Since the FTA test is only qualitative, however, it has potential problems when used to study CSF for the diagnosis of neurosyphilis. These problems do not occur in the use of the FTA-ABS test to diagnose systemic syphilis. To diagnose neurosyphilis, the test should detect local CNS T. Pallidum antibody production in the CSF and not plasma antibody that has leaked into the CSF.

Since the FTA test is so sensitive that it can detect small amounts of T. Pallidum antibody, the possibility of false positive results arising from tiny leakage of blood into the CSF during the lumbar puncture exists. It has been estimated that the CSF in 10% of routine lumbar punctures is grossly contaminated with blood (11) and even higher percentage of specimens would be expected to be contaminated with microscopic amounts of blood. Thus, the usefulness of the CSF-FTA test to diagnose neurosyphilis could be seriously impaired if it reacted to small amounts of plasma antibody passing into CSF.

The following study was undertaken to determine how much FTA reactive blood is necessary to convert normal CSF to CSF-FTA reactive (12).

METHOD

Serum from a patient with active syphilis was used to contaminate normal CSF. The study serum had an FTA-ABS reaction of 3+ and a rapid plasma reagin (RPR) titer of 1:256. Normal CSF was obtained from 18 patients who had nonreactive CSF-FTA and serum FTA-ABS tests. The serum was serially diluted to make the following concentrations : 10, 5, 1, 0.5, 0.1, 0.05, 0.01, 0.005 and 0.001 μl serum per 1 ml CSF. The diluted samples were then coded and a CSF-FTA test was performed as described by Duncan and Associates (6) using T. Pallidum antigen and FITC-antihuman globulin conjugate (Laboratory Branch, Center for Disease Control; Atlanta, Georgia). Each sample was analyzed three different times by an experienced technician who was not aware of the final serum concentration in CSF and scored following the guidelines of the Venereal Disease Research Laboratory, USPHS, Atlanta, Georgia (13).

In addition, a 21 year old male was studied with early secondary syphilis. The blood RPR titer was 1:256 and the FTA-ABS test was 4+ reactive. The CSF had 1 lymphocyte/mm^3, 22 mg/dl protein,

78 mg/dl glucose, non-reactive CSF, Venereal Disease Research Laboratory (CSF-VDRL) test, and non-reactive CSF-FTA test. We considered this patient not to have neurosyphilis and wondered how much of his own serum would be required to convert his CSF-FTA test to reactive. The patient's own serum was diluted into his CSF and CSF-FTA tests were performed once on the serial dilutions, as previously described.

RESULTS

The scoring of the three different CSF-FTA tests on each sample were in close agreement and never varied more than a scoring of 1+. The results of the tests are presented in Table 1.

DISCUSSION

These results suggest that the CSF-FTA test is very sensitive to small amounts of blood contamination. The high titered serum and serum from the patient with secondary syphilis converted the CSF-FTA test to reactive with the equivalent of only 0.8 µl and 0.008 µl of blood per ml of CSF. Both amounts of blood contamination are below the level of detection by visual inspection (14). In the latter situation, the CSF-FTA test would have become falsely positive with a CSF cell count of only 42 RBS/mm^3.

The possibility of a false positive CSF-FTA test on the basis of plasma transudation into the CSF also exists. Although the blood-brain-CSF barrier is normally quite impermeable to immunoglobulins, experimental studies have shown opening of this barrier during seizures, (15, 16) hepatic coma, (17) and blood osmotic changes (18).

TABLE 1

MINIMAL AMOUNT OF FTA-ABS REACTIVE BLOOD IN 1 ML OF

CSF THAT WILL RESULT IN REACTIVE CSF-FTA TEST

	High titered FTA + serum	Secondary syphilis patient's serum in his own CSF	
Amount of serum *	0.5 µl	0.005	µl
Amount of blood *	0.83 µl	0.0083	µl
Amount of protein *	1.5 mg	0.015	mg
Number of RBC/mm^3 *	4,200 RBC	42	RBC

* Based on a red cell count of 5 x 10^6 RBC/mm^3

Diseases such as peripheral neuropathy, meningitis, uremia, etc., commonly are associated with elevated lumbar CSF protein levels which may in part be due to plasma transudation into the CSF. In this study, reactive CSF-FTA tests occurred when the protein in normal CSF was elevated to a total of 190 mg/dl by addition of serum. However, the CSF in the patient with secondary syphilis became CSF-FTA reactive when the protein was raised from 22 mg/dl to 23.5 mg/dl. Had this patient had another cause to elevate his CSF protein and immunoglobulin levels, his CSF-FTA test might well have given a false positive reaction.

Qualitative antibody tests appear to have very limited usefulness in testing CSF. Since there are no known CNS infections in which antibody appears exclusively in the CSF, qualitative tests do not permit a distinction between CSF antibody which originated from plasma or from both plasma and the CNS. Quantitative tests, however, do allow methods of determining whether local CNS antibody production has occurred. The published methods generally compare CSF and serum antibody titers for a series of different antibodies (19, 20, 21, 22) or compare the CSF/serum ratios of IgG or albumin (23, 24, 25). These methods also minimize the chances of yielding false positive results, should there be leakage of blood or plasma into the CSF.

There are now several quantitative tests to detect T. Pallidum antibodies (T. Pallidum hemagglutination test (26), the microhemagglutination test for T. Pallidum, (27) and the ELISA-TP test (28)). These methods could be adapted to test CSF and they should avoid many of the potential problems inherent in the CSF-FTA test for the diagnosis of neurosyphilis.

REFERENCES

1. Cutter, P.W.P., Watters, G.V., Hammerstad, J.P. : The origin and turnover rates of cerebrospinal fluid albumin and gamma-globulin in man. J. Neurol. Sci. 10 : 259-268, 1970.
2. Rosenthal, F.D., Soothill, J.F. : An immunochemical study of proteins in cerebrospinal fluid. J. Neurol. Neurosurg. Psychiat. 25 : 177-181, 1962.
3. Jaffe, H.W. : The Laboratory diagnosis of syphilis : New concepts. Ann. Int. Med. 83 : 846-850, 1975.
4. Harris, A., Bossak, H.M., Deacon, W.E. et al. : Comparison of the fluorescent treponemal antibody test with other tests for syphilis on cerebrospinal fluids. Brit. J. Vener. Dis. 36 : 178-180, 1960.

6. Duncan, W.P., Jenkins, T.W., Parkam, C.E. : Fluorescent treponemal antibody-cerebrospinal fluid (FTA-CSF) test. A provisio-
nal technique. Brit. J. Vener. Dis. 48: 97-101, 1972.
7. Wilkinson, A.E. : Fluorescent treponemal antibody tests on cerebrospinal fluid. Brit. J. Vener. Dis. 49 : 346-349, 1973.
8. Garner M.J., Bachhouse, J.L.: Fluorescent treponemal antibody
tests on cerebrospinal fluid. Brit. J. Vener. Dis. 47:356-358,
1971.
9. Duncan, W.P., Kuhn, V.S.F.: Reactivity of treponemal and non-
treponemal tests with cerebrospinal fluid from syphilitic chim-
panzees. J. Infect. Dis. 125:61-65, 1972.
10. Escobar, M.R., Dalton, H.P., Allison, M.J.: Fluorescent antibody tests for syphilis using cerebrospinal fluid : Clinical
correlation in 150 cases. Am. J. Clin. Pathol. 53:886-890,
1970.
11. Solomon, P. : The diagnosis in spinal fluid contaminated by
blood : The bloody tap. New Eng. J. Med. 212:55-57, 1935.
12. Davis, L.E., Sperry, S.: The CSF-FTA test and the significance of blood contamination, (in preparation).
13. Venereal Disease Research Laboratory : Manual of test for
syphilis - 1969. Public Health Service Publication ≠ 411,
U.S. Government Printing Office, Washington D.C., 1969.
14. Izzat, N.N., Bartruff, J.K., Glicksman, J.M. et al. : Validity of the VDRL test on cerebrospinal fluid contaminated by
blood. Brit. J. Vener. Dis. 47:162-164, 1971.
15. Siemes, H., Siegert, M., Hanefeld, F. : Febrile convulsions
and bloodcerebrospinal fluid barrier. Epilepsia 19:57-66,
1978.
16. Lorenzo, A.V., Shirahinge, I., Liang, M. et al.: Temporary
alteration of cerebrovascular permeability to plasma protein
during drug-induced seizures. Am. J. Physiol. 223: 268-277,
1972.
17. Livingstone, A.S., Potvin, M., Goresky, C.A.et al.: Changes
in the blood-brain barrier in hepatic coma after hepatectomy
in the rat. Gastroenterology 72:697-704, 1974.
18. Hicks, J.T., Albrecht, P., Rapoport, S.I.: Entry of neutralizing antibody to measles into brain and cerebrospinal fluid
of immunized monkeys after osmotic opening of the blood-brain
barrier. Exp. Neurol. 53:768-779, 1976.
19. Norrby, E., Link, H., Olsson, J.: Comparison of antibodies
against different viruses in cerebrospinal fluid and serum
samples from patients with multiple sclerosis. Infect & Immun. 10:688-694, 1974.
20. Cappel, R., Thiry, L., Clinet, G.: Viral antibodies in the
CSF after acute CNS infections. Arch. Neurol. 32:629-631,
1975.
21. Deibel, R., Schryver, G.D.: Viral antibody in the cerebrospinal fluid of patients with acute central nervous system infections. J. Clin. Microbiol. 3:397-401, 1976.

22. Mac Callum, F.O., Chinn, I.J., Gostling, J.V.T.: Antibodies
    to Herpes simplex virus in the cerebrospinal fluid of patients
    with herpetic encephalitis. J. Med. Microbiol. 7:325-331,
    1974.
23. Ganrat, K., Laurell, C.: Measurement of IgG and albumin con-
    tent of cerebrospinal fluid, and its interpretation. Clin.
    Chem. 20:571-573, 1974.
24. Roberto-Thomson, P.J., Esiri, M.M., Young, A.C.et al.: Cere-
    brospinal fluid immunoglobulin quotients. Kappa/lambda ratios,
    and viral antibody titers in neurological disease. J. Clin.
    Path. 29:1105-1115, 1976.
25. Tourtellotte, W.: On cerebrospinal fluid immunoglobulin-G
    (IgG) quotients in multiple sclerosis and other diseases. J.
    Neurol. Sci. 10:279-304, 1970.
26. Robertson, D.H.H., McMillan, A., Young, H. et al.: Clinical
    value of the treponema pallidum haemagglutination test. Brit.
    J. Vener. 51:79-82, 1975.
27. Cox, P.M., Logan, L.C., Norins, L.C.: Automated quantitative
    microhemagglutination assay for treponema pallidum antibodies.
    Appl. Microbiol. 18: 485-489, 1969.
28. Veldkamp, J., Visser, A.M.: Application of the enzyme-linked
    immunosorbent assay (ELISA) in the serodiagnosis of syphilis.
    Brit. J. Vener. Dis. 51:227-231, 1975.

IMMUNOCYTOLOGICAL CSF ALTERATIONS AND BRAIN TUMORS

H. Wiethölter

Institute of Brain Research, University of Tübingen,
Tübingen, F.R.Germany

The presence of a cell-mediated immune response in connection
with brain tumors is no longer a matter of speculation (2, 5, 9).
The histomorphological criteria are round cell infiltrates in
primary and secondary brain tumors (6, 7, 11). A lymphocytic reaction therefore was also to be expected in the context of the cytological evaluation of cerebrospinal fluid (CSF).

Our investigation therefore ought to confirm the suspicion
that lymphocytic reactions in the CSF may occur in conjunction
with brain tumors (cf. 8). The following questions arose in this
context :
1. What is the frequency of occurrence for lymphocytic reactions
   in the CSF in connection with brain tumors?
2. Do tumors accompanied by a lymphocytic reaction in the CSF
   have any histomorphological characteristics?
3. How should such lymphocytic reactions in the CSF occurring in
   conjunction with brain tumors be interpreted?

Those CSF specimens were selected for evaluation out of
15,400 specimens collected between 1969 and 1976 for which histologic specimens of operated brain tumors were available. Specimens
from 202 patients were acquired in this way. Positive demonstration of tumor cells was possible in 18 cases (8.9%). The cell
picture was normal in 71 cases (35.0%). A monocytoid reaction
was described 73 times (36.1%). A lymphocytic and/or lymphomono-
cytic reaction was demonstrable in 40 of the patients (19.8%).
During the course of routine diagnostic procedures, this immuno-
reaction was interpreted as a bacterial meningitis or meningoencephalitis in 16 cases (Fig. 1), even though the lack of plasma cells

271

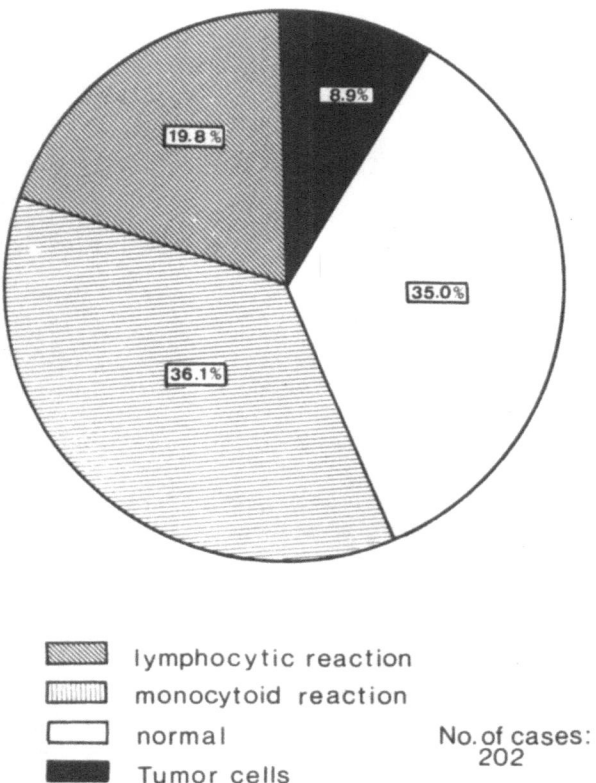

lymphocytic reaction
monocytoid reaction
normal   No. of cases:
Tumor cells   202

Fig. 1. CSF reactions with brain tumors

together with the appearance of stimulated round cells was a typical
feature of this type of reaction.

    Correlation of lymphocytic reaction in the CSF with various
types of tumors showed that a lymphocytic reaction was present in
50% of the glioblastomas (cf. 3) but only 24.1% of the meningiomas.
On the other hand, this investigation revealed no signs of an im-
munoreactive event with secondary brain tumors (Fig. 2); lymphocytic reactions in such CSF however are observed relatively frequent
as we know from experience.

    This amazingly high frequency of lymphocytic reactions led
us to question whether this reaction was dependent on histomorphological or local factors. Histologic sections from 40 tumor specimens with confirmed lymphocytic reactions in the CSF therefore
were compared with 40 other tumor specimens (control group) for

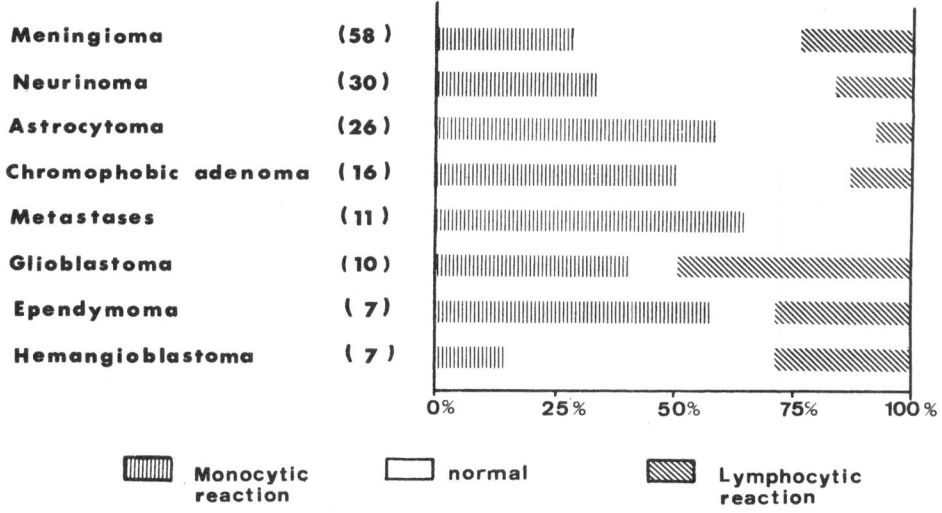

Fig. 2. Cytological reactions in CSF with histologically verified brain tumors

which a monocytoid reaction or a normal CSF cell picture had been established. The following criteria were noted :
1. Localization of tumor;
2. Proximity of tumor to CSF space;
3. Extent of vascularization;
4. Necrosis in tumor;
5. Histological demonstration of lymphocytic infiltrate in the section.

No definite correlation could be **established** concerning the localization of the tumor and its proximity to the CSF space, although pleocytosis in association with tumors located close to the CSF space was mentioned repeatedly (4). The findings however were different when the last three criteria were compared in the two groups of tumors.

The histomorphologic findings for both groups of tumors are presented in Fig. 3. Lymphocytic infiltrate was demonstrated in 20 of the tumors (50%) that were accompanied by a lymphocytic reaction in the CSF and in only 12 tumors of the control group. Comparison of the frequency of necrosis (22 and 9) and the extend of vascularity (19 and 9) revealed distinct differences. As might be expected, two or more of these criteria were observed more frequently in the first group of tumors than in the control group. A lympho-

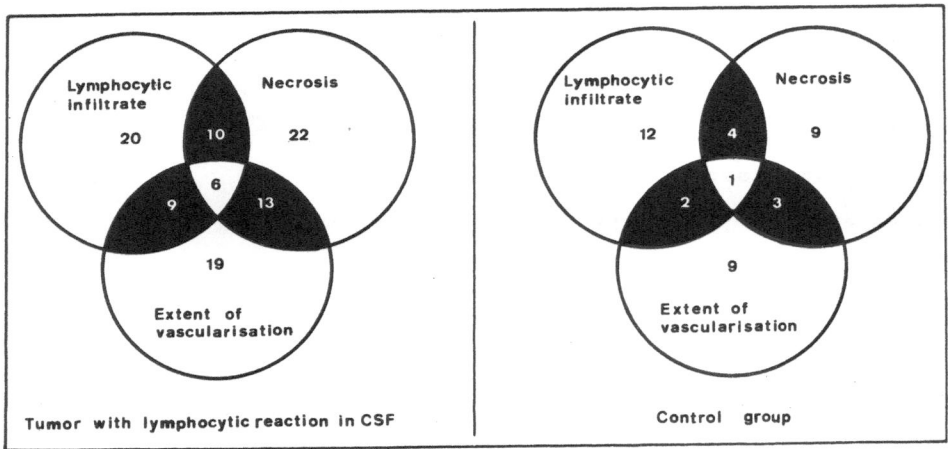

Fig. 3. Histomorphologic criteria in brain tumors

cytic infiltration together with necrosis was demonstrated in
10 cases in the first group, but only 4 cases in the control group.
The differences between the two groups tend to indicate that a
lymphocytic reaction of the CSF occurs more frequently in tumors
with necrosis and pronounced vascularization. As might be expected, a lymphocytic reaction in the tumor itself is more often
accompanied by a lymphocytic reaction in the CSF.

Which interpretation permits the determination of a lymphocytic reaction in the CSF with brain tumors and which antigens
induce it·: tumor-specific or non tumor-specific antigens? A tumor-specific immune response is always mentioned when lymphocytic,
perivascular or diffuse infiltrations are observed in tumors (1, 6).
These infiltrations, as a cell-mediated immunity to tumors, consist
primarily of subpopulations of T lymphocytes. Stavrou and coworkers (10) were able to establish that a high percentage of T
lymphocytes with gliomas, for example, is indicative of tumor-specific and/or tumor-associated antigens.

The absence of plasma cells (B lymphocyte series) in the CSF
cell pictures we examined may, to a certain extent, allow the
interpretation of lymphocytic reactions in the CSF as cell-mediated immune responses. The lymphocytic infiltration and the reaction in the CSF were not just limited to gliomas; they were also
demonstrated to a slight degree with meningiomas, ependymomas,
angioblastomas, and neurinomas (cf.2).

On the other hand, the correlation of necrosis and pronounced vascularization in the tumor with a lymphocytic reaction in the CSF at least indicates that other non tumor-specific antigens (e.g., products of decomposition) may also be responsible for the CSF reaction. The lymphocytic reaction frequently observed following neurosurgical procedures should also be interpreted accordingly. As might be expected, plasma cells are often demonstrable in this context.

In summary, it may be stated that:
1. lymphocytic reactions in the CSF were observed relatively frequently (approximately 20%) in connection with brain tumors. The possibility of such a lymphocytic reaction ought to be considered in the differential diagnosis from abacterial meningitis.
2. The lymphocytic CSF reaction may be considered to a certain extent, as a cell-mediated immune response to tumor antigens.

REFERENCES

1. Di Lorenzo, N., Palma, L., Nicole, S.: Lymphocytic infiltration in long-survival glioblastomas : possible host's resistance. Acta Neurochir. 39, 27-33 (1977).
2. Levy, N.L., Mahaley, M.S., Day, E.D.: In vitro demonstration of cell-mediated immunity to human brain tumors. Cancer Res. 32, 477-482 (1972).
3. Maunoury, R., Vedrenne, C., Constans, J.P.: Infiltrations lymphocytaires dans les gliomes humains. Neurochirurgie 3, 213-222 (1975).
4. Patzold, U., Engelhardt, P., Haller, P.: Liquorbefunde bei Hirngeschwülsten. Nervenarzt 46, 183-188 (1975).
5. Pees, H.W., Seidel, B.: Cell mediated immune response of patients with meningiomas defined in vitro by a (3 H) proline microtoxicity test. Clin. exp. Immunol. 24, 310-316 (1976).
6. Ridley, A., Cacanagh, J.B.: Lymphocytic infiltration in gliomas : evidence of possible host resistance. Brain 94, 117-124 (1971).
7. Schiffer, D., Croveri, G., Pautasso, C.: Frequenza e significato degli infiltrati linfo-plasmacellulari nei gliom umani. Tumori 60, 177-184 (1974).
8. Seyfeddinipur, N., Häring-Krämer, C.: Hirntumoren mit meningo-enzephalitischer Verlaufsform. Diagnostik 6, 465-469 (1973).
9. Shimizu, T., Kito, K.L., Yamazaki, N. et al.: Immunological investigation of brain tumor patients. Neurol. Med. Chir. (Tokyo) 1611, 337-347 (1976).
10. Stavrou, D., Anzil, A.P., Wiedenbach, W., Rodt, H.: Immunofluorescence study of lymphocytic infiltration in gliomas. Neurol. Sci. 33, 275-282 (1977).
11. Takeuchi, J., Barnard, R.O.: Perivascular lymphocytic cuffing in astrocytomas. Acta Neuropath. (Berl.) 35, 265-271 (1976).

STUDY OF HUMORAL IMMUNITY IN CEREBROSPINAL FLUID OF PATIENTS INFECTED WITH SCHISTOSOMIASIS

M.El-Sawy, H.Abaza, N.Hammouda, Y.El-Gohary and M.El-Fatatry

Faculty of Medicine, University of Alexandria, Egypt

Schistosoma ova deposited in the nervous system initiate a granulomatous reaction forming a space occupying lesion leading to pressure atrophy and degeneration of the nerve cells (1). Ghazi (2) demonstrated an incidence varying from 26.7 % to 71.09 %.

Clinically neurological manifestations may be asymptomatic. Severe neurological manifestations such as sensory and vasomotor disturbances, epilepsy and Korsakoff psychosis, meningitis (3) and transverse myelitis (4) may occur.

The present work aims at assessment of the immunological reactions and immunoglobulin patterns in serum and C.S.F. in hepatosplenic schistosomiasis with and without neurological symptoms.

MATERIAL AND METHODS

The present study was conducted on 22 cases suffering from active Schistosoma mansoni and/or haematobium infection and six control subjects. Patients were divided into three groups :
- Group 1. : 6 cases, with early hepatosplenic schistosomiasis.
- Group 2. : 10 cases, with advanced hepatosplenic schistosomiasis having portocaval collaterals and/or portosystemic encephalopathy.
- Group 3. : 6 cases, with active schistosomiasis having nonspecific neurological disturbances in the form of gradual compression with sensory level not related to a special disease entity.

Fasting serum and C.S.F. specimens were taken on which circumoval precipitin test (COP) by method of Shoeb et al. (5); indirect haemagglutination test, IHA (Behring Work) and immunoglobulins (6) were done.

RESULTS

Table 1 : illustrates results of COP, IHA tests and immunoglobulins levels in various groups studies.

TABLE 1

COP, IHA tests and immunoglobulins in serum and CSF in schistosomiasis (Mean $\pm$ S.D.)

Group	COP % positive		IHA % positive		IgA mg %		Ig G mg %		IgM mg %	
	serum	CSF	serum	CSF	serum	CSF	serum	CSF	serum	CSF
controls	–	–	–	–	120 ±14.8	1.04 ±0.64	925 ±74.2	1.70 ±0.62	203 ±77.5	0
Grp 1	50	16.7	100	16.7	186 ±43.9	1.61 ±0.76	786 ±301.4	6.12 ±4.12	324 ±132.4	0.27 ±0.10
Grp 2	50	10	100	20	259 ± 183	0.99 ±0.58	1767 ± 959	5.25 ±51.3	486 ±45.6	2.19 ±1.64
Grp 3	20	0	80	0	1096 ± 678	0.7 ±0.29	1341 ± 927	0	640 ± 374	0.24 ±0.12

DISCUSSION

Our results showed that COP and IHA tests were found to be simultaneously positive in serum and CSF of 45 % of all groups collectively, whereas serum IHA alone was positive in 95 % of cases. The COP was simultaneously positive in serum and CSF in 9 % of cases whereas IHA test was positive in serum and CSF in 14 %. Such findings point to less sensitivity of COP than IHA test in diagnosis of schistosomiasis. Both tests, however, were negative in CSF of cases with neurological manifestations.

Normally CSF does not contain IgM (7) since this type of immunoglobulins has a high molecular weight and cannot traverse the blood brain barrier. The presence of IgM and high levels of IgG and IgA suggests the probable presence of local formation of specific antibodies in the nervous system initiated by cerebrospinal invasion.

The fact that IHA test is positive in CSF suggests the presence of antiworm antibodies, since the red cells used in the test are sensitized by the adult worm antigen. Ghazy (2) demonstrated invasion of worms to CNS through migration of worms into the valveless vertebral venous system (8).

It seems that the positive reaction of these tests and the high immunoglobulin levels depend rather on the presence of a possible shunt between the portal and vertebral venous systems. In support of such view is the presence of high concentration of immunoglobulins in CSF of subjects with portal hypertension in quantities proportional to those present in the serum of the same patients.

REFERENCES

1. Bayoumi, M.L. (1939) : Bilharzial myelitis. J. Egypt. Med. Ass., 8 : 457.
2. Ghazy, A.A. (1974) : Studies on the changes in the lumbo-sacral spinal cord in schistosomal infection. M.D. Thesis Tanta Fac. Med. Egypt.
3. Day, H.B., and Kenawy, M.R. (1936) : A case of bilharzial myelitis : Trans. Roy. Soc. Trop. Med. Hyg., 30 : 223.
4. Lyra A. (1945) : An enquiry into the ectopic lesions in schistosomiasis. Amer. J. Trop. Med., 28 : 175.
5. Shoeb, S., Basmy, K., Kaseeb, N. and El-Ghonemy, M. (1967) : The value of the circumoval precipitin test : J. Egypt. Med. Ass. 50 : 564.
6. Mancini, G., Carbonara, A.O. and Heremans, J.F. (1965) : Immunochemical quantitation of antigens by single immunodiffusion. Immunochemistry 2, 235.
7. Riddoch, D. and Thompson, R.A. (1970) : Immunoglobulin levels in CSF, Br. Med. J. 1 : 396.
8. Mansour, S.E. (1966) : Observations on the relation between the portal and vertebral venous system in portal hypertension. Egypt. Orth. J. 1 : 54.

RESTRICTED HETEROGENEITY OF THE IgG IN NEUROLOGY

A. Lowenthal

Born-Bunge Foundation, Department of Neurochemistry,
U.I.A., Wilrijk, Belgium

Restricted heterogeneity of the cerebrospinal fluid (CSF)
γ globulins was discovered through the use of agar gel electrophoresis. That discovery came at the end of an extensive procedure
which was technical as well as theoretical. Many problems had
to be tackled, only some were solved. First, we shall refer to
the technical problems, then to the neurological diseases in
which restricted heterogeneity is found, then deal with physiopathological problems and finally make a suggestion regarding
terminology.

Apart from the classic distinction made between albumin and
globulin, electrophoresis allowed to identify three globulins,
α , β , and γ . Electrophoresis on paper revealed in CSF a
prealbumin and a predominance of the β globulins. The differences between the CSF electropherogram and that of the serum
immediately gave rise to a number of questions :

1) do the fractions described really all exist or does electrophoresis produce artefacts, particularly in the case of CSF
   which has to be concentrated? Does electrophoresis and
   concentration lead to the loss of certain fractions?

2) what causes the qualitative and quantitative differences in
   CSF observed in pathological conditions? In pathological CSF,
   anomalies are noted in the α region or in the γ region.
   The distinction can be done between a normal pherogram, a
   pherogram of the α type, a pherogram of the γ type and a
   serum type like pherogram. These modifications can be associated with increases of total protein. Colloidal reactions
   employed up to 1950, made it possible to distinguish different
   types of anomalies in the albumin/globulin ratio. Whilst the

colloidal reaction made it possible to distinguish neurosyphilis from multiple sclerosis (MS), paper electrophoresis did
not, and yielded only one and the same information : increase
of γ globulins in both diseases. In our hands, since 1957,
electrophoresis on agar gel revealed a fractionation of the
γ globulins, later called "oligoclonal reaction".

3) thus we arrive at the third and last question : how can we
   explain these modifications in the CSF? Are they the result
   of serum modifications and therefore of a general modification?
   Could we rather contemplate more specific modifications which
   arise in some organ, for example the central nervous system?
   Can we maintain and prove that some CSF proteins, and particularly some γ globulins, are synthetized in the central nervous system? These various questions will be discussed.

THE TECHNICAL PROBLEM

At the first meeting devoted to the study of CSF protein
electrophoresis at Hamburg in 1953, these problems were already
discussed, for example the study of CSF protein concentration.
It can be said that the answers have yet to be found. These
problems will only be resolved when a method of study has been
found for CSF proteins without prior concentration. This may
be possible with Kerenyi's (1) method using silver staining.
The pherograms obtained by this method confirm the major characteristics obtained by agar gel electrophoresis for pre-concentra-
ted CSF. Kerenyi's method is certainly a method for the future.
It is still technically difficult. A study on a larger scale is
advised. Isofocalization, as applied by Delmotte (2) points in
the same direction, although more sensitive, it is less direct
than Kerenyi's method. Other methods show indirectly modifications which were not shown by paper electrophoresis : immunoelectrophoresis confirms that the fractionation of γ globulins,
shown by electrophoresis in agar gel, is not an artefact.

We want to point out that only techniques that show fractionation of γ globulins, this means oligoclonal reaction or restricted heterogeneity of γ globulins, are the only adviced. Glasner's
(3) method can be used to study non concentrated CSF but, until
now could not be used to show in a direct way the oligoclonal
reaction. Glasner is currently trying to improve his technique.

MODIFICATION OF γ GLOBULINS IN DISEASES

The second problem to consider is the fact that in so many
different diseases modifications of the γ globulins are apparent.
This has been a subject of discussion ever since CSF proteins
have been studied by electrophoresis on paper, and even before.

As early as 1942, Kabat (4) proved, by free electrophoresis, that the CSF γ globulins increase in myeloma, neurosyphilis and multiple sclerosis. These are physiopathologically very different diseases.

Electrophoresis on paper, already enabled to ascertain that γ globulins could increase, concurrently with the total protein or in an isolated way as in MS and SSPE. The first type of modification could be observed in meningitis. Attempts have been made to obtain more precise information regarding these anomalies by the study of glucidograms; all they showed, was that there could be differences in the field of γ globulins. To our knowledge, nothing more was added, by lipidograms, whilst enzymograms of LDH for example, revealed the existence of other fractions than those one could see by ordinary electrophoresis.

In fact, it was the use of agar gel electrophoresis that enabled us (5) to take a big step forward. In a series of articles and papers published from our laboratory, we showed in the years 1955 to 1961, that there are two types of patterns at the γ globulin level : a diffuse increase of γ globulins of the serum type, and an increase with fractionation. In the first case, there is nearly always an increase of total proteins and of the absolute concentration of γ globulins. In the second case, total proteins may be normal or increased and the relative concentration of the γ globulins is increased or normal. Electrophoresis in agarose and in cellulose acetate confirm these results but are technically less valid. Immunoelectrophoresis through anomalies of the IgG curve enables to reach similar conclusions. The increase of the γ globulins of the serum type (serum like) is found in bacterial meningitis, cerebral tumours, diabetes, Buillain-Barré syndrome, myxoedema.... Moreover in a few cases of Guillain-Barré's syndrome, fractionation of the γ globulins has also been reported. The serum like type seems to be due to an increase in the permeability of the hemato-encephalic barrier. We shall not elaborate on this.

Fractionation of the γ globulins, or rather of the IgG's, can be seen in cases where the serum pherogram remains normal as in multiple sclerosis, neurosyphilis, chronic meningitis, although in some cases of multiple sclerosis fractionation of the serum may also be found (fig. 1).

Fractionation of the CSF IgG's is seen in other diseases concomitantly with the fractionation of the serum γ globulins: in SSPE, in tripanosomiasis, in necrotic encephalitis, in collage. nosis and in myelomas, that is to say in infectious chronic diseases, in chronic and acute viral nervous system diseases, in diseases related to neoplasm or in acute immune processes.

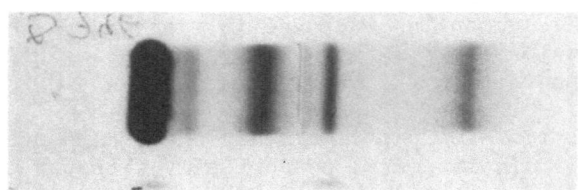

Fig. 1

We have been able to observe this oligoclonal reaction in
ataxia telangiectasia in almost experimental conditions (6) : in
this disease patients are treated by intramuscular injections of
γ globulins for an IgA deficiency, and one notices in the CSF
and in the serum a fractionation of γ globulins, similar to
the one observed in SSPE or in MS.

A similar fractionation has been observed in animals suffering from sheep's visna (7) or dog's distemper. Finally, in
experimental hyperimmunization, similar pictures are seen in the
serum (8). Up to now, we do not know whether CSF has ever been
examined in experimental hyperimmunisation.

Fractionation of the IgG's in CSF is thus not specific of
a disease state. This fractionation appears more frequently in
CSF as in serum. One can assume that in collagenosis or myeloma,
or in ataxia telangiectasia, the fractionation is due to a generalized disorder of the protein metabolism. What must we think
of diseases like SSPE or necrotic encephalitis which are essentially, if not exclusively neurological and where the oligoclonal
reaction is seen in the serum and in CSF? Is there question of
generalized anomalies? Can one go as far as assuming that serum
anomalies reflect what is happening in the central nervous system
and that some serum proteins originate in the central nervous
system? And above all, what can we think of multiple sclerosis
or neurosyphilis, where the CSF anomaly is not always accompanied
by serum modifications? Can the absence of serum anomalies be
put down to technical reasons, for example are these serum
anomalies not quantitatively sufficiently pronounced to be visible?
Above all we wish to underline the fact that fractionation of
immunoglobulins is found in acute and chronic, viral or bacterial,
meningeal or encephalitic diseases. We would like to state that
the anomalies of the IgG's , are in trypanosomiasis and perhaps
certain cases of MS, associated with anomalies of the IgM :
quantitative analysis did show only exceptionally in CSF other
immunoglobulins than the IgG. Sometimes one finds IgM.

DEFINITION OF THE OLIGOCLONAL REACTION

The third problem to consider is the definition of the oli-goclonal reaction. When we saw the fractionation of γ globulins for the first time, we only described it. Others put different labels on it. Some tried to define their nature. Link (11) tried to find whether the ration κ/λ was modified in CSF containing fractionated γ globulins. In other words he tried to find whether homogeneous antibodies were present in these fluids as observed in myeloma. This problem has been tackled in different laboratories : one cannot say that only one type of light chain prevails in these CSF. They are mostly κ , sometimes λ light chains. Vandvik's research reached the same conclusion with his elegant cross immunoelectrophoresis technique; this was demonstrated to be true for MS as well as for SSPE (12). In fact it is only the study of the aminoacid sequence of the variable portion of the SSPE serum immunoglobulins, a study only performed on one fraction until now, but in 7 patients already, that leads to believe that we are dealing with homogeneous antibodies (9). This is a major indication. Vandvik, by affirming that the oligoclonal fractions are IgG_1, moves in the same direction (13).

The presence of 2 to 7 fractions of IgG in the CSF or the serum remains to be solved. We have to add that in SSPE the different antibody fractions are probably measles antibodies as shown by us through isolation and also by Vandvik's qualitative analysis of different fractions. The complexity of the fractionation could also reflect the complexity of the viral antigens which induce those reactions.

WHERE DO THESE ANTIBODIES ORIGINATE ?

After sophisticated calculations, many authors affirm that these IgG originate in the central nervous system or, at least, are formed intrathecally. This is supported by the demonstration, with immuno-histochemical methods, of the presence of specific antibodies in sections of MS and SSPE brains (10). With these methods, antibodies are found in glial cells which might be lymphocytes which moved into the central nervous system. Is it then an immunological phenomenon of the nervous tissue? Can this phenomenon explain the appearance of fractionated γ globulins, hence from the same antibodies in SSPE serum? Even more so, because we know that in myeloma and ataxia telangiectasia, treated with parenteral γ globulins, the γ globulins in CSF and in serum are fractionated. In these cases we are probably dealing with the passage of fractionated IgG from the serum to the CSF. One should also mention here that in myasthenia gravis, fractionated IgG in the CSF were described.

RELATIONSHIP BETWEEN FRACTIONING OF IgG AND NEUROLOGICAL PHENOMENA

A last physiopathological problem to be dealt with, is the relationship between the fractionation of the IgG and the neurological phenomena. It has often been mentioned that there is a particular sensitivity of the central nervous system to the immunological phenomena, for example in encephalitis due to eruptive fevers. Can one believe, however, that the hyperimmunisation noted in SSPE, affects the central nervous system? Nothing of that kind has been noted in experimental hyperimmunisation in animals. It is possible that these animals have not been long enough under observation.

TERMINOLOGY

To conclude, we wish to discuss the terminology. First, one talked only of the increase of the γ globulins as shown by electrophoresis in the CSF of some diseases. We have shown that some of these increases are due to a fractionation of γ globulins, later identified as IgG's. By comparison with myeloma, one called at one time the fractions M-components. The first time we showed pherograms of SSPE serum to internists, they asked whether they were not myelomas. Finally one talked of oligoclonal reaction. The few examinations of immunoglobulins formed by CSF lymphocytes in culture, could also show the oligoclonal fractionation. No formal proof of an oligo or monoclonal synthesis was given until now. So far the comparison with experimental hyperimmunisation in animals and ataxia telangiectasia seems to us much more valid. The serum pherograms are similar in SSPE, experimental hyperimmunisation and ataxia-telangiectasia. One can generally talk of 2 predominant fractions and 5 associated ones. In SSPE and experimental hyperimmunisation, the antibodies content is greatly increased in the serum. The serum fractions can be, in both cases, at least partly, precipitated by the antigens. Finally the sequence of the variable region of the heavy and light chains, shows that in both cases (9), in experimental hyperimmunisation and in SSPE, we are dealing with homogeneous antibodies. For these reasons we think that we have, at least for SSPE, and envisage it for other diseases, to refer to a hyperimmune reaction leading to the formation of homogeneous IgG or IgG of restricted heterogeneity, as mentioned in the experimental work. This means that in diseases where this phenomenon is observed in CSF and, above all in those where it is observed in serum and in CSF, the immunological reaction is strong perhaps, either through intense or repeated or persistant stimulations. One wonders if this hyperimmunisation only develops in an abnormal genetic field. Some have looked for these genetic anomalies in MS and SSPE or in experimental diseases. It is certain that the immunological reaction observed in SSPE, that

is to say the hyperimmunisation observed in this disease, is
not a normal one. The presence in the CSF of IgG fragments, κ
and λ free chains, points in this direction. To our knowledge
there has been no quantitative determination made of the free
κ or λ chains or of other fragments of IgG molecules in
experimental hyperimmunisation.

We do not regard calling the reaction leading to the
formation of fractionated immunoglobulins, restricted heterogeneity, a simple verbal formula. We wonder wether it has not
also a physiological significance. The restricted heterogeneity
of the IgG is observed in many neurological diseases and points
to the existence of an hyperimmunisation process. The physiopathological meaning of this process has to be discussed. The
knowledge of this hyperimmunisation concept can assist us to
tackle the study of MS and SSPE, by new methods inspired by
experimental immunology. Amongst other approaches we could
conjecture that if we isolated the specific antibodies in these
diseases, what is technically possible, could we not trace the
antigen which in MS is still unknown? The discovery of factors
which can control or influence experimental hyperimmunisation
could, on the other hand, open the door to therapeutic trials
in these diseases, and more particularly in MS.

CONCLUSIONS

1. the fractionation of the CSF γ globulins, we described 20
   years ago, is not specific of a disease, but of a hyperimmune
   process,
2. this hyperimmunization leads to restricted heterogeneity of
   the IgG, or synthesis of homogeneous antibodies. Owing to
   amino-acid sequence of high variable region of the IgG's light
   and heavy chains such homogeneous antibodies have been found
   in SSPE serum,
3. restricted heterogeneity of the IgG's could be a pathological
   immune reaction, related perhaps to a genetic background,
4. restricted heterogeneity was first seen in the CSF and is
   very often associated with neurological disorders,
5. central nervous system could be more sensitive to this immunological reaction, than other tissues.

ACKNOWLEDGEMENT

This study has been supported by grants from the Belgian
National Fund for Medical Scientific Research (grant nr 30033),
the Belgian Ministry of Education and Culture and the "Universitaire Instelling Antwerpen".

REFERENCES

1. Kerenyi, L. and Pallyas F. A highly sensitive method for
   demonstrating proteins in electrophoretic, immuno-electropho-
   retic and immunodiffusion preparation. Clin. Chim. Acta 38,
   465, 1972.

2. Delmotte, P. Comparative results of agar electrophoresis and
   isoelectric focusing examination of the γ globulins of the
   cerebrospinal fluid. Acta Neurol. Belg. 72, 226, 1972.

3. Glasner, H. Die diagnostische Bedeutung der Mikrozonenelektro-
   phorese des nicht eingeengten Liquor cerebrospinalis. Dtsch.
   med. Wschr. 103, 1173, 1978.

4. Kabat, E.A., Landow, H. and Moore, D.H. Cerebrospinal Fluid
   Electrophoresis. Proc. Soc. exp. Biol. 49, 260, 1942.
   Kabat, E.A., Moore, D.H. and Landow, H. Electrophoretic
   study of proteins in CSF and their relationship to the serum
   proteins. J. Clin. Invest. 21, 7571, 1942.

5. Karcher, D., van Sande, M. and Lowenthal, A. Microelectrophoresis in agar gel of the proteins of the cerebrospinal
   fluid and central nervous system. J. Neurochem. 4, 135, 1959.

6. Lowenthal, A. The problem of cerebrospinal studies in multiple
   sclerosis. In Multiple Sclerosis, a clinical conspectus.
   Ed. E.J. Field, MTT Press Ltd. p. 207, 1977.

7. Sigurdsson, B., Karcher, D., van Sande, M. and Lowenthal, A.
   Electrophoresis of the serum and the CSF proteins in sheep
   neurological diseases. Protides of the Biological Fluids,
   8th Colloquium, Bruges, 1960. Elsevier, Amsterdam, p. 110,
   1961.

8. Janssens, J. Homogene konijnen antilichamen tegen Micrococus
   Lysodeikticus. V.U.B. Faculteit Wetenschappen. Proefschrift
   licentiaat in de scheikundige wetenschappen, Sept. 1972.

9. Strosberg, A.D., Karcher, D. and Lowenthal, A. Structure and
   idiotype of human homogeneous antibodies. Fed. Proc. (abstr.)
   969, 1975.

10. Prineas, J.W., Raine, C.S., Connell, F. and Wright, R.G.
    Bound immunoglobulin G in chronic multiple sclerosis plaques.
    11th World Congress of Neurology, Excerpta Medica, Amsterdam,
    300, 1977.

11. Link, H. and Muller, R. Arch. Neurol. 25, 326, 1971.

12. Vandvik, B. and E. Norrby. Oligoclonal IgG antibody response
    with central nervous system to different measles virus antigens
    in SSPE. Proc. Nat. Sci. USA Vol. 70, N°4. pp 1060,
    1973.

13. Vandvik, B. Gel-precipitating measles virus antibodies in SSPE
    Relation to oligoclonal IgG proteins in the CSF and serum, and
    the occurrence of two separate fractions of antibody to
    virus nucleocapsids. Acta Path. Microbiol. Scand. Sect. C.
    85 : 324, 1977.

OLIGOCLONAL IMMUNE RESPONSES IN THE CENTRAL NERVOUS SYSTEM (CNS)

IN CONNECTION WITH VIRUS INFECTIONS AND CNS DISEASES OF UNKNOWN

ETIOLOGY

E. Norrby

Department of Virology, Karolinska Institute of
Medicine, Stockholm, Sweden

The central nervous system (CNS) displays a degree of appa-
rant independence from other parts of the organism as concerns
immunological functions. These functions can be analysed both
from the viewpoint of humoral and cell-bound immunity. This presentation will deal only with the former kind of immune response.

One of the unique characteristics of the CNS humoral immune
response is the tendency it shows to display oligoclonal characteristics of the immunoglobulins produced. The reasons for the
occurrence of this phenomenon are unknown and thus open for speculation. By definition all immunoglobulins produced display homogenous migration characteristics upon electrophoretic fractionation. As a consequence two factors decide whether an immune response is classified as polyclonal or oligoclonal. These two
factors are the number of clones of antibodies produced and the
resolution of the fractionation technique employed. Although
oligoclonal IgG is a term of convenience it is a useful concept.

We have studied the appearance and evolution of oligoclonal
IgG in different selected diseases in the CNS by use of three
different techniques. These techniques are :
(a) Characterization of the distribution of specific antibody
activities after electrophoretic separation of immunoglobulins.
(b) Absorption-elution of immunoglobulins with specific antigen(s).
Antibody activities and electrophoretic mobility characteristics
of immunoglobulins remaining after absorption and appearing in low
pH eluates have been determined.
(c) Characterization of specific antibody activities of different

populations of oligoclonal IgG by an imprint electroimmunofixation technique.

By use of these different techniques it is possible to evaluate the occurrence of antibodies against a specific antigen in
a smaller or larger fraction of oligoclonal immunoglobulin. A
discussion of the appearance and evolution of oligoclonal immunoglobulins preferably can be divided to concern acute and subacute
to chronic diseases of either defined or undefined etiology.

ACUTE TO PROLONGED DISEASES OF DEFINED ETIOLOGY

Acute measles encephalitis generally is described as being
of the postinfectious type (1). The evidence for this is the time
interval between rash and development of encephalitis (usually
5 days), histopathological changes (demyelinating alterations,
absence of inclusion-body-bearing cells) and finally the sparse-
ness with which viruses has been isolated from brain tissue. However certain isolations of the virus have been made both from
brain tissue and from cells in the cerebrospinal fluid (CSF).
The protein content of CSF from patients with acute measles encephalitis has been described generally to be increased. Almost
no data are available on the characteristics of CSF proteins and
very few serological studies have been performed. We have studied
one case of acute measles encephalitis in which a production of
oligoclonal IgG detectable in CSF developed over 20 days after
the debute of the disease (2). Antibody studies of serum and
CSF revealed that there was a local production of measles antibodies in CNS simultaneously with the occurrence of oligoclonal IgG.
It was assumed but not proven that the oligoclonal IgG carried
measles antibody specificity. Both the appearance of oligoclonal
IgG and the intrathecal production of measles antibodies were
transient phenomena. They were no longer demonstrable at 4-5
months after the debute of the disease concomitant with an improvement of the clinical conditions.

Lyon et al. (3) recently described a case of acute measles
encephalitis of the delayed type. No virus was isolated but
measles cytopathic changes were detectable and serological studies
revealed a local production of measles antibodies in the CNS.
Results of electrophoretic characterization of CSF proteins were
not described. The patient died of sequelae relating to a commu-
nicating hydrocephalus.

Taken together it seems that current evidence favours the
occurrence of two different forms of acute measles encephalitis.
One form may be of the postinfectious kind, whereas the other form
would be due to a direct attack of virus on CNS tissue. The border between cases of the acute delayed encephalitis caused by a

direct attack by the virus, e.g. the kind of encephalitis seen in
immunosuppressed children and subacute sclerosing panencephalitis
(SSPE) may be poorly demarcated.

One childhood virus disease showing a high frequency of CNS
complications is mumps. We have analysed the CNS immunology of
this disease in two different studies. In a study together with
Vandvik and collaborators (4) 10 children with mumps meningitis
were examined. All cases showed pleocytosis which lasted for
weeks and in a few cases examined for months. Early samples of
CSF ($\leq$ 2 weeks after appearance of disease)showed a normal protein pattern or moderate transudative changes. In later samples,
oligoclonal IgG patterns were detected in 4 out of 10 patients.
In some cases oligoclonal IgG was detectable even in the absence
of a marked increase in CSF protein content. In 2 patients CSF
samples were available 11 and 12 months after onset of disease.
Bands of oligoclonal IgG were still detectable although they were
less pronounced than in early samples. A local production of mumps
virus-specific antibodies was demonstrated by analysis of antibody titers in CSF and serum. The bands of oligoclonal IgG were
found to represent locally produced mumps virus-specific antibodies (5).

In a second study together with Frydén and Link (6) 19 young
adult patients with mumps meningitis and 19 patients with meningitis of some other etiology (defined in 10 cases as being due to
infections with herpes simplex virus, varicella-zoster virus,
ECHO virus, influenza virus and mycoplasma pneumoniae) were investigated. Repeated samples of serum and CSF were collected, in
some cases up to a year or more after the onset of disease. All
patients had pleocytosis during the early phase of the disease.
At one month after onset about 2/3 of the patients in both groups
still showed pleocytosis. More than 3 months after onset all 7
patients with mumps lacked pleocytosis but 2 out of 4 in the control group still showed pleocytosis. Damage to the blood-brain
barrier was found in 2/3 of early samples and about 1/3 at one
month after onset. Oligoclonal IgG was detected in 7 patients in
each group i.e. at a frequency corresponding to that of the afore
mentioned study group. In most cases oligoclonal IgG was present
at the first time of CSF sampling but in 2 patients with mumps
meningitis an evolution from polyclonal to oligoclonal IgG was
observed. The production of oligoclonal IgG appeared durable
in many cases. In the 7 patients with mumps one patient did not
show oligoclonal IgG in the CSF at one year after the disease, but
4 other patients available for sampling still displayed oligoclonal IgG. In two cases this was still detectable at 30 months
after debut of the disease. In the second group of meningitis
cases caused by other agents than mumps persistent production of
oligoclonal IgG for more than one year was found in 3 out of 7
patients.

A local production of mumps virus antibodies within the CNS
was shown in 7 out of 19 patients. Out of these 7 patients 6 showed a local production of IgG within the CNS and in 4 cases this
IgG was oligoclonal. The only parameter among those discussed
which seemed to influence prognosis was duration of damage to the
blood brain barrier.

Altogether about 1/3 of patients with mumps meningitis show
a production of oligoclonal IgG within the CNS and in many of
these cases a local production of mumps antibodies can also be
demonstrated. In the few cases studied it has been shown that
oligoclonal IgG carries mumps antibody activity. In a number of
cases an evolution from polyclonal to oligoclonal IgG has been
found and in several cases the production of oligoclonal IgG has
been durable. It remains to determine whether this prolonged
production of oligoclonal IgG may reflect a tendency for mumps
virus to cause a persistent silent infection.

Herpes simplex virus encephalitis shows a very variable clinical course. Laterre et al. (7) have mentioned that in some cases with protracted disease oligoclonal IgG can be identified.
We have studied the case of HSV encephalitis in a 3 year-old,
which turned fatal after 46 days of illness (8). In the early
stage of the disease transudative protein changes were found in
the CSF. 27 days after onset an oligoclonal IgG pattern started
to emerge and it became increasingly pronounced during the remaining phase of the illness. It was shown that the locally produced
oligoclonal IgG carried virus-specific activity (5). A neutral
extract of brain proteins contained oligoclonal IgG with a pattern
and antibody specificity corresponding to that of the CSF sample
collected just before the death of the patient.

SUBACUTE TO CHRONIC DISEASE OF DEFINED ETIOLOGY

The local immune response in the CNS of patients with SSPE
has been extensively studied (9, 10, 11, 5). The results obtained can be summarized as follows :
(a) Most cases show a very pronounced production of oligoclonal
IgG within the CNS. The band pattern changes in a dynamic way
with time. In repeated samples it can be shown that bands of
IgG are added during the course of the disease, but also that occasionally certain bands may disappear. IgG of restricted heterogeneity partly matching that produced in the CNS may also be detected in serum.
(b)The bands of oligoclonal IgG to a major extent represent measles virus-specific antibodies.
(c) There is a tendency for bands of oligoclonal IgG carrying
a certain, specific antibody activity to occur in a certain region
of the electropherogram. It might be noted that the purified nu-

cleocapsid preparations used in previous studies now have been
shown to include both nucleocapsid and matrix components. Thus
antibody activities in different parts of the electropherogram
detected by the use of this kind of antigen in complement fixation
tests may in fact carry different antibody activities.

Recently we have examined a case of progressive rubella panencephalitis (PRP) (12). The occurrence of a marked production
of oligoclonal IgG and of free light chains of the lambda type
in CSF was shown. The latter finding was interpreted to indicate
the occurrence of asynchrony in the synthesis and assembly of
oligoclonal IgG molecules. Evidence was further obtained that
the oligoclonal IgG observed in CSF and to a certain extent in
serum carried rubella virus-specific antibody activity. The
major part of the virus-specific IgG in the CNS was locally produced.

In summary it can be stated that the accumulation of antigens
of infectious agents in connection with CNS disease readily mounts
a local oligoclonal IgG response. In many cases an evolution
from polyclonal to oligoclonal IgG is observed. This most likely
comes about by a selection for clones of cells producing antibodies of high avidity by the continuing presence of antigen. The
overall majority of the oligoclonal IgG appears to carry antibody
activities against different antigens of the etiological agent.
The production of oligoclonal IgG is dynamic and the observed band
pattern changes in relationship to the development of the disease.
In cases when antigen stimulation ceases the production of oligoclonal IgG gradually wanes.

ACUTE CNS DISEASE OF UNDEFINED ETIOLOGY

The Guillain-Barré (G-B) disease is a polyradiculo-neuropathy
of unknown etiology. It has been noted with relative frequency
to be proceeded by an infection or an immunization. Recently
it was found in the US that the risk to contract G-B disease increased about 5-10 times in connection with administration of an
inactivated vaccine against swine influenza virus. The time interval between vaccination and debute of the disease was about 17
days. No reports have been given on possible immunoglobulin changes in the patients with vaccine-related G-B disease.

In collaboration with Link and Wahren (13) we have studied
a material of 24 G-B patients. Repeated serum and CSF samples
were collected. In spite of the classical criteria on G-B disease,
i.e. the albumino-cytological dissociation, we found a late developing pleocytosis in many cases. More than 50 % of the cases
showed moderately increased cell counts in CSF and in some cases
the number of cell exceeded $50/mm^3$. The pleocytosis developed

somewhat later in relationship to the debute of the disease than in cases of acute viral meningitis. All but 2 (only late samples were available from these 2) displayed evidence of damage to the blood-brain barrier. In 5 out of 11 cases examined, the damage remained for more than 4 months.

The influx of serum proteins into the CNS complicated, but did not completely prevent, the analysis of locally produced immunoglobulins. Comparative protein analysis (determination of the CSF-IgG index) showed a local production of IgG in 15/24 patients. Eight and 6 patients also showed a local production of IgA and IgM, respectively. The highest frequency of occurrence of locally produced immunoglobulins was encountered at 2-4 months after the debute of the disease, except in the case of IgM, which occurred earlier. All 6 patients with increased CSF-IgM had pleocytosis. Ten patients had oligoclonal IgG in CSF and this occurred more frequently in patients with pleocytosis. Five patients also had detectable oligoclonal IgG in serum and in 4 of these the band patterns was identical in serum and in CSF. The fifth patient had a difference in band patterns in serum and CSF indicating a local production within the CNS of at least some of the homogeneous IgG. Disappearance of oligoclonal IgG during the time of observation was found in 4 out of 10 patients. In the remaining 6 patients the production of IgG persisted at least 3 months and in one case more than 13 months. The possible occurrence of certain virus infections has been studied in these patients. Three patients showed evidence (occurrence of IgM) for primary Epstein-Barr virus infections and 2 for primary CMV infection. There was no relationship between the assumed primary infection and pleocytosis in the CSF. The antibody specificity of oligoclonal IgG remains to be determined. No local production of antibodies to measles virus, rubella virus, adenovirus, and poliovirus was encountered. A search for the possible occurrence of a production of a specific antibody should be encouraged.

Another example of an acute disease occasionally associated with production of oligoclonal IgG in the CNS is optic neuritis. After exclusion of acute optic neuritis of known cause two categories remain; patients that produce or do not produce oligoclonal IgG in their CNS. The possible value of this phenomenon in making predictions concerning the risk for development into multiple sclerosis (MS) has been discussed. Somewhat conflicting data have been obtained. In studies by Stendahl et al. (14) the presence of oligoclonal IgG was found to correlate to the occurrence of genetic markers characteristic for multiple sclerosis (MS). However, in another study by Sandberg-Wohlheim (personal communication) no good correlation was found and in some patients a development of bands of oligoclonal IgG during the early phase of the disease was encountered. It seems that a production of demonstrable oligoclonal IgG generally remains remarkably stable similar to the situation in MS.

A local production of antibodies to measles (15) and also
other viruses (Vandvik et al. to be published) in the CNS have
been found in many patients with optic neuritis and oligoclonal
IgG.

CHRONIC DISEASE OF UNDEFINED ETIOLOGY

The disease of overwhelming importance in this category is
MS. Immunoprotein phenomena relating to this disease are discussed in many contributions in this book volume. The following is
only a summary of my own interpretations of available data.

(a) The production of oligoclonal IgG within the CNS generally
is demonstrable at the debute of the disease. Once this production
has been initiated, it appears to proceed in a rather monotonous
fashion over long periods of time.
(b) The oligoclonal IgG can be shown to include up to 4 or more
locally produced virus-specific antibodies, which however represent only a small fraction of the total amount of the oligoclonal
IgG (16, 17, 11, 18). Thus the oligoclonal IgG seems to carry
a broad spectrum of different antibody specificities.
(c) Oligoclonal IgG may also be detected in serum of MS patients.
Generally this oligoclonal IgG is concealed by the simultaneous
occurrence of larger quantities of polyclonal IgG. However, by
use of absorption-elution techniques oligoclonal virus-specific
antibodies may be extracted (11).
(d) No virus has been reproducibly isolated from CNS tissue of
MS patients or otherwise identified in such tissue.

Taken together these data indicate that the persistent production of oligoclonal IgG might not be due to the continuing
presence of a broad spectrum of viral and other antigens but rather
to some lack of balance in immune regulation.

The general picture is that of a polyclonal B cell activation.
The reason why antibodies of certain specificities e.g. against
measles virus antigens occur relatively more frequently among
the oligoclonal IgG is not known. Possibly there may be two different explanations. The first one is the fact that certain viruses,
e.g. measles virus, has a tendency to associate with CNS tissue
and therefore leave an imprint in this tissue in the form of dormant sensitized B cells. Another factor that may be of importance
is the phenomenon of maturation of enveloped viruses via budding
from the cytoplasmic membrane. The expression of a set of virus-
specific antigens at the cell surface (possibly in physical conjunction with histocompatibility antigens) may mobilize qualities
of the immune response different from that activated by products

from replication of a naked virus. The non-specific activation
of clones of sensitized B cells theoretically could be based on
either some general polyclonal activation as mentioned above, but
possibly also an activation of these clones in connection with
some massive activation of other clones of sensitized B cells
reacting against a particular set of antigens. If MS is a disease
relating to unbalanced immune regulation, possibly something might
be learnt from comparative analysis of a similar kind outside
the CNS. Such diseases include e.g. active chronic hepatitis,
connective tissue diseases such as lupus erythematosus and others.
It might be noted that in these diseases an increase of serum IgG
including virus-specific antibody titers may be encountered. It
is not known whether the immunoglobulins produced may have a restricted heterogeneity but this problem can now be approached by
use of the imprint electroimmunofixation technique.

In one study of synovial fluid from a patient with a special
form of rheumatoid arthritis, oligoclonal IgG was encountered (19).
Like in the case of MS CSF a small fraction of this oligoclonal
IgG was found to be oligoclonal measles virus-specific antibodies.
It is hoped that by making analogies between different immunoregu-
lation diseases we may eventually resolve the enigma of the pathogenesis of the MS disease.

REFERENCES

1. Norrby, E. (1975), Measles virus infection in the central nervous
   system. In "Dynamic aspects of hostparasite relationships".
   Vol. II. (Ed. A. Zuckerman) John Wiley & Sons, N.Y.
2. Sköldenberg, B., Carlström, A., Forsgren, M. and Norrby, E.
   (1976). Clin. Exp. Immunol. 23, 451.
3. Lyon, G., Ponset, G., and Lebon, P. (1977). Ann. Neurol. 2, 322.
4. Vandvik, B., Norrby, E., Steen-Johnson, J. and Stensvold, K.
   (1978a). Eur. Neurol. 17, 13.
5. Nordal, H.J., Vandvik, B., and Norrby, E. (1978a). Scand. J.
   Immunol. 7, 381.
6. Frydén, A., Link, H., and Norrby, E. (1978). Infect. Immunity.
   In press.
7. Laterre, E.C., Stevens, A., and Lamy, M. (1973). Excerpta Med.
   296, 1973.
8. Vandvik, B., and Norrby, E. (1978). Arch. Neurol. In press.
9. Vandvik, B., and Norrby, E. (1973). Proc. Natl. Acad. Sci. 70,
   1660.
10. Norrby, E., and Vandvik, B. (1975). Med. Microbiol. Immunol.
    162, 63.
11. Vandvik, B., Norrby, E., Nordal, H., and Degré, M. (1976).
    Scand. J. Immunol. 5, 979.
12. Vandvik, B., Weil, M.L., Grandien, M., and Norrby, E. (1978b)
    Acta Neurol. Scand. 57, 53.

13. Link, H., Wahren, B., and Norrby, E. (1978). Infect. Immunity, In press.

14. Stendahl-Brodin, L., Link, H., Möller, E., and Norrby, E. (1978). Acta Neurol. Scand. 57, 418.

15. Link, H., Norrby, E., and Olsson, J.E. (1973). New Engl. J. Med. 289, 1103.

16. Norrby, E., Link, H., Olsson, J.-E., Panelius, M., Salmi, A.G. and Vandvik, B. (1974). Infect. Immunity 10, 688.

17. Norrby, E. (1978). Progr. Med. Virol. 24, 1.

18. Nordal, H.J., Vandvik, B., and Norrby, E. (1978b). Scand. J. Immunol. 7, 473.

19. Vandvik, B., Mellbye, D.J., and Norrby, E. (1977). Ann. Rheum. Dis. 36, 302.

OLIGOCLONAL VIRUS ANTIBODIES IN HEALTHY ADULTS AND NEUROLOGICAL PATIENTS

H.J. Nordal [+], B. Vandvik [x] and E. Norrby [o]

+ Institute of Immunology and Rheumatology, State Hospital, Oslo, Norway; x Department of Neurology, Ulleval Hospital, Oslo, Norway; ° Department of Virology, Karolinska Institute, Stockholm, Sweden

A sensitive technique (imprint electroimmunofixation, IEIF) for the electrophoretic characterization of virus-specific antibodies was developed: Serum and concentrated cerebrospinal fluid (CSF) are fractionated by agarose gel electrophoresis. Virus antigen-containing gel plates are then incubated in direct contact with the electrophoresis gel for 30 minutes. After separation of the gels the electrophoresis gel is fixed and stained with Coomassie Brilliant Blue. The antigen-containing gel is thoroughly washed in saline, incubated in a buffer containing I^{125}-labelled rabbit anti-human Ig antibodies, washed again, dried and autoradiographed.

IEIF was used to study serum and concentrated CSF samples, adjusted to an IgG concentration of 5 g/l, from various adult donors. Electrophoretically restricted antibodies against antigen preparations of measles, rubella, mumps, and herpes simplex viruses, was found in some normal sera. These sera had all a "polyclonal" γ-globulin distribution and were collected from healthy adult donors. This indicates that in the late convalescence phase after infections caused by these viruses, the production of oligoclonal virus antibodies is a normal phenomenon.

The electrophoretic distribution of virus-specific antibodies in CSF was studied in samples with a normal electrophoretic protein distribution, collected from neurological patients with no known demyelinating or infectious central nervous system (CNS) disease. In these CSF samples patterns of antibody bands closely resembling those of the matching serum samples were found. This was in contrast to the findings in 4 patients with infections of the CNS caused by the 4 viruses studied, and with a local synthesis of

oligoclonal IgG. By means of the IEIF technique a selective increase
of oligoclonal antibodies, specific for the causative organism, could
be demonstrated in CSF from the patient. The oligoclonal virus antibodies generally corresponded to the oligoclonal IgG populations,
demonstrable by Coomassie Brilliant Blue staining, in the CSF. The
antibody activity was clearly higher in the CSF than in the serum
samples adjusted to similar concentrations of IgG, compatible with
a local synthesis of virus-specific antibodies against the causative
organism in the CNS. In these patients the antibody activity was
higher in the CSF than in serum in all electrophoretic fractions.
However, demonstration of higher antibody activity in a single
electrophoretic fraction should in principle be sufficient to state
that local antibody synthesis occurs.

The occurrence of oligoclonal antibodies against measles,
rubella, mumps, and herpes simplex viruses was studied in serum and
in concentrated CSF samples collected from 10 multiple sclerosis
(MS) patients in a chronic progressive state of the disease.

Oligoclonal virus antibodies could be demonstrated in serum and
CSF from 9 of the patients. There was no direct correspondence
between the patterns of antibody bands and the patterns of IgG bands
of the CSF (Fig. 1). Thus oligoclonal antibody populations frequently occurred in electrophoretic mobility areas where no IgG-bands
were demonstrable by protein staining.

In most cases the CSF samples exhibited a larger number of and
more intensely stained antibody bands than the serum samples. The
patterns of antibody bands in matching serum and CSF samples,
adjusted to similar concentrations of IgG, were analysed with
respect to local antibody synthesis in the CNS according to the
criterion proposed above. Local synthesis of oligoclonal antibodies
against at least one of the viruses was concluded to occur in 9 of
the 10 patients. Local antibody synthesis was most frequently seen
for measles antibodies. A simultaneous synthesis of antibodies
against all 4 viruses studied was seen in 1 patient, against 3
viruses in 4 patients and against 2 viruses in 1 patient.

All patients with demonstrable oligoclonal IgG in the CSF had
evidence of local antibody synthesis against at least 1 virus.
However, local synthesis of oligoclonal virus antibodies was also
seen in 2 of the 3 patients studied with electrophoretically normal
γ-globulin distribution of the CSF.

These data may indicate that the local synthesis of virus-
specific antibodies in the CNS of MS patients is elicited by another
mechanism than the physical presence of viruses as immunogens in the
brain of the patient. The significance of the local production of
these antibodies in MS patients is therefore quite uncertain. An

important goal for future
research is to clarify whether
virus-specific antibodies may
be produced as a cophenomenon
in an intense humoral immune
response localized to the CNS.
Although the data obtained
from the 4 patients studied
with various viral infections
of the CNS did not provide
evidence for such a mechanism,
this problem should be studied
in a larger number of patients.
The identification of the
specificities of the major
oligoclonal IgG populations in
the CSF of MS patients is
another important goal for
future work.

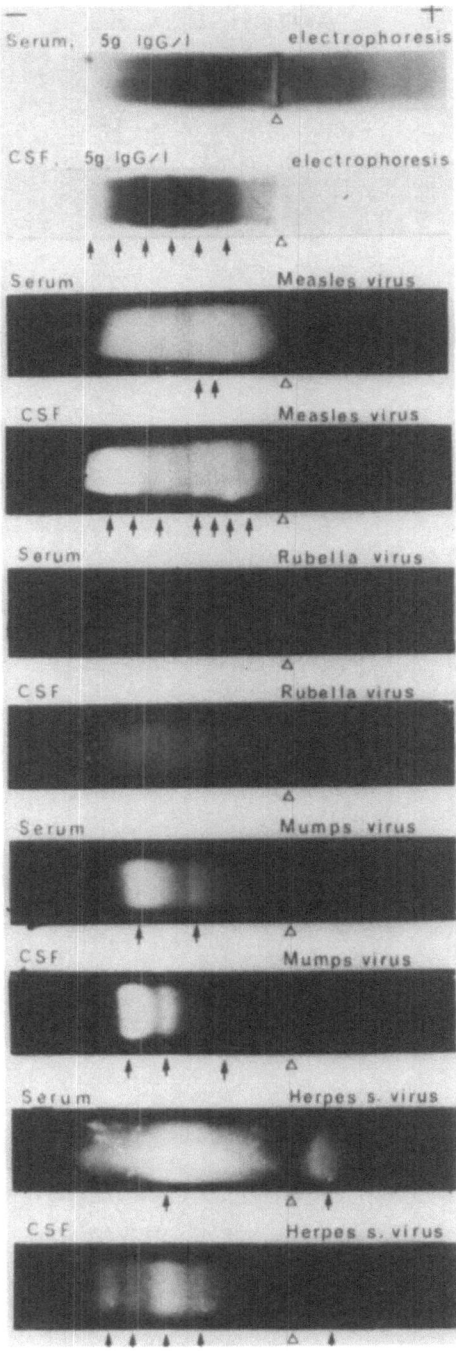

Fig. 1. Electrophoretically
restricted virus-specific
antibodies in serum and concentrated cerebrospinal fluid
(CSF) from a patient with
multiple sclerosis demon-
strated by imprint electroimmunofixation (IEIF). The
reference electrophoreses
of protein cathodal to
transferrin, stained with
Coomassie Brilliant Blue,
of serum and of concentrated
CSF are shown in the upper
part of the figure. Negative
copies of autoradiograms of
virus antigen-containing gels
are shown below. Arrows
indicate bands seen in the
reference electrophoreses
and in the autoradiograms.
Triangles indicate the
position of the sample
application slits.

IMMUNOGLOBULIN STRUCTURE AND FUNCTION : IDIOTYPY AND THE OLIGO-

CLONAL RESPONSE

M. Siegelman and J.D. Capra

Department of Microbiology, Southwestern Medical School,
Dallas, Texas, U.S.A.

INTRODUCTION

Through a study of the myeloma proteins of man, and induced
antibodies and myeloma proteins in other species, a comprehensive
understanding of the relationship of the structure of immunoglobulin molecules and their function is emerging. The domain hypothesis, originally proposed by Edelman in the late 1960's is now on
firm experimental ground (1). The variable domain, consisting
of V_H and V_L is the area of the antigen binding site (2, 3). This
is a pocket or groove in the three-dimensional structure which is
lined by the hypervariable regions (4-6). A large body of experimental data indicates that the idiotypic determinants generally
derive from the structures of the hypervariable regions and thus,
by inference, antibody combining site. An Fc region can be produced from each immunoglobulin class and certain defined biological functions can be ascribed to it. Furthermore, the Fc region
of each class has a distinctly different biological activity. In
the IgG and IgM class, each of the separate Fc domains has been
isolated and separately tested for biological activity. Complement fixing regions, and neutrophil, macrophage, and mast cell
binding areas of the immunoglobulin molecule are known in general
terms (7).

THE VARIABLE REGIONS AND THE COMBINING SITE

Localization of the Antibody-Combining Site

Initial studies of IgG placed the antigen-binding portion
of the molecule in the Fab region (8). The binding site was more

specifically localized when the Fab fragment of a mouse myeloma
protein with anti-DNP (dinitrophenol) activity was shown to maintain this antibody activity after further cleavage by pepsin. The
peps in cleavage product contained 260 residues and consisted of
the amino terminal domains of the light and heavy chains (9, 10).
Thus the V-regions alone possess full antibody activity.

                          The Variable Regions

     The unique characteristic of immunoglobulins, which sets them
apart from all other molecules studied to date, resides in the fact
that their variable region structures differ not only from species
to species but within individuals of the same species as well.
Extensive amino acid sequence data indicates that the variable
region extends from the N terminus through approximately 1/2 of
the light chain and 1/4 of the heavy chain (7, 11). The amino
terminal domains of both the light and heavy chains are characterized by this variability and are termed variable regions, V_L
and V_H, respectively.

     Subgroups. Several light- and heavy-chain variable regions
have been totally sequenced and partial sequences are available
for many others. Although there is great variability among V-
regions and no two proteins from different human individuals have
been identical, they may be assembled into subgroups based on both
antigenic and amino acid sequence similarities. An understanding
of the variable region subgroups is important to appreciate fully
the distinctions and interrelationships between idiotypy and cross-
idiotypic specificity.

     Each type of immunoglobulin constant region has an exclusive
set of variable regions, i.e., V_K for kappa-type light chains, V_L
for lambda-type light chains, and V_H for all classes of heavy
chains. At the present time, four subgroups of human kappa, four
of human lambda and three of human heavy chains have been defined.
However, the number, and significance of V-region subgroups is an
area of intense controversy.

     Based on sequence studies of human myeloma proteins, three
subgroups of heavy-chain variability have been defined (12-14).
One of these subgroups (V_HIII) is present in at least 13 other
mammals. The distribution of heavy chain subgroups and light-
chain types among heavy-chain classes and subclasses is not uniform. In addition, the kappa to lambda ratio of light-chains
associated with the four subclasses of human IgG ranges widely
from 1.1 to 8 (5). The V_HIII subgroup accounts for 20 % of IgG
heavy chains from normal human serum, but is the major subgroup
of serum IgA, being utilized by 75 % of alpha chains (16).

TABLE I

DISTRIBUTION OF THE V_HIII SUBGROUP

AMONG IMMUNOGLOBULIN CLASSES (HUMAN)

	From Myelomas	From Pooled Serum
IgG	18 % (5/28)	25 %
IgA	67 % (20/30)	75 %
IgM	27 % (9/33)	24 %
IgD	14 % (1/7)	ND[*]
IgE	71 % (5/7)	ND

[*] Not Done

These data have been published previously in a study which attempted
to define the relationship between the variable and constant regions
of immunoglobulin, and to provide information concerning the pairing requirement for heavy- and light-chain variable regions. It
was shown that while all classes of immunoglobulin can be associated
with each of the variable region subgroup, certain clear preferen-
ces existed both in the myeloma proteins and in pool of immunoglobulin. These findings were interpreted to place a major constraint
on germ-line theories of antibody formation which generally assume
random pairing of heavy- and light-chains (the P x Q hypothesis).

The Extent of Variability. Despite the great variability of
the variable regions as a whole, there are short stretches of both
the light and heavy chains which are invariant. The position of
the disulfide loop of human kappa chains, for example, is invariant,
and the immediately adjacent residues show a very low level of
variability. Thirteen human myeloma heavy chain variable chain
regions have been completely sequenced to date. About 65 % of
the positions in human heavy chains of the V_HIII subgroups exhibit
limited variability over the amino terminal 120 residues. Seven-
teen of these residue positions or 14 % of the V-region are absolutely invariant in all subgroups (18).

Within the more constant portion or framework of the variable
regions are several hypervariable regions which maintain about
80 % sequence difference. This astonishing level of variability
prompted the first suggestions that these regions embody the
equally variable combining specificities of antibodies. Light
chains have three such regions, starting at positions 28, 50 and

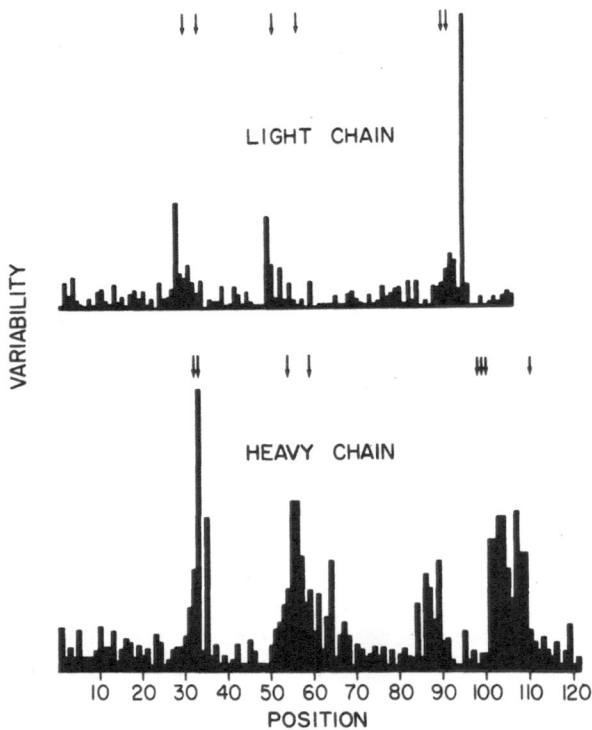

Figure one : Variability of the human light- and heavy-chain
variable regions plotted according to the method of Wu and Kabat
(19). The arrows indicate positions in which affinity labels
have been localized.

96 (19) and extending approximately 10 residues each. The first
second, and fourth hypervariable regions have been identified in
rabbit, but the region of the third appears uniform and may be
correlated with allotype (2).

Affinity-Labeling Studies

It is beyond the scope of this communication to review the
extraordinary studies done by affinity-labeling which document
the localization of the affinity labels to the hypervariable
regions. However, these studies have unequivocally established
the final leg of the tripartite arrangement between the antibody
combining site, hypervariable regions, and idiotypic determinants.

IDIOTYPY AND CROSS IDIOTYPIC SPECIFICITY

In 1955, Slater, Ward and Kunkel (21) immunized rabbits with
human myeloma proteins and observed that when the rabbit anti-
serums were absorbed with normal human serum or a series of myeloma
proteins of similar class and light chain type, the antisera
continued to react with the immunogens. They further showed,
that with the exception of the immunizing agent, the antisera
would not react with any other myeloma proteins tested and rea-
soned that each myeloma protein contained within its structure
specific determinants that were unique unto themselves. These
they termed the "individual antigenic specificies" of myeloma
proteins.

Later, Oudin in France (22) and Williams and Kunkel (23) in
the United States extended these observations to include induced
antibodies. Oudin showed that rabbit anti-Salmonella antibodies
contained what he termed "idiotypic determinants". Simultaneously,
Kunkel and his colleagues demonstrated that human antibodies to
certain red cell antigens contained unique determinants. Soon,
there was substantial agreement that the two phenomena, namely
"individual antigenic specificity" and "idiotypy" were measuring
much the same parameter and "idiotypy" is now used to describe
this general phenomenon.

Cold Agglutinins

An important conceptual advance in our understanding of idiotypy, and the first evidence that the idotypic determinants might
relate directly to the antibody–combining site, came from a study
on human IgM cold agglutinins by Williams et al. (24). By using
appropriately absorbed idiotypic antisera, cross-idiotypic reactions among proteins with similar binding specificities was demonstrated. Thus, antibodies raised in rabbits to certain human IgM
cold agglutinins, after absorption with a pool of IgM proteins
without cold agglutinin specificity, reacted in double–diffusion
tests with certain other IgM cold agglutinins. Employing several
of these antisera, most human IgM cold agglutinins could be grouped
into one of three groups. The relationship between these "cross-
idiotypic groups" and the precise specificity of the individual
cold agglutinins was not appreciated at the time. However, with
the elucidation of the structure of the I determinant and careful
specificity studies by Feizi and Kabat, certain patterns have
emerged (25).

Such idiotypic cross-reactions are rarely reactions of total
identity. Thus, true idiotypic specificity is said to exist only
for the actual immunizing cold agglutinin since absorption of the
idiotypic antiserum with other cold agglutinins will not remove

all the antibody, as indicated by the finding that reactions with the immunizing cold agglutinin can still be demonstrated subsequent to the absorption.

The importance of this observation is that it necessitated a broadening of the concept of idiotypy to include weakly cross-reacting systems. In addition, the relationship of idiotypy to the combining site itself became apparent.

Since then, monoclonal and oligoclonal responses of the anti-I, anti-i, anti-Pr, and anti-Gd specificity have been extensively studied. Amino acid sequence work on these IgM proteins has indicated a diversity in variable region subgroups, although clear associations are evident. There is a clear sequence restriction in that the I cold agglutinins have been $V_K III$ whereas the i cold agglutinins have been $V_K I$. The anti-Pr cold agglutinins have been $V_K IV$, and the $V_H III$ subgroup has been seen almost exclusively in the anti-Pr and anti-Gd antibodies (see Table II).

These studies provide an important extension of the principles of idiotypy to cross idiotypic specificity. However, they raise a provocative point which has still not been thoroughly analyzed nor addressed. That is, how can one be absolutely sure that these idiotypic cross-reactions do not represent anything more than subgroup specific antigenic determinants ? Thus, for example, since it appears to be clear that within a cross specificity group there is, with few exceptions, only a single V_H and V_L subgroup represented, the possibility exists that the cross-specificity is not at all related to the combining site of these molecules,

TABLE II

CLASS, LIGHT CHAIN TYPES AND V-REGION SUBGROUPS

OF HUMAN COLD AGGLUTININS [*]

			SUBGROUP	
SPECIFICITY	CLASS	L CHAIN	V_H	V_L
I	IgM (14/15)	K (15/15)	$V_H I$ (4/4)	$V_K III$ (11/13)
i	IgM (12/12)	K (10/11)	$V_H I$ (3/4)	$V_K I$ 2/3
Pr	IgM (2/2)	K (2/2)	$V_H III$ (2/2)	$V_K IV$ (2)
Gd	IgM (2/2)	K (2/2)	$V_H III$ (2/2)	$V_K I$ (1/2)

[*] Data compiled from references 26-28.

but to antigenic determinants which reside on the "framework"
which might be produced by the unique combinatorial association
of a particular V_H and V_L pair.

Recent studies in our laboratory have been directed toward
a dissection of these relationships. In particular, we have
recently been able to render three separate antisera idiotypically
specific (by immunodiffusion analysis) by absorption with a
single myeloma protein. Thus, for example, in one case, an
antiserum was raised to an IgAl, V_HIII, V_KI human myeloma protein.
When this antiserum was absorbed with a second human IgAl myeloma
protein of identical V-region heavy and light chain subgroup,
the antiserum was idiotypically specific. Similar studies should
be done with the cold agglutinins and anti-gamma globulins. Thus,
rather than absorbing the antisera with a random pool of myeloma
proteins, or with small amounts of normal human serum, a specific
absorption with molecules of defined subgroups and/or sequence
should be done. Such experiments should allow one to dissect
out the distinction between "framework" antigenic determinants
which may contribute to cross-idiotypic specificity, and the
"combining site" specificities themselves.

Anti-gamma Globulins

Cross-idiotopic specificity was extended to the monoclonal
IgM anti-gammaglobulins by Kunkel et al. (29, 30). Utilizing
haemagglutination-inhibition assay system, clear-cut results
were obtained for the IgM anti-gammaglobulins and patterns of
cross reactivity very similar to those among the IgM cold agglutinins were seen. The method of preparing the antisera is illustrated in Figure 2. At the time these studies were done, it
was not possible to absorb the antisera with proteins of defined
V-region subgroups as noted above. Utilizing these reagents,
Kunkel et al. (29, 30) were able to divide the human anti-globu-
lins into two major cross idiotypic groups and further, that a
general relationship existed between these cross specificities,
heavy and light chain variable region subgroups, and anti-gamma-
globulin specificity.

These studies were important in extending the concept of
cross idiotypic specificity to another human system but more
importantly, in this instance, large amounts of material were
now available for structural studies. Our laboratory was fortunate
enough to be able to obtain enough serum from two such patients
(Lay/Pom) in order to do the complete amino acid sequences of
the variable regions of both heavy and light chains. These
studies which have been extensively documented elsewhere (31, 32)
are notable for several reasons, but for our purposes here,

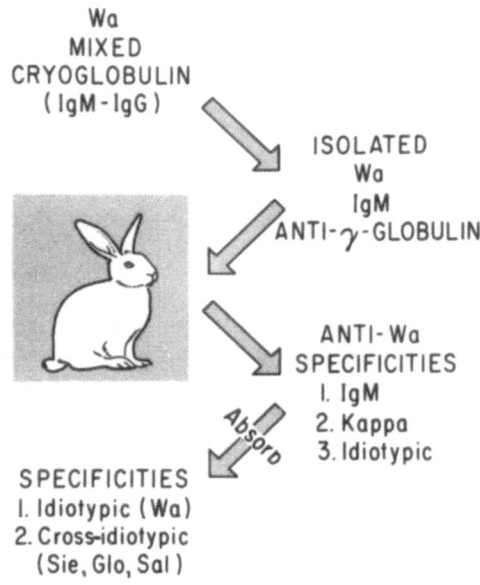

Figure two : Illustration of the method of preparing antisera
with cross-idiotypic specificity for anti-gammaglobulins.

they illustrate the relationship between the hypervariable regions
and the idiotypic specificity. While these proteins have eight
amino acid differences in the framework structures of their
heavy chain variable region, and 27 amino acid differences in the
variable regions of their kappa chains (which incidentally belong
to two different V-region subgroups), four of the six "combining
site" hypervariable regions are identical, a fifth differs by
a single residue (Ala-Ser) while the sixth is quite different.

Other Human Diseases with Monoclonal

or Oligoclonal Responses with Cross Idiotypic Specificity

A number of studies have demonstrated that other human diseases are associated with oligoclonal responses; in many instances,
these represent "monoclonal" proteins in which cross idiotypic
specificity can be demonstrated. An excellent example of these
are the Rh antibodies. Natvig et al. (33), utilized IgG Rh anti-

bodies from several patients immunized through Rh incompatible
pregnancy or by deliberate immunization. Anti-idiotypic antisera
were raised in rabbits and the antisera were absorbed with IgG and
normal human sera. By hemagglutination-inhibition, it was demonstrated that individual antigenic specificity could be demonstrated
for most of these anti-Rh antibodies, but more importantly, cross
idiotypic specificity was demonstrated. It was further shown that
the idiotypic sites could be blocked by combination of univalent
fragments of anti-Rh antibodies and red cell antigens. These
authors were unable to quantitate how much of the Rh antibody
population in each patient contained the idiotype (it should be
noted that in the A/J anti-arsonate system, approximately 60 %
of the immune response represents material with cross idiotypic
specificity (34)). A second important observation in the Rh system
is that in human immunology, at least, it represents the first
example of an IgG antibody with cross idiotypic specificity. This
is particularly important in view of the findings in SSPE and
multiple sclerosis where IgG is the major immunoglobulin. Amino
acid sequence as well as variable region subgroup determinations
have been done on the Rh antibodies and these have illustrated a
significant degree of V-region subgroup restriction in all instances.
The heterophil antibody of infectious mononucleosis and the anti-
gammaglobulins of the IgG type in Waldenstrom's hypergammaglobulinemic
purpura are among other human antibodies in which oligoclonal responses have been demonstrated to generate an idiotypic reagent which
can be absorbed to render it cross idiotypically specific.

        SSPE and the Oligoclonal Response in the Central Nervous System

        We now turn to matters of more direct interest to the topic of
this symposium, oligoclonal responses in diseases of the central
nervous system. Since this will be the subject of several individual papers, this will serve as no more than an overview of the
basic observations in CNS oligoclonal responses, the lines of pur-
suit followed in these investigations, and in particular, how our
knowledge of the structure of immunoglobulins has and can be
brought to bear to study and possible intervene in these disease
processes.

        The major questions to be kept in mind are 1) what is the site
of synthesis of the restricted antibody response and what are the
sources of its induction, maintenance and regulation; 2) what
structural features do the oligoclonal molecules share, and how
reproducible are these features in individuals presenting with the
same symptomatology; 3) what is the specificity of these antibody
populations, and do they arise by chronic, specific antigenic
stimulation, or phenomena more akin to polyclonal activation, and
4) what role do these molecules play, if any, in the pathogenesis
of these diseases?

Site of Synthesis. The first indication of a selective elevation of gammaglobulin levels in cerebral spinal fluid was reported
by Kabat et al. in 1942 in patients with multiple sclerosis and
neurosyphilis using the Tiselius "free flow" electrophoresis (35).
The advent of the simple technique of filter paper electrophoresis
in the 1950's sparked considerable interest in CSF proteins and
reports of elevation of gammaglobulins in other inflammatory diseases with levels of gammaglobulins accrued (36).

With the establishment of the observation of elevated CSF
gammaglobulin levels in MS and other CNS diseases, attention
turned to the source of these additional gammaglobulins. Kabat
et al. had suggested that synthesis occurred locally in the CNS
with subsequent diffusion into the CSF (35). The first solid evidence for local synthesis of the elevated gammaglobulins was
reported by Frick and Sheid-Seydel (37-39) based on studies on the
exchange of I^{131} labeled albumins and gammaglobulins between vascular and CSF compartments, which demonstrated that in normal subjects and those with blood-brain barrier damage, all CSF albumin
and gammaglobulin derived from the circulation. In marked contrast,
up to 92 % of CSF gammaglobulin in patients with MS with elevated
gammaglobulin originated from an extravascular source, strongly
implicating the CNS and/or CSF as that source. Such observations
have since been confirmed and extended to SSPE and Herpes simplex
virus encephalitis (40-42). Further corroboration of local synthesis in MS patients was supplied by Tourtellotte and Parker (43-45),
who demonstrated a concomitant increase in gammaglobulin in brain
tissue of MS patients. The definitive proof that local synthesis
occurred was provided by Sandberg-Willheim et al. who demonstrated
synthesis in vitro of IgG by CSF cells from a number of MS patients
(46, 47). Further suggestive evidence, was based on lowered serum
to CSF antibody ratios (48, 37) in MS and SSPE and other CNS diseases
served to generalize this observation. Recently, Vandvik and
Nordal using immunofluorescent staining showed that elevated CSF
IgM in a patient with chronic meningoencephalitis, was associated
with the presence of IgM on the surface of lymphocytic cells of
the CSF (49). That this IgM might have been passively acquired,
however, was not excluded.

The Restricted Response. Evaluation of relative heterogeneity
of protein mixtures was made possible by the introduction of protein chemistry techniques allowing superior resolution of protein
species. Techniques such as agar gel electrophoresis established
that the gammaglobulin fraction of normal CSF was considerably
more heterogeneous than hitherto recognized (50). Further studies
indicated that, like serum IgG, the IgG of normal CSF was electrophoretically heterogeneous or polyclonal in nature (51). Several
investigations using agar gel electrophoresis of CSF revealed that
IgG of CSF from patients with MS and other CNS diseases had electrophoretic patterns indicative of less heterogeneity, i.e., composed

of fewer bands. In fact, Laterre et al. (52) in a comprehensive study of patients with neurological disorders found a more striking correlation between restricted gammaglobulin electrophoretic patterns and cases of MS than with elevation of CSF gammaglobulin. SSPE, to be the subject of considerable more discussion here later, was another CNS disease noted to be associated with elevated CSF gammaglobulin by Bucher and co-workers (53), and was shown to manifest a similar oligoclonal electrophoretic pattern by Booy (54), Karcher et al. (55), Lowenthal (56) and Laterre (50). These earlier studies set the stage for the characterization of the oligoclonal bands with respect to immunoglobulin subclass and light chain isotype.

The occurrence of selective IgA, IgD or IgE elevations in the CSF has not been reported. Local synthesis of IgM in the CNS, as judged by selected increases of this class in CSF, may occur in African trypanosomiasis, neurosyphilis and some bacterial meningites. The status of the homogeneity of these proteins in these conditions has not been established.

However, there is at least one instance describing restricted IgM bands in a patient with chronic meningoencephalitis. For the conditions that we are interested in, the major emphasis will be on the IgG class of immunoglobulins. The majority of the discrete electrophoretic bands in the gammaglobulin in CSF has been identified as IgG. In a careful study of these bands using counter immunoelectrophoresis on CSF of patients with CNS infections and MS, relatively few of these putatively homogeneous bands were homogeneous for light chain type. Most of the IgG bands reacted with both kappa and lambda chain antisera, and the relative content of kappa and lambda varied from band to band (57). Evidence was also presented that CSF in a variety of neurologic disorders contained free light chains, that is, certain bands reacted with light chain antisera, but none of the class specific antisera. Provided that kappa-lamdba diversity in single bands does not reflect free light chain contamination, this observation of microheterogeneity within as well as between bands suggests that these bands are the product of more than single clones. The significance of the finding of free light chains is not clear. They could be due to proteolytic action on locally synthesized immunoglobulin or to a breakdown of synchronous synthesis in the immunoglobulin producing cells. It would be of interest to determine whether the free light chains derived from the same clones as bands representing whole immunoglobulin, or arise independently.

Subclass restriction of the CSF IgG has also been examined by Vandvik et al. (58). The IgG subclass distribution of normal CSF resembles that of the matching normal sera by the criteria of immunoelectrophoresis and hemagglutination-inhibition. A striking difference in patients with MS and SSPE in CSF and brain extract

samples was abnormalities in the IgGI precipitate arcs, and relative decrease in IgG2, 3, and 4 precipitates. The results are consistent with a displacement of CSF IgG into the IgGI subclass in
these conditions. The predominance of certain subclasses of IgG
has also been noted in several other immune responses; Rh factor,
certain carbohydrates, diphtheria toxin, tetanus toxin, isohemagglutin A, and anti-thrombin factor VIII. The significance of
these restrictions is not clear, but a simple possibility may be
the linkage of antibody V-regions of certain specificities to certain C-regions for their biological function and the proper elimination of particular foreign substances. It should also be noted
that IgGI is the predominant subclass and if a few clones are stimulated to proliferate, they may be most likely of this subclass.

Specificity and Oligoclonal Responses. Further studies of
the oligoclonal band centered on the search for the specificity of
these antibody populations. The local synthesis of measles-specific antibody in CSF of SSPE patients has been established by the
lowered serum to CSF antibody ratios. This knowledge stimulated a
study of specificity of oligoclonal bands for different viral products. Bands separated by preparative electrophoresis were tested
for various viral antibody activities : neutralization, hemolysin
inhibition, hemagglutination-inhibition and activity against nucleocapsids. In one patient, particularly pronounced separation of
activities into separate electrophoretic bands was noted. Since
these bands were also homogeneous for light chain type, the authors
suggest that they may represent monoclonal proteins (59). Furthermore, it appears that certain bands with defined antibody specificities tend to migrate similarly in electropherograms. This is
evocative of a situation of possible cross reactive idiotypes and
should be a major thrust of future studies. Nucleocapsid activity
was quantitatively the most marked, owing either to the immunogenicity of this viral component or its excess production in CNS during SSPE.

Viral specific antibodies have also been isolated from CSF in
both SSPE and MS as viral-antibody complexes, with subsequent acid
elution of these antibodies at different pH's (60). The results
showed that different oligoclonal IgG proteins differed in the pH
required to disassociate them from their complexes. These eluates
could be analyzed further for viral product specificity. Homogeneous electrophoretic bands corresponding to IgG bands in the original material could also be identified. This kind of detailed
analysis correlating elution, specificity, and electrophoretic
variation, allows a careful dissection of the oligoclonal proteins
and such preparative approaches open the way to primary structural
studies as well as development of anti-idiotypic reagents. Another
observation in this study merits mention. Though most, if not all
CSF IgG from SSPE patients was absorbed by virus, only a portion
of the IgG in the CSF from MS patients is virally absorbed. Thus,

while the immune response in SSPE seems clearly to be induced by
a viral agent, the source of induction of the response in MS
remains an enigma.

PERSPECTIVES

Idiotypic reagents could be developed as primary specific
tools to tag cells which are responsible for the production of predominant clones. The first order of business would be to demonstrate the idiotypic identity of predominant immunoglobulin clones
and the Ig borne by lymphocytes in the CSF and, for that matter,
their analogues in serum. Whether these antibody species are due
to increased clonal proliferation or hypersecreting plasma cells
could then be assessed. A handle on what portion of Ig secreting
cells in the CSF are devoted to synthesis of these predominant
idiotypes could also be gained. By way of speculation, might certain clones proliferate for lack of proper idiotype – anti- idiotype
control imposed by the lack of a "network" balance in the restricted
compartment of CSF, or might suppressor T cell activity be excluded
in this compartment? The latter question might be approached with
in vitro mixing experiments between CSF cells of normal and
afflicted individuals. The former possibility opens avenues of
study focusing on the influence which infusion of anti-idiotype
might have on the course of these diseases. In the absence of animal
models, these studies would be rather stringently restricted if
common idiotypes are found not to dominate in different individuals
with the same disease.

The advances briefly outlined above in the analysis of immunoglobulins in CNS disorders leave the field ripe for a deeper analysis of the oligoclonal response and a more precise structural characterization of the molecules present in these conditions. Initial
attempts to develop idiotypic probes have begun. Nordal et al.
(61) produced an antiserum recognizing an idiotypic determinant
associated with a nucleocapsid specific electrophoretically
restricted band in CSF of an SSPE patient. This antiserum did not
react with other oligoclonal proteins in the same patients' CSF
or with serum, or CSF from four other SSPE and 10 MS patients.
Idiotypic identity of matched serum and CSF oligoclonal bands was
established and blockage with viral antigens suggested the site
specific nature of the anti-idiotype. Further studies would provide information on whether the heterogeneity and electrophoretic
bands is also reflected in idotypic heterogeneity as well, and
would hopefully unearth shared idiotypes, conceivably even diagnostic idiotype. If the latter is borne out, clues to the etiology
of these diseases may soon be forthcoming.

ACKNOWLEDGEMENTS

Supported in part by grants from the National Institutes of
Health (AI-12127) and the National Science Foundation (PCM-76-22411)
and by a Training Grant (CA 09082) award by the National Cancer
Institute to the Graduate Program in Immunology.

REFERENCES

1. Edelman, G.M., Cunningham, B.A., Gall, W.E., Gottlieb, P.D.,
   Rutishauser, U. and Waxdal, M. Proc. Nat. Acad. Sci. U.S.A.
   63:78, 1969.
2. Givol, D. Proc. Nat. Acad. Sci. U.S.A. 70:1585, 1973.
3. Edelman, G.M. and Gall, W.E. Ann. Rev. Biochem. 38:415, 1969.
4. Poljak, R.J., Amzel, L.M., Chen, B.L., Phizackerley, R.P. and
   Saul, F. Proc. Nat. Acad. Sci. U.S.A. 71:3440, 1974.
5. Schiffer, M., Girling, R.L., ELy, K.R. and Edmundson, A.D.
   Biochemistry, 12:4620, 1972.
6. Segal, D.M., Padlan, E.A., Cohen, G.H., Rudikoff, S., Potter,
   M. and Davies, D.R. Proc. Nat. Acad. Sci. U.S.A. 71:4298, 1974.
7. Nisonoff, A., Hopper, J.E. and Spring, S.B. The Antibody Molecule. Academic Press, 1975.
8. Porter, R.R. Biochem. J. 73:119, 1959.
9. Inbar, D., Hochman, J. and Givol, D. Proc. Nat. Acad. Sci.
   U.S.A. 69:26, 1972.
10. Hochman, J., Inbar, D. and Givol, D. Biochem. 12:1130, 1973.
11. Capra, J.D. and Kehoe, J.M. Adv. in Immunol. 20:1, 1975.
12. Wang, A.C., Pink, J.R.L., Fudenberg, H.D. and Ohms, J. Proc.
    Nat. Acad. Sci. U.S.A. 66:657, 1970.
13. Kohler, J., Shimizu, A., Paul, C., Moore, V. and Putnam, F.W.
    Nature 277:1318, 1970.
14. Capra, J.D. Nature 230:61, 1971.
15. Schur, P.H. In "Progress in Clinical Immunology" (R.S.
    Schwartz, Ed) Vol I, p. 192, Grune and Stratton, New York,
    1972.
16. Capra, J.D. and Kehoe, J.M. J. Immunol. 114:678, 1975.
17. Capra, J.D. and Klapper, D.G. La Riceria 6:39, 1976.
18. Capra, J.D. Proc. Roy. Soc. Med. Symposium, Rockefeller,
    University, 1975.
19. Wu, T.T. and Kabat, E.A. J. Exp. Med. 132:211, 1970.
20. Mole, L.E., Jackson, S.A., Porter, R.R. and Wilkinson, J.M.
    Biochem. J. 124:301, 1971.
21. Slater, R.J., Ward, S.M. and Kunkel, H.G. J. Exp. Med. 101:
    85, 1955.
22. Oudin, J. Proc. Roy. Soc., Ser. B, 166:207, 1966.
23. Williams, R.C. and Kunkel, H.G. Arthritis Rheum. 6:665, 1963.
24. Williams, R., Kunkel, H.G. and Capra, J.D. Science 161 :
    379, 1968.
25. Feizi, T. and Kabat, E.A. J. Exp. Med. 135:1247, 1972.

26. Capra, J.D., Kehoe, J.M., Williams, R., Feizi, T. and Kunkel H.G. Proc. Nat. Acad. Sci. U.S.A. 69:40, 1972.
27. Wang, A.C., Fudenberg, H.H., Wells, J.V. and Roelcke, D. Nature: New Biol. 243:126, 1973.
28. Riesen, W.F., Majaniemi, I., Huser, H., Braun, D.G. and Roelcke, D. Scand. J. Immunol. 8:145, 1978.
29. Kunckel, H.G., Agnello, V., Winchester, R.J. and Capra, J.D. J. Exp. Med. 137:331, 1973.
30. Kunkel, H.G., Winchester, R.J., Joslin, F.G. and Capra, J.D. J. Exp. Med. 139:128-136, 1974.
31. Capra, J.D. and Kehoe, J.M. Proc. Nat. Acad. Sci. U.S.A. 71:845, 1974.
32. Capra, J.D. and Klapper, D.G. Scand. J. Immunol. 5:677, 1976.
33. Natvig, J.B., Kunkel, H.G., Rosenfield, R.E., Dalton, J.F. and Kochwa, S. J. Immunol. 116:1536, 1976.
34. Nisonoff, A., Tung, A.S. and Capra, J.D. Critical Factors in Cancer Immunology, Miami Symposium, Academic Press, 85, 1975.
35. Kabat, E.A., Moore, D.H. and Landow, H.J. Clin. Invest. 21:571, 1972.
36. Yahr, M., Goldensohn, J.S. and Kabat, E.A. Ann. N.Y. Acad. Sci. 58:613, 1954.
37. Frick, E., and Scheid-Seydel, L. Klin. Wshr. 36:66, 1958(a).
38. Frick, E. and Scheid-Seydel, L. Klin. Wshr. 36:857, 1958(b).
39. Frick, E. and Scheid-Seydel, L. Klin. Wshr. 38:1240, 1960.
40. Cutler, R.W.P., Merlen, E. and Hammerstad, J.P. Neurology 18, Part 2, 129, 1968.
41. Cutler, R.W.P., Watters, G.V. and Hammerstad, J.P. Sci 10 : 259, 1978.
42. Cutler, R.W.P., Watters, G.V., Hammerstad, J.P. and Merlen, E. Arch. Neurol. (Chic.) 17:620, 1967.
43. Tourtellotte, W.W. and Parker, J.A. Sci. 154:1044, 1966.
44. Tourtellotte, W.W. and Parker, J.A. Nature (Lond.) 214:683, 1967.
45. Tourtellotte, W.W., Parker, J.A., Herndon, R.M. and Andros C.V. Neurology 18, Part 2, 117, 1968.
46. Sandberg-Wollheim, M. Sand. J. Immunol. 3:717, 1974.
47. Sandberg-Wollheim, M., Zetterman, O. and Muller, R., Clin. Exp. Immunol. 4:401, 1969.
48. Fraser, K.B. Brit. Med. Bull. 33:34, 1977.
49. Vandvik, B. and Nordal, H. Eur. Neurol. 17:23, 1978.
50. Laterre, E.C. Arscia, Bruxelles, 1965.
51. Link, H. Acta Neurol. Scand. 43, suppl. 28:1, 1967.
52. Laterre, E.C., Callewaert, A., Heremans, J.F. and Sfaeko. Neurology, 20:982, 1970.
53. Bucher, T., Matzelf, D. and Pette, D. Klin. Wschr. 30:325, 1952.
54. Booy, J. Folia Psychiat. Neurol. 62:37, 1959.
55. Karcher, D., Van Sande, M. and Lowenthal, A. J. Neurochem. 4:135, 1959.
56. Lowenthal, A. Agar Gel Electrophoresis in Neurology. Elsevier, Amsterdam, 1964.

57. Vandvik, B. Scand. J. Immunol. 6:913, 1977.
58. Vandvik, B., Natvig, J.B. and Wiger, D. Scand.J. Immunol.
    5:427, 1976.
59. Vandvik, B. and Norrby, E. Proc. Nat. Acad. Sci. 20:1060,
    1973.
60. Vandvik, B., Norrby, E., Nordal, H.J. and Degre, M. Scand.
    J. Immunol. 5:979, 1976.
61. Nordal, H.J., Vandvik, B. and Natvig, J.B. Scand. J. Immunol.
    6:1351, 1977.

STRUCTURAL STUDIES OF IMMUNOGLOBULINS FROM PATIENTS AFFECTED BY SUBACUTE SCLEROSING PANENCEPHALITIS

A.D. Strosberg [+], F. Bollengier [+], N. Mahler-Rabinovitch [+],
H. Valdimarsson [x] and A. Lowenthal [+o]

+ Free University of Brussels (V.U.B.) Belgium
o University of Antwerp (U.I.A.) Belgium
x St. Mary's Hospital, London, U.K.

SUMMARY

Homogeneous immunoglobulin fractions were isolated from sera from several patients affected by subacute sclerosing panencephalitis. In one case, a large amount of plasma was obtained by plasmaphoresis. The major immunoglobulin G fractions were purified by ammonium or sodium sulfate precipitation followed by DEAE-ion exchange chromatography and preparative column isoelectric focusing. Measles antibody activity was verified by inhibition of hemagglutination and precipitin reaction with measles or SSPE virus preparations.

Amino acid sequence determinations of the light and heavy chains and of their peptides confirm the homogeneity of the isolated antibody fractions. A comparison of the light chains amino terminal sequences between themselves and with myeloma proteins indicate that SSPE light chains often belong to a variable region subgroup intermediary between the V_KII and the V_KIII subgroup of chains. An unusually high proportion of SSPE heavy chains belongs to the unblocked V_HIII subgroup.

INTRODUCTION

The initial description of electrophoretically homogeneous immunoglobulin fractions in subacute sclerosing panencephalitis (SSPE) by Lowenthal in 1964 has since been confirmed by several

319

groups of investigators (1, 2). Criteria for homogeneity have
included single electrophoretic mobility in agar, agarose and
polyacrylamide, a narrow range of isoelectric points, antibody
activity restricted to only one of the antigenic subfractions of
measles virus preparations, the presence of either κ or λ light
chains and only G1 heavy chains in isolated fractions of SSPE
immunoglobulins (3, 4).

A first report of structural homogeneity of SSPE immunoglobulin by the criteria of amino acid sequence determination was
published recently (5). In that work we compared three homogeneous
immunoglobulin fractions isolated from a single patients with
SSPE. In the present publication we substantiate our initial
observations by extending them to immunoglobulins from several
other SSPE patients.

MATERIALS AND METHODS

Serological techniques. Serum samples were obtained from
patients who clinically and serologically manifested SSPE.

Isoelectric focusing in polyacrylamide gel slabs was performed as reported previously. Immunoglobulin fractions were purified
by liquid isoelectric focusing with a LKB 440 ml column run at
4°C. A stabilizing gradient of 0-40 % sucrose was used with carrier ampholytes at a concentration of 1 % in the pH range 8-9, 5.
Details of the procedure have been published elsewhere (7).

Ion exchange chromatography. Twice ammonium sulfate (35 %)
precipitated SSPE immunoglobulins were dialyzed overnight against
0.005 M PO_4 buffer, pH 8, and applied to a 5-ml DEAE-cellulose
column, equilibrated with the same buffer. Proteins were eluted
with a 0.005 M to 0.500 M PO_4 buffer gradient.

Preparation of heavy and light chains. Purified SSPE immunoglobulins were mildly reduced and alkylated according to the procedure of Fleischman et al. (8) with 0.1 M 2-mercaptoethanol and 0.11
M iodoacetic acid in 0.4 M Tris-HCl. Heavy and light chains were
separated by Sephadex G-100 gel filtration in 1 N acetic acid and
proteins were dialysed against water and lyophylized.

Sequence determination. Amino terminal sequence determination was performed with a Beckman 890C sequenator, as described
previously (9). A 0.1 M Quadrol buffer system was employed
throughout. PTH amino acid derivates were identified by gas
liquid chromatography (10), and by thin-layer chromatography on
polyamide sheets (11) by the original method but for the substitution of BPBD (Packard, Downers Grove, Ill.) by BBOT (Packard)

as suggested by D. Klapper (personal communication). The identification of the PTH amino acid derivatives was confirmed by HI
hydrolysis (18) and subsequent amino acid analysis on a Durrum amino
acid analyzer.

RESULTS

A number of immunoglobulin components from individual SSPE
patients were purified using ammonium or sodium sulfate precipitation followed by DEAE-cellulose ion-exchange chromatography and
preparative column isoelectric focusing. This last technique
was applied to the serum of patient Fau (figure 1).

The resulting fractions were examined on polyacrylamide slab
gel isoelectric focusing (figure 2). The isolated immunoglobulins
were partially reduced and alkylated and the light and heavy
chains were separated by gel chromatography on Sephadex G 100.

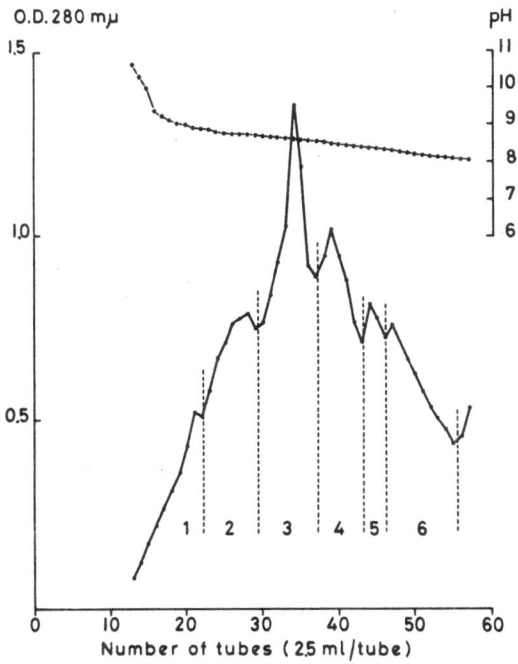

Figure 1 : Preparative isoelectric focusing of the IgG fraction
           of serum Fau.

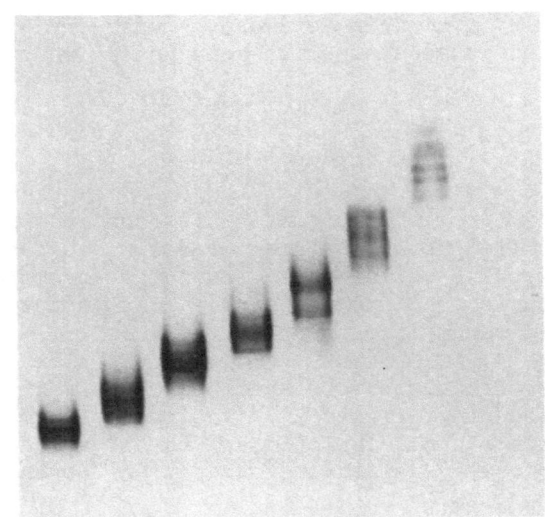

Figure 2: Analytical isoelectric focusing of SSPE immunoglobulin
           fractions from patient Fau, prepared on column focusing

     Both type of chains were submitted to automated Edman degra-
tion. Amino terminal sequences of two light chains presented in
figure 3, are compared to model myeloma sequences.

     Three more L chains, L Rom, L Deb and L Sch were sequenced
for 10 or 11 residues. They all were identical to the Fau sequence,
with either a Met or a Leu residue at position 4.

                            DISCUSSION

     The results reported above, together with those published
earlier (5) confirm that immunoglobulins present in serum of SSPE
patients may be of sufficient restricted heterogeneity to permit
a simple fractionation procedure followed by straight forward
sequence determination. Since cerebrospinal fluid immunoglobulins
share idiotypic determinants with the serum proteins it is likely
that the CSF proteins also would be amenable to structural studies,
provided sufficient amounts of material could be prepared.

     The striking similarities between the five SSPE L chains we
have analyzed so far do suggest that the SSPE immunoglobulins are
drawn from a small subpopulation of the large variety of immuno-

```
              10        20        30              37
               |         |         |               |
         DIVMTQSPLSLPVTPGEPASISCRSSQDLS var var LNWYL

V_KII    ─────────────────T──A──V─  ─   ─   ─────

LFAU     ─ L ──── ST-SA-V-(R)──(-)──6─  Q   Y  -A─Q

LGOE     ─ L ──── A─S────(R)-L─────────  ─   ─   ─────

V_KIII   E ─ L ──── GT-SLS──R─L──────S-N var var ────Q
```

A line indicates identity with the top model sequence.
D=asp, N=asn, T=thr, S=ser, E=glu, Q=gln, P=pro, G=gly, A=ala,
C=cys, V=val, M=met, I=ile, L=leu, Y=tyr, F=phe, W=trp, K=lys,
R=arg, H=his.

Figure 3 : Amino terminal sequences of two SSPE light chains, L
Fau and L Goe, compared to the V_KII and V_KIII prototype sequences
derived from myeloma light chains.

globulins normally present in serum. A comparison of the highly
conserved amino terminal sequence with that of the three prototype subgroup light chain sequences computed from known sequences
of human myeloma light chains confirms indeed that the SSPE chains
belong to an intermediary group which displays a typical V_KII
substitution (Asp in position 1), a typical V_KIII substitution
(Ser in position 12) and two substitutions not frequently encountered in each of the two groups of chains : an Ala or a Ser
residue in position 9 and an Ala or a Val residue in position
13.

We had previously reported that the SSPE heavy chains are
frequently found with an unblocked N terminal residue, a characteristic of the V_KIII subgroup which represents only 20 % of
chains of normal immunoglobulins.

We also report here for the first time the sequence of the
first hypervariable region of an SSPE light chain. A comparison
of hypervariable regions from several chains is necessary before
any conclusion can be drawn as to the existence of a characteristic
set of variable regions present in SSPE immunoglobulins.

ACKNOWLEDGEMENTS

Mr. I. Caplier and V. Lion provided expert technical assistance. The amino acid compositions were kindly determined by Mrs.
M. Van der Linden. The constant support of Dr. L. Kanarek is
gratefully recognized. This work was made possible by funds from
NATO, the Concerted Actions and the Belgian F.G.W.O.

REFERENCES

1. Lowenthal, A. : Agar gel Electrophoresis in Neurology, Elsevier Publishing Co., Amsterdam (1964).

2. Vandvik, B. and Norrby, E. : Oligoclonal IgG antibody response in the central nervous system to different measles virus antigens in subacute sclerosing panencephalitis. Proc. Natl. Acad. Sci. 70, 1060 (1973).

3. Vandvik, B., Natvig, J.B. and Norrby, E. : IgG1 subclass Restriction of Oligoclonal Measles Virus-Specific IgG Antibodies in Patients with Subacute Sclerosing Panencephalitis and in a Patient with Multiple Sclerosis. Scand. J. Immunol., 6, 651 (1977).

4. Bollengier, F., Rabinovitch, N. and Lowenthal, A. : Oligoclonal immunoglobulins, light chain rations and free light chains in cerebrospinal fluid and serum from patients affected with various neurological diseases. J. Clin. Chem. Clin. Biochem. 16, 165 (1968).

5. Strosberg, A.D., Karcher, D. and Lowenthal, A. : Structural homogeneity of human subacute sclerosing panencephalitis antibodies. J. of Immunol. 115, 157 (1975).

6. Awdeh, Z.L., Williamson, A.R. and Askonas, B.A. : Isoelectric focusing in polyacrylamide gel and its application to immunoglobulins. Nature : 219, 66 (1968).

7. Strosberg, A.D., Jeffery, R.A., Freier, L.J. and Connolly, W.J.: Accelerated liquid isoelectric focusing using a direct current source that maintains constant power. Analyt. Biochem. 69, 76 (1975).

8. Fleischman, J.B., Porter, R.R. and Press, E.M. : The arrangement of the peptide chains in γ-globulin. Biochem. J., 88, 220 (1963).

9. Brauer, A.W., Margolies, M.N. and Haber, E. : The application of 0.1 M quadrol to the microsequence of proteins and the sequence of tryptic peptides. Biochemistry. 14, 3029 (1975).

10. Pisano, J.J. and Bronzert, T.J. Analysis of amino acid phenylthiohydantoins by gas chromatography. J. Biol. Chem., 244, 5597 (1969).

11. Summers, M.R., Smythers, G.W. and Orozlan, S. : Thin-layer chromatography of sub-nanomole amounts of phenylthiohydantoin (PTH) amino acids on polyamide sheets. Analyt. Biochem. 53 624 (1973).

12. Inglis, A.S., Nicholls, P.W. and Roxburgh, C.M. : Acid hydrolysis of phenylthiohydantoin of amino acids. Aust. J. Biol. Sci. 24, 1247 (1971).

13. Strosberg, A.D., Marescau, B., Thielemans, K., Vray, B., Karcher, D. and Lowenthal, A. : Cross-idiotypic specificity

among immunoglobulins in subacute sclerosing panencephalitis and multiple sclerosis. Proc. Nato Advanced Study Institute in Neurological Diseases. Antwerp, 1978 (This volume).

INSIGHTS GAINED FROM THE STUDY OF HOMOGENEOUS RABBIT ANTIBODIES

E. Haber, M.N. Margolies and L.E. Cannon

Cardiac Unit, Departments of Medicine and Surgery,
Massachusetts General Hospital and Harvard Medical School,
Boston, Mass., U.S.A.

The immune system is characterized by a remarkable diversity of
antibody specificities. The massive body of experimental data accumulated by Landsteiner (34) attests to the fact that nearly any complex
organic molecule may act as an antigenic determinant and that antibodies may readily differentiate among structures which differ only
slightly. The capacity to recognize a unique molecule within a
complex mixture has been exploited extensively in recent years in
the development of specific and sensitive radioimmunoassays (59).

Investigators early recognized the difficulty of reconciling
a vast number of potential antibody specificities with the present
understanding of the size of the immunoglobulin gene pool and conventional concepts of protein synthesis. If there really were 10^7 or
10^8 different antibodies, each represented by a unique germ line
gene, a very substantial part of the mammalian genome would have
to be occupied by the information relevant to the immune system.
Several proposals were advanced in an attempt to circumvent this
obvious problem. Talmadge (54) suggested that the specificity
of an individual antiserum was really generated by the sum of the
specificities of a multiplicity of component antibodies. Each of
the components would have a broad or more general specificity and
exquisite selectivity could only be attained by summing the properties of many individual antibodies. The demonstration that the
selectivity and specificity of antibody mixtures in sera was also
characteristic of either elicited antibodies (18) or antigen binding
myeloma proteins (45) characterized by complete molecular homogeneity
rendered this explanation of diversity unlikely. Another attempt
at simplification postulated that each antibody combining site was
characterized by multiple specificities (46). According to this
hypothesis a single antibody molecule might serve multiple and diverse

functional requirements. The realization that the antibody combining
site was comprised of both the variable region of the heavy and the
light chain gave rise to still another hypothesis : individual heavy
or light chains might combine with a variety of different partners and
thereby generate a very large number of specificities perhaps limited
only by the number of permutations and combinations possible.

Since there are clearly a variety of mechanisms that could
account for the vast number of antibody specificities observed
without invoking a multiplicity of antibody molecules or their
component polypeptide chains, it would seem relevant to address a
question which may have a less ambiguous answer: how many variable
light and heavy polypeptide chain sequences are there? This question cannot be answered by such data as that of Klinman and his
colleagues (31) who estimated that the adult mouse has in excess
of 10^7 antibody forming clones. If random assortment of light and
heavy polypeptide chains variable regions were allowed, this number
of unique antibodies could be accounted for by 3.3×10^3 light chain
and 3.3×10^3 heavy chain variable region sequences. V region genes
accounting for this number of polypeptide chains would occupy less
than 2% of an average human chromosome (48).

Two recent lines of evidence bear directly on the number of
different variable regions and appear on the surface to be contradictory. Tonegawa and colleagues (55), utilizing nucleic acid hybridization techniques, have clearly shown that there is only one copy
for the gene encoding for the variable portion of the lambda chain
in the mouse. Weigert and colleagues (57), however, have sequenced
8 lambda variable region phenotypes. It is of interest that none
of these phenotypes correspond exactly to the embryonic gene sequence
as it would be translated. Leder (33) enumerated kappa chain
variable region genes in the embryonic genome. While many more
were found than the single lambda V region gene, the number appears
relatively restricted and can by no means account for all the mouse
kappa phenotypes sequenced thus far. Thus nucleic acid hybridization
studies point to a relatively small number of variable region genes
that are amplified by some as yet unknown process to a much larger
number of phenotypes.

A quite contradictory finding is the observation that variable
region phenotypes (idiotypes) are inherited and may even be mapped
in the genome. Indeed Potter (45) is now willing to call these V
region "isotypes". Thus in contrast to nucleic acid hybridization
studies, a large number of germ line genes specifying variable
regions are suggested.

A direct attack on the question of whether there are few or
many variable region phenotypes would simply be to enumerate V
region sequences. One could determine how often identities occurred
among myeloma proteins or count antibodies which appeared in all

members of a given strain ("public" phenotypes). Evidence indicates
that neither myeloma proteins (45) nor antibodies characterized both
by idiotypic identity and occurrence in different individuals(26)
are a representative sample. Nisonoff (26) showed that when the
ARS phenotype common to all A/J mice was suppressed, each individual
mouse would produce antibodies specific for the ARS antigen and
manifesting a unique idiotype not found in any other mouse, hinting
at a vast potential diversity. Our own approach has been to examine
the amino acid sequences of elicited antibodies to relatively simple
antigens in the rabbit (17, 18, 19, 35). We elected to impose
antigen as the only selective force in order to determine the number
of variable region sequences which might appear during the course
of conventional immunization.

The Immune Response to Pneumococcal Vaccines

The ability to obtain large amounts of antibodies that are
monoclonal or greatly restricted in heterogeneity through hyperimmunization of rabbits with bacterial vaccines has provided material
for detailed structural characterization of specific elicited antibodies (32, 17). Although immunization with other antigens rarely
yields sufficient amounts of homogeneous antibody for complete
sequence analysis, improved methods of purification and advances
in sequencing technology now permit extended sequence studies of
antibodies of a variety of specificities. We examined the amino
acid sequences of rabbit antibody V region utilizing data obtained
in our laboratory as well as that reported by others (see figures).

Type III or Type VIII pneumococcal vaccines are employed as
antigens in our laboratory. Most of the antibodies produced are
specific for the capsular polysaccharide of the organism. The
structures of type III(S3) and type VIII (S8) polysaccharides have
been determined (25) and found to be relatively simple. Both are
unbranched linear polymers. S3 is comprised of a repeating disac-
charide, while S8 is a repeating tetrasaccharide (Fig. 1).

Restricted responses are quite frequent among outbred rabbits
(10). Of 40 animals immunized with type VIII vaccine, 38 produced
a restricted response at some time during the course of a one-year
study (a restricted response was defined as one to four discrete
bands in the gamma-globulin region on cellulose acetate electrophoresis of anti-serum). Of 30 animals immunized with type III vaccine,
29 produced a restricted response. Considerable variability in the
general patterns of response was noted. In certain rabbits a single
antibody component was present at varying concentrations throughout
the period of study. When more than one antibody was produced,
quantitative variations within the antibody population were often
observed with time. In other instances, the quantitative relationship among a small number of antibody components was preserved

TYPE III

(Glucuronic Acid–1,4β-Glucose–1,3β–Glucuronic Acid–1,4β-Glucose)$_x$1,3β–

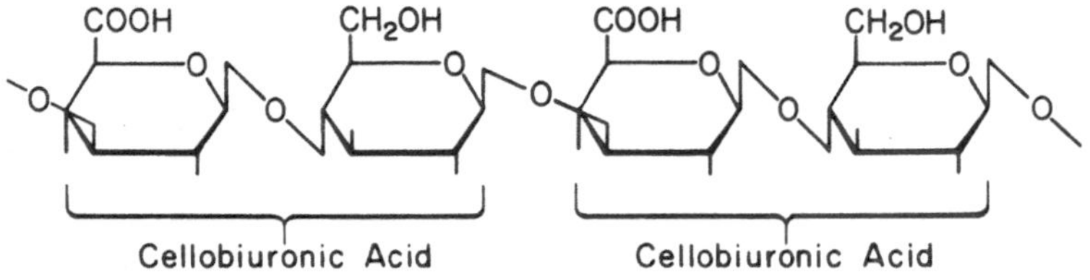

| COOH | CH$_2$OH | COOH | CH$_2$OH |

Cellobiuronic Acid   Cellobiuronic Acid

TYPE VIII

(Glucuronic Acid–1,4β-Glucose–1,4β–Glucose–1,4α–Galactose)$_x$1,4α–

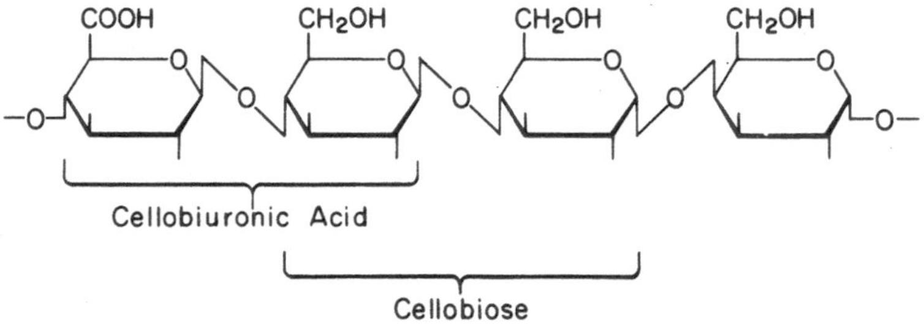

| COOH | CH$_2$OH | CH$_2$OH | CH$_2$OH |

Cellobiuronic Acid

Cellobiose

Figure 1. Structure of the type III and type VIII pneumococcal
polysaccharides. (Reprinted by permission, Raven Press, The
Future of Antibodies in Human Diagnosis and Therapy, p.47, 1977).

throughout the immune response, although the overall concentration
of each of the antibodies would vary.

Both affinity chromatography utilizing polysaccharide-protein
conjugates linked to sepharose (12) and ion-exchange chromatography
on DEAE cellulose have been effective in isolating single antibody
components, which may then be examined to determine amino acid
sequence.

Recently, pneumococcal vaccines have also been exploited as
a vehicle to obtain homogeneous antibodies directed against the
hapten, digoxin. An immunogen consisting of digoxin covalently
attached to type III pneumococci was synthesized as outlined in
Figure 2. Rabbits hyperimmunized with this bacterial-hapten conjugate produced substantial quantities of antidigoxin antibodies (up
to 15 mg per ml of serum) which for 25% of the animals were markedly
restricted in heterogeneity. Thus, conjugation of small organic

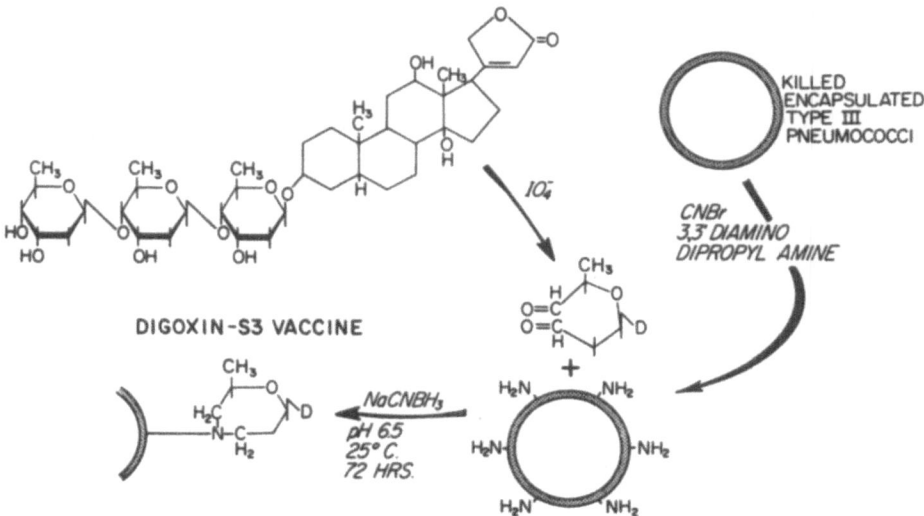

DIGOXIN-S3 VACCINE

Figure 2. Proposed mechanisms for reactions involved in the preparation of digoxin-S3 vaccine. D: = digoxigenin didigitoxose.
Digoxin (digoxigenin tridigitoxose) is oxidized to the vicinal
dialdehyde with sodium metaperiodate. The formalinized type III
pneumococci are activated with cyanogen bromide, and spacer arms
with amino groups are attached using 3,3'-diaminodipropylamine.
The aminated pneumococcus is then reacted with the dialdehyde
derivative of digoxin in the presence of sodium cyanoborohydride.
A rapid selective reduction of a putative iminium ion intermediate
by cyanoborohydride results in the digoxin-S3 vaccine with the
structure shown. (Reprinted by permission, J. Immunology, vol 121,
p.124, 1978).

molecules to bacterial immunogens may provide a general method for
obtaining homogeneous antihapten antibodies in amounts sufficient
for structural studies.

Strategie for Sequence Determination

     Classic methods of amino acid sequence determination are too
timeconsuming to permit comparisons among the primary structures
of a large number of homogeneous Ig heavy (H) and light (L) chains.
Successful automated Edman degradation in the liquid-phase spinning-
cup sequencer results in extended degradations of peptides (15).
Modifications of the programs employed, such as the use of dilute
Quadrol and altered solvent extractions (3), allow for 35 to 63 cycles

of Edman degradation on 5 to 100 nmol of large peptides. Successful extended degradation of small amounts of protein or peptide
require sensitive methods for identification of the PTH-amino acid
recovered at each cycle of degradation. Through the use of a dilute
Quadrol coupling buffer, altered solvent extractions, or the use of
polybrene (30) degradations extending 35 to 63 cycles may be obtained
on 5 to 150 nmol of peptide (Figure 3) (3). Identifications of
phenylthiohydantoin (PTH-) amino acids generated by automated Edman
degradation are obtained by gas-liquid chromatography (3), thin-
layer chromatography on polyamide sheets (53), and more recently
by high pressure liquid chromatography (37, 39). This approach
assures that each PTH-amino acid is identified by at least two independent methods, one of which is quantitative. Quantitative evaluation and confirmation by a second method is critically important for assessing V region homogeneity, especially within hypervariable segments.

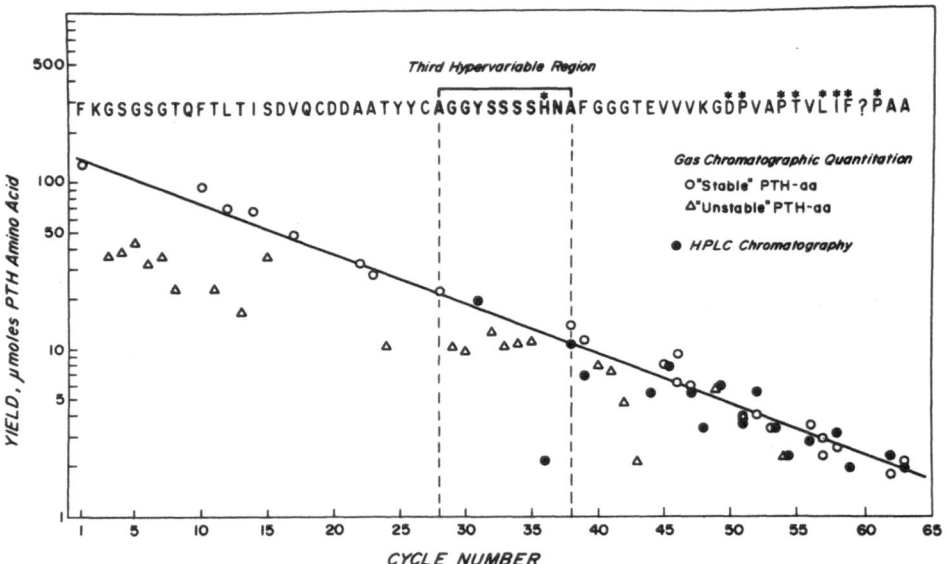

Figure 3. Yields of PTH-amino acids from spinning cup sequencer
degradation employing a 0.1 M Quadrol program on 150 nmol of a 150
residue tryptic peptide obtained from a citraconylated rabbit antibody light chain. HPLC was used for identification beginning after
approximately 30 cycles. Asterisks denote residues which could
be identified only by HLPC, and were not detected either by gas-
liquid chromatography, or by thin-layer chromatography. (Reprinted
by permission, Liquid Chromatography Symposium I, Marcel Dekker
(publisher), in press).

In the L and H chain sequences reported here, only a single amino acid residue was found at each position including the hypervariable regions. This stands in contrast to the results for the pooled L chains of anti-arsonate antibodies elicited in inbred mice (8), or for the antihapten antibodies from inbred guinea pigs (9, 56).

In addition to economy in amounts of antibody and time required to obtain sequence data, extended automated Edman degradation reduces the probability of incorrect sequence alignment caused by inadequate "overlap" sequences. For example, L chain 3368 (see Fig. 4) contains the sequence Asn-Ser-Asn-Asn-Val-Val-Asn-Asn-in the third hypervariable region. The correct assignment of this sequence by classic methods would require long peptides or multiple overlaps. Figures 4 and 5 reveal that there are large differences in chain length among both L and H chains within hypervariable regions (two in the L chain and seemingly only the 3rd in the H chain) that are best assessed by Edman degradation extending through this segment of the L chain. This is especially important, as results of X-ray crystallographic analyses of hapten-binding myelomas (44, 49) reveal that variations in lenght of complementarity segments would be expected to result in marked changes in the size of the antigenbinding site.

To provide large fragments suitable for automated Edman degradation, reproducible methods for cleaving L and H chains into a limited number of peptides have been developed. The strategy for cleavage of rabbit allotype b4 L chains is schematically illustrated in Figure 6. Rabbit antibody b4 L chains contain highly conserved arginine residues at positions 61 and 211. Additional arginines are occasionally found amino-terminal to position 61 but rarely between positions 61 and 98. Arginine residues are not found between positions 98 and 211 in b4 L chains. By restricting tryptic cleavage to arginyl peptide bonds through modification of lysines with citraconic anhydride, a large peptide extending from position 62 to 211 is usually obtained, as well as peptides comprising the amino terminal 61 positions of the L chain. Both the intact L chain and the 62-211 peptide can be sequenced for 40-60 cycles in the automated sequencer. Additional peptides can be generated if necessary by subjecting the purified arginine peptides to tryptic digestion at lysine residues following removal of citraconyl blocking groups.

Sequence analysis of the H chain is more challenging on account of its larger size ($\simeq$ 450 residues vs $\simeq$ 215 residues for L chains) and the presence of an amino-terminal pyrrolidone carboxylic acid residue which is refractory to Edman degradation. As shown in Figure 7, cleavage of rabbit γ -chains with cyanogen bromide produces a fragment, designated C1, containing the amino-terminal 246 residues of the H chain. Many rabbit H chains have a V region

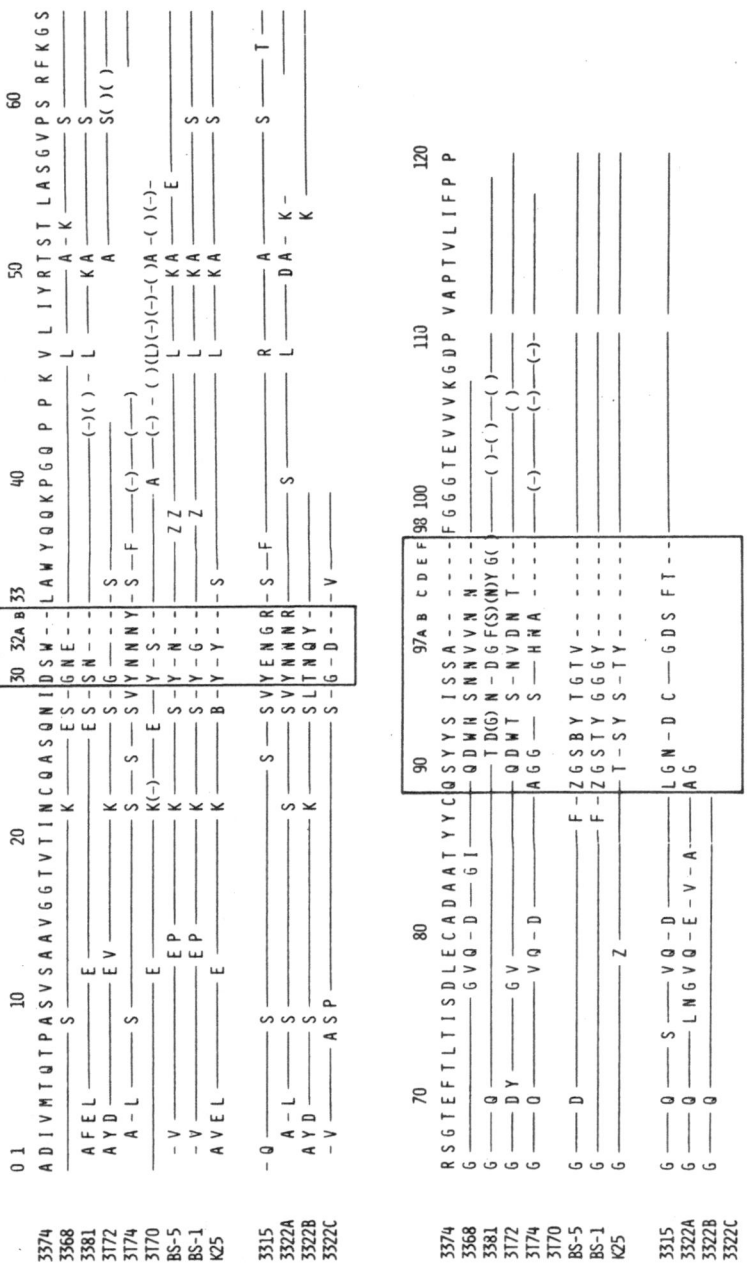

Figure 4. L-chain V region sequences from homogeneous anti-S3 and anti-S8 rabbit antibodies. Amino acid residues are indicated in a single letter code (see Figure 3). Residues in parentheses are tentative assignments and a question mark (?) indicates an unassigned residue. A horizontal line denotes identity with the sequence 3374; a dash denotes a deletion. Position numbering is by homology with the human V$_{KI}$ Ag. Complementarity-determining regions (L1 and L3) are boxed. All the sequences reported here are from our laboratory except BS-1, BS-5, and K25. (20).

Figure 5

Figure 5. H chain V region amino acid sequences of homogeneous and
normal (pool) rabbit Ig. The sequences are arranged according to
group a allotype. A broken line designates a deletion; positions
in parentheses contain tentative assignments or unidentified residues; a horizontal line indicates identity with the topmost sequence. The sequences for 3381, 3374, and 3T72 are from our laboratory.
The data on normal (pool) rabbit Ig; BS-1, BS-5, K25; and 2690 were
reported by others (20). A square corresponds to a cyclised glutamine residue (PCA).

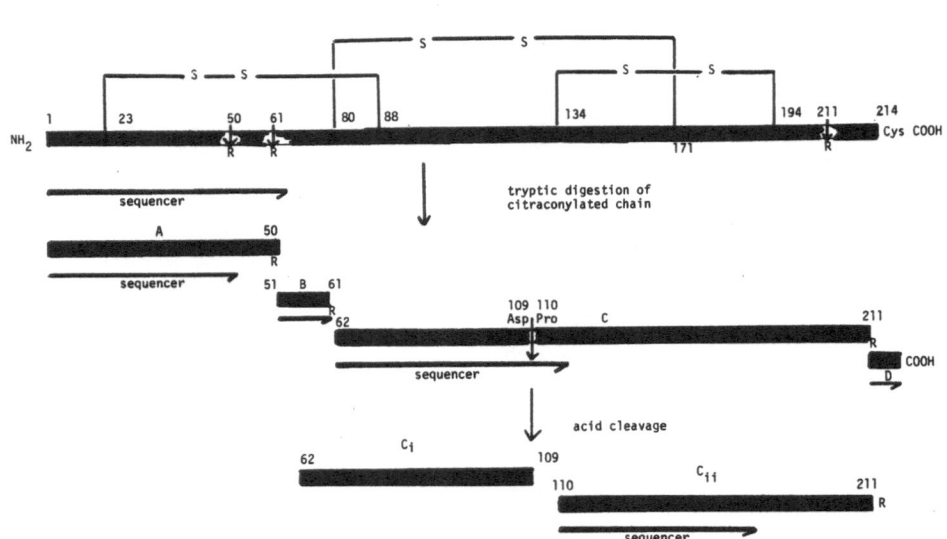

Figure 6. Scheme for sequence determination of rabbit L chains
by automated methods. The L chain is displayed linearly with the
amino terminus at the left. The V domain disulfide bridge (23-88),
and the constant domain disulfide bridge (134-194) are indicated.
The half-cystine residue at position 214 forms a disulfide bridge
with the H chain. An R denotes the position of arginine residues
where trypsin cleaves the citraconylated chain into the daughter
peptides A–D. Each of the peptides A–C may be subjected to automated Edman degradation. Peptide C may be cleaved under mild acid
conditions in b4 L chains between aspartic acid 109 and proline 110
(16). (Reprinted by permission of Raven Press, The Future of Antibodies in Human Diagnosis and Therapy, p. 48, 1977).

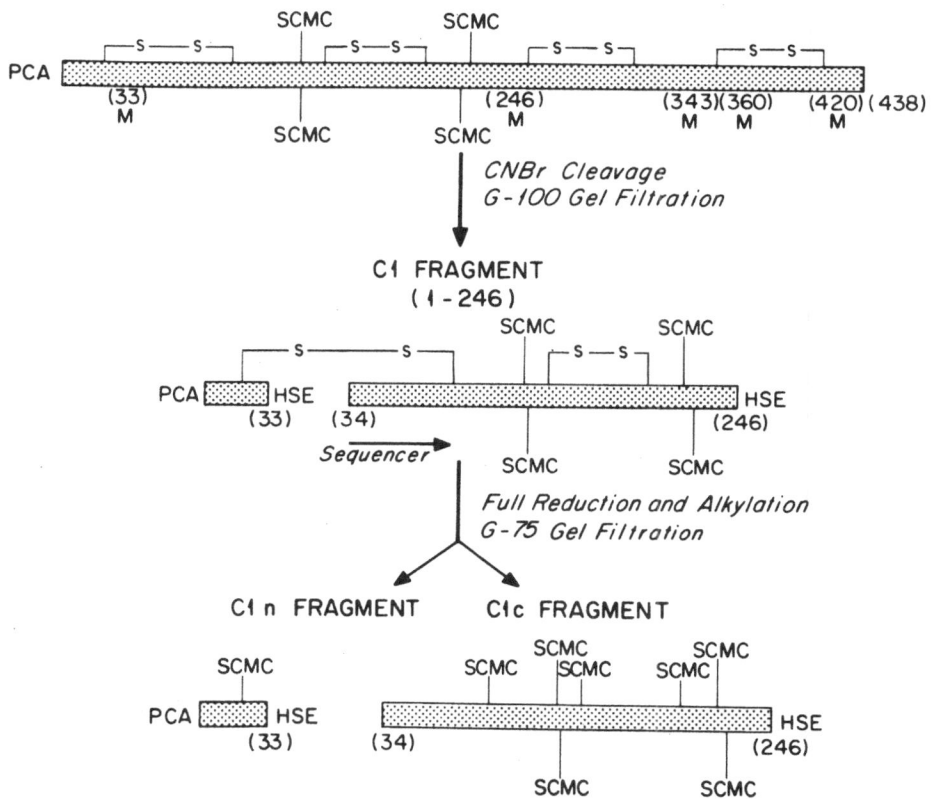

Figure 7a. Strategy for sequence determination of rabbit antibody
H chain V regions by automated methods. The H chain is displayed
linearly with the amino-terminus (pyrrolidone carboxylic acid-PCA)
at the left. Those half-cystine residues, which are reduced and
alkylated in the absence of denaturants, are indicated as SCMC.
The four intradomain disulfide bridges are indicated. The location
of methionine residues is indicated by (M). Cleavage with CNBr yields
a fragment (C1) containing the N-terminal 246 residues with an
internal cleavage (homoserine-HSE, at position 33). This fragment,
when subjected to automated Edman degradation reveals the sequences
beginning at position 34, because the amino-terminal fragment is
blocked to Edman degradation. Following reduction and alkylation
in the presence of denaturants, the C1N fragment (1-33) and the C1C
fragment (34-246) are separated by gel filtration. (Reprinted by
permission, Proceedings of the Basic Science Symposium, American
Society of Microbiology, 1978, in press).

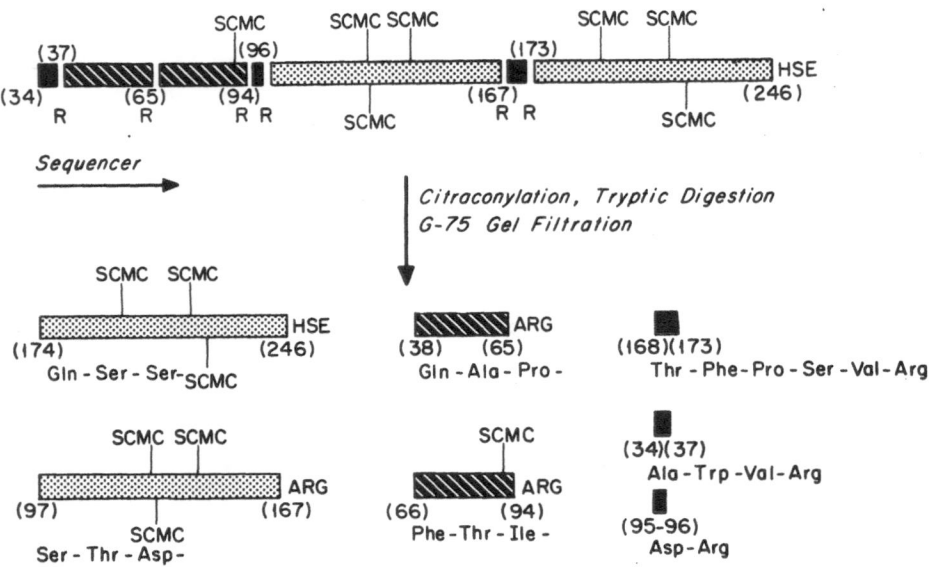

Figure 7b. The positions of arginine residues in the ClC fragment are indicated by R. Following citraconylation of ClC, tryptic arginine peptides are separated by gel filtration. Three mixtures of peptides are obtained as indicated. The amino-terminal sequences of the larger peptides are shown as well as the complete sequences of the smallest peptides. The invariant glutamine residues at positions 174 and 38 are selectively cyclized in acid, permitting Edman degradation of the unblocked member of each pair (97-167, 66-94). The smaller peptides (168-173, 34-37, 95-96) were sequenced following isolation by ion-exchange chromatography. (Reprinted by permission, Proceedings of the Basic Science Symposium, American Society of Microbiology, 1978, in press).

methionine located at position 33 which, when cleaved with cyanogen bromide, results in a free amino terminus at position 34, the fragments 1-33 and 34-246 being covalently linked by the V_H intradomain disulfide bond. Thus, the Cl fragment can be analyzed in the automated sequencer with degradation commencing at position 34. The two fragments 1-33 and 34-246 (ClN and ClC in Figure 7) are then separated by gel filtration following complete reduction and alkylation of Cl. The sequence of the ClN fragment is obtained through analysis of peptides generated by tryptic digestion, hydrolysis with S. aureus protease, and pronase digestion (2, 36). More recently, the sequence of blocked peptides has been simplified by the use of the enzyme pyrrolidone carboxylase (43). The sequence

of the V-region portion of the ClC fragment is solved by analysis
of peptides obtained by tryptic digestion of citraconylated ClC
(Figure 7). Additional overlap peptides are produced as necessary by chymotryptic digestion of ClC (2) or by S. aureus protease
digestion of Cl (38).

Light Chain Variable Region Sequences

Amino acid sequence data for rabbit anti-S3 and anti-S8 antibody V_L regions determined in this laboratory are presented in
Figure 4 with those reported by other investigators. A variability
plot calculated from these data and data reported previously (18)
is given in Figure 8. Examination of these sequence data and the
accompanying variability plot reveals three discrete regions of
increased variability : at the amino-terminus, at positions 29
to 33, and at positions 89 to 98. Each of these "hypervariable"
regions is also characterized by differences in polypeptide length
as indicated by placement of deletions in the shorter L chains in
order to maintain sequence homology. X-ray crystallographic analyses of human and mouse hapten-binding myeloma Fab fragments
(44, 49) reveal that in the intact antibody the regions 29 to 33
and 89 to 98 of V_L fold together with corresponding segments from
V_H (see below) to form the antigen binding site. Thus, these two
hypervariable regions, by virtue of containing residues that contribute to determining the antigen specificity of the binding site,
are also "complementarity-determining". Hypervariability at the
amino-terminus of the V_L region will be discussed subsequently
(see L-chain framework).

Rabbit K_B L chains demonstrate little variation in sequence
in the region (50-56) homologous to the second L chain hypervariable
region of human and murine kappa chains (Fig. 4). An identical
sequence in this region is found among an S3 antibody 3368 and an
S8 antibody 3315, and also among a streptococcal C antibody 4135
and an M. lysodeikticus antibody 120, which are not shown in the
figure. If this region contributes to the binding site, it may
represent a common feature of antipolysaccharide antibodies; a
corollary of this idea must be that an S3 antibody is distinguished
from an S8 antibody by virtue of residues contributed by other
hypervariable regions of L and/or H chains. An alternative explanation is that this region of the rabbit L chain is not involved
in the antigen-binding site. An examination of binding site
structure of haptenbinding myeloma Fab fragments as determined
by X-ray crystallography supports this contention. The second
L-chain hypervariable region of the phosphorylcholine-binding murine
myeloma McPC 603 does not participate in the binding site; in this
protein there is a large first L chain hypervariable region (49).
In the human lambda New Fab' which binds vitamin K, this region

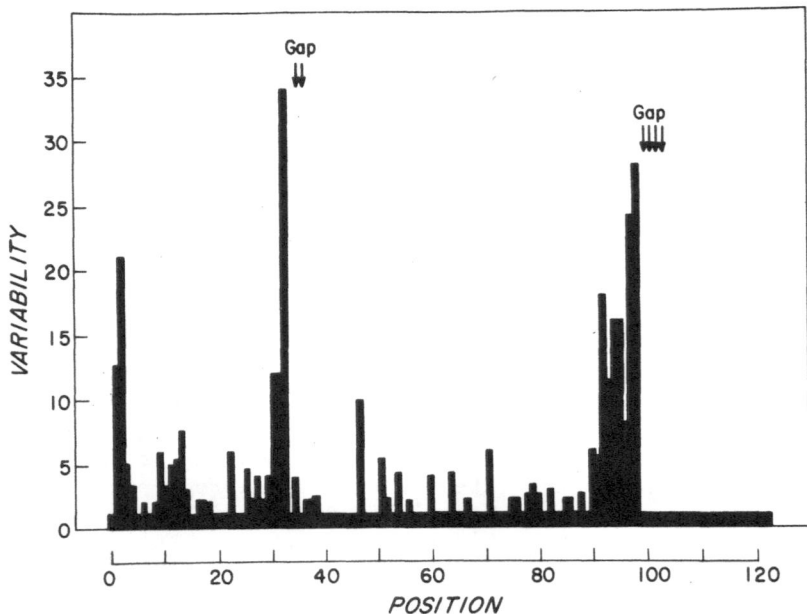

Figure 8. Variability plot according to the method of Wu and
Kabat based on the data from Fig.4 and data reported previously
(18). Variability is defined as the number of different amino
acids at a given position divided by the frequency of the most
common amino acid at that position. The variability at the amino
terminus is lessened when the sequenced are aligned by an objective method. (Reprinted from Proc. Natl. Acad. Sci. USA, 72:
2182, 1975).

is also not involved in binding, perhaps because there is an
adjacent seven-residue deletion in the polypeptide chain (44).
When the position of the alpha-carbons of the V_L kappa dimer REI
are compared with those of McPC 603, this region is superimposable
between the two structures (41), suggesting that it is part of
the "framework". Rabbit kappa chain framework sequences are more
homologous to the human $V_{\kappa I}$ framework than to human $V_{\kappa II}$ or $V_{\kappa III}$.
When a variability plot of human $V_{\kappa I}$ proteins is inspected (27)
significant variability is not seen at positions 50 to 56.
Further generalizations concerning the role of this segment of V_L
in the binding site require the determination of additional sequen-

ces from antibodies of other than carbohydrate specificity and
additional three-dimensional structures.

Presumably, amino acid substitutions within complementarity-
determining regions of the V domain account for the seemingly
unlimited variety of antigen specificities which antibodies may
manifest. Thus, it is not surprising and indeed to be expected
that complementarity-determining regions demonstrate hypervariability (58). However, it is unexpected to find hypervariability
among complementarity-determining regions of antibodies which
have specificity for the same simple antigen. The diversity
among the complementarity-determining regions of the nine anti-S3
antibody L chains shown in Figure 4 is such that no two L chains
share a common complementarity region sequence; nor is it possible
to identify even a single complementarity region position that is
shared among the nine L chains. Can the considerable diversity
found for the complementarity-determining regions of these anti-S3
and anti-S8 antibody L chains be due simply to extensive polymorphisms among allelic V_L region structural genes present in an
outbred population? To evaluate the possible role of such polymorphisms, several antibodies synthesized at the same time by an
individual rabbit were studied (11).

A rabbit (No. 3322) hyperimmunized with type VIII pneumococcal
vaccine produced at one time during the antibody response four
distinct anti-S8 antibody components. Each of these four components was purified by affinity chromatography and together accounted
for greater than 90% of the anti-S8 antibody synthesized by this
rabbit. All four antibodies demonstrated a common subspecificity
in that cellobiose, a constituent of S8 (see Figure 1), could
completely inhibit the binding of the four antibodies to the S8
polysaccharide. The amino acid sequence of the purified 3322
antibodies (3322-A, -B, -C, and -D) are shown in Figure 9 with
that of 3315, an S8 specific antibody, from another rabbit, which
does not bind cellobiose. The three L chains 3322-A, -B, and -C
display unique framework sequences including a difference in chain
length at the amino terminus. Recently, the fourth L chain,
3322-D, was found to have the amino-terminal sequence PCA-Val,
thus representing a fourth framework sequence (24). In addition,
the three L chains 3322-A, -B, and -C demonstrate marked sequence
variability and different lengths within the complementarity-
determining region at positions 29 to 33. The variability in this
region among these L chains isolated from antibodies having a
common subspecificity and obtained from a single rabbit is no
less than that seen among the unselected collection of anti-S3
and anti-S8 L chains shown in Figure 4. If allelic polymorphisms
among V_L structural genes contribute to the diversity of rabbit
anti-S3 and anti-S8 antibody L chains, then this contribution
appears to be minor relative to that of other mechanisms.

```
3315    ALA GLN ILE VAL MET THR GLN THR PRO SER SER VAL SER ALA ALA VAL GLY GLY THR VAL THR ILE
3322A           ALA ─── LEU ─────────────────────────────────────────────────────────
3322B       ALA TYR ASP ─────────────────────────────────────────────────────────────
3322C       ASP VAL ────────────────────── ALA ─── PRO ──────────────────────────────
3322D   PCA VAL


3315    ASN CYS GLN SER SER GLN SER VAL TYR GLU ASN GLY ARG LEU SER TRP PHE GLN GLN LYS PRO
3322A   SER ──────── ALA ────────────────── ASN ─── ASN ───────── ALA ─── TYR ─────────
3322B   LYS ──────── ALA ──────────── LEU THR ASN GLN TYR ··· ─── ALA ─── TYR ─────────
3322C   ─────────── ALA ──────────── ILE GLY SER ASP ··· ··· ─── VAL ─── TYR ───────────
```

Figure 9. Amino acid sequences for positions 0-40 of anti-S8 antibody L chains (11, 24). A line indicates identity with the topmost sequences. Deletions are indicated by broken lines. (Reprinted by permission, Proceedings of the Basic Science Symposium, American Society of Microbiology, 1978, in press).

L-Chain Framework

In contrast to the variability of the complementarity determining regions, the amino acid sequence of the nonbinding-site portion (framework) of rabbit V_L is relatively conserved (with the exception of the three amino-terminal positions), as are the homologous regions in other species. All residues identified by Wu and Kabat (58) that are invariant in myeloma L chains, except for a variation in proline 59, are present in rabbit L chains (35). Examination of the X-ray structures reveals that these residues are required for maintenance of essential features of the three-dimensional structure, such as the constant glycines which define hairpin turns allowing for antiparallel folding of adjacent segments. Whereas invariánt residues indicate positions subject to steric constraints in the three-dimentional structure, variability within the framework indicates positions where changes in amino acid side chains may occur without disturbing the chain folding necessary for immunoglobulin (Ig) function. For example, residue 46 in rabbit L chains exhibits five different amino acid replacements among 11 chains examined.

Another striking example of conservation of overall framework structure is the accomodation of an interdomain disulfide bridge spanning V and C regions in rabbit K_B L-chains (50, 51). The X-ray crystallographic structure of Fab'λ New (44) and the human L-chain dimer Mcg (47) reveals that the homologous residues in these L-chains are located at the correct distance from each other to be consistent with disulfide bridge formation. Thus the interdomain disulfide bridge is not likely to introduce structural constraints interfering with domain folding.

The amino-terminal regions (positions 0-20) is that portion of the rabbit V_L framework for which the greatest amount of sequence data is available (7). Marked variability in this portion of the V_L is unique to rabbit L chains and is not seen among human and murine L chains (6), and it does not contribute to the antigen binding site as indicated by crystallographic analysis. Thus hypervariability is not a sufficient criterion for identifying complementarity-determining residues (35). The hypervariable amino-terminal positions represent positions in the V_L framework where steric variations in amino acid side chains are permitted without interfering with tertiary structure. In Figure 10, we have recorded 66 amino-terminal sequences of rabbit L chains. Antigen specificities represented in this set of sequences are the pneumococcal type II, type III, and type VIII polysaccharides, the streptococcal group-A, group-A-variant, and group-C carbohydrates, the carbohydrate of peptidoglycan cell-wall constituents of M. lysodeikticus, and the protein conjugates of the benzene-arsonate, aminophenyltri-methylammonium, and the benzoate haptens.

The sequences are arranged in Figure 10 to illustrate the occurrence of three different amino-terminal chain lengths in rabbit kappa chains. Light chains having the longest chain length (e.g., 3368) are one amino acid residue longer than L chains having the most common chain length (e.g., 7331-G) and are two residues longer than L chains having the shortest chain length (e.g., 3322-A). In this figure, the sequences have been aligned by arbitrarily placing deletions relative to the longest chain length at the amino-terminal end (positions 0 and 1) of the L chains.

In addition to the occurrence of different chain lengths, this portion of the V_L framework is characterized by increased variability at position 1 (six amino acid residue alternatives)and at position 2 (eight amino acid residue alternatives). The observation that there are 45 unique sequences among the 66 amino-terminal sequences is an additional indication of the diversity among the framework of rabbit V_L. Even among the amino-terminal sequence of L chains associated with the same antigen specificity, considerable diversity is noted. For example, the 18 L chains that are derived from antibodies elicited by the type-III pneumococcal vaccine demonstrate 14 unique sequences. In addition to the occurrence of diverse amino-terminal sequences among L chains associated with the same antigen specificity, there are also numerous instances of identical amino-terminal sequences for L chains associated with very different specificities (e.g., 3413,

Antigen	Antibody Designation	Allo-type	0 5 10 15 20
Pneu III	3368	b4	A D I V M T Q T P S S V S A A V G G T V T
Strep C	K19	b4	———————————— A ————————————
Pneu III	3374	b4	———————————— A ————————————
Pneu VIII	3315	b4	- Q ————————————————————
Pneu III	3T70	b4	——————————— A — E —————————
Pneu VIII	722369	b4	——————————— A — E —————————
Strep Av	K4820	b4	——————————— A — E —————————
Strep Av	K429-1	b4	——————————— A — E —————————
M. Lyso.	1966-1	b6	- E ———————————— E —————————
P̄neu III	3380-3	b4	———————————— A - E P —————
Strep C	4135	b4	———————————— A — E P —————
Strep C	2711	b4	— V ———————— A — E P —————
Strep C	3521	b4	- N ————————— P — G ———————
Ap-BGG	7331-G	b4	A ? ————————————————————
Strep C	K20	b4	A — Z — A ————————————————
Strep C	4182-1	b9	A L ——————————— T ? ———————
Strep Av	K429-7S	b4	A L — E — A —————————————
Strep C	2461-Ib	b4	A L - L - Z — A —————————
Strep Av	K6-89	b4	A L - L - Z — A —————————
M. lyso.	153B	b4	A L ————————— P - E V ——— B ———
P̄neu III	3T75	b4	- V ————————————————————
Pneu VIII	2388-S	b4	- V ———————— A ———————————
Pneu III	722714-T	b4	- V ———————— A — E —————————
Pneu III	722714-G	b4	- V ———————— A — Q —————————
Strep C	4136	b4	- V ———————— A ? - E ———————
Pneu VIII	3322-C	b5	- V ————————— A - P ———————
Pneu III	3T76	b4	- V ———————— A ——— E P —————
Pneu VIII	2348-3	b4	- V ———————— A ——— E P —————
Pneu III	K17	b4	- V ———————— A ——— E P —————
Pneu III	BS-1	b4	- V ———————— A ——— E P —————
Pneu III	BS-5	b4	- V ———————— A ——— E P —————
Pneu VIII	325	b4	- V — Z — A ——— Z P ———————
Pneu III	724812-P	b4	———————————— A ——— E P —————
Pneu VIII	3322-B	b5	A Y D —————————————————
Pneu VIII	2388-C	b4	A Y D —————————————————
Strep A	3547	b4	A Y D —————————————————
Ap-BGG	7331-F2	b4	A Y ? —————————————————
Ap-BGG	7331-E	b4	A Y ——— A —— ? ———————————
Pneu III	3382	b4	A Y D ———————— A — E V ———
Pneu III	3T72	b4	A Y D ———————— A — E V ———
Strep A	3013-III	b4	A Y D — Z — A ——— T V —————
Pneu VIII	2388-2Aa	b4	- P — L ———————— P —————————
M. lyso.	1966-II	b6	- P — L ——————————— E ———
P̄neu III	K25	b4	A V E L —— A — E —————————
Pneu III	3381-2	b4	A F E L —— A — E —————————
M. lyso.	120	b4	A F E L ——————— E —————————
S̄trep C	2869-2	b9	A V - L ——————————— ? ———
Rp-Ed	134	b5	A V - L - Z - A - P ——— P ———
Strep C	2461-1	b4	A F Z — Z —— A — T - P ———
Strep C	2461-1a	b4	A A Z L - Z —— A — Z P ———
Ab-BGG	2717	b4	V E - L ———————— P ———————
Strep C	2990	b4	————————— P T A - Z P ———
Pneu III·	724812-G	b4	A V ——— V — A V - Q E V ———
Pneu VIII	3322-A	b4	A - L —————————————————
Pneu III	3T74	b4	A - L —————————————————
Pneu II	BS-6	b4	A - L —————————————————
Strep C	4153-I	b9	V ——————————— T ——— E ———
Strep C	4153-II	b9	V ——————————— T K —— E ———
Strep C	2869-1	b9	- L ————————— T ? —— E ———
M. lyso.	161	b4	—————————— K - V P — B ———
M̄. lyso.	166	b4	—————————— K - V P — B ———
R̄p-BGG	4140-4	b4	—————————— K - V P — B ———
Strep Av	K9-106	b4	—————————— K - V P — B ———
Strep C	3413	b4	————————— ? - K - V P — D ———
Strep A	3113	b4	——————————— ? - V —— D ———
Strep C	2690	b4	——————— Z ——— ? - V P —— P —

Fig. 10

Figure 10. Amino-terminal sequences of rabbit antibody kappa
chains. Amino acid residues are expressed in the single-letter
code. A question mark (?) designates an undetermined residue.
A line indicates identity with the top sequence (3368). Position
numbering is based on the human $V_K I$ prototype Ag. Sources for
the sequence data are referenced in Cannon et al (6). Pneu II,
Pneu III, and Pneu VIII designate the pneumococcal type II,
type III, and type VIII capsular polysaccharides, respectively.
M. lyso designates the carbohydrate and peptidoglycan cell-wall
constituents of M. lysodeikticus. Strep C, Strep A, and Strep Av
designate the streptococcal group-C, group-A and group-A variant
carbohydrates. Rp-BGG, Ap-BGG, and Ab-BGG designate the bovine
Ig conjugates of the benzenearsonate, aminophenyltrimethylammonium,
and benzoate haptens, respectively. Rp-Ed is the edestin conjugate
of the benzenearsonate hapten. (Reprinted by permission of Cold
Spring Harbor Symposium on Quantitative Biology, XLI : 652, 1977).

←————————————————————

K9-106, 4140-4, and 161 in Figure 10). These findings preclude
a definitive correlation between antigen specificity and V_L
framework sequence. If, as suggested by Cohn et al. (14) each
framework sequence reflects a germ-line gene, then the great
diversity of this set of L-chain amino-terminal sequences derived
from antibodies specific for a limited set of antigens requires
an impressively large germ-line gene repertoire.

    Because L-chain amino-terminal sequences are frequently used
to designate subgroups (21, 4, 28) and in gene-counting calculations (14), it is important to determine whether relationships
inferred by analysis of the amino-terminal 21 positions of the
L chain may be extrapolated to the complete framework of V_L.
If residue differences in the amino-terminal portion of these L
chains are predictive of differences in their complete frameworks,
then, for a given pair of L chains, the total number of framework
differences should be about five times greater than the number of
differences in the amino-terminal 21 positions of the two L chains.
This clearly is not the case for many of the L chains. For example,
based on their amino-terminal sequences, the 3368, 3374, and 3315
L chains should differ by only five to ten residues in their complete framework sequences; in fact, they differ by two to three times
this number. Other L chains with substantial differences in
amino-terminal sequence (BS-1, BS-5, or 4135 compared to K25,
3381, or 120) have very similar sequences in the remainder of their
frameworks (see Haber et al. 1977a for a review of these sequences).
For example, BS-1 and 3381 differ at seven positions in the amino-
terminal 20 residues (Fig. 9), but they differ at only five
positions in the remaining 80 positions of the framework. These
discrepancies between amino-terminal sequence and complete framework sequence place an important constraint on the use of amino-
terminal sequences as markers for germ-line V-region genes in the

rabbit, as well as suggesting that attempts to delineate subgroups
among rabbit L chains by analysis of amino-terminal sequences is
at best misleading.

When more limited sequence data were available, posttransla-
tional degradation was suggested as a possible mechanism for
amino-terminal variability in rabbit L chains. Perusal of the
data in Figure 10 indicates that it is quite impossible to convert
any of the longer sequences into a shorter sequence simply by
amino-terminal deletion (7).

Heavy Chain Variable Region Sequences

It may be argued that the antigen specificity of the antibody
molecule is determined principally by the H chain V region, and
that the failure to find homologous binding site structures among
anti-S3 and anti-S8 antibody L chains reflects the secondary importance of L chains in determining antigen binding function.
Are the complementarity-determining regions of rabbit antibody H
chains as diverse as those of L chains? To answer this question
we have determined V_H region amino acid sequences for three anti-S3
antibody H chains. These data and V_H region sequence data reported by other investigators are given in Figure 5. A variability
plot calculated from these data is shown in Figure 11. X-ray
crystallographic analyses have identified three complementarity-
determining regions within V_H which, in these rabbit H chains,
correspond to positions 29 to 34, postions 49 to 60 and positions
95 to 106 (44, 49). Examination of V_H sequences for rabbit antibodies (Figure 5) and the V_H variability plot (Figure 11) reveals
discrete segments of hypervariability at precisely these locations.
In contrast to rabbit V_L regions which demonstrate differences
in length in both complementarity-determining regions, these V_H
region sequences differ in length only in the complementarity-
determining region at position 95 to 106. Although there is little
sequence homology in the third complementarity-determining region
among these V_H regions, certain positions within the first and
second complementarity-determining regions are highly conserved;
for example, tyrosine at position 31 and methionine at position
33 within the first complementarity-determining region and isoleucine
at position 50, tyrosine at position 58, and alanine at position
59 within the second complementarity-determining region. These
residues predominate at the indicated positions among the homogeneous antibody V_H regions (Figure 5). Amino acid substitutions
at these positions are physicochemically conservative, e.g., valine
for methionine at position 33, leucine for isoleucine at position
50. Since these conserved amino acids occur in the V_H regions
associated with different antigen specificities, these residues
are not likely to contribute directly to antigen-binding. Padlan
(42) has noted similar conservation at the homologous positions

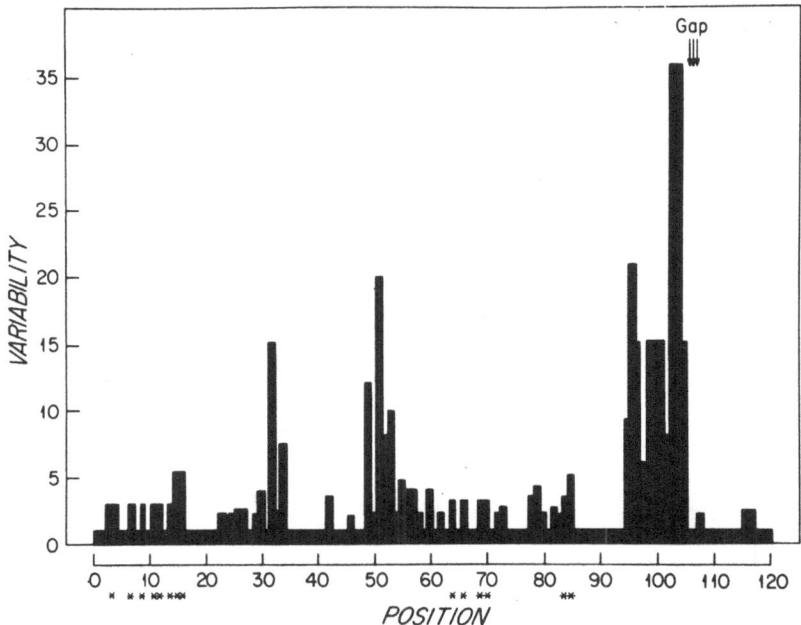

Figure 11. Variability plot for rabbit antibody V$_H$ region sequences calculated from the data in Figure 5. An asterisk denotes
the location of an allotypic correlate (36). (Reprinted by permission, Proceedings of the Basic Science Symposium, American
Society of Microbiology, 1978, in press).

among the V$_H$ regions of murine and human myeloma Igs having unrelated
or unknown antigen specificities. Based on the crystallographic
model of the McPC 603 binding site, he proposed a structural role
rather than a complementarity-determining function for residues
at these positions. When complementarity-determining positions
within the regions 29 to 34 and 49 to 60 are examined (Figure 5
and Figure 11), the variability encountered is comparable to that
found in the complementarity region at positions 29 to 33 among
rabbit anti-S3 and anti-S8 V$_L$ regions (Figure 8). Likewise the
variability in the third complementarity determining region of
V$_H$ is comparable to that of the homologous region in V$_L$ (compare
Figure 8 and 11). Clearly the extensive diversity found among
the complementarity-determining regions of rabbit antibody L chains
is also manifest among H chains.

Allotype	Ig Designation	4 GLU	7 GLY	9 ARG	11 12 VAL THR	14 15 16 GLY THR PRO	64 GLY	66 PHE	69 70 SER LYS	73 THR	84 85 THR GLU
a1	120	—	—	—	— —	— — —					
	Pool IgG	—	—	—	— —	— — —	—	—	— —	—	— —
		—	—	—	— —	— GLY SER	—	—	— —	—	— —
	BS-5	—	—	—	— —	THR PRO GLY	—	—	— —	—	— —
a2	K25	LYS	GLU	GLY	PHE LYS	THR ASP THR	SER	SER	THR ARG	ASX	ALA GLN
	BS-1	LYS	GLU	GLY	PHE LYS	THR ASP THR	SER	SER	THR ARG	ASX	ALA GLX
	2690	LYS	GLU	GLY	PHE LYS	THR ASN THR	SER	SER	THR ARG		
	Pool IgG	LYS	GLU	GLY	PHE LYS	THR ASP THR		SER	THR ARG		ALA ALA
a3	Pool IgG	—	—	ASP	— LYS	— ALA SER	—	—	— —	—	ALA ALA
a neg	Pool Ig	VAL	—	GLY	— —	GLN GLU GLY SER					

Figure 12. Amino acid sequence correlates of group a allotype
(36). All amino acid substitutions in the rabbit V_H that differ
between at least two of the group a allotypes are listed. Residues in hypervariable regions are excluded. A line indicates
identity with the amino acid in the top sequence. References
for the sequence data are given in the legend to Figure 5.
(Reprinted by permission of J. Immunology, 119 : 290, 1977).

Heavy Chain Variable Region Allotypes

Rabbit Ig V_H regions are of interest not only because they
contribute to the antigen specificity of antibodies but also on
account of the presence of V_H region antigenic determinants, the
group a allotypes, which are inherited in an autosomal, codominant
manner (29). The existence of conserved, inherited markers within
the V_H region is difficult to reconcile with the multiplicity of
diverse V_H complementarity-region structures associated with even
the simplest antigens (Fig. 5). Examination of the framework sequences for the V_H regions in Figure 5 reveals a high degree of
sequence conservation for V_H regions associated with a given group
a allotype, and secondly, multiple framework positions that differ
between two or more V_H allotypes. These structural correlates of
the serologically defined group a allotypes are tabulated in
Figure 12. Of the 15 positions shown, amino acid residues differing among all three allotypes are found only at positions 9, 15
and 16. Two of the three H chains studied in our laboratory

(3374 and 3381) have identical amino acid residues at all positions
identified as allotypic correlates; whereas the third H chain (3T72)
differs from 3374 and 3381 only at positions 15 and 16 (Figure 12).
All three H chains were found to express the al allotypic specificity in direct binding assays (36). Inhibition assays utilizing
antiallotypic antibodies prepared against the purified 3374 anti-
doby revealed that 3381 and 3374 were allotypically indistinguishable. However, 3T72, which contains the variant sequence at positions 15 and 16, was found to be deficient relative to 3374, 3381
and normal rabbit al Ig is a major determinant of the al allotype
in that its inhibition of the 3374-antiallotype antibody reaction
was less than 15%. Normal rabbit al Ig and homogenous antibodies
3374 and 3381 completely inhibited this reaction. It may be
concluded, therefore, that V_H residues 15 and 16 constitute or
contribute to a major determinant of the al allotype (36).

Relationship of Hypervariable-Region Sequence to Binding Affinity

and Antigen Specificity

     The sequence diversity seen among H and L chain complementa-
rity regions of S3 antibodies suggests that the relatively simple
S3 antigen (Fig. 1) must interact with these antibodies in a
number of different ways. Figure 13 indicates that the range of
binding affinities for a hexasaccharide subunit of the polysaccharide (three cellobiuronic acid units) ranges over three orders of
magnitude (38). With respect to L-chain complementarity-determining regions, there does not appear to be a strict correlation
between the size of the complementarity region and binding affinity. It is of considerable interest, however, that the apparent
size of the combining site, as revealed by differences in affinity
for tetrasaccharide, hexasaccharide, and octasaccharide, respectively, appears closely related to affinity (Cannon et al,
unpublished data). An antibody of the lowest affinity, such as
3368, binds the tetrasaccharide, hexasaccharide, and octasaccharide
with equal affinity. Antibodies of somewhat higher affinity,
such as 3374 and 3381, bind the hexasaccharide with greater affinity than they do the tetrasaccharide, but they do not discriminate between octasaccharide and hexasaccharide. Antibody 3T72,
which has a still higher affinity, is capable of discriminating
among all three oligosaccharides. The apparent relationship
between the affinity of an antibody and the size of the oligo-
saccharide discriminated may be explained in terms of the number
of possible atomic contracts. This observation is anologous to
that made by Amzel et al. (1), who showed that the human myeloma
protein New binds vitamin K_1 with greater affinity than menadione,
the difference being accounted for by the atomic interactions
of an additional phytyl chain present in vitamin K_1.

Amino Acid Sequences in Complementarity-determining Regions

	First hv Region 23 30 32a b 33	Third hv Region 90 97a b c d e f	K_O (LM^{-1})	Discrimination
3368	C Q A S E S I G N E - - L	C Q Q D W N S N N V V N N - - - F G G	2×10^4	$(S3)_8 = (S3)_6 = (S3)_4$
3374	Q N - D S W - - -	S Y Y S I S S A - - - - - -	2×10^5	$(S3)_8 = (S3)_6 > (S3)_4$
K-25	Q B - Y S Y - - -	T Y S Y - S T Y - - - - - -	2.8×10^5	————
BS-1	Q ——— Y S G - - -	- Z G S T Y G G G Y - - - - - -	1.4×10^6	————
BS-5	Q ——— Y S N - - -	- Z G S B Y T G T - - - - - -	————	————
3381	E ——— S - W - - -	- S T D G N S D G F S - Y G ?	3×10^6	$(S3)_8 = (S3)_6 > (S3)_4$
3T74	S - Q - - V Y - N N Y -	- A G G Y S - S S H N A - - -	7×10^6	————
3T2	Q ———— S W - - -	——— T - S ———— D - T - - - -	1×10^7	$(S3)_8 > (S3)_6 > (S3)_4$
3T70	N - Y S S - - -	————————————————	1.2×10^7	————

Figure 13. Light-chain complementarity-region sequences and binding properties of antipneumococcal type-III polysaccharide antibodies. The sequence data are from Figure 4. Affinity constants (K_O) for BS-1 and K25 were reported by Huser et al. (23); affinity constants for the remaining antibodies were previously reported (38). Discrimination is a measure of the relative capacity of the tetra-, hexa-, and octasaccharide subunits ($S3_4$, $S3_6$, and $S3_8$) of the S3 polysaccharide to inhibit the binding of anti-S3 antibody to iodinated S3 polysaccharide. (Reprinted by permission of Cold Spring Harbor Symposium on Quantitative Biology, XLI : 654, 1977).

Homogeneous Hapten Specific Antibodies

In order to determine if diversity among V_L and V_H regions specific for the same antigen is unique to polysaccharide specific antibodies, we have examined the V_L regions of antibodies specific for digoxin (60). The amino-terminal sequences for two antidigoxin antibody L chains elicited in rabbit 302 and 303 are shown in Figure 14. These V_L regions differ in framework sequence at several positions (positions 2-4, 19, 20, 22, 27) and also demonstrate little homology in the complementarity-determining region at positions 29 to 33. Both L chains share a common amino-terminal chain length as well as the same complementarity-determining region length. Additional sequence data should reveal whether these common features are truly associated with specificity for digoxin. Nevertheless it appears likely that the V region sequence diversity documented for rabbit anti-S3 and anti-S8 antibodies also exists among rabbit antibodies directed against haptens.

DISCUSSION

The marked heterogeneity of antibodies elicited by conventional immunization has retarded detailed structural studies on this representative set of immunoglobulins. We are now able to test whether generalizations concerning immunoglobulin sequence made from myeloma proteins are appropriate. Rabbits respond to immunization with pneumococcal type III or type VIII vaccines, or to these vaccines carrying additional haptenic determinants with a restricted antibody response. An individual animal may produce only a single antibody or only a small set of antibodies, but these antibodies differ greatly among one another in affinity, apparent size of the combining site, and most importantly, amino acid sequence of the complementarity regions of both the L and the H chains. This diversity can be seen even among L chains from a single rabbit manifesting the same L chain allele, effectively excluding genetic polymorphism as the explanation of diversity. No two rabbits have been found (among 35 L chains and 9 H chains in which complementarity regions have been examined) that produce the same antibodies in response to a given antigen. This suggests that the repertoire of antibody combining sites, expressed as complementarity region amino acid sequences, is extremely large. Indeed each animal may have one or more unique solutions to the problem of how best to bind an antigenic determinant. We can confidently answer the question of whether there are a large number of heavy and light chain variable region phenotypes in the affirmative. If the variable region sequences specific for the simple antigens we have examined are as diverse as is apparent from the data presented here, then the total number of complemen-

E. HABER ET AL.

Antibody 0 1 2   10   20
  303   - - I E M T Q T P S P V S A A V G G T I S
  302   - - A V L ——————————————————————————— V T

                          30   32 a b 33
  303   I N C Q S S K S V Y T N D F L(S)W Y Q Q K
  302   —S( )—— Q —— N( )N D —( )———

Figure 14. Amino terminal amino acid sequences of isolated L
chains from purified antidigoxin antibodies 303 and 302 (60),
given in the one-letter code. A line indicates identity with
the amino acid directly above it. Residues in parentheses are
those for which the PTH—amino acid could be identified by only
a single method. A blank in parentheses indicates a position
at which a residue has not be identified. Broken lines at
positions 0 and 1 indicate deletions with respect to the longest
rabbit L chain sequences. (Reprinted by permission of J. Immunol.
121 : 127, 1978).

tarity determining sequences for all antigens must be very large
indeed.

    In any given rabbit only a small number of clonal products
are observed, yet antibody binding affinity can vary over three
orders of magnitude among individual rabbits (Fig. 13). This
excludes the affinity of B cell receptors as the sole determinant
of clone choice if all animals were to have the same repertoire.
Rather it suggests that each animal does not have the same library
of precursor cells specific for a given antigen.

    How different are these individual antibodies? The V-region
frame work is relatively conserved. This is particularly striking
in the H chain, where framework, variation for a given allotype is
minimal(36). If the above allotypes indeed represent isotypes,
the quantitative expression of which is modulated by other controlling genes, as suggested by Strosberg (52) and Mudgett-Hunter
et al. (40) then it appears that framework sequences associated
with a given allotype are coded by recently diverged genes or
allelic forms of a single gene. The marked differences among the
a1, a2, and a3 allotypes suggest that they are products of genes
that diverged earlier. Within these highly conserved frameworks
associated with a given allotype, considerable variability is

found in complementarity regions. These show no linkage to framework structure. Indeed, among the H chains sequences thus far
examined, the greatest similarity between complementarity-region
sequences is found between two chains (K25 and BS-5, Fig. 5) that
have framework sequences belonging to two different allotypes.

   If framework sequences alone are examined, the H-chain data
suggest a limited number of genes. The L-chain framework data,
however, indicate far more diversity. The frequency of unique
sequences even in the segment comprising the amino terminal 20
residues and the absence of identities in 10 complete V_L sequences available suggest that a relatively large number of genes
must be postulated. In an attempt to examine the relationship
between framework-and complementarity-region sequences in the L
chain, two sets of framework sequences exhibiting considerable
similarity were selected. The L chains of the S3-specific
antibodies BS-1 and BS-5 demonstrate some degree of conservation
in both framework (3 residue differences in 100 positions) and
complementarity region sequences (5 differences in 11 positions)
(Figure 4). Differences in sequence between the complementarity
region of these two L chains are markedly less than those seen
in the population of S3 antibodies. Thus in this example, similar
complementarity regions are associated with similar framework
sequences. The second set of L chains presents quite a different
picture (3381, K25, and 120; see Haber et al. (18)). Although
these L chains are being compared because of conservation of
similar framework sequences (six to eight residue difference),
the complementarity regions are very different. Not only are
there very substantial amino acid sequence differences (there
is only one position where all three chains have a residue in
common), but L chain 3381 is six residues longer that K25 and
120 in the region 89 to 98. Thus very similar framework phenotypes
may be associated with vastly different complementarity-region
structures.

   When all the available sequence data from rabbit antibodies
are analyzed to test for correlation between complete framework
sequence and combining-site sequence, a general lack of correlation is seen (18, 6). It is of particular interest that even when
a highly inbred population of rabbits was immunized with a very
simple antigen (polyrhamnose) and antibodies were selected by a
very rare L-chain framework (isoleucine amino terminus occurs only
in 3 % of normal rabbit L chains), each antibody elicited still
showed a unique L-chain complementarity region (4, 5).

   An additional indication of complementarity-region diversity
as compared with framework is the finding of a significant difference in the frequency of 1-, 2-, and 3-base-change events and
of deletions or insertions that occur in these two regions (Table
1). Note that amino acid differences that occur in the framework

are due predominately to single-base-change events. In the
complementarity regions, double mutations and deletions or insertions account for the majority of residue differences. This
suggests that the nature of the selective pressure that generates
variability in these two regions is likely to be different.

    This complex picture, characterized by 1) a multiplicity
of combining sites specific for a relatively simple antigen
(though individual animals respond in a mono-or pauciclonal
manner), 2) a lack of correlation between framework and complementarity-region structures, and 3) a difference in apparent
mechanism of diversification of framework and complementarity-
region sequences, is difficult to reconcile with models in
which all information is carried in the germ-line. If evolutionary diversification of framework and complementarity regions
occurred and diversification of the framework was constrained
by selection for essential structural features, some evidence
of an association between framework and complementarity-region
sequences should be seen. The absence of such linkage argues
against a simple germ line hypothesis.

    How can these observations be reconciled either with inheri-
tance of idiotypes, or with the evident linkage of framework and
hypervariable region structures in other systems (13, 22)? In
every instance where 1) inherited V-region structures, 2) a simple
association between complementarity regions and antigen, or 3) an
association of framework- and complementarity-region sequences
has been demonstrated, the antibodies studied were either myeloma
proteins or antibodies that showed idiotypic identity among different individuals of the same strain. These are conveniently
named "public phenotypes". It is difficult not to agree that
these public phenotypes may be the expression of germ-line genes.
It is evident that germ-line gene product must be selected when
the criterion for selection is the inheritance of phenotype.
It is not so obvious why myeloma proteins for the most part appear to be the expression of germ-line genes. Perhaps oncogenic
induction occurs prior to somatic diversification of Ig V-region
genes.

    By analogy, the unique antibodies characteristic of each
individual are conveniently called "private phenotypes". All
the antibodies described in this paper that have simply been selected by antigen fall into this class.

    It is likely that the private phenotypes represent the vast
majority of elicited antibodies. The observations of Nisonoff
(26) indicate that in the course of ordinary immunization it is
rather difficult to find an inherited (or public) phenotype, and
that when one is found and specifically suppressed, the antibody
response is carried by a variety of other antibodies unique to the

individual animal (private phenotypes). These private phenotypes
almost certainly represent the product of somatic diversification
suggested by the studies of Tonegawa and colleagues (55). Certainly occasional expression of germ-line antibody genes will
be found, but these are likely to be a very small minority of
the total antibody population, most antibody variable regions
being the product of a somatic diversification process. Thus
the limitless number of combining sites of amino acid sequences,
which may be seen among antibodies to simple antigens such as
S3 and S8, simply indicate 1) that there are many alternative
ways for an antibody to bind a given antigenic determinant, and
2) that substantial somatic diversification of light and heavy
chain variable regions and subsequent clonal selection permits
the expression of most effective alternative structures for
specific antigen binding.

ACKNOWLEDGEMENT

Supported by NIH grants AI 04967 and HL 19259 and a Grant-
in-Aid from the American Heart Association.

* Work performed during tenure as an Established Investiga-
tor of the American Heart Association.

+ Present address:Rosensteil Basic Medical Science Center
and Department of Biology, Brandeis University, Waltham, MA
02154.

REFERENCES

1. Amzel, L.M., Poljak, R.J., Saul, F., Varga, J.M., and Richards,
   F.F. : The three-dimensional structure of a combining region-
   ligand complex of immunoglobulin New at 3.5 A resolution.
   Proc. Nat. Acad. Sci. 71:1427, 1974.
2. Andrews, D.W., Cannon, L.E., Rosemblatt, M.S., Margolies, M.N.
   and Haber, E. : The heavy chain variable region sequence of
   a rabbit homogeneous antipneumococcal type III polysaccharide
   antibody. Fed. Proc. (abstr) 36:742, 1977.
3. Brauer, A.W., Margolies, M.N., and Haber, E.: The application
   of 0.1 M Quadrol to the microsequence of proteins and the sequence of tryptic peptides. Biochemistry 14:3029, 1975.
4. Braun, D.G., and Jaton, J.-C.: The amino terminal sequence of
   antibody light chains: evidence for possible inheritance of
   structural genes. Immunochemistry 10:387, 1973.
5. Braun, D.: Light chain hypervariable region sequences of
   rabbit antibodies elicited by group A-variant streptococcal
   vaccines. In, The Future of Antibodies in Human Diagnosis
   and Therapy. (E. Haber and R. Krause, eds.) Raven Press,

New York, 1977.

6. Cannon, L.E., Margolies, M.N., Strosberg, A.D., Chen, F.W., Newell, J. and Haber, E.: Diversity among rabbit antibody light chain amino terminal sequences. J. Immunol. 117:160, 1976.

7. Cannon, L.E., Margolies, M.N., Strosberg, A.D., Chen, F.W., Newell, J., and Haber, E.: Computer analysis of the variable region sequences of rabbit antibody light chains. Fed. Proc. 35:314, 1976b.

8. Capra, J.D., Tung, A.S., and Nisonoff, A.: Structural studies on induced antibodies with defined idiotypic specificities. J. Immunol. 115:414, 1975.

9. Cebra, J.: Relationship among sequences of hypervariable regions, V_H framework and ligand binding specificities of antihapten antibodies from inbred guinea pigs. In, Antibodies in Human Diagnosis and Therapy (E. Haber and R. Krause, eds) Raven Press, N.Y. 1977, pp 79-82.

10. Chen, F.W., Strosberg, A.D., and Haber, E.: Evolution of the immune response to type III and type VIII pneumococcal polysaccharides. J. Immunol. 110:98, 1973.

11. Chen, F.W., Cannon, L.E., Margolies, M.N., Strosberg, A.D., and Haber, E.: Purification, specificity and hypervariable region sequence of anti-pneumococcal polysaccharide antibodies elicited in a single rabbit. J. Immunol. 117:807, 1976.

12. Cheng, W.C., Fraser, K.J., and Haber, E.: Fractionation of antibodies to the pneumococcal polysaccharides by affinity chromatography. J. Immunol. 111:1677, 1973.

13. Claflin, J.L. and Rudikoff, S.: Uniformity in a clonal repertoire: a case for a germ-line basis of antibody diversity. Cold Spring Harbor Symposia on Quantitative Biology XLI:725, 1976.

14. Cohn,M., Blomberg, B., Geckeler, W., Raschke, W., Riblet, R., and Weigert, M.: First order considerations in analyzing the generation of diversity. In, The Immune System-genes, receptors and signals. (E.E. Sercarz et al. eds.) Academic Press, N.Y. 1974, p.89.

15. Edman, P. and Begg, G.: A protein sequenator. Eur. J. Biochem. 1:80, 1967.

16. Fraser, K.J., Poulsen, K., and Haber, E.: Specific cleavage between variable and constant domains of rabbit antibody light chains by dilute acid hydrolysis. Biochem 11:4974, 1972.

17. Haber, E.: Antibodies of restricted heterogeneity for structural study. Fed. Proc. 29:66, 1970.

18. Haber, E., Margolies, M.N., and Cannon, L.E.: Origins of antibody diversity: insights gained from amino acid sequence studies of elicited antibodies. Cold Spring Harbor Symposium on Quantitative Biology. XLI:647, 1977a.

19. Haber, E., Margolies, M.N., and Cannon, L.E.: The structure of the framework and complementarity regions of elicited antibodies. In, The Future of Antibodies in Human Diagnosis

and Therapy (E. Haber and R. Krause, eds), Raven Press, N.Y. 1977b.

20. Haber, E., Cannon, L.E., and Margolies, M.N.: Structure of the variable regions of the light and heavy chains of homogeneous rabbit antibodies: the problem of origin of antigen combining site diversity. Basic Science Symposium (Am. Soc. Microbiology, pub), in press.

21. Hood, L., Eichmann, K., Lackland, H., Krause, R.M. and Ohms, J.J.:Rabbit antibody light chains and gene evolution. Nature 288:1040, 1970.

22. Hood, L., Loh, E., Hubert, J., Barstad, P., Eaton, B., Early, P., Fuhrman, J., Johnson, N., Kronenberg, M., and Schilling, J.: The structure and genetics of mouse immunoglobulins: an analysis of NZB myeloma proteins and sets of Balb/c myeloma proteins binding particular haptens. Cold Spring Harbor Symposium on Quantitative Biology. XLI:817, 1976.

23. Huser, H., Haimovich, J. and Jaton, J.-C.: Antigen binding and idiotypic properties of reconsituted immunoglobulin G derived from homogeneous rabbit anti-pneumococcal antibodies. Eur. J. Immunol. 5:206, 1975.

24. Johnstone, A.P., Kindt, T.J.: Amino terminal sequences of blocked κ chains from homogeneous rabbit antibodies. Febs. Letts. 77:65, 1978.

25. Jones, J.K.N., and Perry, M.B.: The structure of type VIII pneumococcus specific polysaccharide. J. Am. Chem. Soc. 79:2787, 1957.

26. Ju, S.-T., Owen, F.L., and Nisonoff, A.: Structure and immunosuppression of a cross reactive idiotype associated with anti-p-azophenylarsonate antibodies of strain-A mice. Cold Spring Harbor Symposium on Quantitative Biology. XLI:699, 1976.

27. Kabat, E.A., and Wu, T.T.: Attempts to locate complementarity determining residues in the variable positions of light and heavy chains. Ann. N.Y. Acad. Sci. 190:382, 1971.

28. Kindt, T.J., Thunberg, A.L., Mudgett, M., and Klapper, D.G.: A study of V region genes using allotypic and idiotypic markers. In, The Immune System-Genes, receptors, signals (E.E. Sercarz, et al, eds.) Academic Press, N.Y., 1974, p.69.

29. Kindt, T.J.: Rabbit immunoglobulin allotypes: structure, immunology, and genetics. In, Adv. In Immunology (F.J.Dixon and H.G. Kunkel, eds.) vol 21, Academic Press, N.Y. 1975, pp. 35-81.

30. Klapper, D.G., Wilde, C. III, Capra, J.D.: Automated amino acid sequence of small peptides utilizing polybrene. Anal. Biochem. 85:126, 1978.

31. Klinman, N.R., Sigal, N.H., Metcalf, E.S., Pierce, S.K., and Gearhart, P.J.: The interplay of evolution and environment in B-cell diversification. Cold Spring Harbor Symposium on Quantitative Biology XLI:165, 1976.

32. Krause, R.M.: The search for antibodies with molecular uniformity. Adv. Immunol. 12:1, 1970.

33. Leder, P., Honjo, R., Seidman, J., and Swan D.: Origin of immunoglobulin gene diversity: the evidence and a restriction-modification model. Cold Spring Harbor Symposium on Quantitative Biology, XLI:855, 1977.

34. Landsteiner, K.: The specificity of serological reactions. Harvard University Press, Cambridge, Mass. 1945.

35. Margolies, M.N., Cannon, L.E., Strosberg, A.D., and Haber, E.: Diversity of L chain variable region sequences among rabbit antibodies elicited by the same antigens. Proc. Nat. Acad. Sci. 72:2180, 1975.

36. Margolies, M.N., Cannon, L.E., Kindt, T.J., and Fraser, B.: The structural basis of rabbit V_H allotypes: serologic studies on a1 H chains with defined amino acid sequence. J. Immunol. 119:287-293, 1977.

37. Margolies, M.N. and Brauer, A.W.: Protein microsequencing using high pressure liquid chromatography of phenythiohydantoin amino acids. J. Chromatog. 148:429, 1978.

38. Margolies, M.N., and Haber, E.: Amino acid sequence of a rabbit homogeneous antipneumococcal type III polysaccharide antibody heavy chain variable region. Fed. Proc. 37:1852A, 1978b.

39. Margolies, M.N., and Brauer, A.W.: Quantitative identification of phenylthiohydantoin amino acids by high pressure liquid chromatography during extended automated Edman degradation. In, Liquid Chromatography Symposium I (Marcel Dekker, Publisher), in press.

40. Mudgett-Hunter, M., Yarmush, M.L., Fraser, B.F., and Kindt, T.J.: Rabbit laten group a allotypes: characterization and relationship to nominal group a allotypic specificities. J. Immunol. in press.

41. Padlan, E.A., and Davies, D.R.: Variability of three-dimensional structure in immunoglobulin. Proc. Nat. Sci. 72:819, 1975.

42. Padlan, E.: Structural implications of sequence variability in immunoglobulins. Proc. Nat. Acad. Sci. 74:2551, 1977.

43. Podell, D.N., and Abraham, G.N.: A technique for the removal of pyroglutamic acid from the amino terminus of proteins using calf liver pyroglutamate amino peptidase. Biochem. Biophys. Res. Comm. 81:176, 1978.

44. Poljak, R.J., Amzel, L.M., Chen, B.L., Phizackerley, R.P., and Saul, F.: The three dimensional structure of the Fab' fragment of a human myeloma immunoglobulin at 2.0 A resolution. Proc. Nat. Acad. Sci. 71:3440, 1974.

45. Potter, M.: Antigen binding myeloma proteins. Adv. Immunol. 25:145, 1977.

46. Richards, F.F., Konigsberg, W.H., Rosenstein, R.W. and Varga, J.M.: On the specificity of antibodies. Science 187:130, 1975.

47. Schiffer, M., Girling, R.L., Ely, K.R., and Emundson, A.B.: Structure of a λ-type Bence Jones protein at 3.5 A resolution. Biochem. 12:4620, 1973.

48. Smith, G.P.: The variation and adaptive expression of antibo-

dies. Harvard University Press, Cambridge, Mass. 1973.

49. Segal, D.M., Padlan, S.A., Cohen, G.H., Silverton, E.W., Davies, D.R., Rudikoff, S., and Potter, M.: The structure of McPC 603 Fab and its hapten complex. In, Progress in Immunology (L. Brent and J. Holborow, eds). vol 2. North Holland Publishing Company, Amsterdam, 1974, pp. 93-102.

50. Strosberg, A.D., Fraser, K.J., Margolies, M.N. and Haber,E.: Amino acid sequence of rabbit pneumococcal antibody. In Light chain cysteine-containing peptides. Biochem. 11:4978, 1972.

51. Strosberg, A.D., Margolies, M.N., and Haber, E.: The interdomain disulfide bond of a homogeneous rabbit pneumococcal antibody light chain. J. Immunol. 115:1422, 1975.

52. Strosberg, A.D.: A possible control by regulatory allelic genes of allotypic expression. Biochem. Soc. Trans. 4:41, 1976.

53. Summers, M., Smythers, G., and Oroszlan, S.: Thin-layer chromatography of subnanomole amounts of phenythiohydantoin (PTH) amino acids on polyamide sheets. Anal. Biochem. 53: 624, 1973.

54. Talmadge, D.W.: Immunological specificity. Science 129, 1643, 1959.

55. Tonegawa, S., Maxam, A.M., Tizard, R., Bernard, O., and Gilbert, W.: Sequence of a mouse germ-line gene for a variable region of an immunoglobulin light chain. Proc. Nat. Acad. Sci. USA 75:1485, 1978.

56. Trischmann, I., Dugan, E., and Cebra, J.: A comparison of the heavy chain variable regions of different anti-dinitrophenyl (DNP) antibodies raised in inbred guinea pigs. Fed. Proc. 34: 970, 1975.

57. Weigert, M., and Riblet, R.: Genetic control of antibody variable regions. Cold Spring Harbor Symposium on Quantitative Biology. XLI:837, 1976.

58. Wu, T.T. and Kabat, E.A.: An analysis of the sequences of the variable regions of Bence Jones proteins and myeloma light chains and their implications for antibody complementarity. J. Exp. Med. 132:211, 1970.

59. Yalow, R.S.: Radioimmunoassay: a probe for the fine structure of biologic systems. Science 200:1236, 1978.

60. Zurawski, V.P., Novotny, J., Haber, E., and Margolies, M.N.: Antibodies of restricted heterogeneity directed against the cardiac glycoside digoxin. J. Immunol. 121:122, 1978.

CIRCULATING IMMUNE COMPLEXES IN NEUROLOGICAL DISORDERS

P.L. Masson

Unit of Experimental Medicine, International Institute
of Cellular and Molecular Pathology, University of
Louvain, Brussels, Belgium

INTRODUCTION

Immune complexes (IC) have been detected in the blood of
patients with multiple sclerosis (1, 2, 3), Guillain-Barré syndrome (1, 3), optic neuritis (1), subacute sclerosing panencephalitis (4), and amvotrophic lateral sclerosis (5). However,
little is known of the pathogenic role of these IC, the nature
of their antigens (Ag), the reasons for their occurrence or
their possible clinical significance. Some information can be
obtained from observations made in systemic or non-neurological
diseases with circulating IC.

EXPERIMENTAL IC DISEASE OR SERUM SICKNESS

When a patient is injected with large amounts of a foreign
protein, e.g. horse anti-tetanus serum, he may develop, within
8-10 days, serum sickness which is characterized by fever, adeno-
pathies, urticaria, arthritis and proteinuria. Dixon (6) reproduced these phenomena experimentally by injecting heterologous
proteins into rabbits. About 10 days after the injection, just
before the appearance of free Ab, the elimination rate of the Ag
suddenly increases. At that time, histological examination shows
inflammatory reactions in the renal glomeruli, vessel walls, synovial membranes and choroid plexus, with deposits of immunoglobulins (Igs), Ag, and complement factors detectable by immunofluorescence.

Lampert et al. (7) used horse ferritin as Ag to cause serum sickness in mice (20 mg of ferritin intraperitoneally twice

361

weekly for more than 4 weeks). Using electron microscopy, they
were able to see deposits of IC in the choroid plexus and renal
glomeruli of these animals, the IC being easily recognized by
their ferritin content. Involvement of the choroid plexus was
less severe than that of renal glomeruli. IC deposits were found
within the extracellular, perivascular space.

Not all animals within the same species develop serum sickness after injections of high doses of Ag. The appearance of
lesions depends upon the immune response of the animal. A minimal response is necessary, but the production of large amounts
of Ab can prevent the disorder. Apparently, the lesions are due
to IC which are not eliminated because they do not reach the
critical size capable of triggering the endocytosis by macrophages. Ag excess or low affinity of the Ab could explain the small
size of the complexes. The delayed clearance of IC could, therefore, be considered as a relative immunodeficiency.

DETECTION AND DETERMINATION OF IC

More than twenty techniques have thus far been proposed for
the detection or determination of IC in the blood. If this effort to develop new procedures indicates the great interest raised by IC, it suggests also that the ideal test has still to be
developed. Such a test, in addition to being easy, sensitive
and reproducible should be able to detect all kinds of IC and
to provide information on their composition. As IC differ in
size, Igs involved, and content of complement components and
rheumatoid factor (RF), the ideal test should include several
reagents with different specificities. Therefore, we have tried
to develop a method in which at least two reagents could be used,
i.e. human RF and Clq. As these reagents display a strong agglutinating activity, techniques based on agglutination appeared
to us particularly suitable. We first set up a manual test based on the agglutination of IgG-coated particles (latex). The
results were expressed as dilution titres at which the patient's
serum was still capable of inhibiting the agglutination activity
of RF or Clq (8). To improve the precision and accuracy of the
test and to facilitate its application, an instrumental system
was developed. This system, which is suitable for various immu-
noassays (9, 10) is called PACIA for Particle Counting ImmunoAssay. It uses a modified blood cell counter to count the free
particles which are reduced in number by agglutination. The
technique has been completely automated to analyze many samples,
each with several agglutinators. Nowadays these agglutinators
are whole rheumatoid serum or mouse serum. The latter contains
an agglutinator which is still not completely identified but
presumably corresponds to Clq. It has a specificity, with regard

to the size and antibody content of IC, similar to that of human Clq. The murine agglutinator has the great advantage of
not requiring any purification (11).

To prevent interference by agglutinating factors present
in the samples, the latter are all treated with dithiothreitol,
which is then oxidized before the test with hydrogen peroxide
to avoid inactivating the agglutinator. In the automated method
the inhibition is expressed in equivalents of heat-aggregated
IgG. The murine agglutinator recognizes IC different from those reacting with rheumatoid sera (12). Correlation between the
results obtained with rheumatoid serum and those with mouse serum was observed only when sera from patients with the same
disease (breast cancer, Crohn's disease, systemic lupus erythematosus, leprosy) were considered. When the results relating
to different diseases were mixed up, no significant correlation
was obtained.

ROLE OF IC IN DISEASE

IC have been implicated in human disease following their
identification in the tissues where lesions are found and by
comparison with similar damage produced by serum sickness. In
most types of glomerulonephritis, arthritis and vasculitis there are good reasons to believe that IC play a determinant pathogenic role (55). Some forms of urticaria, erythema nodosa, uveitis, haemolysis and trombocytopenia could also be due to IC.
It is often very difficult to distinguish between damage due
to IC or to autoantibodies, the more so in that the two mechanisms
are frequently associated.

In neurological diseases the role of IC is still very obscure. Nevertheless, some neuropsychiatric complications of systemic lupus erythematosus (SLE) could be due to the deposits of
IC in the choroid plexus. Involvement of the central nervous
system in SLE is secondary only to nephritis as the major cause
of morbidity and mortality in the natural history of the disease. The reported frequency of such involvement varies from 25
to 75 %. The many neurologic manifestations of SLE include seizures, psychosis, delirium and cranial nerve palsies. Hemiparesis, chorea, tremor and peripheral neuropathy are less frequent.

Hyaline (often calcified) deposits are common in the stroma
of the human choroid plexus. Their origin from trapped IC was
suggested after finding aggregates of Igs within the choroid
plexus stroma in patients with SLE (13) and in (NZB x NZW) hybrid mice with spontaneous autoimmune disease similar to human

SLE (14). However, a clear correlation between the pathologic findings and the neurological disorders is still lacking. The study of Atkins et al. (13) was limited to two SLE patients and controls; SLE patients without neurological manifestations were not examined. In a more recent study, including two patients with SLE and a control without SLE, IC deposits were found in the choroid plexus of the SLE patient who had presented neurological signs (personality changes, seizures, multiple neuropathies) (15).

The vasculitis also due to IC could explain by impairment of the blood circulation some neurological dysfunctions found in SLE. Another plausible pathogenetic mechanism is the occurrence of lymphocytotoxic Abs which react with brain tissues. Serum from most patients with SLE contains Abs (mainly IgM) directed at heterologous and autologous lymphocytes. They are cytotoxic to both T and B-cells. The antigenic determinants have not yet been defined but some are present in brain tissue which is capable of absorbing more than 90 % of the lymphocytotoxic activity of some SLE sera. Although lymphocytotoxic Abs occur in the sera of a majority of patients with SLE, the cytotoxic capacity was found to be greater in the sera of those patients with neurological disorders, and also in those with haematologic abnormalities (16). The observation that complement factors, especially $C4$, are decreased in the cerebrospinal fluid of SLE patients with neurologic or psychiatric signs confirms the immunological origin of the brain lesions (17), but does not tell us whether autoantibodies or IC cause the neurological damage.

Deposits of IC in the choroid plexus could lead to spinal fluid changes that may be responsible for neurologic and psychiatric disturbances seen in patients with chronic and acute infections. Such deposits have been found, for example, in mice chronically infected with lymphocyte choriomeningitis virus (18).

Discussion of the role of IC in SLE leads us to multiple sclerosis as the latter can be mimicked to some extent by neurological forms of SLE. Fulford et al. (19) described six patients in whom the clinical picture suggested possible multiple sclerosis but who had some laboratory evidence of SLE. They suggested the name "lupoid sclerosis" for this group. Few clinical features of SLE were present, however, and the predominant neurological picture was a slowly progressive spastic paraplegia. Since that publication, a few other isolated cases have been reported (20, 21, 22, 23). The occurrence of SLE and multiple sclerosis in identical twins has also been reported (24). As the major pathogenic mechanism in SLE is related to IC, the possibility of the involvement of IC in demyelinisation, observed in multiple sclerosis or Guillain-Barré syndrome, must be examined. The detection of IC in the blood of 30 to 70 percent of patients with multiple sclerosis or Guillain-Barré syndrome (1, 2, 3) cannot be taken as an argument for this hypothesis. As we shall see later, circulating IC are quite common and could be just secondary to any autoimmune process. However, the existence of this autoimmune process is still not clearly demonstrated. We should know whether the Igs found in the demyelinated plaques are there because they react with an autoantigen present in the myelin or in the oligodendrocytes or because of the affinity of IC for some of these structures. The relationship of multiple sclerosis or Guillain-Barré syndrome with viral infections is compatible with both mechanisms, the viral antigens being present in the IC or incorporated in the membranes, or having triggered autoimmune reactions.

The most frequent neurologic disorders are presumably related to circulatory insufficiency caused by arterio-sclerosis. This justifies a few words on the possible pathogenic role of IC in the development of the atheroma plates. Is has been shown repeatedly that induction of arteriosclerosis by a cholesterol-rich diet was markedly accelerated by serum sickness. It seems that the damage caused by IC to the endothelium, like that due to hypertension, allows platelet factors and beta-lipoproteins to gain access to the media. Under the joint action of these factors the smooth muscles proliferate and form the plaques (25). In this context, the observations by Delire et al. (26), that babies fed on cow's milk have circulating IC, is particularly interesting, especially when the results of autopsies done by Osborn (27) are considered. In this study there was a significant correlation between coronary lesions and the fact that the subjects had been fed on cows' milk.

LOCALIZATION OF IC

In most IC diseases the deposits are found on the basal membrane of capillaries or larger vessels. In the kidney, a receptor for the complement factor C3b has been found on the glomerular basement membrane (28). As IC generally contain C3b, their accumulation in this tissue could be explained by the existence of this receptors. However, it is possible that some IC are formed in situ. According to Izui et al. (29), DNA has a particular affinity for the glomerular basal membrane, and the DNA-antiDNA complexes found in SLE would be formed after the deposit of Ag. Those present in the circulation would be different and apparently did not contain DNA as Ag (30).

Another possible explanation for the deposits of IC on basal membrane would be the affinity of polymerized IgG for collagen. This hypothesis is suggested by a recent observation of

Eeckhout et al. (31) who reported that collagen from guinea pig
skin was capable, like Clq, of agglutinating human IgG-coated
particles. As collagen and certain parts of the Clq molecule
have similar structures, it is tempting to draw a parallel between the reactions of Clq and collagen with Igs.

Myelin extracts would also be capable of binding Igs by
their Fc-region. This was shown by immunofluorescence as well
as by absorption of Ab directed against Ag unrelated to the myelin extracts.

Removal of myelin basic protein from the brain extracts almost totally abolished the reaction (32). In our laboratory,
C. Sindic has observed that the basic protein agglutinated
IgG-coated particles, confirming the interaction of IgG with the
basic protein (unpublished). Such interaction will be facilitated when the IgG molecules are polymerized by their combination with Ag. It is therefore possible that some of the serum
factors that demyelinate neurological tissue in culture or inhibit their myelination process (33, 34, 35, 36) as well as those
blocking the neuro-electric conduction (37, 38) correspond to
IC. Such factors have been found in patients with multiple sclerosis as well as with a great variety of neurological disorders.

The deposition of IC requires a local increase of vascular
permeability. The injection of IC into mice or guinea pigs results in IC deposits only if a vasodilatation is produced by
injecting histamine, or by degranulating the basophils or mast
cells and platelets which will increase the vascular permeability. It is worth mentioning here that in IC diseases such as
SLE and rheumatoid arthritis the number of basophils is significantly decreased (39).

INTERFERENCE OF IC WITH THE IMMUNE RESPONSE

By polymerizing the antigens and by their interactions with
the Fc and C3 receptors of macrophages and lymphocytes, IC are
expected to interfere with the development of the immune response. Apparently they do it by blocking either the expression or
the induction of the response. This interference has been observed in cancer where the defense mechanism could be hampered
by the presence of IC (40, 41). We have detected, in the sera
of pregnant women, factors resembling IC and which could play
a role in the tolerance of the foetus by the mother (42).

CLEARANCE OF IC

To be eliminated, IC must reach a critical size which allows them to be picked up by the reticuloendothelial system (43). When there is an excess of Ag or when the affinity of the Ab is low the Ag-Ab network will be too small and its elimination delayed.

RF, which occurs frequently in diseases with circulating IC, could favor the elimination of IC by increasing their size. Van Snick et al. (44) have found that IgM RF enhanced in vitro the attachment and ingestion of heat-aggregated IgG by macrophages. This effect depended upon the integrity of the Fc portion of the IgG antibody. Reduction and alkylation of the aggregated IgG did not modify their interaction with RF but prevented their uptake by macrophages in the absence as well as in the presence of RF. At too high a concentration of RF, its enhancing effect on endocytosis tended to decrease, presumably because the Fc-region of the IgG molecules was masked by RF in excess. Conflicting results were reported on the opsonic effect of RF. Some authors (45, 46) observed that RF inhibited the phagocytosis of antibody-coated particles (red cells or bacteria). It is likely, that with antigens of this size, the only effect of RF was to mask the Fc-region of the Ab involved, so that phagocytosis was inhibited.

NATURE OF ANTIGENS IN IC

A great hope in the study of IC is that, by identification of the Ag, it will be possible to gain access to the cause of the disease. Drugs and infectious (viral, bacterial and parasitic) antigens have been found in IC (55). However, in many disorders, even of infectious origin, IC may contain autoantigens, such as DNA. It has been shown by Izui et al. (47, 48) that endotoxin caused the release of DNA and the production of anti-DNA antibody, presumably by a non-specific mitogenic effect on B lymphocytes. Other products released by bacteria, viruses or parasites could have the same effect. In their work on IC from ITP patients, Lurhama et al. (49) have identified DNA; whereas viral antigens, apparently in free form, were detected by counterelectrophoresis. These viral antigens originated from hepatitis B virus in 48 % of ITP patients, from adenovirus in 14 % and from Epstein-Barr virus in 12 %.

IgG is the main autoantigen of the IC of rheumatoid patients. These IC are made up of self associated IgG with RF activity (50). The small amounts of IC detected by Hay et al. (51) in healthy individuals consisted also of self-associated

IgG. It is likely that any stimulation of the immune system results
in the production of RF, first of IgM and later of IgG nature.
The presence of IgG RF should normally result in the formation of
IgG aggregates, persisting in trace amounts in most normal subjects. It is also likely that complexes consisting of idiotypes
and anti-idiotypes occur after strong immunization. The possible pathogenic role of such complexes is still unknown (52).

As we have seen in a previous section, food antigens can
be found in circulating IC. Food antigens were identified in
the IC of babies fed on cows'milk and in IgA-deficient patients
(53, 54). Whether vascular disorders, such as migraine occurring after ingestion of certain foods, are triggered by the formation of circulating IC should also be considered. It is possible that the formation of circulating IC with food antigens
could play a role in certain forms of postprandial migraine.

CLINICAL APPLICATIONS

Circulating IC can be detected in numerous diseases such
as infections, connective tissue disorders, granulomatosis and
cancer (55). Hence the clinical interest in detecting or determining IC might appear questionable. What is the use of a
test that become positive with a common cold as well as in the
presence of cancer ? At first glace the clinical applications
of the detection of IC are to some extent the same as those of
the erythrocyte sedimentation rate (ERS). However, in some cases the occurrence of IC may precede the inflammatory reaction;
hence the acceleration of the ESR. Some preliminary data suggest that, within a certain clinical context, the detection of
IC could be a useful warning sign.

For example, it has been reported that the vasculitis of
workers exposed to vinyl chloride is due to IC (56). Early detection of such complexes should allow the prevention of this
industrial disease. Delire et al. (57)have observed a close
correlation between the development of perinatal disorders and
the inhibitory activity of cord serum towards rabbit RF. The
occurrence of IC in about 20 % of non-selected neonates has
been confirmed recently (unpublished) by the agglutination inhibition test with human RF and Clq applied to cord blood sera.
Most newborns with IC required particular care in the days following birth. The detection of IC in cord blood could therefore
be useful by announcing perinatal disorders.

Nowadays, the most common application of the determination
of IC is the longitudinal study of various diseases. IC would
be particularly useful for foreseeing the relapse in acute leu-

kemia (58) and could become a useful parameter to monitor the evolution of various tumours (59)(60) or disorders like Crohn's disease (61). However, in multiple sclerosis the frequency of IC did not correlate with the clinical status of the patients (1).

The identification of the antigen present in the IC accompanying infections should facilitate the aetiological diagnosis. However, it would probably be more appropriate to search directly for free antigens from viral or bacterial origin (62, 63). Techniques of great sensitivity are now available which can detect tiny amounts of these antigens. Their discovery and identification in cerebrospinal fluid could be of great help for the aetiological diagnosis of meningitis (64, 65).

CONCLUSIONS

The study of circulating IC is fascinating because of the multiple prospects that it offers. In addition to the possibility of explaining the pathogenesis of various diseases IC could give access to the aetiological agent by identification of the Ag present in certain IC. They lead us also to the fine mechanisms which regulate the immune system, e.g. the anti-idiotype reaction and the production of rheumatoid factor. The clinical application of the IC assay essentially appears as a new probe for assessing the functional state of the immune system, an increase in the level of IC indicating that the body is now facing an antigenic challenge. However, the promising prospects offered by the IC will only be realized when techniques capable of distinguishing the various sorts of IC are available. This hope will presumably be satisfied by the introduction of tests based on the use of several reagents with different specificities.

REFERENCES

1. T.G. Tachovsky, H. Koprowski, R.P. Lisak, A.N. Theofilopoulos and F.J. Dixon, Lancet II, 997 (1976).
2. P. Davous, C.M. Jacque, L. Grangeot-Keros, R. Marteau and N. Baumann, Biomedicine 29, 103 (1978).
3. J.M. Goust, F. Chenais, J.E. Carnes, C.G. Hames, H.H. Fudenberg and E.L. Hogan, Neurology 28, 421 (1978).
4. A.D. Dayan and M.I. Stokes, Brit. Med. J. 2, 374 (1972).
5. M.B.A. Oldstone, L.H. Perrin, C.B. Wilson and F.H. Norris, J.R. Lancet II, 169 (1976).
6. F.J. Dixon, Harvey Lect., 58, 21 (1963).
7. P.W. Lampert, R. Garrett, A. Lampert, Acta Neuropath. 38, 83 (1977).

8. A.Z. Lurhuma, C.L. Cambiaso, P.L. Masson and J.F. Heremans, Clin. Exp. Immunol. 25, 212 (1976).

9. C.L. Cambiaso, A.E. Leek, F. De Steenwinkel, J. Billen and P.L. Masson, J. Immunol Methods 18, 33 (1977).

10. C.L. Cambiaso, H. Riccomi, C. Sindic and P.L.Masson, J. Immunol. Methods, in press (1978).

11. C.L. Cambiaso, C. Sindic and P.L. Masson, submitted.

12. C.L. Cambiaso and P.L. Masson, Prot. Biol. Fluids, 26, in press (1978).

13. C.J. Atkins, J.J. Kondon, Jr., F.P. Quismorio and G.J. Friou Ann. Int. Med. 76, 65 (1972).

14. P.W. Lampert and M.B.A. Oldstone, Science 180, 408 (1973).

15. M.E. Gershwin, L.R. Hyman and A.D. Steinberg, J. Pediat. 87, 588 (1975).

16. H.G. Bluestein and N.J. Zvaifler, J. Clin. Invest. 57, 509 (1976).

17. L.D. Petz, G.C. Sharp, N.R. Cooper and W.S. Irvin, Medicine 50, 260 (1971).

18. P.W. Lampert and M.B.A. Oldstone, Virchows Arch. A Path. Histol. 363, 21 (1974).

19. K.W.M. Fulford, R.D. Catterall, J.J. Delhanty, D. Doniach and M. Kremer, Brain 95, 373 (1972).

20. D.I. Shepherd, A.W. Downie and P.V. Best, Arch. Neurol. 30, 423 (1974).

21. C. Vitale, M.F. Kahn, M. de Sèze and S. de Sèze, Ann. Méd. Int., 124, 211 (1973).

22. W. Cendrowski and M. Stepien , Europ. Neurol. 11, 373 (1974).

23. T. Mizutani, M. Oda, M. Tsuganezawa, H. Abe, C. Ohshio, K. Suzuki and H. Shiraki, J. Neurol. 217, 43 (1977).

24. F.F. Holmes, D.W. Stubbs and W.E. Larsen, Arch. Intern. Med. 119, 302 (1967).

25. R. Ross and J.A. Glomset, N. Engl. J. Med. 295, 369 & 420 (1976).

26. M. Delire, C.L. Cambiaso and P.L. Masson, Nature, 272, 632 (1978).

27. G.R. Osborn, in Le rôle de la paroi artérielle dans l'arthérogénèse, C.N.R.S., Paris (1968) 93.

28. M.C. Gelfand, M.M. Frank and I. Green, J. Exp. Med. 142, 1029 (1975).

29. S. Izui et al., J. Exp. Med. 144, 428 (1976).

30.S. Izui, P.-H. Lambert and P.A. Miescher, Clin.Exp. Immunol. 30, 384 (1977a).

31. Y. Eeckhout, H. Riccomi, C. Cambiaso, G.Vaes and P. Masson, Arch. Intern. Physiol. Biochem. 84, 37 (1976).

32. J.A. Aarli, S.R. Aparicio, C.E. Lumsden and O. Tönder, Immunology, 28, 171 (1975).

33. P.C. Dowling, S.U. Kim, M.R. Murray and S.D. Cook, J. Immunol. 101, 1101 (1968).

34. T. Tabira, H. Def. Webster and S.H. Wray, N. Engl. J. Med. 295, 644 (1976).

35. M.B. Bornstein and C.S. Raine, Neuropathol. Appl. Neurobiol. 3, 359 (1977).
36. J. Ulrich and H. Lardi, J. Neurol. 218, 7 (1978).
37. C.L. Schauf, F.A. Davis, D.A. Sack, B.J. Reed and R.L. Kesler, J. Neurol. Neurosurg. Psychiatry 39, 680 (1976).
38. M. Schmutz, H.P. von Hahn and C.G. Honegger, Eur. Neurol. 15, 345 (1977).
39. J. Benveniste, Nouv. Presse Méd. 2, 703 (1973).
40. H.O. Sjögren, I. Hellström, S.C. Bansal and K.E. Hellström, Proc. Nat. Acad. Sci. 68, 1372 (1971).
41. R.W. Baldwin, M.R. Price and R.A. Robins, Nature, 238, 185 (1972).
42. P.L. Masson, M. Delire and C.L. Cambiaso, Nature 266, 542 (1977).
43. M. Mannik and W.P. Arend, J. Exp. Med. 134, 19s (1971).
44. J.L. Van Snick, E. Van Roost, B. Markowetz, C.L. Cambiaso and P.L. Masson, Eur. J. Immunol. 8, 279, (1978).
45. R.P. Messner, T. Laxdal, P.G. Quie and R.C. Williams, Jr., J. Clin. Invest. 47, 1109 (1968).
46. F.C. McDuffie and H.W. Brumfield, J. Clin. Invest. 51, 3007 (1972).
47. S. Izui, P.-H. Lambert, F.J. Fournié, H. Türler and P.A. Miescher, J. Exp. Med. 145, 1115 (1977b).
48. S. Izui, N.M. Zaldivar, I. Scher and P.-H. Lambert, J. Immunol. 119, 2151 (1977c).
49. A.Z. Lurhama, H. Riccomi and P.L. Masson, Clin. Exp. Immunol. 28, 49 (1977).
50. R.M. Pope, D.C. Teller and M. Mannik, J. Immunol. 115, 365 (1975).
51. F.C. Hay, L.J. Nineham, G. Torrigiani and I.M. Roitt, Clin. Esp. Immunol. 25, 185 (1976).
52. D.A. Rowley, G.W. Miller and I. Lorbach; J. Exp. Med. 148, 148 (1978).
53. F. Damacco, S. Antonaci, L. Scarpioni and L. Bonomo, Prot. Biol. Fluids 26, in press (1978).
54. C. Cunningham-Rundles, W.E. Brandeis, R.A. Good and N.K. Day, Prot. Biol. Fluids 26, in press (1978).
55. WHO, The role of immune complexes in disease, WHO, Geneva (1977).
56. W.A. Milford Ward, S. Udnoon, J. Watkins, A.E. Walker and C.S. Darke, Brit. Med. J. 1, 936 (1976).
57. M. Delire, M.C. Leclercq, C.L. Cambiaso, P.L. Masson and A. Malherbe, in Journées nationales de néonatalogie, A. Minkowski (Ed.), Jean Gaulier, Paris (1975), 39.
58. N.A. Carpentier, G.T. Lange, D.M. Fière, G.J. Fournié, P.-H. Lambert and P.A. Miescher, J. Clin. Invest, 60, 874 (1977).
59. R.D.Rossen, M.A. Reisberg, E.M. Hersh and J.U. Gutterman, J. Nat. Cancer Inst. 58, 1205 (1977).
60. H. Teshima, H. Wanebo, C. Pinsky and N.K.Day, J. Clin. Invest. 59, 1134 (1977).

61. R. Fiasse, A.Z. Lurhuma, C.L. Cambiaso, P.L. Masson, and C. Dive, Gut 19, 611 (1978).

62. D.M. Granoff, B. Congeni, R. Baker, Jr., P. Ogra and G.A. Nankervis, Amer. J. Dis. Child. 131, 1357 (1977).

63. M. Pollack, Infect. Immun. 13, 1543 (1976).

64. H. Käyhty, P.H. Mäkelä and E Ruoslahti, J. Clin. Path. 30, 831 (1977).

65. L. Pifer, S. Elliott, T. Woodard, D. Woods and W.T. Hughes, J. Pediatr. 92, 227 (1978).

PARTIAL PURIFICATION OF MULTIPLE SCLEROSIS SPECIFIC ANTIGENS

S.C. Rastogi, J. Clausen, T. Fog[x], H. Offner and
G. Konat

Neurochemical Institute, Copenhagen, Denmark
x Municipal Hospital, Copenhagen, Denmark

SUMMARY

Antigenic similarities and differences between 6 multiple
sclerosis (MS) brains and 7 non-MS brains autopsy specimens
have been elucidated by crossed immunoelectrophoresis (CIE)
using antibodies prepared by immunization of rabbits with cytoplasmic and microsomal fractions of the brains. The following
data were obtained : 1) a "measles" antigen and two specific
antigens have been purified more than 3000 fold from MS brains
by means of molecular filtration and DEAE cellulose chromatography.
2) all 3 antigens have a molecular weight between 10^5-10^6 daltons
and isoelectric points between 3.5-6.0. 3) "measles" antigen
has been also found in 3 out of 7 non-MS brains, however, it
did not stimulate antibody formation in rabbits in contrast to
measles antigen of MS brain. The significance of the above
mentioned data is discussed in view of the immunological abnormalities previously found in MS patients. It cannot be excluded
that the antigens found represent one or more viral antigens.

INTRODUCTION

Multiple sclerosis (MS) is a neurological disease of unknown
etiology, but epidemiological studies have revealed a statistical significant increased serum measles antibody titer in MS
patients (1, 5). Thus the demyelination process in multiple
sclerosis may be due to a chronic (viral) infection or to immunological abnormalities. A virus infection in the central nervous
system (CNS) may cause formation of new (viral) antigens. However,

373

even an autoimmune process may lead to lysosomal activation and
conformational abnormalities in CNS antigen.

Recently, we demonstrated a measles antigen and a specific
antigen in MS brain cytosole fraction not present in non-MS brain
homogenates (11). In the present paper a method for partial
purification of these antigens and new findings concerning "MS
specific antigens " are described.

MATERIAL AND METHODS

Materials

Chemicals : Measles antigen was prepared from infected vero
cells (10) and human myelin basic protein from MS and non-MS
brains were prepared according to Eylar et al. (7).

Control and MS brains : Brains from 6 patients and 7
non-MS patients (12) were used in the present investigations.
Brains were collected 16 h after death and twelve of them were
immediately frozen (-70°C). MS brain no. 6 was, however,
immediately processed. Macroscopical inspection of all 6 MS
brains revealed plaques mainly in the periventricular area.
Classical microscopical examination revealed in these areas
demyelination. When alive all the patients were clinically
diagnosed as having "certain MS" (13). No plaques were found
in non-MS brains used.

Methods

Immunization of rabbits and preparation of antisera has been
described before (12). Antibodies used were concentrated 3 fold
by precipitating them from antiserum at 2M ammonium sulfate
pH 6.8. The precipitate was dissolved in 0.005 M sodium Na-
phosphate buffer (pH 8.2) and dialyzed against the same buffer.

Fractionation of cytosole : MS and non MS-brain cytosole
were fractionated stepwise by means of Millipore Hi-flux molecular
filtration system. Millipore Pellicone membranes, which retain
particles over a definite size (molecular weight) were used
for filtration. The scheme indicated in Fig. 1 was used.

DEAE-cellulose column chromatography : 10 to 15 mg protein
in 1 ml fraction B (material retained on filter PTHK, Fig. 1)
were applied on a DEAE-cellulose (pH adjusted to 7.2-7.4 after

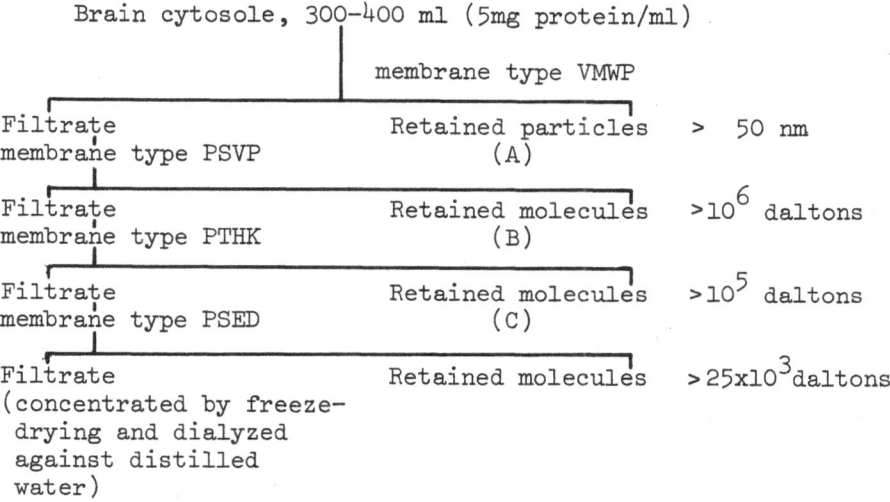

Brain cytosole, 300-400 ml (5mg protein/ml)

membrane type VMWP

Filtrate membrane type PSVP	Retained particles (A)	> 50 nm
Filtrate membrane type PTHK	Retained molecules (B)	$>10^6$ daltons
Filtrate membrane type PSED	Retained molecules (C)	$>10^5$ daltons
Filtrate (concentrated by freeze-drying and dialyzed against distilled water)	Retained molecules	$>25 \times 10^3$ daltons

FIG. 1

washing) column (22 cm x 0.8 cm²). Discontinuous elution was performed with 50 ml batches of distilled water, 0.25 M, 0.5 M,
0.75 M, 1M, 2 M, 3 M sodium chloride solutions (22°). 3.6 ml
fractions were collected on a LKB fraction collector equipped
with UVICORD. The optical density of each fraction was determined at 280 nm. The pooled distilled water eluate (see results)
were concentrated by freeze drying. The fractions eluted in
0.25 M NaCl were concentrated by ultrafiltration through SM 13200
membrane (Sartorius Membranes, Göttingen, W. Germany).

Crossed immunoelectrophoresis (IE) in 1 % agarose was performed as described before (11) except that the buffer was replaced by 0.05 M sodium barbital buffer, pH 8.5. To determine
specificity of MS specific antigens : 1) MS antigen was electrophoresed against MS and non-MS antibodies and vice versa.
2) MS and non-MS antigens were run on the same gel (Tandem crossed IE). 3) intermediate gel-crossed IE (4) of MS antigen against
MS and non-MS antibody containing gels, and finally 4) MS
antigen was electrophoresed against MS antibodies preabsorbed
with various amounts of non-MS antigen (11).

Isoelectricfocussing on LKB PAGE plates (pH range 3.5-9.5)
using a LKB Multiphor no. 2117 apparatus and LKB power supply
2103 was carried out as described in standard method provided
with gels (12).

SDS-PAGE was carried out as described by Agrawal et al. (2).

Protein was determined by the method of Lowry et al.(8).

RESULTS

Crossed IE of measles antigen revealed presence of "measles" antibodies in all antisera isolated from rabbits injected with MS cytosole and MS microsomes. However, none of the antisera prepared from rabbits injected with non-MS cytosole or non-MS microsomes were found to contain measles antibodies.

Fractionation of cytosole by Millipore membranes followed by Tandem crossed IE of fractions revealed that all 6 MS fraction B (molecules between 10^5-10^6 daltons) contained measles antigen (Fig. 2). However, only 3 non-MS brains out of 7 contained the measles antigen.

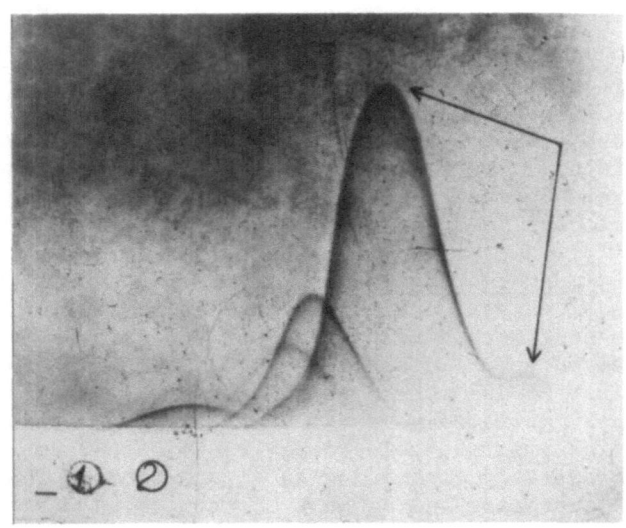

Fig. 2 CIE-tandem technique : Antigens applied in the hole
       below the left. Primary migration from left to the right
       (250 V, 3 H). Secondary migration into the gel containing
       antibody : from below upwardly (50 V, 20 H, 10°C)

       Antigen   Hole 1 : MS Fraction B (250 µg protein)
                  Hole 2 : Measles antigen 400 µg protein)
       Antibody : Anti MS cytosole (45 µl/cm^3 gel)

    Besides measles antigen, crossed IE of MS fraction B versus
anti-MS cytosole revealed two extra immunoprecipitation arcs
compared to crossed IE of the same versus anti-non-MS cytosole.
Crossed IE of fractions B from 7 non-MS brains versus anti-MS
cytosole did not reveal any of these two immunoprecipitation
arcs. Intermediate gel crossed IE, in which MS fraction B was
electrophoresed against gels containing anti-MS cytosole and
anti-non-MS cytosole (in the intermediate gel) also revealed
presence of two extra immunoprecipitates only in the gel containing
anti-MS cytosole. However, crossed IE of non-MS brain fraction
B versus anti-MS/anti-non-MS cytosole absorbed with MS/non-MS
fraction B did nor reveal any immunoprecipitation arcs. Thus,
the two immunoprecipitation arcs shown by MS fraction B (fig 3)
may represent two antigens present in MS brains only.

    An attempt to purify further these antigens from fraction
B by means of Sephadex gel filtration failed. Discontinuous
elution of fraction B on a DEAE-cellulose column with 0-3 M NaCl
revealed two major peaks (Fig. 4) : one eluted in distilled water
(peak 1) and one eluted in 0.25 M sodium chloride (peak 2).
Further elution with increasing concentration up to 3 M sodium
chloride eluted only trace amounts of proteins. The elution
pattern of MS and non-MS fraction B on the DEAE-cellulose column
were identical. Peak 1 from both MS-and non-MS material contained

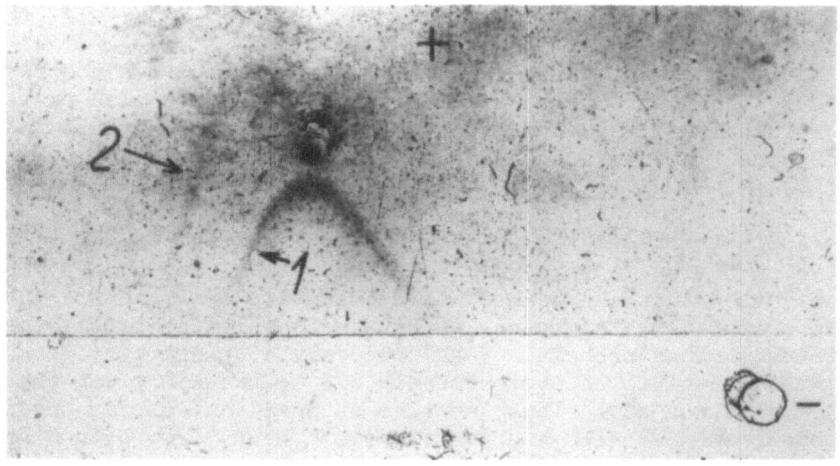

Fig. 3   CIE (For details cf. Legend to Fig. 2)

         Antigen   MS fraction B (250 ug protein)

         Antibody Anti-MS cytosole (45 ul/cm^3 gel) preabsorbed
                   with non-MS fraction B (1.1 mg protein/600 ul
                   antiserum incubated (37°C) for 2 h. Immunopre-
                   cipitate removed by centrifugation.

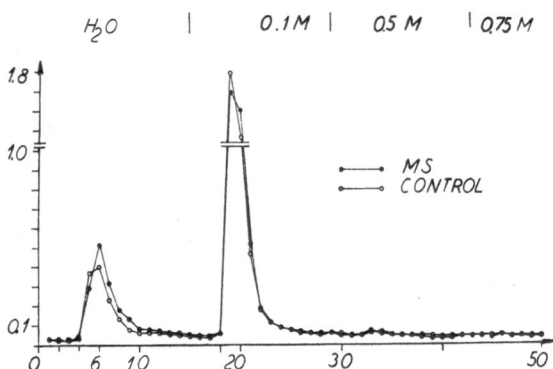

Fig. 4   Elution pattern for DEAE-cellulose column chromatography
          of fraction B (for details cf. the text), 12,7 mg
          protein.

          Ordinate : O.D. at 280 nm

          Abscissa : Fraction no. (3.6 ml)
          The concentration of sodium chloride used for elution
          is indicated on the top.

myelin basic protein (judged by SDS-PAGE and isoelectricfocussing
together with some other proteins).

    Analysis of peak 2 by crossed IE using cross-wise absorbed
antibodies with or without the Tandem technique revealed that
peak 2 contained measles antigen (all MS and 3 non-MS) and the
two MS specific antigens were only present in peak 2 of MS brains
(Fig. 5).

    isoelectricfocussing of peak 2 revealed that isoelectric
point of proteins in this fraction were between 3.5 to 6. SDS-
PAGE revealed that the peak 2 did not contain myelin basic protein.
As the preparation is impure, we have not analyzed it for other
constituents than protein. Total recovery of protein in peak 2
was, thus, found to be approximately 0.3 mg protein/g wet brain
(both MS and non-MS). Thus, measles antigen as well as specific
antigens from MS brains are purified more than 3000 folds starting from the brain.

    We have also been able to prepare peak 2 from the superna-
tant of brain homogenate centrifuged at 1000 g-av for 25 min.
The supernatant was then filtered through Millipore membrane
type GSVP (which retains particles over 220 nm). The filtrate
then is filtered through membrane type VMWP (50 nm) and the
filtrate was further purified as was the case with the cytosole.

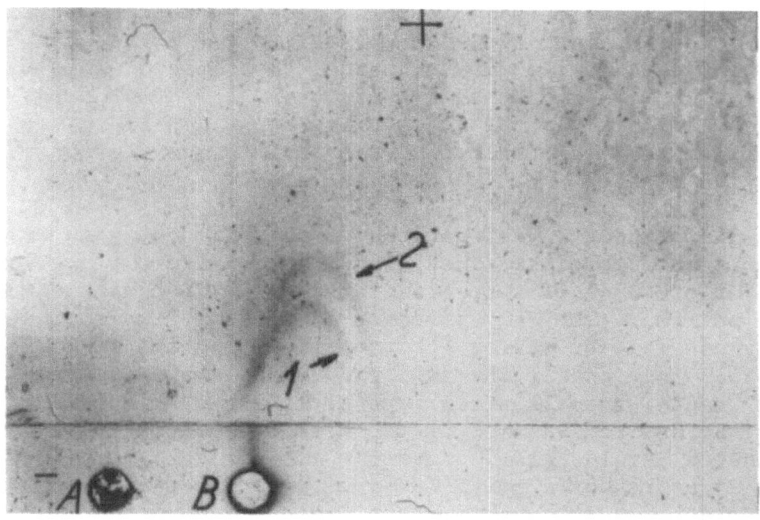

Fig. 5 Antigen A – measles antigen (400 μg protein per hole)
        B – MS peak 2 (150 μg protein)

Antibody – anti MS cytosole (45 μl/cm^3 gel) preabsorbed
           with non-MS peak 2 (1.5 mg protein/600 μl
           antiserum).

Crossed IE of serum and CSF of MS patients versus anti-MS
cytosole or crossed IE of peak 2 versus anti-MS serum or anti-MS
CSF did not indicate presence of either measles or specific
antigens in MS serum or MS CSF.

DISCUSSION

Results of the present investigation demonstrated that a
measles antigen was present in all 6 MS brains studied. The
presence of measles antigen in 3 out of 7 non-MS brains studied
indicated that measles antigen may not be a primary cause of MS.
This is in agreement with Ammitzbøll et al. (3), who showed
the oligoclonal IgG bands of spinal fluid (CSF) occurred significantly related to increased CSF measles antibody titer, but it
was not specific for MS.

Though measles antigen was present in 3 of the non-MS brains,
none of these gave rise to antibody formation in rabbits. Thus,
the antigenic site may still be masked in these brains. In vivo
production of antibody by measles antigen may depend on unmasking
of antigenic sites, which in turn may be achieved by a stimulus

due to other infection(s) or physiological, immunochemical or
genetic abnormalities. The CNS may be looked upon as a closed
compartment with limited immunological capacities. This may
cause measles virus to be activated during different pathological processes, similar to the in vitro isolation of measles
virus of lymphnode cultures of human individuals previously infected with measles (6).

In the present investigation two specific antigens were
found only in MS brains. These findings confirm our previous
reports of presence of a specific antigen in MS brains and a
measles antigen. The demonstration of two specific antigens
was only possible by taking into consideration the following
points : 1) that one of the antigens caused antibody formation
in experimental animals after several months of immunization.
2) that the antibodies used in the present investigation were
concentrated 3 fold, and 3) that the antigen used (fraction B
or peak 2) is rather a purified (enriched) material compared
to cytosole. Our data may explain the early findings of Steiner
(14) that MS-brain tissue may cause increased complement
consumption compared to non-MS tissue.

The peak 2 isolated by DEAE-cellulose column chromatography
of MS fraction B contained measles antigen as well as the two
specific antigens. The isolation of all 3 antigens in the same
fraction at a degree of more than 3000 fold purification may
indicate a close physico-chemical properties e.g. similar isoelectric points of these antigens. The nature of these antigens
has not been defined yet, because the antigens preparation is
still crude. However, they may be : 1) microbiological antigens
(e.g. viral glycoproteins or RNA) or their degradation products,
or 2) complexes of microbiological agent and host antigens, or
3) brain cell proteins with changed conformational state due to
immunological abnormalities in the brain (lysosomal activation).

The peak 2, which contained these antigens was not found
to be contaminated with myelin basic protein. We have also
ruled out the possibility of the specific antigen to be myelin
basic protein by lack of fusion of immunoprecipitates and by
absorption experiments. However, it is not certain if the specific antigens represent conformationally changed complexes
(thus producing new antigen) of other brain proteins with myelin
basic protein, degraded basic protein or modified basic protein.

In a recent report (9) an infectious agent has been isolated
from MS bone marrow cells and that was reported to be producing
cytopathogenic effects similar to paramyxo-viruses. The size of
this infectious agent has been found to be approximately 220 nm.
Our efforts to isolate any specific antigen in the MS cytosole
fraction greater than 50 nm particle-size were unsuccessful.

Thus, if such agent is present in the brain of MS patients it might have been possible to detect it by the immunological methods involved in the present report.

The peak 2 isolated by MS brains has been found to be stimulating AER forming lymphocytes only from MS patients (Offner et al, in preparation).

REFERENCES

1. Adams, J.M. & Imagawa, D.T. (1962) Proc. Soc. Exp. Biol. Med. (N.Y.) 111, 562.
2. Agrawal, H.C., Burton, R.M., Fishman, M.A., Mitchel, R.F. & Prensky, A.L. (1972) J. Neurochem. 19, 2083.
3. Ammitzboll, T., Clausen, J. and Fog, T. (1977) Acta Neurol. Scand. 56, 153.
4. Axelsen, N.H., Kroll, J. & Weeke, B. (1973) Scand. J. Immunol. 2, Suppl. 1, Universitetsforlaget, Oslo.
5. Beck, H.W. & Clausen, J. (1977) Zbl. Bakt. Hyg., 1. Abt. Orig. A, 238, 431.
6. Enders-Ruckle, G. (1965) Arch. ges. Virusforsch. 16, 182.
7. Eylar, E.H., Salk, J., Beveridge, G.C. & Brown, L.V. (1969) Arch. Biochem. Biophys. 132, 34.
8. Lowry, O.H., Rosenbrough, N.J., Farr, A.L. & Randall, F.J. (1951) J. Biol. Chem. 193, 265.
9. Mitchel, D.N., Posterfield, J.S., Micheletti, R., Lange, L.S., Goswani, K.K.A., Taylor, P., Jacobs, J.B., Hoskley, D.J., Salsbury, A.J. (1978) Lancet, ii, 387.
10. Offner, H., Ammitzbøll, T. & Clausen, J. (1973) Acta Pathol. Microbiol. Scand. Sec. b 81, 157.
11. Rastogi, S.C., Clausen, J. & Fog, T. (1978a) Acta Neurol. Scand. 57, 438.
12. Rastogi, S.C., Offner, H., Konat, G. & Clausen, J. (1978b) Acta Neurol. Scand. (in press).
13. Schumacher, G.A. Beebe, G., Kilber, R.F., Kurland, L.T., Kutzke, J.F., McDowell, F., Nagler, B., Sibley, W.A., Tourtelotte, W.W. & Williams, T.A. (1965) Ann. N.Y. Acad. Sci. 122, 552.
14. Steiner, G. (1935) Arch. Neurol. (Chir) 34, 466.

CHARACTERIZATION OF MEASLES SPECIFIC PROTEINS SYNTHESIZED

FROM ACUTELY AND PERSISTENTLY INFECTED CELLS

S. Rozenblatt and O. Pinhasi

Department of Virology, Weizmann Institute of
Science, Rehovot, Israel

INTRODUCTION

Considerable evidence implicates measles virus or a closely-related virus in the rare degenerative neurological disease, subacute sclerosing panencephalitis (SSPE). This fatal disease, occurring in children several years after measles infection, is marked by gross cortical deterioration and loss of function. The sera and cerebrospinal fluid of SSPE patients contain high titers of measles antibodies (2) and paramyxovirus nucleocapsids have been identified in diseased nerve tissue (10). Infectious measles-like virus has been recovered by cocultivation of SSPE brain biopsy material with susceptible cells(4, 7). It has been suggested that this disease results from a persistent measles infection in which persistently infected cells arise that support virus production for extended periods of time without cytopathic effect and cell lysis. Cell lines of persistently infected measles virus have been established (8, 9) and can serve as a model system in order to study virus expression and its relationship to SSPE.

We have initiated studies where the synthesis of measles virus proteins were compared in acutely infected cells and persistently infected cells. We have utilized immunoprecipitation techniques in order to isolate and characterize measles specific proteins. Differences in the electrophoretic mobility of the viral matrix (M) protein were found. The viral M protein in the persistently infected cell lines had a slower electrophoretic mobility than that of the wild type virus M protein in acutely infected cells. The possible role of these altered M proteins are discussed.

MATERIALS AND METHODS

Cells and Viruses

The CV-1 line of African green monkey kidney cells was obtained from Flow Laboratories, Rockville, Maryland. The cells were grown in Dulbecco modified Eagles medium (DME) supplemented with 10 % calf serum. Hela K-11-HG (Cl-11) and K-11A-HG-1 (Cl-A) cell lines persistently infected with measles virus were obtained from R. Rustigian. Cl-11 is a carrier culture, which yields low levels of infectious virus. Cl-A is a "non-yielder" line, derived from Cl-11 following extensive serial passage in the presence of measles anti-sera. The Edmonston strain of measles virus was obtained from B. Fields, and had been plaque-purified twice in monkey CV-1 cells. Stock viral suspension $2x10^6-6x10^6$ PFU/ml was obtained from the pooled fluids of infected cultures with marked cytopathic effect.

Labelling of Cytoplasmic Proteins

Measles cytoplasmic proteins were labelled with (^{35}S) methionine (10-20 μCi/ml) (Amersham) for 1-6 hr in Dulbecco modified Eagle's medium lacking methionine 20 hrs post-infection. After the labelling period the cells were washed with reticulocyte standard buffer (RSB) and cytoplasm was obtained by lysis in RSB containing 0.5 % nonident P-40 (NP-40). Nuclei were removed by centrifugation at 2000 xg for 10 min at $4°C$.

Polyacrylamide Gels

Sodium dodecyl sulfate (SDS) 10 % polyacrylamide gels were prepared according to the Laemli procedure (5). The gels were run for approximately 2hr at 150 V (constant voltage) stained with coomassie blue, dried and either autoradiographed or fluorographed (1).

Immunoprecipitation

Measles specific proteins were immunoprecipitated from ^{35}S-methionine-labelled extracts of measles-infected cells. Cellular products were centrifuged at 12,000 xg for 10 min, prior to incubation with 10 μl of guinea pig anti-measles virus sera for 10 min at $37°C$, followed by incubation for 1 hr at $4°C$. Rabbit anti-guinea pig sera (0.15 ml) was added and the mixture was left overnight at $4°C$. The mixture was diluted to 1.5 ml with cold PBS and centrifuged at 3,000 xg for 15 min ar room temperature. The pellet was washed four times with 1.5 ml of cold PBS and centrifuged. The immunoprecipitates were solubilized in 50 μl electrophoresis buffer and analyzed on SDS polyacrylamide gels..

RESULTS

Measles Virus Proteins from Acutely-Infected CV-1 Cells

Cytoplasmic extracts of ^{35}S-methionine labelled uninfected monkey cells (CV-1 line) and monkey cells acutely infected by measles virus were analyzed by SDS polyacrylamide gel electro-phoresis. It can be seen in Fig. 1 that several new polypeptides appear in the cytoplasm of infected cells with molecular weights estimated as 78,000, 70,000, 60,000, 40,000 and 35,000. This is consistent with previously reported analysis of proteins observed in measles virus infected cells. The 78,000, 70,000, 60,000 and 35,000 polypeptides are very likely the same as the previously described G(glycosylated), P(phosphorylated), N (nucleocapsid) and M(matrix) proteins, respectively (6, 11, 12). In order to further identify and analyse measles virus specific proteins, cytoplasmic extracts were subjected to immunoprecipi-tation with guinea pig anti-measles serum. As seen in Fig. 1, 4 major polypeptides are immunoprecipitated from ^{35}S-methionine labelled infected cell extracts, with molecular weights estimated as 78,000, 70,000, 60,000 and 35,000 again likely the previously designated G, P, N and M proteins. None of these were obtained after reaction of uninfected cells with guinea pig anti-measles sera. In addition, a group of polypeptides are precipitated with molecular weights ranging from 43,000 to 45,000. In our studies we have focused on the four G, P, N and M polypeptides until further analysis of the 43,000 to 45,000 group is completed. The 40,000 MW novel polypeptide seen in infected cells was not immunoprecipitated with guinea pig anti-measles sera; this could mean that this is a non-structural viral protein, or possibly a cellular protein whose synthesis is induced after viral infec-tion.

Measles Protein Synthesis in Persistently Infected Hela Cells

As viral expression in SSPE may be analogous to that in chronically infected cells, we have carried out comparable experiments with two such persistently infected Hela cell lines, Cl-11 and Cl-11A. Both lines were tested for measles antigens by the indirect fluorescent staining technique using guinea pig anti-measles and FITC rabbit anti guinea. Under the conditions used, 95 % of the cells exhibited positive fluorescent staining (Fig. 2).

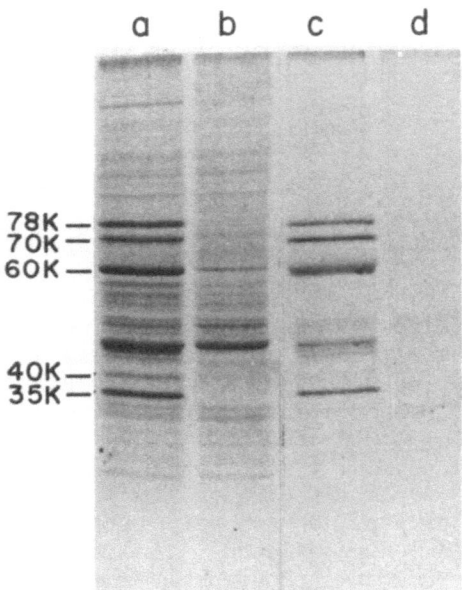

Fig. 1 : <u>Measles polypeptides synthesis in acutely infected cells</u>
Measles infected and uninfected cells were labelled with 35S-
methionine (10 μCI/ml) 24 hr p.i. for 1 hr. Cells were washed
with RSB and extracted with RSB containing 0.5 % NP$_{40}$, and either
directly treated with electrophoresis sample buffer or immunoprecipitated.
a) infected cell extract;
b) uninfected cell extract;
c) guinea pig anti-measles immunoprecipitate of (a);
d) guinea pig anti-measles immunoprecipitate of (b).

        Viral proteins synthesized in the persistent lines were
analyzed by immunoprecipitation as described above for acute
infection. When extracts of 35S-methionine-labelled persistent
lines were subjected to SDS polyacrylamide gels electrophoresis
there was no marked difference in the pattern of polypeptides
synthesized in uninfected Hela cells or lines of Cl-11 or
cl-11A. However, guinea pig anti-measles sera immunoprecipitated
three major polypeptides from Cl-11 and cl-11A but not uninfected Hela extracts, with molecular weights determined as 78,000,
70,000 and 60,000 which comigrate electrophoretically with measles
proteins similarly isolated from acutely infected CV-1 cells
(Fig.3). In addition, a polypeptide which migrated somewhat
slower than the 35,000 (M) protein of infected CV-1 was also
specifically immunoprecipitated.

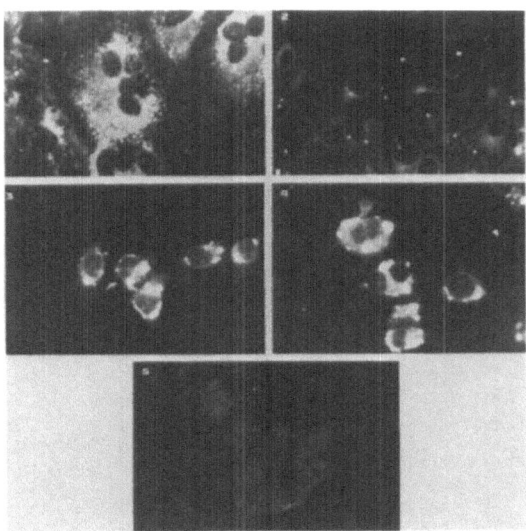

Fig. 2 : Intracellular viral immunofluorescence of Hela cells
The presence of measles specific antigens in acutely and persistently infected cells was determined by the indirect immunofluorescence technique with guinea pig anti-measles sera and fluorescence isothiocyanate conjugated rabbit anti-guinea pig γ globulin.
1. lytically infected CV-1 cells,
2. mock infected CV-1 cells;
3. persistently infected Cl-11;
4. persisteltly infected Cl-11A;
5. mock infected Hela cells.

It has previously been reported that the 78,000 (G) protein
is glycosylated (6, 11, 12). This was confirmed by labelling
infected and uninfected cells with glucosamine, followed by their
extraction, immunoprecipitation of the ^{3}H-glucosamine-labelled
extracts with guinea pig anti-measles sera, only the 78,000 (G)
polypeptide was observed indicating that this is the only glycosylated measles polypeptide (Fig. 4). Similar experiments demonstrated that the 78,000 viral protein immunoprecipitated from
Cl-11 (Fig. 4) and Cl-11A (data not shown) is also glycosylated.

The acutely infected cells and persistently infected cells,
Cl-11 and Cl-11A were analyzed for hemadsorption. Although G
protein (78,000) could be extracted from Cl-11A, the cells were
completely negative for hemadsorption (Fig. 5). This difference
could be due (a) to a slight alteration in the G protein (hemaglu-

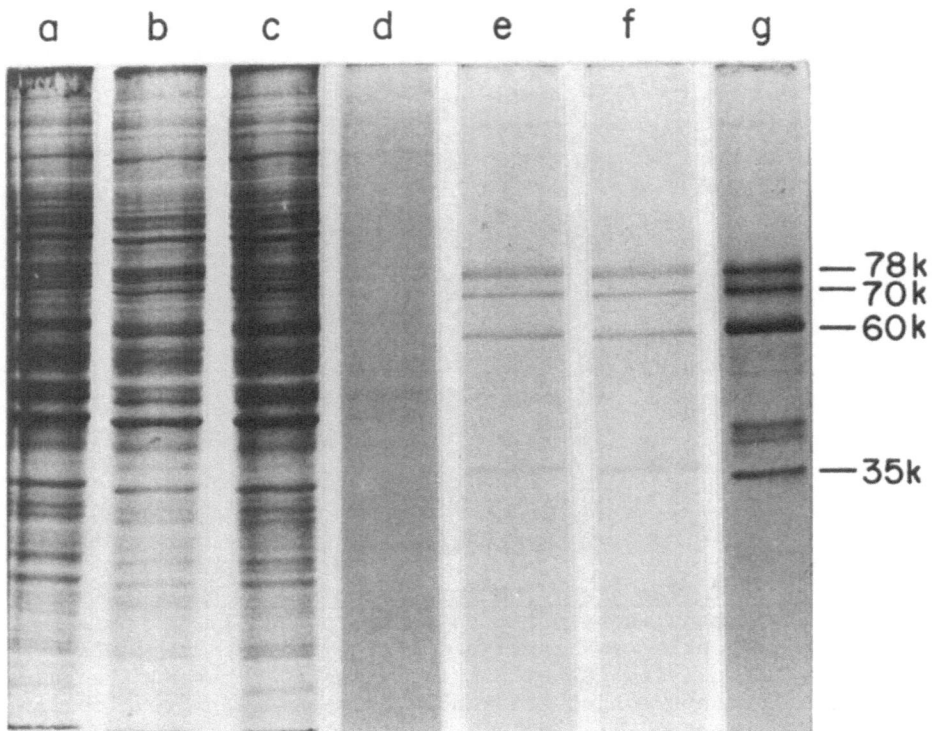

Fig. 3 : <u>Measles polypeptide synthesis in persistently infected</u>
<u>cells.</u>
Persistently infected and uninfected Hela cells were labelled
with ^{35}S-methionine 20 µCi/ml for 1 hr. Cells were washed with
RSB and proteins extracted as described in Fig. 2.
a) uninfected cells extract;
b) persistently infected Cl-11 cell extract;
c) persistently infected Cl-11A cell extract;
d) guinea pig anti-measles immunoprecipitate of (a);
e) guinea pig anti-measles immunoprecipitate of (b);
f) guinea pig anti-measles immunoprecipitate of (c);
g) guinea pig anti-measles immunoprecipitate of lytically infected
   cell extract.

tinin) that we could not detect under conditions that we have
used; (b) modification in host in such a manner that G protein
is not exposed on the cell surface and remains internal; or (c)
the concentration of G protein is not sufficient to interact
with red blood cells.

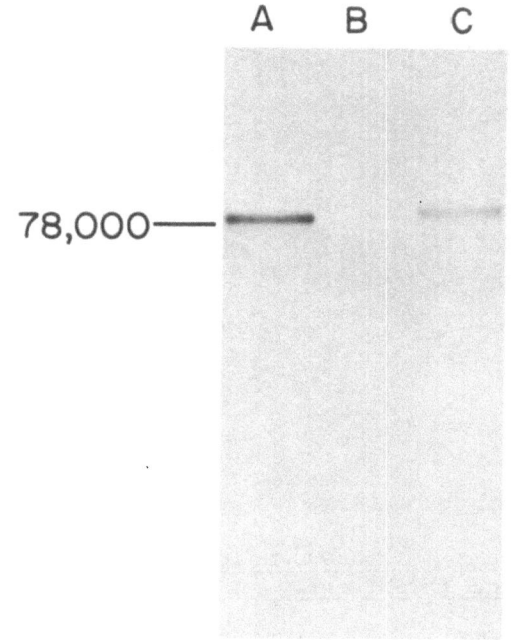

Fig. 4 : <u>Measles glycoprotein synthesis in acutely and persis-</u>
        <u>tently infected cells.</u>
Infected and uninfected cells were labelled with ^{3}H-glucosamine
20 μCi/ml for 4 hr. Cells were washed with RSB and proteins
extracted as described in Fig. 2. Guinea pig anti-measles
immunoprecipitate of (a) acutely infected cells; (b) uninfected
cells; (c) persistently infected Cl-11 cells.

    As reported previously, the 70,000 (P) and 60,000 (N)
proteins are phosphorylated (12). This was confirmed by labelling
infected and uninfected cells and the two persistently infected
cell lines (Cl-11, Cl-11A) with (^{32}P). Measles specific proteins
were extracted immunoprecipitated and characterized as described
in Materials and Methods. The results described in Fig. 6 indicate that P and N proteins are the two major phosphorylated proteins and are modified in persistently infected cells as well
as in acutely infected cells.

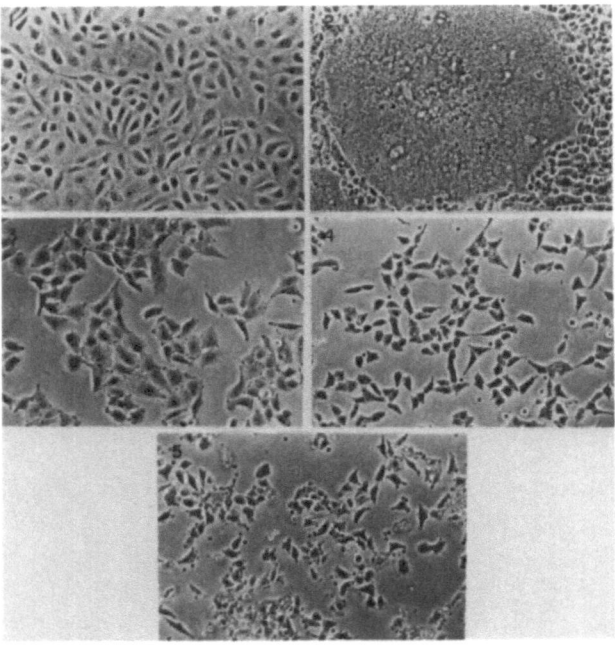

Fig. 5 : Hemadsorption of rhesus monkey erythrocytes to measles
          acutely and persistently infected cells.
1. uninfected CV-1;
2. acutely infected CV-1;
3. uninfected Hela;
4. persistently infected Cl-11A;
5. persistently infected Cl-11.

                              DISCUSSION

        In order to evaluate the involvement of measles virus in
SSPE, we have studied measles virus proteins synthesis in acutely and persistently infected cells. Guinea pig anti-measles
virus sera was used to isolate measles proteins from the cellular products of acutely and persistently infected cells.

        Three major viral specific polypeptides isolated from acu-
tely infected cells, glycoprotein (G); phosphoprotein (P); and
the nucleocapsid protein (N) were indistinguishable by electrophoretic mobility from those purified in persistently infected
cells.

        Experiments were performed in order to find out if differen-
ces in modification of measles virus proteins can account for

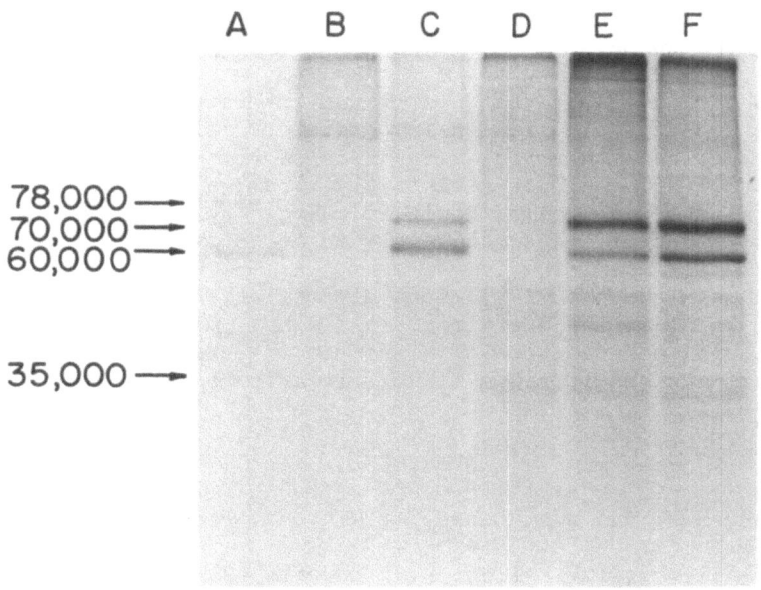

Fig. 6 : Measles phosphoprotein synthesis in acutely and persis-
        tently infected cells
Infected and uninfected cells were labelled with (^{32}P)-100 μCi/ml
for 4 hr. Cells were washed with RSB and proteins extracted
as described in Fig. 2.
Guinea pig anti-measles immunoprecipitates of
a) (^{35}S)-methionine measles acutely infected cells, as marker;
b) uninfected CV-1;
c) acutely infected CV-1;
d) uninfected Hela cells;
e) persistently infected Cl-11;
f) persistently infected Cl-11A cells.

the different cycle response in persistent and acute infection.
Two criterias were used, glycosylation and phosphorylation.
The glycoprotein (G) is glycosylated whether the cells are acutely
infected or persistently infected. In addition, no differences
were observed for the phosphorylated protein, the phosphoprotein
(P) and the nucleocapsid protein (N) were both phosphorylated.

    A striking finding is the difference in the electrophoretic
mobility of the matrix protein (M) noted in our experiments,
and it is particularly interesting in the light of recent reports
of an altered M protein in SSPE virus isolated by co-cultivation

of diseased patients' tissues (3, 13). In a similar fashion
the putative M protein isolated from the persistent lines had
a reduced electrophoretic mobility when compared to the M protein
in lytic infection.

One can speculate that host-virus interaction leads to a
modification of the M protein in persistent infection which
could interfere with normal maturation of the virus. The
defect, however, could be exclusively viral; a mutation in the
M protein gene could also result in changed cellular modification
of the polypeptide and subsequently in defective maturation.

Although phosphorylation and glycosylation did not show
specific labelling of M protein, it did not rule out a post-
translational modification of M protein in persistently infected
cells that can result in a slower migration on acrylamide gels.

REFERENCES

1. Bonner, M.W. and R.A. Laskey. 1974. J. Biol. Chem. 252 :
   1102-1106.
2. Connoly, J.H., I.V. Allen, L.J. Hurwitz, J.H.D. Millar. 1967.
   Lancet 1 : 542-544.
3. Hall, W.W., W. Kiessling, V. ter Meulen. 1978. Nature 272 :
   460-462.
4. Horta-Barbosa, L., D.A. Fuccillo, J.L. Sever. 1967. Nature
   221 : 974.
5. Laemli, V.K. 1970. Nature 227 : 680-685.
6. Mountcastle, W.E. and P.W. Choppin. 1977. Virology 78 :
   463-474.
7. Payne, F.E., J.V. Baublis, H.H. Itabashi, 1969. N. Eng. J.
   Med. 281 : 585-589.
8. Rustigian, R. 1966. J. of Bact. 92 : 1792-1804.
9. Rustigian, R. 1966. J. of Bact. 92 : 1805-1811.
10. Tallez-Nagel, I. and D.H. Harter. 1966. Science, N.Y. 154 :
    899-901.
11. Tyrrel, D.L.J. and E. Norrby. 1978. J. Gen. Virol. 39 :
    219-229.
12. Wechsler, S.L. and B.N. Fields. 1978. J. Virol. 25 : 285-
    297.
13. Wechsler, S.L. and B.N. Fields. 1978. Nature 272 : 458-460.

NEW POLYPEPTIDES IN MEASLES VIRUS INFECTED VERO CELLS

D.A. Vanden Berghe and G. Huybreghts

Department Microbiology, U.I.A., Wilrijk, Belgium

The polypeptide composition of measles virus and the synthesis of virus-specific proteins in CV-1 cells have been extensively analyzed by polyacrylamide gel electrophoresis (1, 2, 3, 4, 5). The different protein patterns of "purified measles virus" reveal similarities but also large differences. Using several previously described methods we failed to prepare measles virus free of cellular proteins (cf.3). The significance of "purified measles virus preparations" must therefore be questioned. Pulse experiments with different cell lines (Vero, BSC-1, HEp-2, Hel) and two different measles virus strains (Edmonston A and B) result in the detection of up to 9 presumable virus specific polypeptides with a MW between 90.000 and 30.000 daltons. According to their MS we find : p81, p73, p67, p62, p58, p51, p43, p41 and p37.

Figure 1 shows the sucrose density gradient centrifugation profile in the last step of virus purification (method according to D. Waters and R. Bussell, 1973). The virus bands at density 1, 19 (fig. 1A) but the cell control (fig. 1B) shows also labelled material of the same density.

The polypeptide composition of the measles virus band (6) on SDS-polyacrylamide gel is shown in fig. 2. Six major polypeptides are clearly separated : 1 : p81, 2 : p73, 3 : p62, 4 : p51, 5 : p43 and 6 : p37.
The major difference between our results and previously described polypeptide composition of measles virus is that the polypeptide p51 migrating between NP (p62) and actin (p43) is very clear compared to the other polypeptides. When labelled amino-acids were added one day after infection and measles virus was harves-

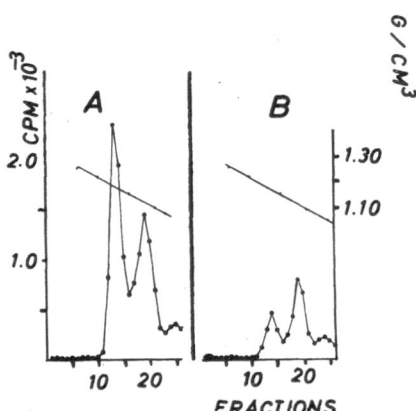

Fig. 1. <u>Preparation of semi-purified measles virus</u>. Vero monolayer cells were infected with Edmonston A measles virus (multiplicity of infection MOI 0.01) and labelled with ^{14}C-L-Valine and ^{14}C-L-Leucine (0,5 μC/ml) after 48h. An uninfected monolayer was used as cell control. CPE was complete 4 days after infection and virus was purified according to the method of Waters D. and Bussell R. (5). The virus pellet was centrifuged in a sucrose density gradient at 106.000 g for 18 hours. 1A Sucrose density gradient of measles virus. 1B cell control.

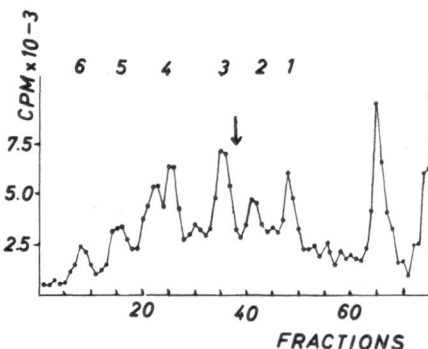

Fig. 2. <u>Polypeptide pattern of ^{14}C)-semi-purified measles virus (fig.1).</u> Protein extraction and polyacrylamide gel electrophoresis was previously described (6). The six measles virus polypeptides are indicated by numbers and bovine albumin by an arrow. Top gel is right.

ted three days after infection the polypeptide pattern of purified
measles is somewhat different. This is illustrated in fig. 3.

Polypeptide p51 is now the most important while p61 and p71
are not all visible. These results suggest a correlation between
the two nucleocapsid polypeptides (p62 and p72) and p51.
We also observed that p51 was accumulated in the nucleus of
measles infected Vero cells two days after infection and that the
intensity of the p51 peak was inversely proportional to the peptide p62.

Fig. 4 shows the polypeptide composition of the nuclei in
flat bed gel. The labelled amino acids were added 1, 2 and 3
days after infection (MOI : 0.1 TCD 50/cell) and the nuclei
were isolated 3 or 4 days after infection. Polypeptides p62 and
p72 are only faintly visible when cells are pulse-labelled 1 day
after infection. In the other cases p62 and p72 became more prominent and p51 disappears. The cell control shows no significant
polypeptides in the same MS regions. To show the exact nature
of the p51 polypeptide we isolated the nucleocapsids by 1% DOC
treatment of the nuclei. In these experiments cells were infected with MOI 0.01, 0.1 and 1.

CPE was complete three days after infection in the case of
MOI 1 while with MOI 0.01 only small multinucleated cells were
visible all over the monolayer.

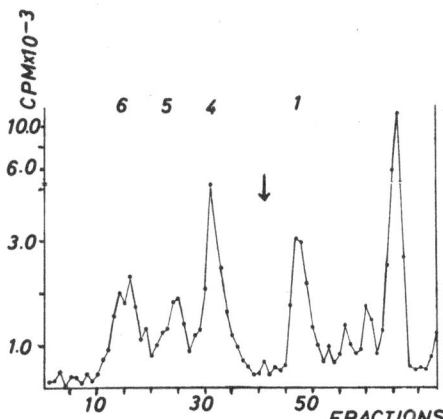

Fig. 3 Polypeptide pattern of (^{14} C)-semi-purified measles virus.
Vero cells were infected with measles virus at MOI 0.01 and the
^{14} C-amino acids were added one day after infection. Virus purification as described under fig. 1 started three days after infection. The measles virus polypeptides are indicated by numbers and
bovine albumin by an arrow.

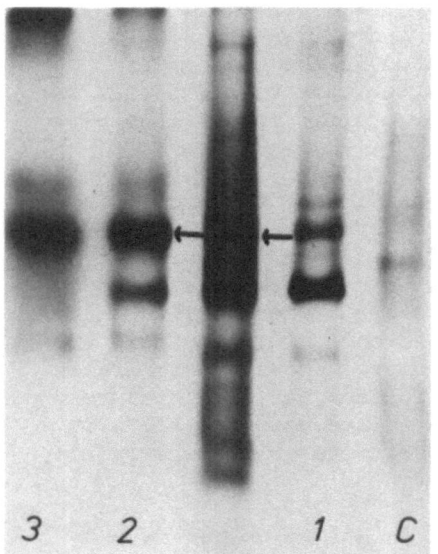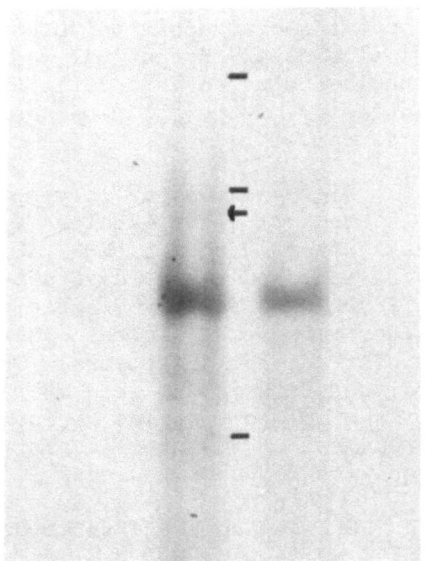

Fig. 4 Flat bed polyacrylamide gel electrophoresis of nuclear
material. Measles infected Vero cells were washed twice with
culture medium and 1 ml RSB was added. Cells were broken by free-
zing (-30°C) and thawing (37°C). The cell suspension is further
treated as described (6). Nucleus associated cytoplasm and nucleus unassociated cytoplasm were prepared. The last sediment
containing the nuclei was centrifuged over 60 % sucrose in RSB
and the nuclear pellet was resuspended in 1 ml RSB. Protein
extraction and flat bed electrophoresis is as described (6, 7),
except that 0.1 % SDS is added in gel and electrophoresis buffer.
The position of the NP (p63) is indicated by an arrow.
4.A.1. Characteristics : MOI 0.01, pulse labelling 24 h after
       infection. Nucleus purification three days after infection.
    2. MOI 0.01, pulse labelling 48 h after infection, nucleus
       purification three days after infection.
    3. MOI 0.01, pulse labelling 72 h after infection, nucleus
       purification four days after infection.
4.B. Characteristics : MOI 0.01, pulse labelling 18 h after in-
     fection, nucleus purification one day later. Two different
     experiments are illustrated.

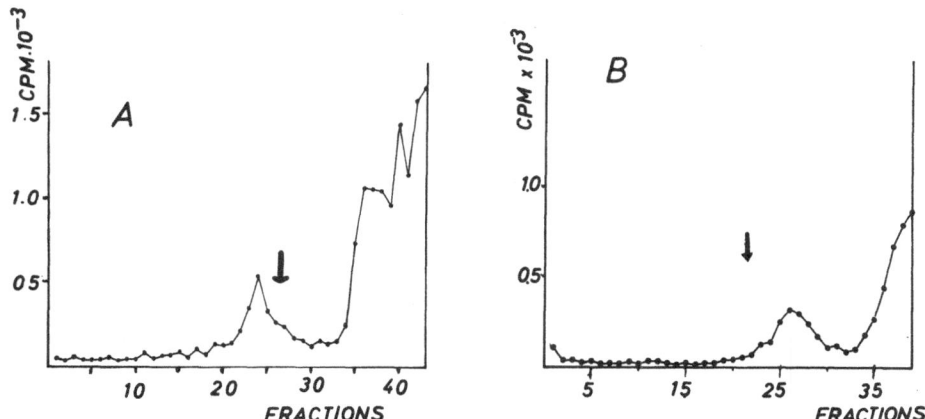

Fig. 5. Sucrose gradient of measles virus nucleocapsids isolated by DOC treatment of the nuclei. Measles infected Vero cells were pulse labelled two days after infection and the nuclei were isolated one day later. The suspension of Vero cell nuclei containing 1% DOC is incubated for 15 minutes at 37°C and layered on 15-30% sucrose as described previously[3](6). Centrifugation at 113.000 g for 2 hours. The position of (^{3}H) -labelled poliovirus (155 S), added as marker particle, is indicated.
5.A. Experiment characteristic : MOI 1
5.B. Experiment characteristic : MOI 0.01

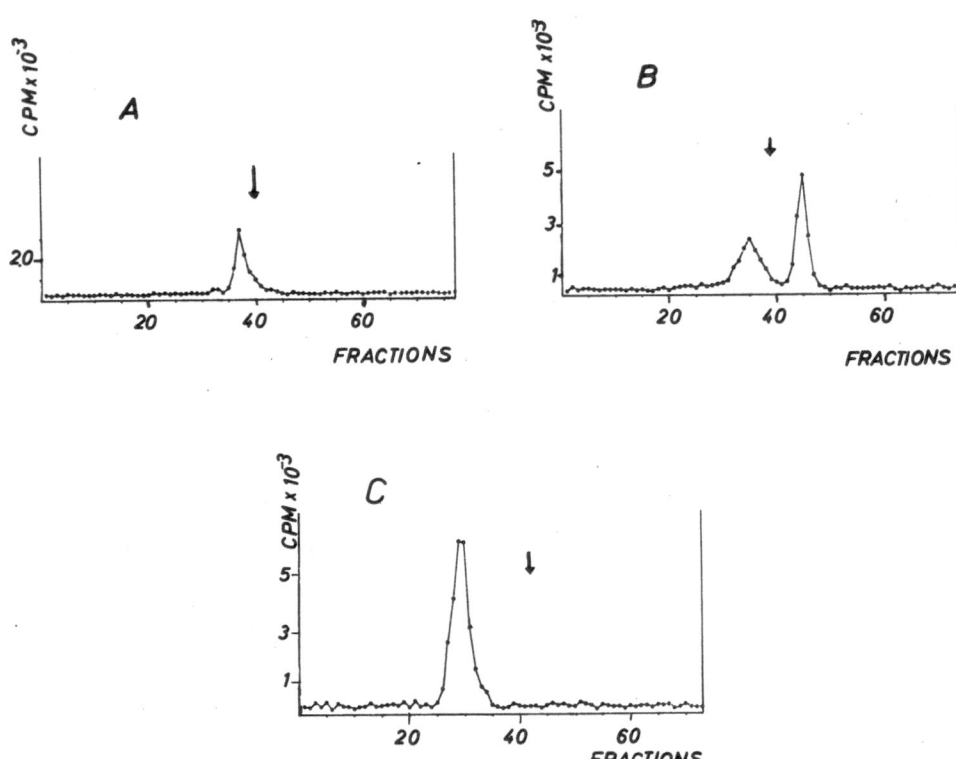

<u>Fig. 6. Polypeptide pattern of measles virus nucleocapsids.</u> Meas-
les virus nucleocapsids prepared as described under Fig. 5. are
analyzed by SDS polyacrylamide gel electrophoresis as described
under Fig. 2. The position of bovine albumin is indicated.
6.A. : MOI 0.1
6.B. : MOI 1
6.C. : MOI 0.01

Fig. 5 shows the sucrose gradient for nucleocapsid isolation after DOC treatment of nuclei. Distinct nucleocapsid peaks are seen with a sedimentation coefficient of $\pm$ 200S for MOI 1 and 0.1 and $\pm$ 100S for MOI 0.01. All these nucleocapsids banded at 1.30 g/cm^3 in CsCl.

Fig. 6 shows the polypeptide composition of the different nucleocapsid species.
Nucleocapsids isolated 3 days after infection with MOI 0.01 contain polypeptide p51 while the other nucleocapsid (MOI 1 and 0.1) patterns in SDS polyacrylamide gel shows the normal p61 and p72 polypeptides.

We conclude that polypeptide p51 is formed early in infection when a low MOI is used or that the NP (p62) is cleaved into a p51 polypeptide under these circumstances.

ACKNOWLEDGEMENT

The authors thank M. Verckens for excellent technical assistance.

REFERENCES

1. Hall, W.W. and Martin, S.J. (1973). J. gen. Virol. 19, 175-188.
2. Schluederberg, A., Chavanisch, S., Lipman, M.B. and Carter, C. (1974). Biochem. Biophys. Res. Commun. 58, 647-651.
3. Mountcastle, W.E., and Choppin, P.W. (1977). Virology, 78, 463-474.
4. Wechsler, S.L. and Fields, B.N. (1978). Virology, 25, 285-297.
5. Waters, D.J. and Bussell, R.H. (1973). Virology, 55; 554-557.
6. Vanden Berghe, D.A. (1973). Bioch. Biophys. Res. Commun., 50, 957-963.
7. Vanden Berghe, D.A. and Pattyn, S.R. (1978) J. gen. Microbiol. in press.

THE FATE OF ANTIGEN-ANTIBODY COMPLEXES ON MEASLES VIRUS-INDUCED

GIANT CELLS

E.L. Hooghe-Peters *

National Institutes of Health, NINCDS, Bethesda,
Maryland, U.S.A.

The importance of different mechanisms of defense (interferon,
antibodies, cell-mediated immunity, macrophages) against viral infection is poorly understood. The various mechanisms of defense
may have both favorable and deleterious effects. The relative
importance of these various mechanisms varies for different viruses
and for different host tissues. We have studied the effects of
antibodies on measles induced giant cells in the absence of complement. Antibodies have been implicated in the induction of persistent infections by measles virus, possibly through the generation of defective viruses (1, 2).

Giant cells resulting from the fusion of measles virus-infected cells, were detected in monolayers of Vero cells, three
days after infection. The monolayers were washed and radioimmunolabeled in the cold using a two layer (sandwich) technique. In
this procedure, cells were first treated with human Ig containing
antibodies to measles virus. This was followed by treatment of
the cells with staphylococcal protein A (SpA) which had been labeled with radioactive iodine. After washing, the cells were incubated at 37° for 0-24 hours and processed for autoradiography.
Following the incubation period, the medium was collected and
assayed for radioactivity. When cells were fixed immediately after
the labeling procedure (0 hours incubation) the distribution of
measles antigen was homogeneous (Figure 1). After incubation at
37° for 5 minutes redistribution of the label resulted in patch
formation (Figure 2).

* Present Address : Département de Morphologie, Institut
  d'Histologie et d'Embryologie, Ecole de Médecine, Genève,
  Switzerland.

The analogy between these observations and similar observations
in other systems (3) was supported by the requirement for divalent
reagents (no patching with Fab fragments) and the temperature-de-
pendency (no patching at 4°). Metabolic energy was not required
since patching took place in the presence of sodium azide. After
one hour of incubation at 37°, redistribution of label was seen to
occur by coalescence of the patches into one or several strands of
antigen-antibody complexes, usually assuming the shape of a ring
(Figure 3). The label did not further redistribute into a polar
cap.

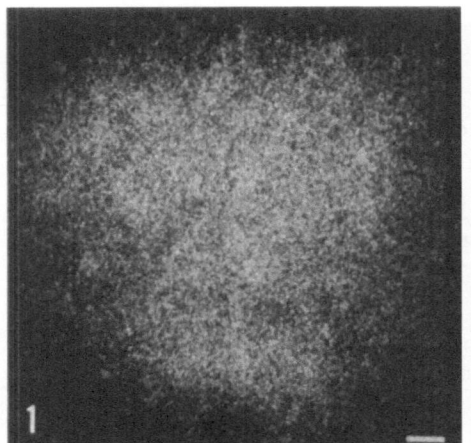 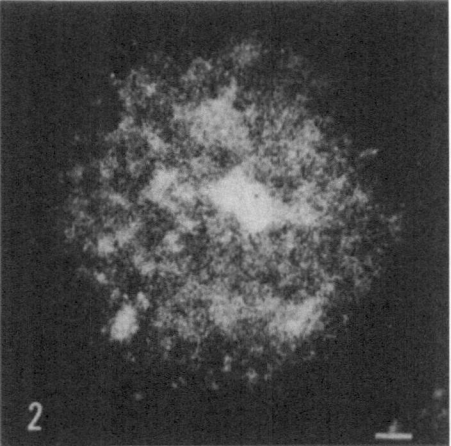

Fig. 1. Dark field radioautogram of measles-infected Vero cells
grown as monolayers. Cells were infected with measles virus at
a low multiplicity of infection (0.005 plaque forming unit/cell).
Two to three days post infection, cell fusion occurs as a result
of the infection. After assessing the presence of giant cells on
the monolayer, cells are incubated with normal human IgG (with
a high antibody titer to measles virus) and then with 125 I Spa
at 4°C, each for 1h. Cells were subsequently fixed. This micrograph shows the distribution of antigenic sites on the cell surface of a typical giant cell. The label (silver grains appearing
as white dots) is distributed homogeneously over the giant cell
surface. Bar = 100 μ.

Fig. 2. Dark field radioautogram of a monolayer of measles virus-
infected Vero cells. Cells were radioimmunolabeled at 4°C as
described in Fig. 1, further incubated for 1 h. at 37°C in pre-
heated medium (capping conditions) and subsequently fixed. Clusters of grains are detected in various areas of the cell membrane.
Bar = 100 μ.

Ring formation observed in the present study was analogous to
cap formation in both its requirements for particular reagents and
in its time course (3). Clearing of the antigen-antibody complexes
proceeded through both shedding into the extracellular medium and
endocytosis. Assaying the release of label into the medium gave
a measure of shedding. After 15 minutes, 12% of the label was
recovered in the medium. After 24 hours, 88% of the label was
recovered in the medium. A portion of the label underwent endocytosis as was demonstrated by electron microscopy (4). While
antigen-antibody complexes were cleared from the surface of the
cell, measles antigens were re-expressed, as was demonstrated by a
second labeling. Thus, it appeared, the antigen(s) studied were
synthesized by the cell and were not cytophilic. The turnover of
measles antigen was rapid, in agreement with previous data (5).
At no point was there a total eclipse of the antigen(s). In fact,
antigenic modulation, which had been observed on measles virus
infected cells, was induced only by prolonged treatment with antibody (6). It is not clear why redistribution of the antigen-
antibody complexes did not follow the usual pattern (leading to
cap formation). It may be envisaged that the cell membrane has
different properties in the center of the syncytium where lysis
is going to occur. Identical redistribution into a ring was induced by antibodies to normal Vero cell antigens. Ring formation

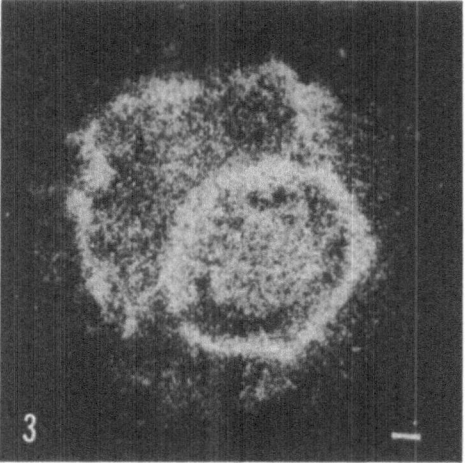

Fig. 3. Dark field radioautogram of cells labeled at 4°C as described in Fig. 1 and incubated under capping conditions for 3 h.
Silver grains cluster to specific configurations, usually resembling
closed ring. In this micrograph, two apparent rings have formed
midway between the center and the periphery (not visible) of the
giant cell. Bar = 100 μ.

was therefore a characteristic feature of the giant cell membrane and not of the viral antigens. Monkey red blood cells hemadsorbed to giant cells also form a ring, as shown by scanning electron microscopy (7). This establishes the presence of the viral antigen on the cell surface. Thus the rings that we describe do not appear to be homologous to the rings formed by the endocytosed antigen-antibody complexes described by Schlessinger et al. (8).

The following factors related to redistribution of antigens are considered to be relevant to clinical situation (1) antigenic modulation (2) shedding of immune complexes (3) endocytosis (and subsequent degradation of viral components).

We have previously shown that antibodies could induce the capping of normal antigens on neurons (9). If dissociated nerve cells in culture can be infected with measles virus, it may be possible to assess the importance of antibody-induced redistribution on the outcome of the infection.

REFERENCES

1. Gould, J.J. & Almeida, J.D. J. Med. Virol. 1, 111, 1977.
2. Rustigian, R. J. Bacteriol. 92, 1805, 1966.
3. Loor, F. Prog. Allergy 23, 1, 1977.
4. Hooghe-Peters, E.L. & Dubois-Dalcq, M. J. Cell Biol. 75, 396, 1977.
5. Ehrnst, A. & Sundqvist, K.G. Cell 5, 351, 1975.
6. Oldstone, M.B.A. & Tshon, A. Clin. Immunol. Immunopath. 9, 55, 1978.
7. Rentier, B., Hooghe-Peters, E.L. & Dubois-Dalcq, M. J. Virol. 1978 (in press).
8. Schlessinger, J., Schechter, Y., Willingham, M.C. & Pastan, I. Proc. Nat. Acad. Sci. U.S.A. 75, 2659, 1978.
9. Hooghe-Peters, E.L. & Hooghe, R. (submitted for publication).

INDUCTION OF INFECTIOUS VIRUS AND VIRAL SURFACE ANTIGEN IN VERO

CELLS PERSISTENTLY INFECTED WITH JUNIN VIRUS

C.E. Coto[+], M.E. Leon[+], L.M. Peralta[o], G. Help[+] and R.P. Laguens[o]

[+] Department of Biochemistry, University of Buenos Aires, Buenos Aires, Argentina
[o] Faculty of Medicine, University of la Plata, Buenos Aires, Argentina

SUMMARY

Persistently infected lines were obtained from surviving Vero cells after a lytic infection with Junin virus. These cell lines eliminated small amounts of infectious virus in a cyclic pattern. Immunofluorescent studies revealed that about 20 % of cells contained cytoplasmic Junin virus antigens and only 4 % showed cell surface associated antigens. Treatment with either actinomycin D or cycloheximide increased the number of cells with surface antigens and induced the appearance of plaque forming virus.

The results suggest that in this system, control of persistant infection is DNA dependent and that active protein synthesis is necessary to maintain the suppressed state of the virus.

INTRODUCTION

One of the main characteristics of Arenaviruses is their ability to produce persistent infections in their natural hosts (1).

Junin virus, one of the members of this group, pathogenic for man and the aethiological of Argentine hemorrhagic fever, does not escape from this general property. Recent evidence has shown that in Calomys musculinus, the most important Junin virus reservoir in nature (2), viral antigen and infectious virus can be demonstrated as long as 18 months after infection by natural routes (3). These facts support the importance of studies pointing to an

405

understanding of the relationship between host and virus. The mechanisms by which virus genetic information is maintained in animals persistently infected with Arenaviruses are not known.

Vero cells are one of the few targets in which Junin virus induces a lytic infection (4). However some cells remained undamaged and from them persistently infected lines can be established (5), (6).

A Vero cell line persistently infected with Junin virus (VRJ), developed in our laboratory, released small amounts of virus in a cyclic fashion (7).

For lymphocytic choriomeningitis virus (LCM), the prototype of the Arenavirus group (1), cyclic infection was postulated as an explanation for the persistence of this virus in mice (8). Rawls (9) stated "that a requirement of this hypothesis is the regulation of virus synthesis that can be mediated through a gene product coded by the virus or the host cell which results in the loss or complete repression of virus genetic information."

In order to find out if a cell host product (s) is responsible for the regulation of persistent infection, the effect of cell metabolic inhibitors on virus induction in Vero cells was studied.

RESULTS

The studies reported were performed on two Vero cell lines persistently infected with Junin virus designated VRJ 3 and VRJ 78. Both were obtained in a similar way with minor variants.

ESTABLISHMENT OF VRJ 3 AND VRJ 78 CELL LINES

VRJ 3 cells : Vero cells grown in 199 medium were infected with Junin virus, attenuated strain XJ Cl 3 at a multiplicity of infection of 0.06. Cytopathic effects (CPE) appeared 2 days later and the maximum virus titer was detected in the supernatant on day 3 p.i. (3.6×10^5 PFU/ml). On the 5th day p.i. the monolayer was almost destroyed, but on day 8 regrowth was observed. Cells were trypsinized on the 18th day p.i. and since that moment once or twice a week.

VRJ 3 cell line was studied during 110 passages. VRJ 78 cell line was obtained similarly to VRJ 3 cell line, only that the cells were left 35 days prior to trypsinization. Afterwards it was passed in average each four days.

CRITERIA USED TO ASSESS PERSISTENT INFECTION

VRJ 3 and VRJ 78 cells were superinfected with Junin virus at different passages. No plaque formation was seen after challenging with different doses of virus while in control cultures virus titers reached normal values. However, VRJ 3 cells were susceptible to Vesicular Stomatitis Virus (VSV), Newcastle Disease Virus (NDV) and Measles virus infection as it is shown in Table 1.

TABLE 1

Susceptibility of VRJ 3 cell line to exogenous virus infection.

Virus	Titer (PFU/ml)	
	Vero	VRJ 3
NDV	8.7×10^3	2.8×10^3
VSV	1.1×10^7	5.4×10^7
Measles	6.8×10^3	7.2×10^3
Junin	7.5×10^7	< 5

CHARACTERISTICS OF VRJ CELLS

Production of infection virus : Supernatants from CRJ 3 cells were assayed for virus infectivity either in Vero cells, using a standard plaque assay revealing plaques on day 7th p.i. or in new-born mice (24-48 hs of age) inoculated intracerebrally. Table 2 shows that infectivity assays performed in culture fluids from passage 3 up to 102 failed to demonstrate the presence of virus by the PFU method. Low levels of virus were detected only by inoculation of new-born mice in the early evolution of the VRJ 3 cell line and later on passages 75, 77, 94, 96 and 101 showing a cyclic pattern of virus production. Thus the cell line was scarcely virogenic. VRJ 78 cell line was non-virogenic in all the passages tested up to the present time.

IMMUNOFLUORESCENT STUDIES

Immunofluorescence procedures were performed for detection of cytoplasmic Junin virus antigen in acetone-fixed VRJ cells and on unfixed cell monolayers for membrane associated antigen.

After many passages infected cells were not morphologically
different from uninfected cells. Analysis of VRJ cells by immunofluorescence using the indirect staining technique revealed
that about 20 % of the cells contained viral antigens. The antigens were located only in the cytoplasm and presented granular
appearance (Figure 1). The number of cells showing positive
membrane fluorescence were 4-5 % (one fifth of those showing intracellular fluorescence) (Figure 2). Superinfection of VRJ cells
with Junin virus did not change the number of cells showing positive immunofluorescence, indicating that resistance of cells
to reinfection is present at the virus entrance. It is interesting that in spite of this fact only 20 % of cells showed fluorescence; the remaining cells were virus unsusceptible.

From these results it is evident that Junin virus is present
generally in a repressed state in VRJ cells.

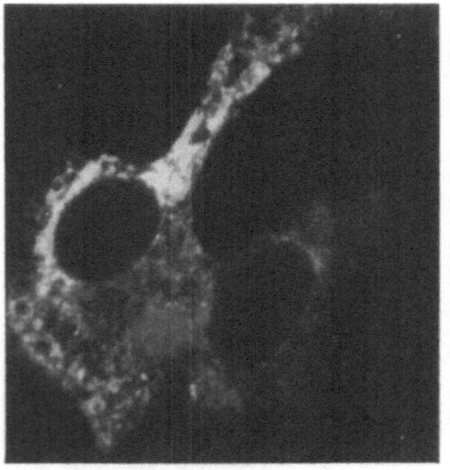 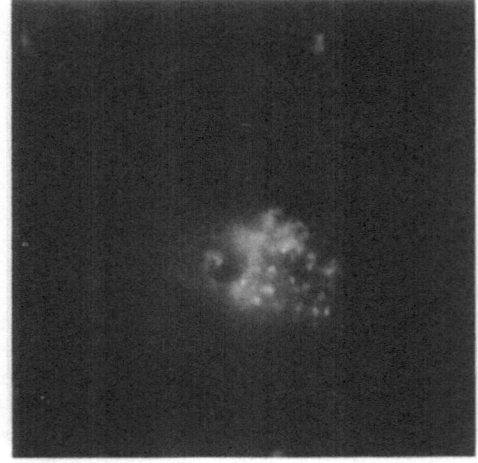

Fig. 1   Fig. 2

Figure 1 : Junin virus antigen inside VRJ 78 cells. Cells were
fixed with acetone and stained with mouse hyperimmune antiserum
ascitic fluid in combination with antimouse total immunoglobulin
serum labelled with fluorescein isothiocyanate.

Figure 2 : Junin virus surface antigen on VRJ 78 cells. Viable
(unfixed) cells were stained as explained in Figure 1.

TABLE 2

Junin virus release from CRJ 3 cells

Cell Passage level	Mice mortality
	(%)
3	88,8 $\neq$
6	50
11, 12, 14, 16, 17	
19, 25, 30	0
64, 66, 67, 68, 70, 72	0
75	16,6
77	44,4
79	0
94	77,7
96	71,4
101	33,4
102	0

$\neq$ Mortality produced by undiluted supernatants from VRJ 3 cells
in 8 or more new born mice.

ATTEMPTS TO INDUCE VIRUS ANTIGENS IN VRJ 78 CELLS BY COCULTIVA-

TION WITH NORMAL VERO CELLS

As only a small percentage of VRJ cells are susceptible to
virus infection and the remaining ones are resistant, it is hard
to demonstrate the presence of releasing virus. Accordingly it
was considered that cocultivation with sensitive Vero cells could
represent a useful model for such a demonstration.

Confluent monolayers of VRJ and Vero cells were trypsinized
and the cell concentration were adjusted to 10^5 cells/ml in 199
medium. Cocultivation was accomplished by mixing these cells in
a proportion of 1 volume to 1 volume and then were seeded in
cover slips. At 72 hours after seeding, cytoplasmic and surface
viral antigens were investigated. Results are summarized in
Table 3. A significant percentage of cells show membrane surface
antigen in cocultivated cultures.

TABLE 3

Induction of Junin virus surface in VRJ 78 cells by cocultivation with Vero cells.

Cell cultures	Fluorescent antigens ≠	
	Cytoplasmic	Surface
	(%)	
$VR_{10}J_{78}$	19	3
$VR_{10}J_{78}$ + Vero	22	14
$VR_{12}J_{78}$	20	4
$VR_{12}J_{78}$ + Vero	26	13

≠ Percentage was determined by counting 500 cells.

ATTEMPTS TO INDUCE VIRUS ANTIGENS BY TREATMENT WITH ACTINOMYCIN D

OR CYCLOHEXIMIDE

In previous work (6) it was shown that treatment of cultures
with actinomycin D was able to induce virus multiplication in persistently infected cultures.

Confluent monolayers of VRJ cells grown in cover slips were
exposed to actinomycin D (AD), an inhibitor of DNA dependent RNA
synthesis at 0.01; 0.5; 1.0 or 1.5 µg/ml and incubated for different times at 37°C (see legend Table 4). Cells at 72 hours
after seeding were treated with AD at the stated concentrations
for 3 or 24 hours. In the first case, the inhibitor was washed
after 3 hours and the cells were further incubated to complete
24 hours and processed for fluorescence staining. No toxic
effects of the inhibitor was observed at the concentration used.
As it can be seen in Table 4, AD treatment for 24 hours induces
the appearance of membrane antigen, independently of the concentration employed. Treatment for only 3 hours at the lowest
concentration of AD (0.01 µg/ml) was unable to induce antigen
synthesis.

In order to find out if the effect of AD was on the nucleic
acid directly or on a final protein product, cycloheximide, a
potent inhibitor of protein synthesis was assayed. VRJ cells
grown in coverslips at 72 hours post-seeding were treated with
50 µg or 100 µg of cycloheximide for 2 or 24 hours and then
processed for immunofluorescent staining. The results of

TABLE 4

Induction of Junin virus surface antigens in VRJ$_{78}$$^{\neq}$ cells by Actinomycin D.

Drug concentration	Time	Immunofluorescence staining	
µg/ml	h	Cytoplasmic(%)	Surface(%)
0	3	19$^{\neq\neq}$	4
0.01	3	20	3
1.0	3	19	10
1.5	3	17	11
0	24	20	4
0.01	24	18	11
1.0	24	18	11
1.5	24	17	11

$\neq$ Cell passage level 13
$\neq\neq$ Percentage was determined by counting 500 cells.

TABLE 5

Induction of Junin virus surface antigens in VRJ$_{12}$78 cells by cycloheximide.

Drug concentration	Time	Fluorescent antigens	
µg/ml	h	Cytoplasmic	Surface
		(%) $\neq$	
0		19	4
50	2	21	10
50	24	19	10
100	2	19	13
100	24	21	10

$\neq$ Percentage was determined by counting 500 cells.

Table 5 show that cycloheximide induces the synthesis of virus
membrane antigen independently of the exposure time. In spite
of the presence of immunofluorescence positive cells, the inoculation of supernatants into new-born mice rendered consistently
negative results.

EFFECT OF AD ON THE INDUCTION OF INFECTIOUS VIRUS

Induction of infectious Junin virus was attempted in cultures of VRJ 3 cell line at non virogenic passages 64, 66, 68, 70
and 72.

Immunofluorescence studies showed that only 3-4 % of cells
which presented membrane associated antigen are the probable virus producers. Accordingly it was thought that virus had to
reach a threshold to be detected by inoculation of the supernatants. A more sensitive method to detect virus could be the
addition of a standard overlay to the VRJ cell monolayer in order
to immobilize budding virus. However, since most cells remained
unsusceptible to virus reinfection it was thought that addition
of a monolayer of normal Vero cells could provide a layer of
sensitive cells to amplify the lytic effect of the small amount
of released virus. Confluent monolayers of VRJ cells grown in
60 cc bottles were covered with 10 ml of 199 medium containing
2×10^6 normal Vero cells. Cultures were incubated for 24 hours
at 37°C to allow Vero cells to settle down and then the cells
were overlaid with agar-containing medium. Seven days later
cells were stained to reveal plaques.

For induction studies, VRJ cell monolayers were treated
with 199 medium containing 0.5 µg/ml of AD for 3 hours. After
that they were thoroughly washed with PBS and overlaid with
agar or with normal Vero cells. Plaques were revealed 7 days
later. No infectivity was found in the supernatants prior to
induction by inoculation into new-born mice. In Table 6 it can be
seen that VRJ cells at passage 72 were spontaneously virogenic,
although the corresponding supernatant failed to kill new-born
mice (Table 2). AD treatment allows the appearance of plaques
in non virogenic cultures except for passage 64, the plaques
were only detected if a monolayer of Vero sensitive cells was
spread over the VRJ cell monolayer.

DISCUSSION

Junin virus produces two types of infection in Vero cells.
The primary infection is a lytic one in which most of the cells
are destroyed with concomitant release of large quantities of

TABLE 6

Recovery of Junin virus from VRJ 3 cells

Cell passage	Days in-vitro	Treatment			
		Agar	Ac.D	Cocultivation	Ac.D+ cocult.
				(PFU/Plate)	
64	226	0	74	0	80
66	234	0	0	N.D.	139
68	240	0	0	0	73
70	248	0	0	0	67
72	255	89	83	110	94

N.D. : not done.

virus. In surviving cells a persistent infection is established
with very little or any infectious virus release. Apparently
this virus would be produced by 3-4 % of the cells showing fluorescent antigen associated to the cell membrane. At the present
time the mechanisms which lead to persistent infection with
Arenaviruses are poorly understood. In our case, interferon is
presumably not the control factor, since VRJ cells can support
the growth of several viruses unrelated to Junin virus. By contrast VRJ cells displayed a state of refractoriness to the replication of exogenous Junin virus, this property of homologous
refractivity is often encountered in persistently infected cells
and is characteristic of the regulated type of persistent infection (11).

With the present evidence it is not possible to explain how
persistent infection is established in Vero cells although our
results permit the interpretation of some facts once the persistently infected line had stabilized.

Induction of infectious virus and surface viral antigen by
either AD or cycloheximide treatment suggests that control of
this persistent infection is a deoxyribonucleic acid dependent
function and that active protein synthesis is necessary to maintain the virus suppressed. The site of block in the synthesis
of infectious virus might be a late maturation step as it has
been demonstrated in persistently infected cultures with Measles
(12, 13) and Mumps (14) viruses.

Our data also show that the infection persists for hundreds
of cell generations with the cells maintaining the potential to
produce infectious virus. This strongly indicates that the viral RNA was copied faithfully and completely in each generation
and its role as messenger for coding viral proteins was also
complete.

REFERENCES

1. Rowe, W.P., Murphy, F.A., Bergold, G.H., Casals, J., Hotchin,
   J., Johnson, K.M., Lehmann Grubbe, F., Mims, C.A., Traub, E.,
   Webb, P.A. (1970). Arenaviruses. Proposed names for a newly
   defined virus group. J. Virol. 5, 651-652, 1970.
2. Sabattini, M.S., Gonzales de Rus, L.E., Diaz, G. and Vega,
   V.R. Natural and experimental infection of rodents with Junin
   virus. Medicina (B. Aires) 37, 53, 149-161, 1977.
3. Martinez Peralta, L., Cossio, P., Sabattini, M.S., Maiztegui,
   J., Arana, R., and Laguens, R.P. Presence of viral particles
   in the salivary gland of calomys musculines infected with
   Junin virus by a natural route. Intervirology (in Press).
4. Coto, C.E.. Junin virus. Prog. Med. Virol. 18, 127-142,
   1974.
5. Boxaca, M. Establecimiento y caracteristicas de una sublinea
   de celulas Vero persistentemente infectadas con virus Junin.
   Medicina (B. Aires) 30 : 50-61, 1970.
6. Coto, C.E.; Damonte, E.B., Help, G.I., Leon, M.E.L. Virological studies of cells chronically infected with Junin virus.
   Medicina (B. Aires) 37, S3, 39, 1977.
7. Help, G.I., Leon, M.E., Coto, C.E. Interference associated
   to cell cultures chronically infected with Junin virus.
   Rev. Soc. Arg. Microbiol. 8, 45-53, 1976.
8. Hotchin, J. The role of transient infection in Arenavirus
   persistence. Prog. Med. Virol. 18, 81-93, 1974.
9. Rawls, W.E., Banerce, S.N., Mc Millan, C.A., Buchmeier, M.J.
   Inhibition of Pichinde virus replication by Actinomycin D.
   J. Gen. Virol. 33, 421-434, 1976.
10. Rutter, G. and Gschwender, H.H. Lymphocytic choriomeningitis
    and other Arenaviruses. Ed. F. Lehmann Grubbe. Springer Ver-
    lag. Berlin pag. 51-59, 1973.
11. Walker, D.L. The viral carrier state in animal cell culture.
    pag. 111-148. In J.L. Melnick (ed) Prog. Med. Virol. vol. 6.
    Karger, Basel.
12. Menna, J.H., Collins, A.R., Flanagan, T. Characterization of
    an in vitro persistent state measles virus infection. Esta-
    blishment and virological characterization of the BGM/MV cell
    line. Infect. Immun. 11, 152-158, 1975.
13. Flanagan, T.D. and Menna, J.H. Induction of measles virus
    Hemagglutinin in a persistently infected nonvirogenic line

of cells. (BGM/MV). J. of Virol. 17, 1052-1055, 1976.
14. Northrop, R.L. Effect of Puromycin and Actinomycin D on a
persistent Mumps virus infection in vitro. J. Virol. 4,
133-140, 1969.

ANTIBODY TO OLIGODENDROGLIA

O. Abramsky[*], D.H. Silberberg, R.P. Lisak, T. Saida
and D. Pleasure

Department of Neurology, University of Pennsylvania,
School of Medicine, Philadelphia, PA, U.S.A.
[*] Department of Neurology, Hebrew University-Hadassah
Medical School, Jerusalem, Israel

Oligodendrocytes, the myelin forming cells of the central
nervous system, were isolated from bovine white matter by trypsinization and sucrose gradient centrifugation, according to the
method of Poduslo and Norton (1). The isolated cells were characterized biochemically by their composition and specific activity
of several enzymes (2), and morphologically by transmission and
scanning electron microscopy (3). Antibodies to oligodendroglia
were induced in rabbits and guinea pigs by injections of isolated
cells in complete Freund's adjuvant, and were demonstrated by
both indirect immunofluorescent technique and in vitro cytotoxic
test (4-6).

Indirect immunofluorescence studies, using fluoresceinated
goat antirabbit or anti-guinea pig immunoglobulin, showed that
rabbit and guinea pig anti-oligodendrocyte sera reacted specifically with the surface of isolated oligodendrocytes in suspension.
The antisera reacted with oligodendroglia in brain sections of
various species, central nervous system tissue cultures and
dissociated cerebellar cells cultures, as well. Other cells,
such as neurons, astrocytes, fibroblasts, neuroblasts, and hepato-
cytes were not demonstrated by this technique. The antisera to
oligodendroglia reacted with oligodendrocytes in suspension,
cultures and sections even after preincubation with purified
myelin, neuroblastoma, grey matter, myelin basic protein, galactocerebroside and non-brain tissue, but not after absorption
with oligodendrocyte fraction or whole white matter. Since anti-
oligodendroglia sera bind only to oligodendroglia and absorptions
with myelin and other brain constituents do not change the speci-

417

ficity, it appears that the membrane antigens responsible for the
immune response do not exist or are hidden in myelin and other
brain cells, and are specific or prominent in oligodendroglia.

Low levels of anti-basic protein antibodies were found by
radioimmunoassay in anti-oligodendroglia sera, and few sera showed
significant anti-galactocerebroside antibody titer by agglutination and radioimmunoprecipitation techniques.

Antisera raised in rabbits against whole white matter,
myelin basic protein or galactocerebroside bound to bovine
oligodendroglia in suspension culture as demonstrated by indirect
immunofluorescence. Absorption of anti-basic protein sera by
either basic protein or whole white matter removed this binding
to oligodendroglia. Absorption of anti-galactocerebroside sera
with galactocerebroside, oligodendroglia or purified myelin
reduced the anti-galactocerebroside titer as well as the binding
to oligodendroglia (7, 8).

Anti-oligodendrocyte serum destroyed oligodendroglia and produced both demyelination and myelination inhibition in mouse
cerebellum cultures. These gliomyelinotoxic effects occurred
several hours after application of antiserum, and were complement
dependent. Axons remained intact. Antiserum to galactocerebroside,
but not antiserum to basic protein, also produced in vitro
demyelination. The myelinotoxic and gliotoxic activities of anti-
oligodendrocyte serum could be removed by prior incubation of
serum with isolated oligodendrocytes, but were only partially
decreased by absorption with purified myelin and not affected by
non-brain tissue. Myelinated mouse dorsal root ganglia cultures
were not affected by the application of anti-oligodendrocyte serum.
These findings suggest that antibodies to more than one brain
antigen can react with oligodendroglia and produce demyelination.

Antibodies to oligodendroglia were demonstrated by indirect
immunofluorescence in the serum of more than 90% of patients with
multiple sclerosis (9, 10). 29% control sera, including sera from
SSPE patients, showed similar response. The antibodies were
absorbed by preincubation of serum with oligodendrocytes or whole
white matter, but not with purified myelin or non-brain tissue,
and the immunofluorescence was blocked in some cases by rabbit
anti-oligodendrocyte serum. These findings suggest that anti-myelin
antibodies are distinct from anti-oligodendroglia antibodies, and
that demyelination could be a result of immunopathologic reaction
directed against oligodendroglia.

REFERENCES

1. Poduslo, S.E., Norton, W.T. : Isolation and some chemical properties of oligodendroglia from calf brain. J. Neurochem. 19 : 727, 1972.
2. Pleasure, D., Abramsky, O., Silberberg, D., Quinn, B., Parris, J., Saida, T. : Lipid synthesis by an oligodendroglial fraction in suspension culture. Brain Res. 134 : 377, 1977.
3. Silberberg, D.H., Sanders, C., Abramsky, O., Saida, T.: Scanning electron microscope observations of isolated oligodendrocytes. J. Neuropathol. Exp. Neurol. 36 : 630, 1977.
4. Abramsky, O., Saida, T., Lisak, R.P., Pleasure, D., Silberberg, D.H. : Immunological studies with isolated oligodendrocytes. Neurology 27 : 342, 1977.
5. Abramsky, O., Lisak, R.P., Pleasure, D., Gilden, D.H., Silberberg, D.H.: Immunologic characterization of oligodendroglia. Neurosci. Lett. 8 : 311, 1978.
6. Saida, T., Abramsky, O., Silberberg, D.H., Pleasure, D., Lisak, R.P., Manning, M. : Anti-oligodendrocyte serum demyelinates cultured CNS tissue. Soc. Neurosci. Abst. 7 : 527, 1977.
7. Lisak, R.P., Abramsky, O., Saida, T., Pleasure, D., Silberberg, D.H. : Immunological studies of antibodies to oligodendroglia and galactocerebroside. Neurology 28 : 392, 1978.
8. Lisak, R.P., Abramsky, O., Dorfman, S., George, J., Manning, M., Pleasure, D.E., Saida, T., Silberberg, D.H. : Antibodies to galactocerebroside bind to oligodendroglia in suspension culture. J. Neurol. Sci. in press.
9. Abramsky, O., Lisak, R.P., Silberberg, D.H., Pleasure, D. : Antibodies to oligodendroglia in multiple sclerosis. Trans. Amer. Neurol. Assoc. 102 : 15, 1977.
10. Abramsky, O., Lisak, R.P., Silberberg, D.H., Pleasure, D.: Anti-oligodendroglia antibodies in patients with multiple sclerosis. New Engl. J. Med. 297 : 1207, 1977.

BRAIN SPECIFIC PROTEINS IN CEREBROSPINAL FLUID

E.R. Einstein

Institute of Human Development/Department of Physiology
University of California, Berkeley, CA, U.S.A.

Although this workshop is dedicated to "Humoral Immunity in Neurological Disease," the discussion of proteins which have their origin either in brain or in both brain and plasma should be described here briefly. The inclusion is justified on the basis that these are potential antigens which may provoke circulating antibodies.

One may assume that the brain specific proteins have some particular (although not yet defined) function in the nervous system. Their presence and possible increase may be characteristic of a particular neurological disease and therefore useful in diagnosis.

Since earlier reports on specific brain proteins of the CNS (1, 2, 3), several other proteins have been assembled in two recent reviews (4, 6). Some of these brain specific proteins have been demonstrated in the cerebrospinal fluid.

For brevity CNS proteins found in the fluid are presented here in table form. The number of references on each CNS protein is rather extensive; therefore, in this short report we limited it to 1-3 references. One reference relates to the protein in the CNS and its properties, the other to its presence in the cerebrospinal fluid. More detailed description and references will appear in Proteins of the Brain and Cerebrospinal Fluid in Health and Disease, by Elizabeth Roboz Einstein (5), with comments by A. Lowenthal and D. Karcher on the usefulness of the techniques in diagnosis of neurological diseases.

TABLE 1

PROTEINS OF THE CSF ORIGINATING IN THE NERVOUS TISSUE

Name of Compound	Origin (Localization)	Author(s)	Reference
Alpha-albumin	normal & patho-logical brain tissue	Karcher D., Zeman W., Lowenthal A., Chamoles N.	Brain Res. 17 : 207, 1970
" "	(demonstrated with IRMA) in CSF	Gheuens J., Lowenthal A., Karcher D., Noppe M.	in Franck et al. (Eds.) Dynamic Properties of Glial Cells. Per-gamon Press (in press, 1978).
glial fibril-lary acidic protein	astrocytes en-riched in MS	Eng L., Lee Y-L., Miles L.E.M.	Anal. Biochem. 71 : 243, 1976.
"	"	Bignami A., Eng L., Dahl D., Uyeda C.T.	Brain Res. 43 : 429, 1972;
"	in CSF of MS	Eng L., Lee Y-L;., Miles L.E.M.	Int. Soc. Neuro-chem. 1975 abstr. 225.

Alpha-albumin and glial fibrillary acidic protein : complete anti-genic identity, biochemical characteristics are close.

S-100	in glial cyto-toplasm, astro-cytes and oli-godendrocytes	Moore B.W.	Res. Commun. 19 : 739, 1965
"	in CSF	Murazio M., Massaro A., Michetti F.	Proc. Int. Soc. Neurochem. 6 : 324, 1977.

TABLE 2

PROTEINS OF THE CSF ORIGINATING IN THE NERVOUS TISSUE

Name of Compound	Origin Localization	Author(s)	Reference
alpha$_2$-glyco-protein	glial cell	Warecka K., Möller H.J. Vogel M.M. Tripatzis I.	J. Neurochem. 19 : 719, 1972
" "	glial cell and CSF	Leonhardt K., Renschler H. Warecka K.	Munch. Med. Wschr. 117 1113, 1975.
14-3-2 pro-tein	neuronal enolase activity	Bock E. and Dissing J.	Scand. J. Immun. 4 : 31, 1975.
14-3-2 pro-tein	neuronal in CSF ?	Marangos P.J., Zomzely-Neu-rath C. Luk D.C. York C.	J. Biol. Chem. 250 : 1884, 1975
2'3'-cyclic nucleotide phosphohydro-lase	myelin	Kurihara T. and Tsudaka Y.	J. Neurochem. 14 : 1167, 1967
" "	in CSF of pa-tients with de-myelinating di-seases	Sprinkle T.J. and McKhann G.M.	Neurocsi. Letts 7 : 203, 1978
" "	" "	Banik N.L., Mauldin L.B. Hogan E.L.	Brain Res./ in press, 1978
Basic myelin protein	white matter	Einstein E.R. Robertson D.M. Dicaprio J.M. and Moore W.	J. Neurochem. 9 : 353, 1962
amino acid se-quence	"	Eylar E.H.	Nat. Acad. Sci. 67 : 1425, 1970
Basic myelin protein	in CSF	Cohen S.R., Brune M.H. Herndon R.M. and McKhann G. M.	in Myelination and Demyelina-tion ed. Palo p. 513, 1978 Plenum Press
Basic myelin fragment	in CSF	Whitaker J.N.	Neurology 27, 911, 1977

We have some searching questions. Is the reason for the small number of non-plasma proteins found in the fluid, that monospecific serum to the particular purified CNS protein has not been made available for preparing antibodies ? Consequently no survey has been conducted. Or is there actually only a limited number of proteins present in the fluid ? Is their appearance in the fluid due to cell destruction, blood-brain-CSF changes, or more closely related to the disease process as are the basic myelin protein, its degradation product and 2'3' cyclic nucleotide phosphohydrolase to multiple sclerosis ? According to Sprinkle and McKhann (7), the increase of this enzyme does not parallel that of the myelin basic protein in the CSF. Is it possible that the release of this enzyme from the myelin signifies a different stage of the disease ?

We have many questions which await an answer. But one could expect that with the use of monospecific antisera to purified brain proteins and application of sensitive immunoradiometric and other assays, the number of brain specific proteins in the CSF will increase greatly in the near future.

REFERENCES

1. Shooter, E.N. and Einstein, E.R. : Proteins of the Nervous System. Annu. Rev. Biochem. 40 : 635, 1972.
2. Rauch, H.C. and Einstein,E.R. : Specific brain proteins. A biochemical and immunological review. In : Ehrenpreis and Kapin (Eds.) Review of Neuroscience, Vol. 1, 1974, p. 283.
3. Carnegie, P.R. and Dunkley, P.R. : Basic proteins of central and peripheral nervous system myelin. In : Agranoff and Aprison (Eds.) Advances in Neurochemistry, N.Y. Plenum Press, Vol. 1, p. 96, 1975.
4. Zomzely-Neurath, C. and Keller, A. : Nervous system specific proteins of vertebrates. A search for functions and physiological roles. Neurochemical Research 2 : 253, 1977.
5. Einstein, E.R. : Proteins of the Brain and Cerebrospinal Fluid in Health and Disease (in preparation).
6. Bock, E. : Nervous system specific proteins. J. Neurochem. 30 : 7, 1978.
7. Sprinkle, T.J. and McKhann, G.M. : Activity of 2'3'-cyclic nucleotide 3'-phosphodiesterase in cerebrospinal fluid of patients with demyelinating disorders. Neuroscience Letters 7 : 203-206, 1978.

LOSS OF A BRAIN-SPECIFIC ANTIGEN (ALPHA$_2$-GLYCOPROTEIN) IN HUMAN GLIAL TUMORS

K. Warecka

Neurological Department, Medical High School Lübeck, Lübeck, F.R.Germany

SUMMARY

137 human brain tumors obtained from operation table have been investigated for their brain-specific antigen content (alpha$_2$-glycoprotein) by means of the rocket immunoelectrophoresis and other immunological techniques. Against one third of the tumors antisera have been made. The antigen has not been showed in malignant glial tumors i.e. in glioblastoma multiform . In all benign glial tumors as in astrocytomas the protein is present, however, in various concentrations, but always in a lower quantity as in normal brain tissue. This partial depletion of the antigen in astrocytomas could be demonstrated immunoelectrophoretically.

Already about 20 years ago the loss or partial depletion of tissue specific antigens has been described by many investigators (16, 17, 18, 6, 7, 8, 9) as well as recently by Warecka (15) and Jacque et al. (3).

This paper is a continuation of our previous work published 1975 (15) showing that in the malignant human brain glial tumors i.e. glioblastoma multiform , the brain-specific antigen namely alpha$_2$-glycoprotein is absent. Contrary in astrocytoma, a tumor of morphologically normal astrocytes, a partial depletion of this antigen could be shown.

425

MATERIALS AND METHODS

137 biopsies or larger specimens of human tumors were obtained in the course of operation and split in two pieces. One portion was immediately frozen for the assay, the second one was used for histology. Their histological diagnoses are shown in Table 1.

Aqueous extracts of 37 tumors were prepared and injected into one rabbit each; antisera against each individual tumor were obtained. Each tumor extract was tested with its own antiserum and with antiserum against alpha$_2$-glycoprotein. Each anti-tumor serum was tested with alpha$_2$- glycoprotein.

100 tumors were examined quantitatively by rocket immuno-electrophoresis of Laurell (1966).

Table 1 : 137 investigated brain tumors [x]

TUMOR	NUMBER OF INVESTIGATED CASES
astrocytoma	12
glioblastoma multiforme	28
oligodendroglioma	5
spongioblastoma	5
medulloblastoma	6
medulloblastoma + brain tissue	1
ependymoma	5
acoustic neuroma	16
meningioma	40
chromophobe adenoma of the hypophysis	4
hemangiopericytoma	1
lymphadenoma + brain tissue	1
metastasis of adenocarcinoma	5
metastasis of melanoma	1
mixed tumors (astrocytes, glioblasts and oligodendrocytes)	2
not classified	5

[x] 37 brain tumors have been investigated by Ouchterlony immunodiffusion. From all of these tumors antiserum was prepared by inoculation of rabbits.
    100 tumors have been investigated by quantitative immunoelectrophoresis (see below).

From 5 normal human brains of patients without any neurological diseases and without any macroscopic changes 10 various areas were cut out and corresponding areas were pooled (see also table III).

Alpha$_2$-glycoprotein was prepared from normal human adult brain by affinity chromatography as preciously described (Warecka et al. 14); antiserum against this antigen was developed in rabbits. The preparation of the antigens, the inoculation of the rabbits, Ouchterlony immunodiffusion, and immunoelectrophoresis were performed as previously described (11).

The purity of the alpha$_2$glycoprotein was tested by Ouchterlony immunodiffusion as well as by Laurell's electroimmunoassay with human antiserum and with anti-transferrin, anti-albumin and anti-gammaglobulinserum.

The purity of the anti-alpha$_2$-glycoprotein serum was tested by both above mentioned methods with albumin, transferrin, gammaglobulin and human serum.

RESULTS

Table II is a short summary of the results of our previous work.

The main publications are cited under the following numbers at the end of the paper (1, 2, 5, 10-15).

Table III shows that the white matter of the brain hemispheres reveals the highest quantities of the alpha$_2$-glycoprotein. In the white matter of the cerebellum the content of the alpha$_2$-glycoprotein is remarkably lower, but the quantities of the alpha$_2$-glycoprotein in the white matter of the cerebellum are still higher than in the chiasma opticum and in the cortex of the brain hemispheres. The lowest quantities of alpha$_2$-glycoprotein were obtained in the substantia nigra.

Table IV shows the quantities of the alpha$_2$-glycoprotein in brain tumors. Two of the tumors (24 and 28) were not classifiable histologically. Tumor 6 (lymphadenoma) and tumor 23 (medulloblastoma) were contaminated with brain tissue, therefore these data are not representative for the tumors. Six of the investigated medulloblastomas do not contain alpha$_2$-glycoprotein (see table I). One medulloblastoma was contaminated with brain tissue. Among the 40 meningiomas the alpha$_2$-glycoprotein was present only in four tumors (see also table I). We do not have any explanation for that. Also glioblastoma multiform 4 contains some quantities of alpha$_2$-glycoprotein. In all of the

Table II : Biochemical and biological properties of the brain
specific alpha$_2$-glycoprotein.

It is soluble in aqueous buffers
It is an acidic glycoprotein
It gives upon SDS - polyacrylamide gel electrophoresis one
prominent periodic acid-Schiff staining band at apparent
M_W 45 000

It contains carbohydrate residues in molar ratio :

glucosamine	6.3	galactosamine	0.8
mannose	1.5	NANA	0.7
glucose	1.4	fucose	0.5
galactose	1.0		

It binds to *Concanavalin A*

SPECIFITY	IMMUNOLOGICALLY SPECIFIC FOR THE WHITE SUBSTANCE OF HUMAN BRAIN
PRESENCE IN :	
a) NORMAL TISSUE	IN BRAIN HEMISPHERES, IN SPINAL CORD, IN N OPTICUS, NOT FOUND IN PERIPHERAL NERVOUS SYSTEM
b) NORMAL CELLS	IN THE GLIA TISSUE , NOT FOUND IN NEURONS
c) TUMORS	FOUND IN ASTROCYTOMA, NOT PRESENT IN GLIOBLASTOMA MULTIFORME
PHYLOGENESIS	COMPLETE OR ALMOST COMPLETE IDENTITY WITH AN EQUI-VALENT PROTEIN OF MACACA MULATTA, SEMIIDENTICAL WITH A BRAIN-SPECIFIC PROTEIN OF RAT AND NO IDENTITY WITH MOUSE BRAIN-SPECIFIC PROTEIN
ONTOGENESIS	APPEARANCE ON 16[h] WEEK OF FETAL LIFE, ON THE TIME OF MYELINATIONGLIA-STAGE

other 27 investigated glioblastomas alpha$_2$-glycoprotein was
absent (see table I). The acousticus neurinoma II contains traces of alpha$_2$-glycoprotein, in contrast, to that in all other of
the 15 acousticus neurinomas where no alpha$_2$glycoprotein was
found. In ependymoma 30 alpha$_2$-glycoprotein was present in
other four investigated ependymomas alpha$_2$-glycoprotein was
absent.

Table V represents the tumors which do not show any reaction to the anti-alpha$_2$-glycoprotein serum. All of the investigated astrocytomas with both immunological methods i.e. by
Ouchterlony immunodiffusion and by quantitative immunoelectrophoresis revealed alpha$_2$-glycoprotein, however, in various quan-

Table III:Presence of alpha$_2$-glycoprotein in various areas of
the brain investigated by quantitative immunoelectrophoresis.

Brain areas [*]	x̄ Rocket height (cm)[**]	α$_2$-Glycoprotein (g/l)	Total protein (g/l)	$\frac{\alpha_2\text{-Glycoprotein}}{\text{Total protein}} \cdot 10^3$
Corpus callo sum	1.97	1.84	61.0	30.16
Capsula interna	2.20	2.08	78.0	26.67
Hemispheres of cerebellum	1.25	1.04	95.0	10.95
Chiasma opticum	1.78	0.41	53.0	7.74
Cortex (pooled from many brain areas)	2.30	0.55	72.0	7.64
Substantia nigra (pedunculi cerebri)	1.38	0.29	98.0	2.96
White substance:				
frontal lobe	3.20	3.20	59.0	54.24
occipital -"-	2.31	2.22	62.0	35.81
temporal -"-	2.61	2.60	87.0	29.89
parietal -"-	3.33	3.36	128.0	26.25

[*] Brain tissue was taken from normal brains and corresponding areas were pooled
[**] Mean value from samples applied in duplicate

tities. The amount of alpha$_2$-glycoprotein in each astrocytoma
was varying, but in general always smaller than the smallest
amount of alpha$_2$-glycoprotein, of all investigated brain areas
of normal brain tissue even smaller than in the substantia nigra,
which normally reveals the smallest quantity (compare table III
with table IV). The comparison of both quotients : the one
alpha$_2$-glycoprotein in astrocytoma (alpha$_2$-GP$_A$) to the total
protein in astrocytoma (TP$_A$) to alpha$_2$-glucoprotein in white
matter of brain (alpha$_2$GP$_{WM}$) to total protein in white matter
of brain TP$_{WM}$)

$$\frac{\text{alpha}_2\text{GP}_A}{\text{TP}_A} \quad : \quad \frac{\text{alpha}_2\text{GP}_{WM}}{\text{TP}_{WM}}$$

Table IV : tumors with presence of alpha$_2$-glycoprotein investigated by quantitative immunoelectrophoreses.

Tumors		$\bar{x}$ Rocket height (cm)	α_x Glycoprotein (g/l)	Total protein (g/l)	$\dfrac{\alpha_x \text{Glycoprotein}}{\text{Total protein}} \cdot 10^3$
Astrocytoma	No.34	0.69	0.10	10.4	9.62
-"-	No.56	0.80	0.13	17.2	7.60
-"-	No.35	0.64	0.09	34.6	2.60
Ependymoma	No.30	1.75	0.40	37.4	10.70
Medulloblastoma + brain tissue	No.23	1.55	0.34	45.0	7.56
Glioblastoma	No. 4	0.74	0.12	65.8	1.82
Acoustic neuroma	No. 11	0.26	trace	7.0	-
Meningioma	No.31	1.48	0.32	100.2	3.19
-"-	No.27	0.85	0.15	78.8	1.90
-"-	No.26	1.10	0.22	249.2	0.88
-"-	No.22	1.02	0.19	233.6	0.81
Lymphadenoma + brain tissue	No. 6	0.51	0.05	40.2	1.24
Not classifiable No.28		1.38	0.29	20.8	13.94
Not classifiable No.24		0.94	0.17	9.0	0.19

showed much higher quantities of alpha$_2$-glycoprotein in the white matter of the brain. Summarizing these data, it is to say that the white matter of the brain hemispheres contains the largest quantities of alpha$_2$-glycoprotein. In astrocytomas and mixed tumors containing mature astrocytes the quantities of alpha$_2$-glycoprotein are varying. The quantities are always lower than in the normal brain tissue. Fig. 1 and 2 show the results of our experiments with quantitative immunoelectrophoresis. Fig. 3 shows the morphological changes of alpha$_2$-glycoprotein precipitation line in astrocytoma.

Summarizing the data obtained with our experiments is to say :
firstly : in every glial tumor containing mature astrocytes the antigenic alpha$_2$-glycoprotein is present.

Table V : Tumor with the absence of alpha$_2$-glycoprotein, number of investigated cases.

Tumor with the absence of alpha$_2$- glycoprotein	number of investigated cases
glioblastoma multiforme	27
oligodendroglioma	5
spongioblastoma	5
medulloblastoma	6
ependymoma	4
acoustic neuroma	15
meningioma	36
chromophobe adenoma of the hypophysis	4
hemangiopericytoma	1
metastasis of adenocarcinoma	5
metastasis of melanoma	1
not classified	3

In this tumors the alpha$_2$-glycoprotein has not been found by either of the two applied methods i.e. by Ouchterlony immunodiffusion and by quantitative immunoelectrophoresis of Laurell.

secondly : the amount of alpha$_2$- glycoprotein is varying in indi-
          vidual astrocytomas, but it is almost always lower as
          in the normal areas of the brain.
thirdly : a partial depletion of this antigen could be shown im-
          munoelectrophoretically in astrocytoma cells (see fig.3)
fourthly : the biochemical changes in tumors anticipate the struc-
          tural changes (see discussion).
in the fifth place : this antigen (alpha$_2$-glycoprotein) is lost
          in malignant glial tumors i.e. in glioblas-
          toma multiform .

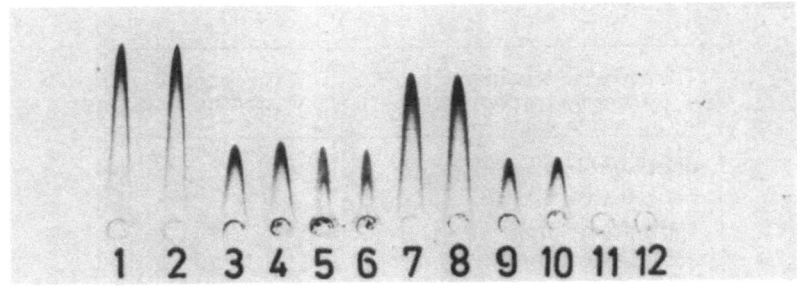

Fig. 1 : quantitative immunoelectrophoreses : the gel plate contains 15 ml of 1 % agarose with 400 µl of monospecific anti-alpha$_2$-glycoprotein serum.
1 + 2 - 0,36g/l alpha$_2$-glycoprotein + 0.13 tris-veronal buffer
          v/v
3 + 4 - astrocytoma 56; 0.13 g/l alpha$_2$-glycoprotein
5 + 6 - astrocytoma 34; 0.10 g/l   - " -
7 + 8 - substantia nigra; 0.29 g/l   - " -
9 + 10 - astrocytoma 35; 0.09 g/l   - " -

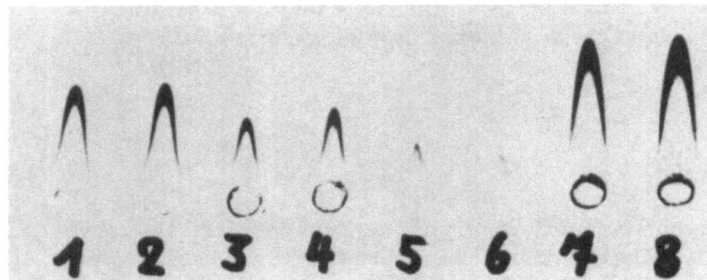

Fig. 2 :
1 + 2 cerebellum; 1.04 g/l alpha$_2$-glycoprotein 1:3 diluted
3 + 4 astrocytoma 35; 0.09 g/l alpha$_2$-glycoprotein
5 + 6 acousticus neurinoma : traces of alpha$_2$-glycoprotein
7 + 8 corpus callosum : 1.84 g/l alpha$_2$-glycoprotein 1:3 diluted

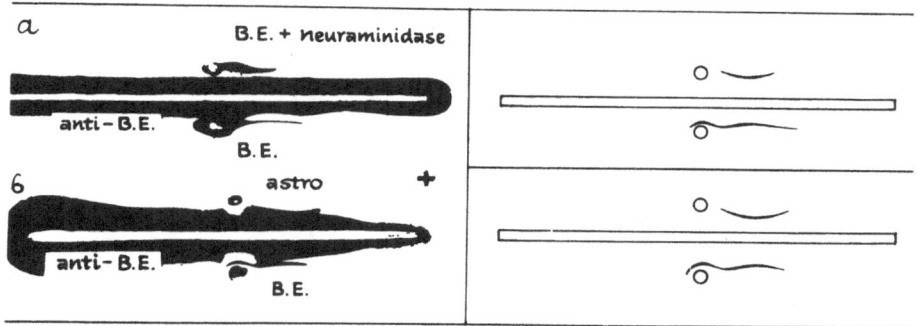

Fig. 3 : immunoelectrophoretic pattern of water extracts of white
matter of brain (B.E.) whithout neuraminidase treatment (a and b :
lower hole), after treatment with neuraminidase (a : upper hole)
and with water extract of astrocytoma (astro) developed with
antibrain serum (anti-B.E.) after absorption with human liver
and human serum (a and b : middle grove). Notice the difference
between the shape of the neuraminidase-treated and untreated preparation (a) and the lack of the semicircle in the antigens (a
and b : upper hole) of the white matter after treatment with
neuraminidase (a) and in astrocytoma (b).

DISCUSSION

Our data show evidently that the brain specific-$alpha_2$-gly-
coprotein is present in all tumors containing mature astrocytes.
The quantities of the antigenic $alpha_2$-glycoprotein are different
in these tumors, probably depending on the biochemical resp. metabolic process going on at least parallel to the malignant transformation of the cell or above this perhaps provoking the dedif-
ferentiation of the cells. The available evidence would merely
suggest that if important proteins are lost, these losses must
occur concomitantly with a metabolic effect, which provides a
cell division. The cell division might be enhanced in several
ways by the loss of appropriate catabolic enzymes.

Furthermore the data could also indicate that the biochemical process anticipates the morphological process : although the
quantities of $alpha_2$-glycoprotein in each particular tumor are
different, the histological picture is still uniform, showing
the presence of mature astrocytes. Moreover, the process of
malignant transformation could be demonstrated immunologically
on the basis of the immunoelectrophoretical picture, which showed
a loss of a part of the precipitation line in the astrocytoma

if compared with the conventional precipitation line corresponding
to the alpha$_2$-glycoprotein. Such destruction of the precipitation line of the alpha$_2$-glycoprotein could be reproduced experimentally by incubating the white matter of the brain with neuraminidase (see fig. 3). So, it could be said that the malignant
transformation from astrocytoma to glioblastoma multiform starts
with destruction of the glycoprotein by loosing NANA.

With other words in astrocytomas a partial depletion of the
antigen is visible (see also quantitative data on Table IV).
Which enzymatic processes are exactly going on could not be answered. The evolutionary process does not end with the formation
of cancer cells, but continues : cancer of low malignancy evolve
into cancer of increasing malignancy. The antigenic alpha$_2$-glyco-
protein is lost in malignant glial tumors i.e. in glioblastoma
multiform. The evidences of the malignant transformation of
astrocytoma to glioblastoma multiform are taken daily from the
catamnesis and observation of neurological patients with brain
tumors.

The loss of specific antigen is one of the attributes of
malignancy. In all probability this is a secondary phenomenon,
but not the primary cause of carcinogenesis. How far these
data could contribute to the immunological theory of formation
of neoplasia it is too early to decide.

ACKNOWLEDGEMENT

I like to express my thanks to Prof. Dr. med. R. Kautzky
and Prof. Dr. med. H. Müller, Neurosurgery Dept. University Hamburg, Federal German Republic for providing me with the tumors
and for the histological diagnoses respectively.

REFERENCES

1. Brunngraber, E.G., J.P. Susz and K. Warecka Electrophoretic
   analysis of human brain-specific proteins obtained by affinity chromatography. J. Neurochem. 22: 181-182, 1974.
2. Brunngraber, E.G., J.P. Susz, J. Javaid, A.Aro and K. Warecka
   Binding of Concanavalin A to the brain-specific proteins obtained from human white matter by affinity chromatography.
   J. Neurochem. 24 : 805-806, 1975.
3. Jacque, C.M., C. Vinner, M. Kujas, M. Raoul, J. Racadot and
   N.A. Baumann, Determination of glial fibrillary acidic protein (GFAP) in human brain tumors. J. Neurol. Sci. 35:
   147-155, 1978.
4. Laurell, C.B. Quantitative estimation of proteins by electrophoresis in agarose gel containing antibodies. Anal. Biochem.

15 : 45-52, 1966.
5. Lange, U. Gehirnspezifische Proteine in normalen und mutanten Mäusen : "Jimpy". Immunologische Vergleichsuntersuchungen mit "Quaking" und anderen Mammalia. M.D. Thesis, Medical High School Lübeck, West Germany.
6. Nairn, R.C., H.G. Richmond, M.G. McEntegart and J.E. Fothergill Immunological differences between normal and malignant cells. Brit. Med. J. II, 1335-1340, 1960.
7. Nairn, R.C., M.G. McEntegart, J.E. Fothergill and I.B. Porteous Specific antibody against gastrointestinal mucosa. Lancet II, p. 109, 1961.
8. Nairn, R.C., J.E. Fothergill, M.G. McEntegard and H.G. Richmond Loss of gastro-intestinal-specific antigen in neoplasia. Brit. Med. J. I, 1791-1793, 1962.
9. Nairn, R.C., J.E. Fothergill and M.G. McEntegard and I.B. Porteous Gastro-intestinal-specific antigen : an immunological and serological study. Brit. Med. J. I, 1788-1790, 1962.
10. Vogel, H.M. Die Lokalisation des gehirnspezifischen alpha$_2$-Glykoproteins in Gehirnzellen. M.D. Thesis, Medical High School Lübeck, West Germany.
11. Warecka, K. and H. Bauer Studies on "brain-specific proteins in aqueous extracts of brain tissue. J. Neurochem 14 : 783-787, 1967.
12. Warecka, K. Immunochemical studies on a water-soluble-brain specific glycoprotein from human and rat brain. Life Sci. 6 : 1999-2002, 1967.
13. Warecka, K. and D. Müller The appearance of human "brain-specific" glycoprotein in ontogenesis. J. Neurol. Sci. 8, 329-345, 1969.
14. Warecka, K., H.J. Möller, H.M. Vogel and I. Tripatzis Human brain specific alpha$_2$-glycoprotein-purification by affinity chromatography and detection of a new component; localization in nervous cells. J. Neurochem. 19 : 719-725, 1972.
15. Warecka, K. Immunological differential diagnosis of human brain tumors. J. Neurol. Sci. 26 : 511-516, 1975.
16. Weiler, E. Die Änderung der serologischen Organspezifität beim Buttergelb-Tumor der Ratte im Vergleich zu normaler Leber. Z. Naturforsch. 7b : 324-326, 1952.
17. Weiler, E. Antigenic differences between normal hamster kidney and stilbestrol induced carcinoma : complement fixation reactions with cytoplasmic particles. Brit. J. Cancer 10 : 533-560, 1956.
18. Weiler, E. Die Änderung der serologischen Spezifität von Leberzellen der Ratte während der Cancerogenese durch p-Dimethyl-aminoazobenzol. Z. Naturforsch. 11b : 31-38, 1956.

NEUROBLASTOMA CYTOSKELETON SHOWN BY IMMUNOFLUORESCENCE

J. Sotelo, B.H. Toh, A. Yildiz and E.J. Holborow

The London Hospital Medical College, London, U.K.

Since the initial work of Loewy (1952) on the biochemical basis of cytoplasmic movement (13), knowledge in this field has increased. We are beginning to understand many of the processes related to cell movement such as cytoplasmic streaming, phagocytosis, cell locomotion, membrane function, cell division, internal transport, and internal structural support (3, 14, 16). At least three different types of fibrillar proteins make up the cellular skeleton : microfilaments, microtubules and intermediate filaments.

INTRACELLULAR FIBRILS

Filament :	Protein :	Diameter
Microfilaments	Actin and myosin	6 nm
Microtubules	Tubulin	10 nm
Intermediate filaments	Skeletin	22 nm

The biochemical isolation of intracellular actin, myosin, tubulin, and skeletin (4, 6, 7, 14) made it possible to produce specific antibodies in rabbits against any of the cytoskeleton proteins (11). Besides some human sera obtained from certain viral,autoimmune and malignant diseases have shown antibodies reactive by immunofluorescence with the intracellular system of skeletal proteins (5, 8, 9, 18, 19) presumably as a result of cellular changes associated with the disorders referred to. The above facts permit the study of the cell cytoskeleton by immunological methods.

Within the nervous system the cytoplasmic fibrillar proteins seem to be associated with synaptic transmission, axoplasmic flow, cell shape, cell development and growth. We examined monolayer cultures of neuroblastoma cells for immunofluorescence reactivity with specific sera containing antibodies directed against different cytoskeletal proteins, looking for their topographic location in the neural cell. Our results showed an elaborate morphology of neurofilaments (intermediate filaments) in the cell body, distributed around the nucleus and extending into the cell processes and as fine linear filaments present throughout the axon. Actin and myosin-like microfilaments were located mainly in the axon growth cone and in microspikes. When neuroblastoma cells were reacted with both human antiintermediate filament antisera and rabbit antiactin or antimyosin antisera, in double fluorochrome studies using rhodamine-fluorescein conjugates, the organization and topographic location of neurofilaments in the cells were found to be different from those of actin and myosin.

The above findings support the concept that actin and myosin microfilaments are related to motility in the growth cone and their presence in the synaptic region could indicate that the contractile proteins system may be involved in the synaptic transmission (1, 12, 20). It is possible that before the onset of axon development the cell makes its filament structure which subsequently migrates from the perinuclear region to the periphery, unwinds, and forms the axon skeleton. This suggestion is supported by the observation that the assembly of cytoskeleton proteins is closely related to neurite extension (10) and that drugs which disrupt microtubules or microfilaments inhibit morphological differentiation of neuroblastoma cells.

Intermediate filaments form a flexible and resistant internal skeleton for the axon (16), this observation sustains the theory that they may be related to enzymatic and chemical axoplasmic transport, which is a major activity of these specialized cell section.

The strong similarities between neurofilament and glial fibrillary protein isolated from multiple sclerosis plaques (2) and the demonstration of neurofilament bundles in nerve cells in disorders such as Wallerian degeneration, Pick's and Alzheimer's diseases, amyotrophic lateral sclerosis and brain tumors (10, 15, 17, 18, 19) suggest that these diseases may be closely related to pathological changes in neurofilament organization.

The physiology and immunopathology of proteins which constitute the cytoskeleton in neural cells raise many questions in the neurosciences and provide an exciting area for research.

REFERENCES

1. Berl, S., Puszkin, S. and Nicklas, W.J. : Actomyosin-like protein in the brain. Science 179 : 441 (1973).
2. Bignami, A., Eng, L.F., Dahl, D. and Jyeda, C.T. : Localization of the glial fibrillary acidic protein in astrocytes by immunofluorescence. Brain Res. 43 : 429 (1972).
3. Buchler, A.G. : Kinetics of cell movement. Sci. Amer. 238 : 68 (1978).
4. Burns, R. : Ciliar dyenins. Nature 269 : 559 (1977).
5. Gabbiani, G., Csank, B.J., Schneeberger, J.C., Kapanci, Y.; Trenchev, P. and Holborow, E.J. : Contractile proteins in human cancer cells. Am. J. Pathol. 83 : 457 (1976).
6. Gilbert, D.S. : Axoplasm chemical composition in Myxicola and solubility properties of its structural proteins. J. Physiol. 253 : 303 (1975).
7. Gilbert, D.S. : 10 nm filaments. Nature 269 : 559 (1977).
8. Holborow, E.J.: The immunobiology of contractile proteins in membrane alterations as basis of liver injury. Ed. by Popper H., Bianchi, L., Reutter, W., MTP Press Ltd. Lancaster England (1977).
9. Holborow, E.J. : Smooth muscle autoantibodies, viral infections and malignant disease. Proc. R. Soc. Med. 65 : 481 (1972).
10. Jorgensen, A.O., Subrahmanyan, L., Turnbul, C. and Kalnins V.I. Localization of the neurofilament protein in neuroblastoma cells by immunofluorescent staining. Proc. Nat. Acad. Sci. 73 : 3192 (1976).
11. Lazarides, E. and Burridge, K. : Anti-actin, immunofluorescent localization of a muscle structural protein in nonmuscle cells. Cell 6 : 289 (1975).
12. Littauer, U.Z., Schmitt, H. and Gozes, I. : Properties and synthesis of tubulin in neuroblastoma cells. J. Natl. Cancer Inst. 57 : 647 (1976).
13. Loewy, A.G. : An actomyosin-like substance from the plasmodium of myxomycete. J. Cell Comp. Physiol. 40 : 127 (1952).
14. Polland, T.D. and Weihing, R.R. : Actin and myosin and cell movement. CRC Critical Reviews in Biochemistry, January 1974.
15. Rewcastle, N.B. and Ball, M.J. : Electron microscopic structure of the "inclusion bodies" in Pick's disease. Neurology 18 : 1205 (1968).
16. Staechelin, A. and Hull, B. : Junctions between living cells. Sci. Amer. 238 : 5 May (1978).
17. Terry, R.D. : Neuronal fibrous protein in human pathology. J. Neuropathol. Exp. Neurol. 30 : 8 (1971).
18. Toh, B.H., Muller, H.K. and Elrick, W.L. : Smooth muscle associated antigen in astrocytes and astrocytomata. Br. J. Cancer 33 : 195 (1976).
19. Toh, B.H., Quist, R., Randell, V.B. and Elrick, W.L. : Increased expression of actin-like protein in human and ethylnitrosurea-induced tumors of the nervous system. Cancer Research

37 : 4280 (1977).

20. Toh, B.H., Cragg, B.C., Sing, S.C. and Koh, S.H. : Brain
    actin demonstrated by immunofluorescence. Exp. Neurol. 58 :
    425 (1978).

IN VITRO ASSESSMENT OF THE CELL-MEDIATED IMMUNE RESPONSE TOWARDS HUMAN GLIOMAS

C. Solheid, J. Dumon and M. Titeca

Born-Bunge Foundation, Department of Neuropathology
and Department of Neurogenetics, U.I.A., Wilrijk, Belgium

INTRODUCTION

Cell-mediated immunity (CMI) towards autologous or homologous tumor cells has been shown in many patients with gliomas — (for review see 1). Most reported studies were carried on using the visual microcytotoxicity assay (MCA) (2), involving the co-culture of peripheral blood lymphocytes (PBL) with anchorage-dependent target cells for 2-3 days, followed by the counting of the target cells that have escaped lymphocyte-mediated destruction and thus still adhere to the substrate. The MCA measures several phenomena, both specific and non-specific, involving different lymphoid cell subpopulations (3).

On the other hand, the chromium ^{51} release assay (CRA) (4) performed in a shorter period of time (4-18 hours) measures "direct" lymphocytotoxic events, involving activity of sensitized cytotoxic T-lymphocytes (CTL) participating in the primary immune response to a given antigen and, as demonstrated recently, "natural" or "spontaneous" cytotoxicity mediated by "natural killer" (NK) lymphocytes (5, 6).

In the first part of this study we have examined the value of the CRA, easy to perform and less time-consuming than the MCA, in the assessment of tumor directed CMI in glioma patients, more especially in the demonstration of a primary immune response. Since this response was not demonstrable in each case, and since the assay did not always discriminate between cytotoxicity patterns of PBL from glioma and non-glioma patients, we investigated, in the second part of this study, whether memory T-cells (MTL) could be demonstrated in the former. This was done by reactivating the PBL through a secondary antigenic stimulus in vitro before performing the CRA.

MATERIALS AND METHODS

Tissue Culture Lines

They originated from biopsies obtained at neurosurgical interventions and cultured in medium containing 85 % Hams'F 10 and 15 % foetal calf serum, supplemented by antibiotics and fungizone. Cells used in this study were derived from glioblastomas, astrocytomas, normal glia, meningiomas, and from secondary brain tumors. In some experiments skin fibroblasts were also used. These cells were used as targets in the CRA.

Isolation of PBL

This was performed by centrifugation on Ficoll-Hypaque. Usually $5x10^5$ - 10^6 PBL were recovered per ml of blood. Granulocyte contamination was below 10 %.

"Direct" CRA

$5x10^3$ Cr^{51} - labelled target cells and $25x10^4$ PBL were mixed in a volume of 0.1 ml in wells of Falcon microtest II plates (3040) and incubated for 4 hours at 37°C. After incubation the radioactivity of the supernatant was determined and the percent specific release calculated by the formula = $\frac{E-S}{T-S}$ x 100, where E = experimental release (in presence of PBL), S = spontaneous release (target cells alone), and T = release after treatment with 2 % triton X.

Activation of PBL or "two-step CRA"

$5x10^3$ glioma or non-glioma cells (activator cells) were plated in wells of microtest II plates; after plating, $5x10^5$ PBL were added and the wells incubated for 44-48 hours. At this time $5x10^3$ Cr^{51} labelled glioma cells (from a glioma cell line selected for sufficient Cr^{51} uptake and low spontaneous release) were added to each well; the microplates were incubated overnight at 37°C. Thereafter radioactivity of the supernatants was determined and the percent specific release calculated as for the direct CRA. In parallel control experiments PBL were incubated without activator cells for the same time period.

In both direct and two-step CRA, percent specific release was considered statistically different from the spontaneous release at $p < 0.05$ as calculated by Students' test.

RESULTS

Direct CRA

In a series of 7 glioma patients, 6 were significantly cytotoxic towards homologous glioma cells; 3 patients with brain metastases were unreactive, but out of 4 non-tumoral patients 3 showed significant cytotoxicity towards glioma and normal glial cells as well. Relying on this assay it was not possible to distinguish between glioma and non-tumoral patients.

Two-step CRA

In these experiments,PBL from glioma and non-glioma patients were incubated either alone or in the presence of glioma cells during 44 hours before adding the labelled glioma cells from the same cell line as the activator cells. In the glioma patients group, 6 out of 7 experiments showed a significant increase in cytotoxicity after co-culture of the PBL with glioma cells, as compared with PBL incubated alone. In the non-glioma patients group, out of 5 experiments, 3 showed unchanged cytotoxicity and 2 showed a significant decrease after co-culture with glioma cells.

Specificity of the Activation

In order to rule out non-specific activating factors due to co-culture of PBL with cultured cells, PBL from glioma and non-glioma patients were co-cultured either with glioma or with non-glioma cells (normal glia, meningioma, brain metastases). The 6 glioma patients studied all showed increased cytotoxicity after activation on glioma cells, as compared with the cytotoxicity achieved after activation on other cells. In the non-glioma patients group, neither activation procedure was able to increase the reactivity of the PBL.

DISCUSSION

From the data obtained with the direct CRA in our human glioma system, it appears clearly that this assay cannot discriminate between disease-related lymphocytotoxicity (reactivity of glioma patients' PBL towards glioma target cells) and natural

cytotoxicity (reactivity of non-glioma patients's PBL towards
glioma and/or non glioma targets). Recent reports have demonstrated that this reactivity of normal subjects towards cultured
cells was not an artifact; moreover, the lymphocyte subpopulation involved in this phenomenon (NK cells) has been partially
characterized (6, 7). It is thus clear that data obtained in
humans with the direct CRA are influenced by too many variables
(K- and NK cell activity, individual susceptibility of cultured
lines to natural killing) and that a more specific effector
system has to be found.

Data from animal tumor models have shown the regression of
primary CTL a few weeks after tumor induction, but the persistence
of memory- T lymphocytes which can be primed by a secondary antigenic stimulus in vitro to generate secondary CTL with increased
and tumor-specific cytotoxicity (8). Therefore we submitted the
PBL of our patients to an antigenic restimulation in vitro by activating them in presence of intact tumor cells before looking
at their cytotoxic potential. It was thereby postulated that a
secondary immune response (increase in cytotoxicity after activation) would only be found in patients with in vivo sensitized
lymphocytes, whereas the natural killing activity would not increase. Our experiments indeed are strongly in favor of the existence of a secondary cell-mediated immune response in our glioma
patients, in the sense that only activation by glioma cells resulted in increased cytotoxicity. Moreover, natural cytotoxicity
displayed by some non-tumoral patients never increased after
activation; in some cases even a significant decrease of reactivity was observed. Our findings support the view that, in human
cancer as a chronic disease, activity of primary CTL as assessed
by the CRA is low (9). However, measurable levels of tumor-specific cytotoxicity can be achieved by providing specific antigenic
reactivation. The two-step CRA appears to fulfill this requirement, allows good distinction between disease and non-disease
related cell-mediated cytotoxicity and can be performed on a
routine basis in the hospital practice.

REFERENCES

1. Mahaley, M.S., Brooks, W.H., Bigner, D.D., Roszman, T.L. and
   Dudka, L. Immunobiology of primary intracranial tumors. I.
   studies of the cellular and humoral general immune competence
   of brain tumor patients. J. Neurosurg. 46, 484-494 (1977).
2. Takasugi, M. and Klein, E. A micro assay for cell-mediated
   immunity. Transplantation, 9, 219-227 (1970).
3. Baldwin, R.W. In vitro assays of cell-mediated immunity to
   human solid tumors. Problems of quantitation, specificity
   and interpretation. J. Nat. Cancer Inst. 55, 745-748 (1975).

4. Cerrotini, J.C. and Brunner, K.T. Cell-mediated cytotoxicity, allograft rejection, and tumor immunity. Adv. Immunol. 18, 67-132 (1974).
5. Scollard, D. Cellular cytotoxicity assays detect different effector cell types in vitro. Transplantation, 19, 87-90 (1975).
6. Kay, H.D., Bonnard, G.D., West, W.H. and Herberman R.B. A functional comparison of human Fc receptor-bearing lymphocytes active in natural cytotoxicity and antibody-dependent cellular cytotoxicity. J. Immunol. 118, 2058-2066 (1977).
7. Herberman, R.B., and Oldham, R.K. Problems associated with study of cell-mediated immunity to human tumors by microcytotoxicity assays. J. nat. Cancer Inst. 55, 749-753 (1975).
8. Wright, P.W., de Landazuri, M.O., and Herberman, R.BB, Immune response to Gross-virus induced lymphoma : comparison of two in vitro assays of cell-mediated immunity. J. nat. Cancer Inst. 50, 947-954 (1973).
9. Currie, G. Immunological aspects of host resistance to the development and growth of cancer. Biochim. Biophys. Acta, 458, 135-165 (1974).

MACROPHAGE-SPECIFIC ANTIGENS

L.I. Persson & L. Rönnbäck

Department of Neurology, Sahlgren Hospital, and
Institute of Neurobiology, University of Göteborg,
Göteborg, Sweden

SUMMARY

An antiserum-specific for mesodermal cells with cross-reactivity with microglia has been prepared by immunizing rabbits with unstimulated rat peritoneal macrophages. The characteristics of the antigens and antiserum are presented. The anti-macrophage antiserum provides one way of positive identification of reactive mesodermal macrophages of a monocytic origin both in nervous tissue and in cerebrospinal fluid.

INTRODUCTION

Monocytes and other mesodermal macrophages form part of the reticulo-endothelial system (RES). Both hematogeneous monocytes, tissue-resident monocytes and other macrophages possess phagocytic properties. Macrophages are also considered to interact with antigens co-operatively with lymphocytes, and thereby play an important role in the development of immunity and immunocompetence.

In spite of the great clinical importance of monocytic macrophages in immunity and phagocytosis, relatively little is known about the inherent properties of the macrophages. Monocytes as well as peritoneal macrophages possess receptors for IgG and complement (3, 5, 7, 11) and high levels of non-specific esterases.

The knowledge of the antigenic properties of monocytic and peritoneal macrophages is sparse and most antisera prepared to macrophages have been found to have low specificity to macrophages and to cross-react with various other cell types, e.g. lymphocytes. In a study by Stinnet et al. (26) one macrophage-specific antigen with a molecular weight of 83,000 Daltons has been characterised.

A monocytic origin of the microglial cells in the normal as well as in the reactive brain has been advocated. In the early phases of brain injuries there is an invasion of polymorphonuclear neutrophilic leucocytes into necrotic areas (2, 15, 16, 23, 27). Later, the neutrotrophilic leucocytes are replaced by invading hematogeneous phagocytic monocytes (21, 27) which develop a morphology similar to that of reactive microglia.

The resident microglial cell is characterized by its morphology and the ability to be impregnated by the Del Rio-Hortega silver carbonate impregnation technique (3). The microglial cell also possesses high levels of non-specific esterases, similar to monocytes (17) and nucleoside phosphatases (24). Some monocytic macrophages in the brain with an esterase activity and a morphology similar to microglia also possess membrane receptors for IgG and complement C'3 (18, 19). All these studies, together with studies using isotope-labeling of cells (1, 12), indicate a monocytic and mesodermal origin of microglia. Further support for this conclusion is given by studies combining several of these techniques (9, 10, 13, 14, 20, 25).

However, in spite of all these excellent studies indicating a mesodermal and probably monocytic origin of microglia, no direct evidence of a specific mesodermal origin exists. One such evidence of an origin from a specific monocytic or macrophage cell line should be the demonstration of microglial antigens specific to monocytes.

Previous studies have shown that neuroectodermal cells, i.e. astrocytes, oligodendrocytes, glioblasts and neurons possess the nervous tissue-specific S-100 protein (4, 8), while the 14-3-2 protein is localised only to neurons (22). The present study was performed as an attempt to obtain an antiserum specific to antigens of monocytic macrophages, and to investigate whether the microglial cells possess these antigens.

PRODUCTION OF ANTISERUM

Rat peritoneal mononuclear macrophages were prepared by rinsing the rat peritoneal cavity with tissue culture medium 199 for 2 min. The cells recovered were centrifuged and washed repeatedly with medium 199. The washed cells were counted in a chamber, and 10^7 cells were suspended in 1 ml saline, frozen and homoge-

nized. One ml homogenate was mixed with an equal volume of
Freund's complete adjuvant and injected into the hind subcutis
of adult rabbits, one ml (10^7 cells) once weekly for 4 weeks.
After an interval of 4 weeks, the rabbits were given an intravenous injection of 10^7 cells without Freund's adjuvant. Ten
days after the intravenous injection, the rabbits were given subcutaneous injections of 10^7 cells with Freund's adjuvant once
weekly for 5 weeks. One month after the last subcutaneous injection, the rabbits were given an intravenous booster injection
of 10^7 homogenized cells without adjuvant. Ten days after the
last injection, the rabbits were bled and serum prepared. The
antiserum was used crude or brought to 2 % by ammonium-sulphate
precipitation, according to Hijmans et al. (8).

DETECTION OF THE ANTIGENS

Antibodies to macrophages were coupled to a cyanogen-bromide-
activated Sepharose 4B column. Homogenates of rat peritoneal macrophages, thymus and spleen were passed the column and the antigens reacted with the antibodies were eluted by lowering of pH.
The eluate was incubated with antibodies against macrophages and
centrifuged. The pellet was dissolved in sodium duodecyl-sulphate
after reduction with 2-mercaptoethanol. SDS electrophoresis in
15 % polyacrylamide gels was performed. At least three bands
with molecular weights of 31,000, 33,000 and 35,000 were revealed
together with the light (m.w. 25,000) and the heavy (m.w. 50,000)
chains of the antibodies added (Fig.1).

CHARACTERISATION OF THE ANTISERUM

A single precipitation band was obtained when homogenized
peritoneal macrophages were tested by double diffusion in 1 %
agar against the antiserum in a concentration of < 1 mg IgG/ml.
When higher concentrations were used, another weak precipitation
band was also observed. Two precipitation lines, one dense and
one weak, were also observed when the antiserum was tested by
double diffusion against homogenized and supernatant solutions
from lung, kidney, spleen, thymus, liver and brain.

LOCALISATION OF THE ANTIGENS

Peritoneal Macrophages

After rinsing the peritoneal cavity with tissue culture medium 199, the medium contained about 95 % small mononuclear round
or ovoid cells of a monocyte-like appearance with a slightly ec-

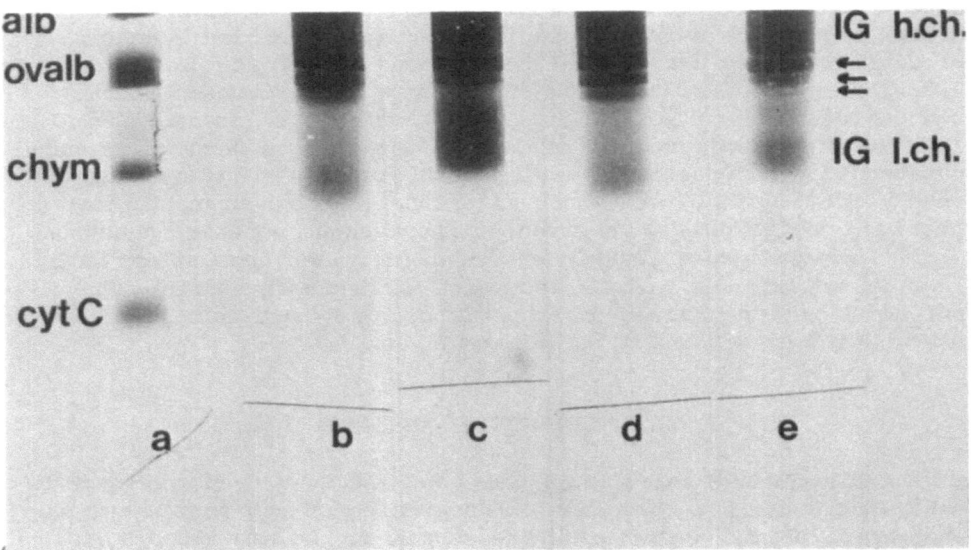

Fig. 1 : SDS electrophoresis in 15 % polyacrylamide gels in 4 mm
(i.d.) glass tubes of
a) standard proteins (albumin,ovalbumin,chymotrypsin,cytochrome C)
b)and c) antigen-antibody mixture of peritoneal macrophages;
d) antigen-antibody mixture of spleen;
e) antigen-antibody mixture of thymus.
At least three protein bands with molecular weights 31,000, 33,000
and 35,000 are seen together with the heavy (50,000 m.w.) and
light (25,000 m.w.) chains of IgG.

centric nucleus, with a cell diameter of 8-15 μm. More than 95 %
of the cells excluded Trypan blue at viability tests. The collected cells were used unfixed or fixed in buffered formaldehyde.
These monocyte-like cells showed an intense fluorescence specific
of TRITC after incubation first with anti-macrophage antiserum
prepared in rabbits, followed by incubation in TRITC-labeled an-
ti-rabbit-IgG produced in goats (Fig. 2 a).

     One to two per cent of the cells in the rinsing solution
were large, flat mesothelial cells with a diameter of 50-60 μm.
These cells showed a weak granular cytoplasmic fluorescence of
TRITC after incubation. 3-4% of the cells in the tissue culture
medium after peritoneal rinsing were made up by neutrophilic leucocytes which showed no specific fluorescence after incubation.

     After injection of 3 ml of liquid paraffin intraperitoneally,
an exudate was collected 5 days after the injection. Fifty per

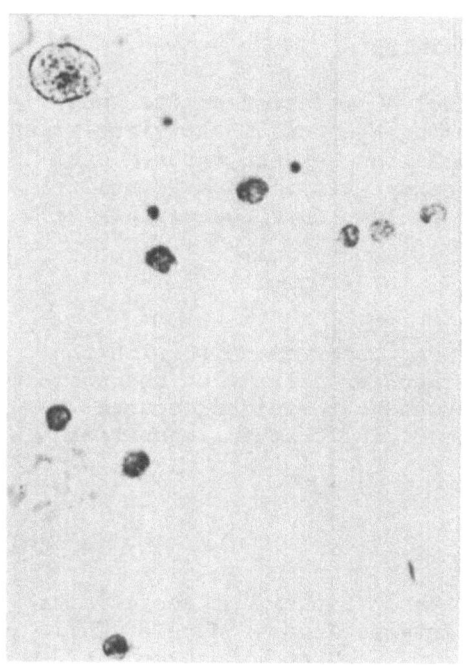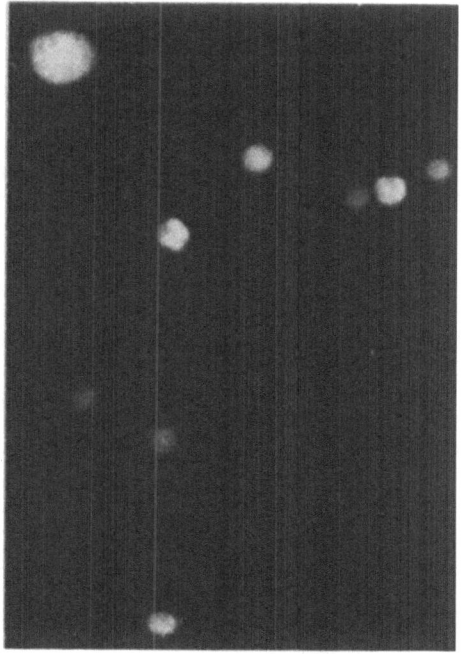

Fig. 2a : Formaldehyde-fixed rat peritoneal macrophages showing
an intense naphthol AS-MX phosphate esterase activity, indicating
an origin of monocytic.   x 640.

Fig. 2b : The esterase-positive mononuclear peritoneal macrophages and one flat large peritoneal mesothelial cell of Fig. 2a
after incubation with rabbit anti-macrophage antiserum, followed
by incubation in TRITC-labeled goat anti-rabbit IgG.   There is
an intense fluorescence of TRITC, indicating presence of macrophage antigens reactive with the antiserum.   x640.

cent of the cells in the peritoneal exudate after paraffin injection consisted of polymorphonuclear leucocytes. These cells showed no specific fluorescence of TRITC after incubation with antiserum to peritoneal macrophages. Mononuclear phagocytes, making
up 50 % of the cells in the peritoneal exudate, showed a very intense cytoplasmic fluorescence of TRITC after incubation with the
antiserum. No nuclear fluorescence was observed in any of the
experiments.

     There was no difference among the cells with respect to the
distribution or the intensity of the fluorescence of TRITC, irres-

pective of whether the peritoneal cells were incubated without
prior fixation or after fixation with formaldehyde.

Enzyme Histochemistry

Enzyme histochemistry of naphthol AS-MX-esterase i.e. unspecific esterases or ali-esterases, using Fast Red TR as visualizing
diazonium salt, showed a close correlation between intense esterase activity and intense anti-macrophage activity as visualized
by the fluorescence of TRITC in mononuclear macrophages (Fig. 2).

Liver

Specific fluorescence of TRITC was observed neither in the
liver parenchymal cells, nor in the Kupffer cells with the antiserum used. However, macrophages around arteries and central
veins showed an intense fluorescence of TRITC after incubation
with the antiserum.

Thymus

Scattered clusters of cells at the periphery of the germinal
centres of the follicles showed an intense fluorescence of TRITC
in the experiments performed (Fig. 3). The stroma macrophages
showed no specific fluorescence with the antiserum used. The
morphology and appearance of anti-macrophage positive cells in
the thymus were similar to those of dendritic cells and to monocytes in the spleen, but the tendency to form clusters was especially marked in the thymus.

Peripheral Blood

Rat monocytes showed a positive reaction against the TRITC-
labelled anti-macrophage antiserum. Neutrophilic leucocytes,
thrombocytes and lymphocytes showed no fluorescence.

Spleen

In the unfixed as well as in the formaldehyde-fixed sections
of the spleen there was an intense cytoplasmic fluorescence of
TRITC in numerous small, ovoid or slightly fusiform cells, similar to monocytes, after incubation with anti-macrophage antiserum.
(Fig. 4.). These cells were situated both in the red and in the
white pulp, especially at the border between the white and the
red pulp and often lining entering blood vessels. No specific

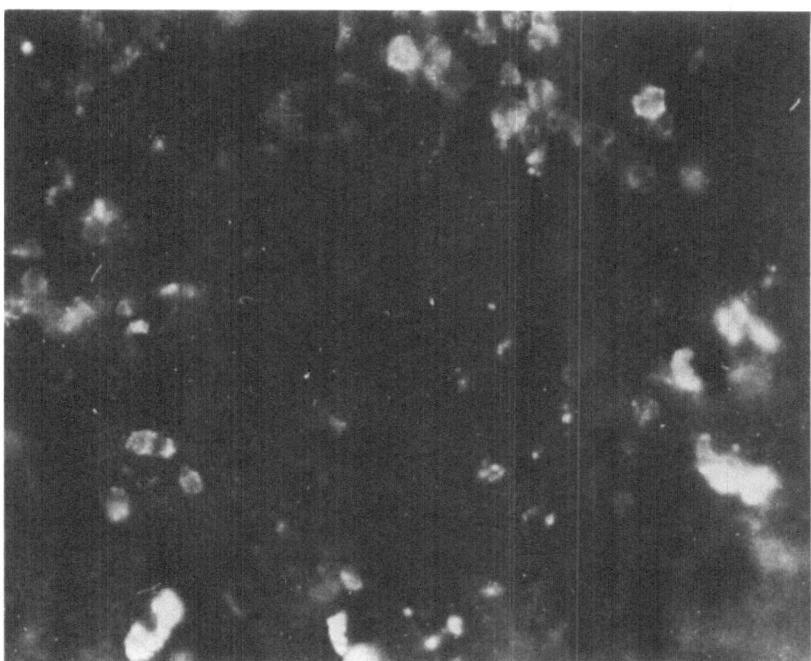

Fig. 3 : Rat thymus incubated with anti-macrophage antiserum.
Numerous macrophages at the periphery of a germinal centre show
an intense fluorescence. Only few fluorescent macrophages are
observed within the central part of the germinal centre. No specific fluorescence is observed in thymocytes or in reticular cells.
The shape of the anti-macrophage positive cells is similar to
that of dendritic cells. Formaldehyde fixation.   x 500.

activity was observed in siderophages (lining cells) or fibroblasts.

                            Brain

     A few macrophages situated along the larger vessels in non-
injured brain showed positive reaction against the anti-macrophage
antiserum. The adventitia of large vessels both in the cerebrum,
cerebellum and the leptomeninges contained a few cells with specific fluorescence of TRITC. No endogeneous parenchymal cells
showed positive reaction against the TRITC-labelled antimacrophage
antisera.

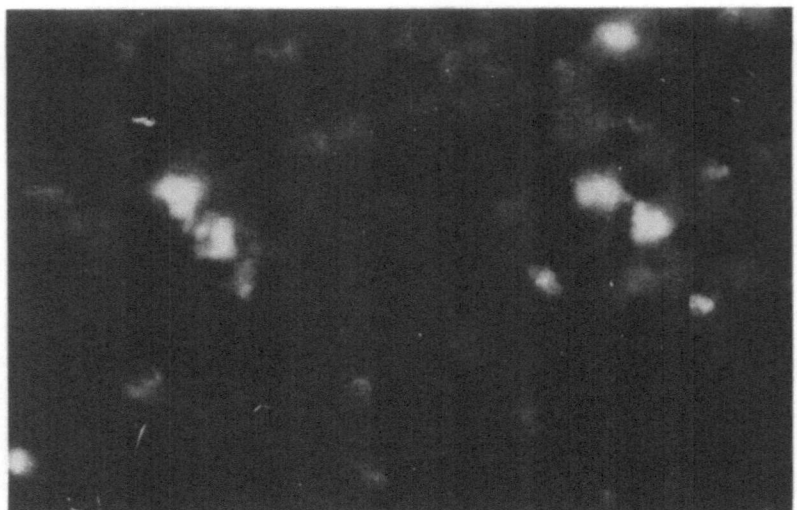

Fig. 4 : Rat spleen incubated with anti-macrophage antiserum.
Multiple macrophages show specific fluorescence indicating macrophage antigens reactive with the antiserum. Siderophages (lining
cells) and stroma connective tissue cells show no specific fluorescence. Formaldehyde fixation.   x 800.

Cerebral Stab Wounds

Two to eight days after cerebral stab injury there were
numerous mononuclear cells showing a specific fluorescence of
TRITC within 300 µm from the edge of the wound. (Fig. 5). Anti-
macrophage-serum-positive cells showed an ovoid of fusiform appearance with a few slender processes. The small elongated nucleus of these cells showed no specific fluorescence. Invading
polymorphonuclear phagocytic cells showed no reaction with the
anti-macrophage antiserum.

DISCUSSION

The study performed indicated that mononuclear macrophages,
irrespective of their location in blood, peritoneum, thymus, leptomeninges, in spleen or around blood vessels in various organs
share antigens specific to this monocytic line of macrophages.
The same antigenic properties were also revealed in microglial
cells in the brain. There was a close correlation between high
activity of unspecific naphthol phosphate-esterases as demonstra-

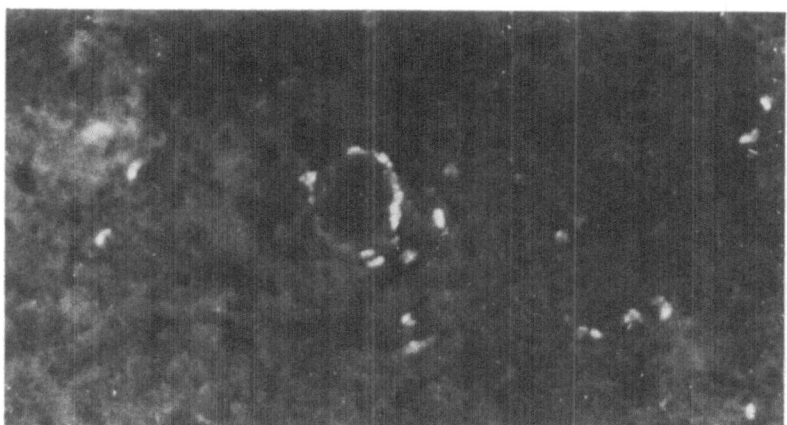

Fig. 5 : Cerebral stab wound of a rat 2 days after injury, 200
µm from the centre of the wound. Numerous cells are located
around a venule in the centre, with an intense fluorescence of
TRITC. A few fluorescent microglia-like macrophages are observed
in neuropil. Formaldehyde fixation.   x 320.

ted by enzyme histochemistry and intense fluorescence of TRITC
after incubation with rabbit-antiserum to macrophages, followed
by incubation with TRITC-labeled goat-antirabbit IgG. The
antiserum produced showed no cross-reaction to neutrophilic leucocytes, to lymphocytes, or to other connective tissue cells.
SDS electrophoresis showed at least 3 bands with M.W. 31,000,
33,000 and 35,000, respectively. Whether these bands constitute
3 different antigens or are subunits of one protein is under
further investigation.

    The present method of identification of mononuclear monocytic
macrophages provides one way of positive identification of monocytic macrophages, irrespective of their location in different
organs. It also provides a simple way to analyse the origin of
monocytic phagocytes, including microglial cells, both in normal
and in reactive brain.

ACKNOWLEDGEMENTS

    The present study was supported by Tore Nilson's Foundation
for Medical Research, the Fylgia Foundation, the Anna Ahrenberg
Foundation and the Medical Faculty of Göteborg.

REFERENCES

1. Adrian, E.K., Walker, B.E. J. Neuropath. exp. Neurol. 21, 597-604 (1962).
2. Coen, E. Beitr. path. Anat. Physiol. 2, 107-128 (1888).
3. Del Rio-Hortega, P., Penfield, W. Cerebral cicatrix. Bull. Johns Hopkins Hospital 41, 273-303 (1927).
4. Haglid, K.G., Hamberger, A., Hansson, H.-A., Hydén, H., Persson, L.I., Rönnbäck, L. J. Neurosci. Res. 2, 175-191 (1976).
5. Heusser, C.H., Andersson, C.L., Grey, H.M. J. exp. Med. 145, 1316-1327 (1977).
6. Hijmans, W., Schuit, H.R.E., Klein, F. Clin. exp. Immunol. 4, 457-472 (1969).
7. Huber, H., Fudenberg, H.H. Int. Arch. Allergy 34, 18-31 (1968).
8. Hydén, H., McEwen, B. Proc. Nat. Acad. Sci. (U.S.A.) 55, 354-358 (1966).
9. Kitamura, T. Acta path. Jap. 23, 11-26 (1973).
10. Kitamura, T., Tsuchihashi, Y., Tatebe, A., Fujita, S. Acta Neuropath. (Berl.) 38, 195-201 (1977).
11. Knutson, D.W., Kijlstra, A., van Es, L.A. J. exp. Med. 145, 1368-1381 (1977).
12. Konigsmark, B.W., Sidman, R.L. J. Neuropath. exp. Neurol. 22, 643-676 (1963).
13. Ling, E.A., Paterson, J.A., Privat, A., Mori, S., Leblond, C.P. J. Comp. Neurol. 149, 43-72 (1973).
14. Ling, E.A., Leblond, C.P. J. Comp. Neurol. 149, 73-82 (1973).
15. Matthews, M.A., Kruger, L. J. Comp. Neurol. 148, 285-312 (1973).
16. Matthews, M.A., Kruger, L. J. Comp. Neurol. 148, 313-346 (1973).
17. Oehmichen, M. Acta Histochem. (Jena) 47, 289-304 (1973).
18. Oehmichen,M., Huber, H. J. Neuropath. exp. Neurol. 35, 30-39 (1976).
19. Oehmichen, M., Grüninger, H., Saebisch, R., Narita, Y. Acta Neuropath. (Berl.) 23, 200-218 (1973).
20. Paterson, J.A., Privat, A., Ling, E.A., Leblond, C.P. J. Comp. Neurol. 149, 83-102 (1973).
21. Persson, L.I. Virchows Arch. B Cell Path. 22, 21-37 (1976).
22. Persson, L.I., Rönnbäck, L., Grasso, A., Haglid, K.G., Hansson, H.-A., Dolonius, L., Molin, S.-O., Nygren, H. J. Neurol. Sci. 35, 381-390 (1978).
23. Schultz, R.L., Pease, D.C. Amer. J. Path. 35, 1017-1042 (1959).
24. Sjöstrand, J. Acta physiol. Scand. 67, 219-228 (1966).
25. Skoff, R. J. Comp. Neurol. 161, 595-612 (1975).
26. Stinnett, J.D., Kaplan, A.M., Morahan, P.S. J. Immunol. 116, 273-278 (1976).
27. Tschistowitsch, T. Beitr. pathol. 23, 321-350 (1898).

OLIGOCLONAL IgG BANDS AND MEASLES ANTIBODIES IN MULTIPLE SCLEROSIS
(MS) CSF AND BRAIN EXTRACTS

P.D. Mehta, A. Kane, H. Thormar and H. M. Wisniewski

New York State Institute for Basic Research in Mental
Retardation, Staten Island, New York, U.S.A.

SUMMARY

Although measles antibodies are found in CSF and brain extracts of a few MS patients, quantitation data demonstrated that
the measles specific IgG is less than 5% of the total IgG, indicating that the major portion of oligoclonal IgG is not synthesized
against measles virus. Individual oligoclonal bands were isolated
from 2 MS brain extracts with measles antibody titers. The results
showed that measles HI, CF and neutralizing activities were found
in all isolated oligoclonal fractions and the titers were proportional to the IgG concentration.

INTRODUCTION

The antigens responsible for the synthesis of oligoclonal
bands in MS have not been identified. However, a number of studies
(1-4), using different serological methods, have shown a greater
frequency of measles virus antibody in CSF of MS patients than in
the control group, indicating a possible role of measles virus in
the etiology of MS. Thus, the object of the present investigation
was to quantitate the amount of measles specific IgG in CSF and
brain extracts from MS patients with significant measles antibody
titers, and to determine if measles activity is present in one or
more specific bands or is distributed throughout all oligoclonal
bands.

MATERIALS AND METHODS

Collection of Samples

CSF and autopsy brain tissues from MS patients and controls
were obtained from Dr. H. Schutta, Downstate Medical Center,
Brooklyn, N.Y.

Brain Extracts

Brain tissues were washed with 0.15 M NaCl, thinly sliced,
homogenized with PBS pH 7.4, centrifuged and concentrated as described previously (5).

Isolation of Oligoclonal IgG Bands

Individual oligoclonal bands from MS brain extracts were isolated by the combination of repeated gel filtration on Sephadex
G-200 column and preparative isoelectric focusing procedures as
previously described (5). The homogeneity of the bands was examined by agarose gel electrophoresis (6).

Virological Techniques

The measles antibody titers in CSF and brain extracts were
determined by hemagglutination inhibition (HI), complement fixation
(CF) and neutralization tests (6).

Quantitation of Measles Specific IgG

CSF and brain extracts were suitably absorbed with concentrated preparation of cell associated measles virus and noninfected Vero cell cultures respectively. The IgG from absorbed and
unabsorbed samples were quantitated by radial immunodiffusion
method and the measles specific IgG as a % of the total IgG was
determined as previously described (6).

RESULTS AND DISCUSSION

The measles HI and neutralizing antibody titers in CSF and
brain extracts are shown in Table 1. Although 10% of the CSF's
had significant titers (32-128), none of them showed more than 5%
measles specific IgG. Similar results were seen in neutral pH MS

brain extracts. In contrast, SSPE patients had significantly high measles specific IgG contents in both CSF and brain extracts (6).

Table 1

Measles Virus Antibodies in CSF and Brain Extracts

of MS and Controls[a]

Group	Sample	No. of Patients Tested	No. Positive	% Positive	Measles Antibody Titers	Measles Specific IgG (% of the Total IgG)
MS	CSF	41	20	49	2–8(15)[b]	<5
					16–128(5)[b]	<5
	Brain Extract	7	2	30	100–200[c]	<5
Controls	CSF	30	4	13	2–8	<5
	Brain Extract	5	–	–	<2–4	<5
SSPE	CSF	9	9	100	64–256	30–60
	Brain Extract	6	6	100	128–1024[c]	40–80

[a]Controls consisted of patients having neurological disorders other than MS and SSPE such as CNS tumors, headaches, degenerative disease, optic atrophy, etc.
[b]Number inside parenthesis represents the No. of CSF's out of the total positives.
[c]Antibody concentration is expressed at an IgG concentration of 1 mg/ml.

In addition, the electrophoretic analysis (7) between CSF and brain extracts absorbed with measles virus and those absorbed with noninfected Vero cells, respectively, showed no significant differences in their oligoclonal band patterns. Thus our results suggest that the major portion of oligoclonal bands synthesized in MS are not measles specific.

Since only a small portion of IgG from MS CSF and brain extracts were measles specific, it was of interest to see if measles antibody activity is associated with all oligoclonal bands or is restricted to one or more specific bands. IgG fractions were

initially isolated by Sephadex G-200 column chromatography. About
5 mg of partially purified IgG was subjected to isoelectric focusing column and the elution profile is shown in Fig. 1. The purity
of the individual oligoclonal bands is shown in Fig. 2. The three
oligoclonal IgG's starting from the cathode had isoelectric points
of 8.8, 8.3 and 8.0, respectively.

Measles HI and CF antibody activities were found in all oligoclonal IgG's and the titers were proportional to the IgG concentration. These results are somewhat different from those observed
in SSPE CSF and brain extracts, where uneven distribution of measles
antibody activities against different measles viral antigens was
seen in isolated oligoclonal bands (5,8).

ACKNOWLEDGMENTS

This work was supported in part by a grant from the National
Multiple Sclerosis Society (Grant No. RG 1189-A-1).

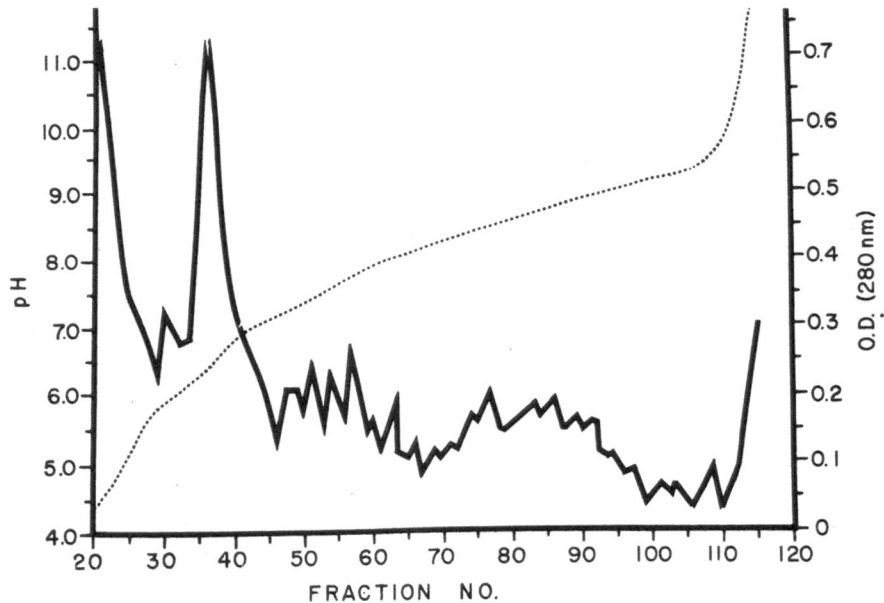

Figure 1. The isoelectric focusing profile of an MS brain IgG in
pH 7-10 gradient range. Fraction Nos. 55-100 showed precipitin
line in Ouchterlony test against anti human IgG serum. Selective
fractions were pooled, dialyzed, concentrated and run in agarose
gel electrophoresis.

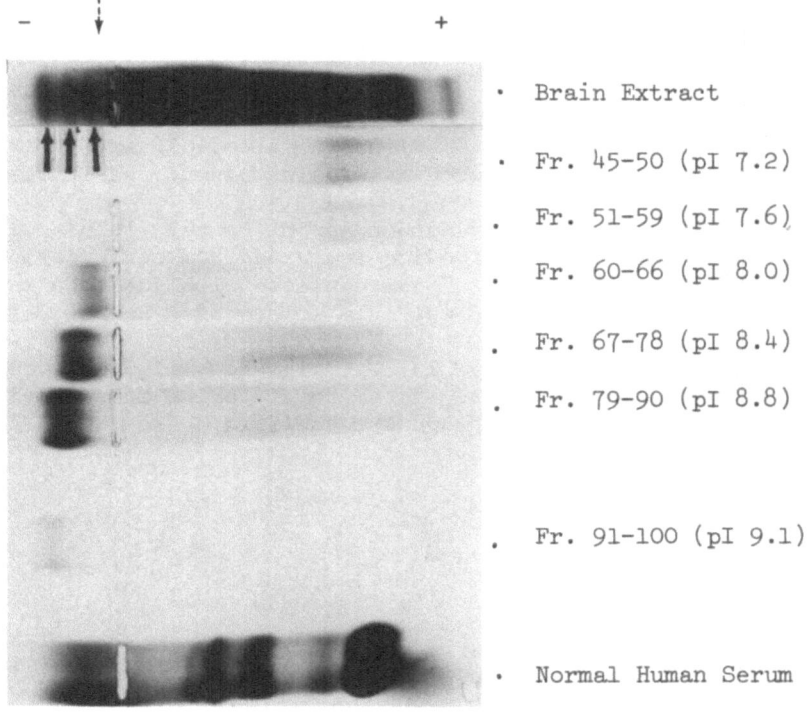

- Brain Extract
- Fr. 45-50 (pI 7.2)
- Fr. 51-59 (pI 7.6)
- Fr. 60-66 (pI 8.0)
- Fr. 67-78 (pI 8.4)
- Fr. 79-90 (pI 8.8)
- Fr. 91-100 (pI 9.1)
- Normal Human Serum

Figure 2. Agarose gel electrophoretic patterns of the MS brain extract and IgG fractions isolated by isoelectric focusing technique as shown in Fig. 1. The solid arrows denote the oligoclonal bands, whereas the broken arrow on the top represents the point of application.

REFERENCES

1. Brown, P., F. Cathala, D.C. Gajdusek and C.J. Gibbs, Jr. 1971. Measles antibodies in the cerebrospinal fluid of patients with multiple sclerosis. Proc. Soc. Exp. Biol. Med. 137:956.
2. Haire, M. 1977. Significance of virus antibodies in multiple sclerosis. Brit. Med. Bull. 33:40.
3. Norrby, E., H. Link and J.E. Olsson. 1974. Measles virus antibody titers in cerebrospinal fluid and serum from patients with multiple sclerosis and controls. Arch. Neurol. 30:285.
4. Vandvik, B. and M. Degre. 1975. Measles virus antibodies in serum and cerebrospinal fluid in patients with multiple sclerosis and other neurological disorders with special reference to measles antibody synthesis within the central nervous system. J. Neurol. Sci. 24: 201.

5. Mehta, P.D., A. Kane and H. Thormar. 1976. Relationship between homogeneous IgG fractions and measles virus antibody activities in subacute sclerosing panencephalitis brain. J. Immunol.
117:2053.
6. Mehta, P.D., A. Kane and H. Thormar. 1977. Quantitation of
measles virus specific immunoglobulins in serum, CSF and brain extract from patients with subacute sclerosing panencephalitis. J.
Immunol. 118:2254.
7. Vandvik, B., E. Norrby, H. Nordal and M. Degre. 1976. Oligoclonal virus-specific IgG antibodies isolated from cerebrospinal
fluids, brain extracts and sera from patients with subacute
sclerosing panencephalitis and multiple sclerosis. Scand. J. Immunol. 5:979.
8. Vandvik, B. and E. Norrby. 1973. Oligoclonal IgG antibody
response in the central nervous system to different measles virus
antigens in subacute sclerosing panencephalitis. Proc. Natl. Acad.
Sci. 70:1060.

CHARACTERIZATION OF THE HUMORAL IMMUNE RESPONSE WITHIN THE CNS BY IMMUNOFIXATION

H. Link, M. Laurenzi and A. Fryden

Department of Neurology, University Hospital
Linköping, Sweden

SUMMARY

Agarose gel electrophoresis and subsequent immunofixation revealed one or more bands consisting of IgG, IgA, IgM free Lambda chains and free Kappa chains in 39, 1, 1, 7 and 0, respectively, of 39 consecutive multiple sclerosis CSF specimens. A predominance of IgG Kappa bands was found in 30 of them, of IgG lambda bands in 5. 27 CSF specimens also displayed IgG Kappa and Lambda present in the same band, probably due to microheterogeneity.

The oligoclonal reaction demonstrable in CSF in acute aseptic meningitis and Guillain-Barré syndrome is dominated by IgG Lambda. A selection of the oligoclonal immune response within the CNS depending on etiology may be proposed.

INTRODUCTION

The occurrence of oligoclonal immunoglobulins (Ig) in cerebrospinal fluid (CSF) due to Ig synthesis within the CNS is a well known phenomenon in multiple sclerosis (MS) and may also be found in acute aseptic meningitis and Guillain-Barré syndrome (GBS). Sometimes, uncertainty exists regarding the presence of bands, and they have hitherto only been incompletely characterized regarding inter alia class and light chain type. Therefore, immunofixation after agarose gel electrophoresis was applied.

463

MATERIALS AND METHODS

39 consecutive patients with clinically definite MS and 10 patients with uncomplicated acute aseptic meningitis and oligoclonal reaction demonstrable by agarose gel electrophoresis of CSF were included.

Agarose gel electrophoresis was performed on preformed agarose gel (Panagel slide, Millipore Biomedica, Acton, MA, USA). For immunofixation, cellulose acetate strips dipped in specific antiserum were applied to the gel surface immediately after electrophoresis (2). During 1 hour of incubation, specific immune complexes are formed as insoluble precipitates. Proteins not precipitated were then removed by washing and absorption on filter paper, whereupon the plate was dried and stained. The band pattern was compared with that obtained at routine agarose gel electrophoresis run in parallel.

TABLE 1

Relation between light chain type of oligoclonal CSF IgG bands, CSF Kappa/Lambda ratio and CSF IgG index in 39 MS patients.

Oligoclonal IgG	CSF Kappa/Lambda ratio			CSF IgG index	
	>1.7 (n=14)	0.7-1.7 (n=20)	<0.7 (n=2)	>0.70 (n=35)	≤0.70 (n=4)
Kappa only (n=10)	5	5	0	8	2
Lambda only (0)	-	-	-	-	-
Predominance of Kappa (n=20)	9	9	1*	19	1
Predominance of Lambda (n=5)	0	3	1*	4	1
Same number of bands with Kappa and Lambda (n=4)	0	3	0	4	0

* Band consisting of free Lambda chains present

RESULTS

Immunofixation revealed 1 - 10 IgG bands (mean 5 bands) in all 39 MS CSF and 1 - 2 bands with the same mobility in 4 of the corresponding serum specimens. Bands consisting of IgA and IgM were found in CSF from one patient each. Bands were always found on the cathodic side of the application slit but in 16 case 1 - 2 bands also migrated on the anodic side. Bands consisting of free Lambda chains only were found in CSF in seven cases, while bands with free Kappa chains only were not identified.

Table 1 shows that IgG Kappa bands only were found in 10 of the 39 MS patients, and a predominance of IgG Kappa bands in an additional 20, while a predominance of IgG Lambda bands was observed in only 5 and only IgG Lambda bands in none. In 27 of the patients one or more IgG bands containing Kappa as well as Lambda were identified. IgG Kappa bands only were found in presence of a normal CSF Kappa/Lambda ratio (0.7 - 1.7), indicating that the determination of this ratio is less useful for diagnostic purposes. An abnormally low CSF Kappa/Lambda ratio (0.7) was found in 2 of the MS patients, both had bands consisting of free Lambda chains. A normal CSF IgG index (0.70) in the presence of an oligoclonal reaction was found in 11 %.

The bands found in CSF in aseptic meningitis consisted of IgG in all 10 patients, IgM in 2 of them and free Lambda chains also in 2 of them. In contrast to the findings in MS, IgG Lambda bands only were found in two patients, and a predominance of IgG Lambda bands in 3.

DISCUSSION

Agarose gel electrophoresis and subsequent immunofixation can be recommended for confirmation of an oligoclonal reaction in CSF and for characterization of oligoclonal Ig regarding class and light chain type. Oligoclonal IgA and IgM can be found in CSF in MS, oligoclonal IgM also in aseptic meningitis. The humoral immune response within the CNS in MS is dominated by intrathecal synthesis of IgG Kappa, in aseptic meningitis and Guillain-Barré syndrome (1) of IgG Lambda. These observations need to be confirmed on greater patient material. If they are correct, a selection of the oligoclonal immune response within the CNS depending on the etiological agent can be proposed.

ACKNOWLEDGEMENT

This work has been supported by the Swedish Medical Research Council (Project no. 3381).

REFERENCES

1. Link, H., Wahren, B. and Norrby, E., Prolonged pleiocytosis
   and immunoglobulin changes in the CSF of patients with Guillain-Barré syndrome and acute and reactivated CMV and EBV infections. Submitted to Infection and Immunity.
2. Ritchie, R.F. and Smith, R., I. General principles and application to agarose gel electrophoresis. Clin. Chem.
   497-499, 1976.

EFFECTS OF SERUM FACTORS UPON MYELIN ORGANIZATION IN ORGANOTYPIC CULTURES OF NERVOUS TISSUE

C.S. Raine and M.B. Bornstein

Albert Einstein College of Medicine
Bronx, N.Y., U.S.A.

INTRODUCTION

Recent studies (1-3) have shown that when myelinated, organo-typic cultures of central nervous system (CNS) tissue are exposed to heated (complement-inactivated) anti-whole CNS antiserum from rabbits with acute experimental allergic encephalomyelitis (EAE), myelin sheaths are not destroyed, but oligodendroglia are stimulated to produce profuse, aberrant arrays of their processes and the periodicity of myelin sheaths acquires a unique morphology. The same serum in the presence of complement demyelinates the tissue within the first few hours of exposure (4,5). In addition, there appears to be a specific effect of EAE serum on CNS elements. These changes are associated with the binding of antibody to the myelin sheaths (6). To test whether similar abnormalities could be induced in the peripheral nervous system (PNS), the present study involved cultures of PNS and CNS tissue exposed to heated and unheated serum from rabbits with experimental allergic neuritis (EAN), induced by challenge with PNS tissues in complete Freund's adjuvant (CFA). Similar swellings in PNS myelin occurs on exposure to complement-inactivated EAN serum while intact EAN serum demyelinates. Some of the changes resemble those accompanying the neuropathy which occurs in certain hypergammaglobulinemic disorders and these might indicate that humoral factors have significant effects upon the maintenance of myelin in its normal state.

MATERIALS AND METHODS

Serum: Adult New Zealand albino rabbits, weighing between 3 and 4 kg, were sensitized with 0.4 ml (0.1 ml in each footpad) of

an emulsion made up of 1 part bovine spinal nerve roots, 1 part
saline and 2 parts CFA. Between 12 and 14 days post-inoculation,
animals became quadriparetic and were exsanguinated under anesthesia.
The serum was separated under sterile conditions, divided into
aliquots and stored at -90°C until use.

Cultures: Myelinated cultures of mouse dorsal root ganglia
(DRG), sometimes in combination with spinal cord fragments, were
maintained by techniques standard in these laboratories (7). For
the present experiments, cultures were used between 28 and 40 days
in vitro (DIV). Experimental cultures were exposed for periods of
time ranging up to 14 days to normal nutrient medium containing
25% unheated EAE serum or to 25% of the same EAN serum which had
been complement-inactivated (heated at 56°C for 30 mins). To examine the reversibility of the changes, some cultures were exposed
to unheated and heated EAN serum for 1-2 weeks then returned to
normal feeding solution. Control cultures were fed normal nutrient
medium or nutrient containing 25% normal rabbit serum. Cultures
were observed in the living state and at selected timepoints after
exposure to EAN serum, were prepared for ultrastructural study (8).

RESULTS

The myelin sheaths in cultures of mouse DRG began to demyelinate with 72 hours of exposure to unheated EAN serum. This progressed to total- demyelination by 7 days. Initially, affected myelin sheaths displayed a transient swelling of the superficial lamellae and, with time, this progressed deeper into the sheath. The
widened lamellae then fragmented and were transformed into a vesicu-
lated network (Figure 1). The degenerating myelin was phagocytosed
by the ensheathing Schwann cells (9). By 8 days' exposure, no intact
PNS myelin could be seen. Neurons and other PNS elements were not
affected. CNS myelin in attached spinal cord fragments was also
destroyed.

Exposure to unheated EAN serum for 7-14 days followed by removal
of the offending serum from the nutrient medium led to remyelination
of some internodes in 1-2 weeks.

Heated (complement-inactivated) aliquots of the same myelinotoxic EAN serum had a distinctly different effect upon PNS myelin
in cultures. Most apparent perhaps, was its failure to demyelinate
the tissue during a 16 day exposure to 25% concentrations. Instead,
the myelin sheaths underwent a gradual transformation into a swollen
state, highly reminiscent of the response in CNS cultures exposed
to heated EAE serum (1,2). After about 4 days' exposure to heated
EAN serum, PNS myelin sheaths demonstrated an elongation and widening of the outer mesaxon within which 4 lamellar components
(instead of the usual 2) could be discerned (Figure 2). This

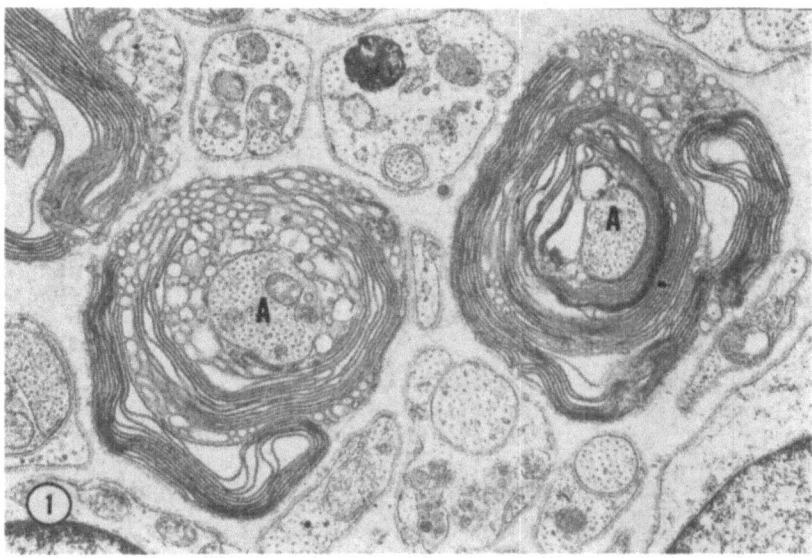

Figure 1: DRG culture exposed to intact EAN serum for 96 h. Note how the myelin sheaths of two fibers (axons at A) have been trans- formed into swollen lamellar and vesicular networks. X 16,000.

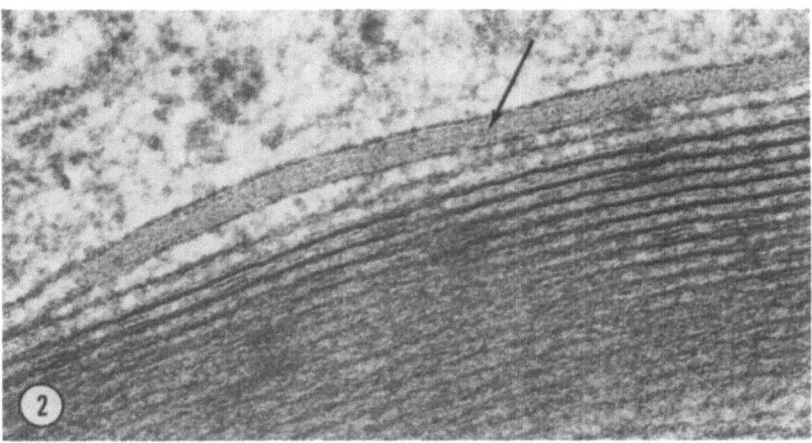

Figure 2: DRG culture exposed to heated (complement-inactivated) EAN serum for 96 h. The outer mesaxon of this PNS myelin sheath is swollen and 4 leaflets (arrow), instead of the usual 2, are in the position of the presumptive intraperiod line. X 150,000.

doubling of the leaflets continued into the outer layers of myelin
in the space normally occupied by the bilamellar intraperiod line.
The periodicity of the myelin sheath was increased from the usual
11.7 nm (approximately) to about 23 nm. With increase in exposure
time, deeper layers of myelin became widened but rarely was the
entire PNS sheath involved (Figure 3).   Unlike the oligodendrocyte
in CNS cultures exposed to heated EAE serum (1-3), Schwann cells in
heated EAN-treated cultures were not stimulated to produce vast
amounts of redundant, aberrant myelin, but some axons possessed
thicker than normal myelin sheaths, perhaps an indication of hypermyelination.   The basal laminae of PNS fibers in cultures exposed
to both unheated and heated EAN serum, were markedly thickened
(Figure 3).

Some PNS cultures were exposed to heated EAN serum for 2 weeks
after which they were returned to normal nutrient medium. Even after
2 weeks' return to normal conditions, the swollen myelin failed to
revert completely to its normal periodicity (Figure 4).   CNS tissue
also displayed myelin swelling in the presence of heated EAN serum.

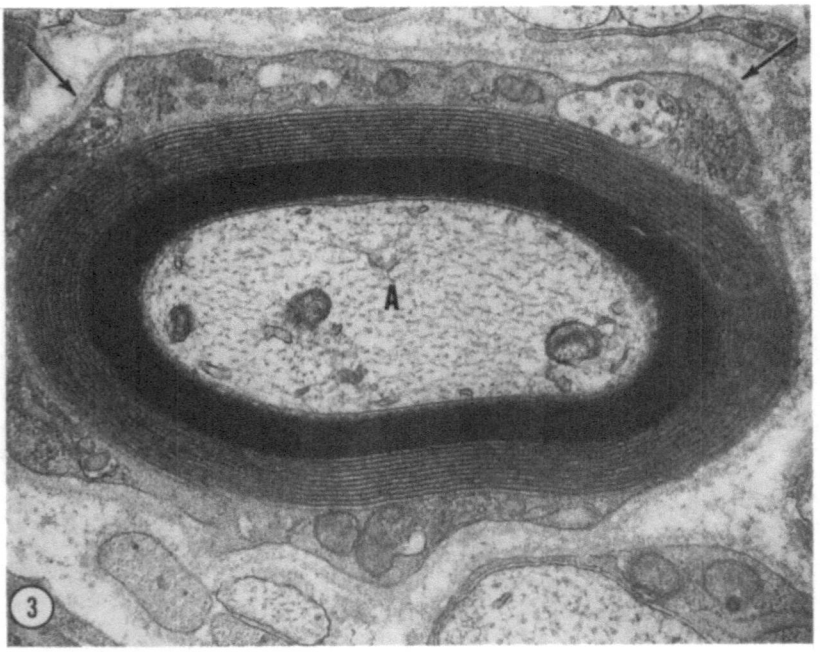

Figure 3: DRG culture, 16 days' exposure to heated EAN serum. The
outer myelin lamellae of this PNS fiber display widening to 23 nm.
Deeper layers possess the normal 11.7 nm spacing. The basal lamina
(arrows) is thickened. Axon at A.   X 32,000.

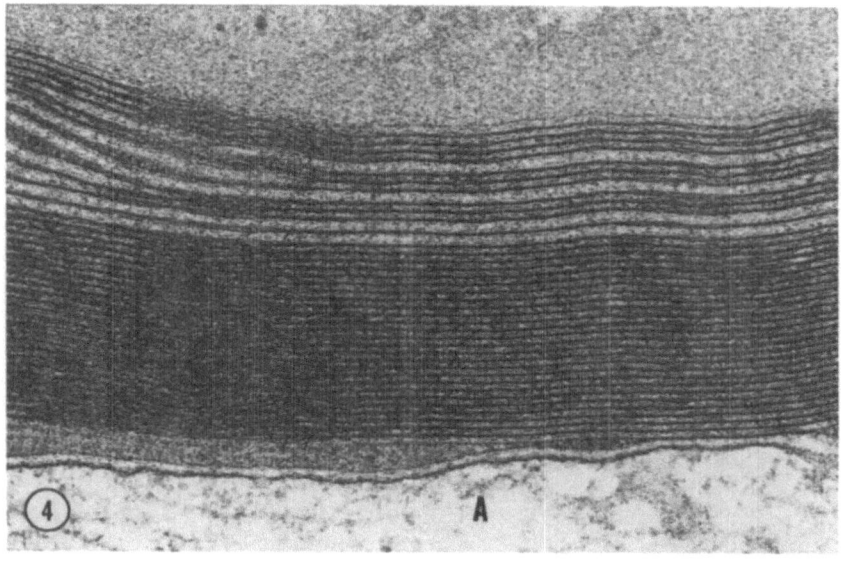

Figure 4: DRG culture, 14 days' exposure to heated EAN serum followed by 14 days' normal feeding. The myelin sheath shows an incomplete return to the normal periodicity. Axon at A. X 65,000.

DISCUSSION

    The present study, reported in full elsewhere (9), has demon-
strated that, like heated myelinotoxic EAE serum, potent heated EAN
serum causes a transformation of myelin into a swollen structure.
This transformation involved a doubling of its normal periodicity
and the appearance of 4 leaflets at the normally bifilar intraperiod
line. Apparently, therefore, some serum component is responsible
for this structural change. Recent immunocytochemical studies on
heated EAE serum and swollen CNS myelin in vitro have shown a concomitant binding of IgG in the position of the intraperiod line
(6). Whether the additional leaflets are structural entities or
some serum component precipitated by the preparative techniques is
not known.

    Exactly how complement-inactivated serum factors interact with
myelin and the myelinating cell is not known. The initial rapid
myelin swelling produced in the presence of whole serum might expose
previously concealed antigenic sites upon which anti-CNS antibodies
might then act. Evidently, the process of heating at 56°C for 30
min., a procedure believed to deplete C3a (10), is sufficient to
arrest the myelinolytic process at an early stage. Since local

macrophages fail to restore the serum to its potent state by producing C3 (11), it may be suggested that in some way, macrophages
in these cultures which began as embryonic tissue, may not have acquired or developed the capacity that mature macrophages possess
in vivo.

In CNS cultures exposed to complement-inactivated EAE serum,
oligodendroglia produce a profusion of aberrant processes while
simultaneously leaving naked many axons which would normally be
ensheathed (2,3). This caused us to speculate as to the possibility
that the immunologic factor responsible for this faulty myelination
had stimulated the myelinating oligodendroglia to elaborate myelin
but that the putative signal for ensheathing the axon had been
interrupted. A similar profusion of redundant myelin was not apparent in PNS explants exposed to heated EAN serum. However, evidence for hypermyelination, as suggested by thicker than normal
myelin sheaths, was sometimes encountered. The relative absence of
redundant aberrant myelin in PNS cultures in the present situation
might be related to the 1:1 relationship between Schwann cells and
myelin internodes. In the CNS, the oligodendrocyte is reputed to
maintain up to 50 internodes of myelin at some distance from the
cell body and the heavily committed myelinating cell might have
difficulty in adjusting the thickness of its internodes as more
myelin is formed. Consequently, there might be accumulation of
aberrant myelin not associated with axons in the CNS. However, in
the PNS, the Schwann cell can probably adjust more readily by modi-
fying the thickness of its single myelin sheath itself.

Previous studies on EAE serum demonstrated its specificity for
CNS tissue (1,12). EAN serum, on the other hand, affects both PNS
and CNS myelin. It is believed that this lack of specificity of
EAN serum is related to some antigens in PNS myelin being unique to
the PNS and others which are shared with CNS myelin. This aspect,
and the relevance of the present findings to previous PNS demyelinating studies in vitro and in vivo, have been discussed previously
(9).

The action of serum factors, specifically gammaglobulins, upon
peripheral myelin is not unprecedented. In the human peripheral
neuropathies associated with macrogammaglobulinemia (13-15) and
Waldenström's syndrome, the major described alterations have been
thicker than normal myelin sheaths (hypermyelination) and a dramatic increase in myelin periodicity - appearances virtually identical to those described here to occur in vitro. Whether the myelin
abnormalities in situ are related to binding of antibody to the
intraperiod line, as is apparently the case in vitro (6), remains
to be demonstrated. That the bound immunoglobulin in vitro might
be related to specific myelin antigen is likely but preliminary
studies in these and other laboratories indicate that myelin basic
protein alone is not implicated. The thickening of PNS fiber basal

laminae and the incomplete return of the normal myelin periodicity after removal of heated EAN serum, are probably also indicative of bound immunoglobulin, the specificity of which awaits clarification.

In conclusion, it appears that the demyelinating effect of anti-nervous system serum on nerve tissues in culture can be arrested at an early stage by inactivating complement that may be present in the nutrient medium. Some Schwann cells and oligodendroglia may simultaneously be stimulated to produce an excess of myelin. This represents one of the first demonstrations of possible interactions between the immune system and nervous system development and also suggests a combined immunological-tissue culture approach to the analysis of cell interactions in myelinogenesis.

ACKNOWLEDGMENTS

Supported in part by USPHS grants NS 08952 and NS 11920; and National Multiple Sclerosis Grant, RG 1001-B-12.

REFERENCES

1. Bornstein, M.B. and Raine, C.S. Lab. Invest. 35:391-401, 1976.
2. Raine, C.S., Diaz, M., Pakingan, M. and Bornstein, M.B. Lab. Invest. 38:397-403, 1978.
3. Diaz, M., Bornstein, M.B. and Raine, C.S. Brain Res. (in press).
4. Bornstein, M.B. and Appel, S.H. J. Neuropath. Exp. Neurol. 20:141-157, 1961.
5. Raine, C.S. and Bornstein, M.B. J. Neuropath. Exp. Neurol. 29:177-191, 1970.
6. Johnson, A.B., Raine, C.S. and Bornstein, M.B. Lab. Invest. (submitted).
7. Bornstein, M.B. In: Tissue Culture Methods and Applications, edited by P.F. Kruse, Jr. and M.K. Patterson, Jr., Academic Press, New York, pp. 86-92, 1973.
8. Raine, C.S. In: Progress in Neuropathology, Vol. 2, edited by H.M. Zimmerman, Grune and Stratton, New York, pp. 27-68, 1973.
9. Raine, C.S. and Bornstein, M. Lab. Invest. (submitted).
10. Alper, C.A. In: Structure and Function of Plasma Proteins, Vol. 1, edited by A.C. Allison, Plenum Press, New York, p. 202, 1974.
11. Allison, A.C. Immunol. Rev. 40:3-27, 1978.
12. Bornstein, M.B. and Raine, C.S. Neuropath. App. Neurobiol. 3:359-367, 1977.
13. Sluga, E. Wiener Klin. Wochenschr. 82:667, 1970.
14. Propp, R.P., Means, E., Deibel, R., Sherer, G. and Barron, K. Neurology (Minneap.) 25:980-988, 1975.
15. Julien, J., Vital, C., Vallat, J.-M., Lagueny, A., Deminiere, C. and Darriet, D. Arch. Neurol. 35:423-425, 1978.

THE ENHANCING EFFECT OF MULTIPLE SCLEROSIS BRAIN HOMOGENATES ON THE ACTIVE E ROSETTE FORMING LYMPHOCYTES

H. Offner, G. Konat, S.C. Rastogi, T. Fog, and J. Clausen

Neurochemical Institute, Copenhagen, Denmark

The ability of a lymphocyte to bind sheep red blood cells in the form of a rosette is one of the specific T-cell markers. A subpopulation of T-cells which possesses high affinity receptors for SRBC and forms rosettes rapidly is referred to as active E rosette.

The active E rosette test (AER) was adapted recently as an in vitro assay and correlated with the delayed hypersensitivity. In this assay, antigen sensitive T cells are measured by the in vitro exposure of lymphocytes to trace amounts of antigen. The increase in active E rosettes after antigenic stimulation is indicative of the sensitivity to the antigen. Hashim et al. (1) using AER test have shown the increased number of rosettes after basic protein stimulation of lymphocytes from guinea pigs with experimental allergic encephalomyelitis. Also a significant increase in the percent of active E rosettes was detected after in vitro exposure of lymphocytes from patients with multiple sclerosis and other neurological diseases to basic protein (2, 3).

Coded samples of peripheral blood from 42 MS patients and 96 other neurological patients were studied for their active rosette formation after antigenic stimulation with homogenates of MS and control brains.

PREPARATION OF BRAIN HOMOGENATE

3-4 g frontal and occipital lobe (both white and grey matter) from a brain were mixed and 25 % homogenate was prepared in 0.14 M sodium chloride. The homogenate was centrifuged (4°) for 25 min.

at 1000 g and the supernatant was used as an antigen for the assay.
Protein was determined by the method of Lowry et al. (4).

ACTIVE E ROSETTE TEST

The active E rosette forming cells were assayed by a modification of the method described elsewhere (5, 6, 7). Peripheral
lymphocytes were isolated employing lymphoprep (Nyegaard Co., Oslo)
gradient, washed twice with medium 199 and resuspended (4 x 10^6
cells/ml) in medium 199 containing fetal calf serum. Sheep red
blood cells (SRBC) in Alsevar's solution were washed three times
with medium 199 and suspended in medium 199 to a concentration of
1 % (v/v).

For each test, 0.25 ml lymphocyte suspensions were aliquoted
into glass tubes, mixed with 10 µl medium containing antigen dilutions and incubated for 15 min. at 22°C (Ag-AER). As a control,
lymphocyte suspensions 0.25 ml was incubated with 10 µl medium in
the absence of added antigen (AER). Following incubation, 0.25 ml
SRBC were added and cells centrifuged at 200 g for 3 min. The
pellet, immediately, was resuspended and counted. A lymphocyte
was classified as an active E rosette if three or more SRBC adhered
to its surface. Each sample was run in duplicate and at least
300 cells were counted in each slide. Cell viability determined
by Trypan blue exclusion was always more than 90 %.

To overcome a technical problem of resuspension of lymphocyte
E rosettes we designed a simple apparatus (Fig. 1). The apparatus
consists of cylindrical tubes holder (with 6 positions) which is
subjected to a combined, swinging rotation motion by a system of
2 synchronous electrical motors. The holder swings vertically
up and down in the plane of its axis from horizontal position to
about 22 degree. By means of gearbox the motion of the holder
is set to 12 full swings and one rotation per minute. The resus
pension time of 3 min. was found to be most satisfactory.

Statistical evaluation was performed by calculating standard
deviation and level of significance by Student's T-test and "chi-
square" test.

Dose-response experiments were performed to determine the
optimum concentration of antigen for use in assay. The dose of
MS brain supernatant giving the maximum increase in AER after 15
min. incubation with MS lymphocytes was 2.3 µg protein/0.25 ml.
Significant but lesser increase were also observed with 23 µg and
0.23 µg as compared to unstimulated lymphocytes.

The results are expressed as ratios of the average antigen
stimulated AER over non stimulated cells from the same patient.

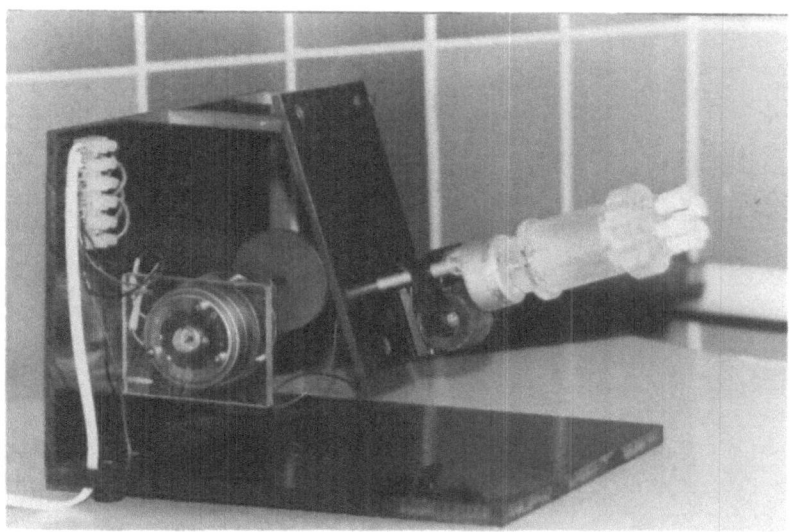

Fig. 1. Apparatus for resuspension of lymphocyte E rosettes.

Lymphocytes from MS and ON patients were tested against 8 brain homogenates (4 controls and 4 MS).

The results are expressed as ratios of the average antigen stimulated active E rosettes (Ag-AER) over non-stimulated lymphocytes from the same patient (AER). Changes in AER greater than 15 % of the control value after antigen stimulation were considered as positive.

Of 34 patients with definite diagnosis of MS, 30 showed ratio Ag-AER/AER higher than 1.15, when their lymphocytes were incubated with MS brain homogenate (mean 1.40 + 0.20) (Table 1). Four MS patients gave negative results. Of 2 probable MS cases, 1 was positive in AER test (mean 1.26). Of 6 possible MS patients, 6 were positive (mean 1.31). Four MS patients responded also to control brain, but the response was lower that that to MS brain. The difference between Ag-AER/AER of MS lymphocytes with MS and control antigen was significant at the level p<0.001. The Ag-AER/AER ratio for neurological controls was 1.11 + 0.39 and 1.10 + 0.42 with MS and control brain respectively. Of 96 neurological patients, 7 responded to MS antigen and 8 to control antigen in AER test. Response of 4 OND was higher with MS brain than with control brain. These 4 cases were more or less severe Lymphocytes from patients with multiple sclerosis and other neurological disorders incubated for 15 min. at 22°C with 2.3 µg pro-

TABLE 1

Subjects	Ag-AER/AER with MS antigen	Positive response	Ag-AER/AER with control antigen	Positive response
MS Definite (34)	1.40+0.20	30 (88%)	1.07+0.21	3 (8.8%)
MS Probable (2)	1.26	1 (50%)	1.08	0 (0%)
MS Possible (6)	1.31+0.15	6 (100%)	1.03+0.10	1 (16.6%)
Other neuro- (96) logical	1.11+0.39	7 (7.3%)	1.10+0.42	8 (8.3%)

tein/0.25ml of MS and control brains and assayed for AER. The
ratio is calculated from the formula Ag-AER/AER and represents the
mean + SD.

alcoholics. The difference between Ag-AER/AER ratio of MS and
OND with MS antigen was significant at the level p < 0.001.

The present results indicate the existence of an antigen in
MS brains to which lymphocytes of MS patients responded in active
E rosette test. The assay requires minimal amount of material
and blood and no sophisticated laboratory equipment. The test is
rapid and can be completed in one day. The apparatus for resuspension of E rosettes has proved a standardized and reproducible
method and reduces the source of error in the test. This immunological test is not a "specific MS reaction", however, the majority of MS cases are positive. In this way this test together
with other laboratory and clinical approximations to the diagnosis (spinal fluid, periphlebitis retinae, evoked potentials) may
be an important aid in the diagnostic armentary. Further studies
in patients with hepatic disease may possibly contribute to an
explanation, why young alcoholics show this anomaly. Furthermore
cases of neuroimmunological diseases, lupus erythematosus disease, Guillain-Barré will be studied as well as the possible influence of corticoids or other immunosuppressive drugs will be explored.

Further, our preliminary results (on 17 MS and 16 OND patients) indicate that there are two antigens in brain homogenates
to which MS patients respond in the AER-test. One is identical
with myelin BP. The second is purified 3000X but is still unidentified. Purification and concentration was achieved by filtration
of brain cytosole on millipore and molecular filters. One antigen
was found in the 25000 filtrate and was identical to myelin BP.

The other antigen had a molecular weight between 10^5 - 10^6 daltons. It could be eluted as a second peak on a DEAE-cellulose column (Rastogi et al., preceeding paper).

Using myelin crude BP as the antigen, the dose response curve showed a maximum response at 0.1-5.0 pg of antigen/test. With MS myelin BP, lymphocytes from MS patients showed a positive response in all of the cases, compared with 40% of OND patients. With myelin crude BP from control brains, MS patients were 75% positive and OND were again 40% positive. However, there was a marked difference between MS patients and controls, the optimum response of MS lymphocytes to MS BP was obtained at a much lower concentration than their response to control BP (some 10 x lower) whereas control lymphocytes achieved their optimum responses with the same concentration of both antigens.

Using peak 2 as an antigen, so far, only MS patients (except one with amyotrophic lateral sclerosis) have shown a response. Optimal antigen concentration in the AER-Test was 1-50pg. Tandem crossed immunoelectrophoresis of MS peak 2 and MS myelin BP versus anti MS brain cytosole absorbed with control peak 2 revealed that one of the two arcs present in peak 2 fused with one of the 2 arcs for MS BP. This may explain why MS BP reacts at lower concentration and in all MS patients as compared with control BP. It seems probable that there are two antigens in crude MS BP, one of these BP and the other is also contained in MS peak 2. In control BP however, there is only one antigen which is BP.

The nature of the peak 2 antigens in MS has not yet been determined. It is presumably an abnormal protein of high molecular weight which may be a brain protein modified by viral infection or by demyelination process.

REFERENCES

1. Hashim, G.A., Lee, D.H., Pierce, J.C. : Neurochem. Res. 2, 99-109 (1977).
2. Hashim, G.A., Lee, D.H., Pierce, J.C., Braun, C.W., Fitzpatrick, H.F. : Neurochem. Res. 3, 37-48 (1978).
3. Offner, H., Rastogi, S.C., Konat, G., Clausen, J. : J. Neurol. in Press (1978).
4. Lowry, O.H., Rosebrough, N.J., Farr, A.L. and Rundall, F.J. : J. Biol. Chem. 193, 265-271 (1951).
5. Smith, R., Kerman, R., Ezdinli, E. and Stefani, S. : J. Immunol. Methods 8, 175-184 (1975).
6. Felsburg, P.J., Edelman, R. Immunology 118, 618-629 (1977).
7. Offner, H., Konat, G., Raun, N.E., Clausen, J. : Acta Neurol. Scand. 57, 380-384 (1978).

FURTHER STUDIES ON THE ELUTION OF IMMUNOGLOBULIN FROM MULTIPLE SCLEROSIS BRAIN

D. Gilden and T. Tachovsky

Multiple Sclerosis Research Center of the Wistar Institute and Department of Neurology, University of Pennsylvania, Philadelphia, Pa, U.S.A.

ABSTRACT

Multiple sclerosis (MS) and control brain slices were repeatedly washed with phosphate buffered saline (PBS) then treated for 90 seconds with an acetic acid solution pH 2.5 with citrate-phosphate-borate buffers ranging in pH from 2.2 to 11.6. The protein concentrations of PBS washes and neutralized eluates were determined, and the eluates were assayed for Ig by competition microradioimmunoassay using rabbit anti-human $F(ab')_2$. Successive PBS washes reduced extracellular protein to a very low level. Equivalent quantities of protein were recovered from seven MS and six non-MS brain samples after both PBS washing and acetic acid elution. However, the amount of protein needed for 50% inhibition of ^{125}I-IgG binding to anti-human $F(ab')_2$ was less than 25 μg/ml in 7 of 9 samples of MS brain tissue in contrast to 3 of 12 samples of non-MS brain. Myelin basic protein did not inhibit the competition of unlabelled IgG with ^{125}I-IgG for anti-human $F(ab')_2$; IgG was a more effective competitor than IgA or IgM. It was possible to elute Ig from human brain at various pHs ranging from 2.2 to 11.6. At pHs 5.2 and 8.5, the distinction between MS and normal brain as determined by elution of Ig was greatest.

INTRODUCTION

There is satisfactory evidence that immunoglobulin (Ig) is present in multiple sclerosis (MS) brain (1, 2, 3). However, this Ig has not yet been isolated for chemical and biological analysis. This is partly due to the paucity of unfixed MS brain

481

tissue available for study. Also, because it is not possible to routine perfuse human brain in situ, material eluted from homogenized brain tissue is not likely to be free of serum protein.

Nevertheless, Link found discrete gamma bands by agar gel electrophoresis in 6 of 10 water-soluble brain protein preparations, and IgG was isolated by ion exchange chromatography and gel filtration (4). Increased concentrations of IgG and IgA and a significant difference in the ratio of these two Ig to albumin were found in MS brain compared with controls that included two Jakob-Creutzfeldt diseases brains.

Vandvik later demonstrated oligoclonal measles virus-specific IgG in cerebrospinal fluid (CSF), brain extracts and sera from patients with subacute sclerosing panencephalitis and MS (5). An increase of oligoclonal IgG after absorption-elution with measles virus antigens was seen in a brain plaque extract from one MS brain but not in six of the MS CSF samples studied. Bands of IgG were detected in the eluates from the MS brain homogenates and four of the MS CSF samples.

Using immunofluorescent technique, Simpson et al. originally demonstrated that IgG in MS brain is both cell-bound and extracellular (1). Much, but not all, of the specific immunofluorescence was quenched by repeated brain washing. The quantity of extracellular Ig is greater than cell-bound Ig due to the large quantities of Ig in the serum.

Initial efforts were designed to demonstrate removal of cell-surface Ig from human brain. The technique devised was artificial absorption of antibody against 2-4 dinitrophenol (DNP) to hapten-conjugated brain and elution of the antibody at pH 2.5 (6). Less than 1 ng of anti-DNP antibody could be eluted and detected. Similar techniques were then applied directly to MS and control brain tissue, and a significant difference was demonstrated in the Ig eluted from MS compared with control brain (7). Further studies, including an attempt to determine the optimum pH for elution, are described in this paper.

MATERIALS AND METHODS

Preparation and Elution of Brain Tissue

In all but one experiment, 10 g of grossly normal subcortical white matter (WM) was dissected from both MS and control (normal or non-MS neurologically diseases) human brain. Seven brains were from cases of pathologically proven MS, one from a patient with Jakob Creutzfeldt disease, and five from humans who died after trauma or drug intoxication. Razor thin slices were hand cut from the entire mass. The sliced tissue was placed in Petri dishes and washed using 5 liters of phosphate-buffered saline (PBS) pH 7.1, and finally rinsed in 3 ml of PBS. The 3-ml rinse was labelled "PBS wash" and kept at 4°C and then assayed for Ig. The brain tissue was then washed for 90 seconds in 3 ml of 0.5 M a ic acid, pH 2.5, containing Pepstatin 50 ug/ml (to preserve brain tissue form enzymatic digestion) (8) and 0.004 M epsilon aminocaproic acid. The eluate was immediately neutralized with 0.3 - 0.4 ml of 6 M K_2CO_3.

In one experiment, 8-5 g sections of WM were cut from both MS and normal brain, and following PBS washing, brain tissue was treated with citrate-phosphate-borate buffers ranging in pH from 2.2 to 11.6, and containing Pepstatin and epsilon aminocaproic acid as described above. The elution was repeated three times. All eluates were maintained at 4°C until assayed for Ig. Protein concentrations were determined by the method of Lowry et al. (9).

Antiserum

In order to facilitate assay of all isotypes, hyperimmune serum to $F(ab')_2$ fragment of human IgG was prepared in rabbits and kindly supplied by Dr. Walter Gerhard of the Wistar Institute. The globulin fraction of this serum was prepared by precipitation with 50% ammonium sulfate.

Myelin Basic Protein

Myelin basic protein that had been extracted from human cerebellum using established methods (10, 11) was kindly supplied by Dr. Sheldon Miller of the Wistar Institute. This material gave a single band on SDS-polyacrylamide gel electrophoresis.

Human Immunoglobulin

Human IgG was prepared from outdated whole blood by precipitation with ammonium sulfate at 50% of saturation. The IgG was then isolated by chromatography on DEAE-cellulose (DE52, Whatman) equilibrated with 0.005 M KPO_4 buffer, pH 7.9. The purified IgG was rendered 7S by centrifugation at 100,000 x g for 90 minutes; the upper one-third of the sample in the centrifuge tube was removed and labelled 7S IgG. A single batch of IgG was used for all the experiments described. The IgG was labelled with $Na^{125}I$ by the Chloramine T method (12). IgM was purchased from Cappel Laboratories, Dowingtown, Pa., and chromatographed on Sepharose 4B (Pharmacia) prior to use. IgA was purchased from Calbiochem and chromatographed in Sephacryl S-200 (Pharmacia) prior to use.

Competitive Microradioimmunoassay

All specimens were coded in double blind fashion before testing. The microradioimmunoassay was performed with minor modification as described by Rosenthal et al. (13). One hundred μl of a 1:2500 dilution of rabbit anti-human $F(ab')_2$ of IgG in Barbital buffer (μ=0.2), pH 8.6, was added to wells of polyvinyl microtiter plates (Cooke Engineering Company, Alexandria, Va.), and the plates were incubated overnight at $4°C$. The antiserum was removed by inversion of the plate, and 200 μl of a 1% bovine serum albumin (BSA) solution in barbital buffer was added. The plates were incubated an additional 90 minutes at room temperature; immediately prior to use the plates were inverted to remove the BSA solution.

Brain eluates were clarified by centrifugation at 8000 x g for 2 minutes in a Brinkmann microfuge before use. Brain eluates, IgG, and competing substances were then diluted in 0.01 M KPO_4 buffer, pH 7.5, containing 0.15 M NaCl, 0.01 M NaN_3 and 0.1% (W/V) BSA. Fifty μl of either eluate, IgG, or other competing substances (IgA, IgM or myelin basic protein) was added to triplicate wells, and immediately thereafter 50 μl of ^{125}I-labelled IgG (specific activity 10 μCi/μg, 10,000 cpm/well) was added. After 4 hours at room temperature, the plates were inverted and rinsed three times with the diluting buffer. The wells were then removed separately and counted in an intertechnique gamma spectrometer. A standard inhibition curve using unlabelled IgG was performed in each assay. Fifty percent inhibition of binding for all experiments was always between 5 to 15 ng/well.

Calculations

Results of the competition microradioimmunoassay were normalized and plotted as protein concentration vs. percent inhibition of binding; 50% inhibition values were read directly from the curves. The percent Ig was calculated by dividing the concentration of brain eluate necessary for 50% inhibition of binding by the concentration of 7S IgG necessary for 50 % inhibition of binding in a standard curve. In some experiments, limiting dilutions of brain washes and eluates failed to reach zero percent inhibition. Thus, the percent inhibition was normalized by averaging the values obtained at a protein concentration of 1 μg/ml. The percent inhibition was then calculated by substracting the average percent inhibition at 1 μg/ml from the maximum binding value and dividing the experimental value by this new normalized maximum binding value.

RESULTS

Maximum binding of ^{125}I-human IgG to rabbit anti-human F(ab')$_2$ occurred at a 1:2500 dilution of the rabbit gamma globulin; 75% of the input counts were bound to the polyvinyl wells.

In each experiment, a standard inhibition curve was performed. Concentrations of unlabelled 7S human IgG necessary to inhibit 50% of binding of ^{125}I-human IgG to rabbit anti-human F(ab')$_2$ ranged from 5 to 15 ng/well.

In order to establish that washing of brain slices with large amounts of PBS had successfully removed extracellular protein, and had not selectively removed protein from either MS or non-MS brain, in some experiments tissue slices were washed five times with 1 liter of PBS each time. After each 1-liter wash, the tissue was suspended in 3 ml of PBS. The PBS was then removed and labelled "PBS wash", and the brain tissue was washed three times with 3 ml of 0.5 M acetic acid, pH 2.5. The protein concentrations of PBS washes and acid eluates of samples from two different non-MS and one MS brain are shown as example in Table 1. Equivalent quantities of protein were recovered after PBS washing from both MS and non-MS brain. Successive PBS washes resulted in a diminution in the amount of protein recovered in the 3-ml samples. After acetic acid elution of both MS and non-MS brain, the concentration of protein increased. Again, there was little difference in the concentration of protein eluted from either MS or non-MS brain (Table 1).

Repeated PBS washings reduced the inhibitory activity of both MS and non-MS brains in the competitive microradioimmunoassay to a low but constant level (data not shown). Acetic acid washes, on the other hand, contained measurable amounts of Ig. Figure 1 shows the μg/ml of protein needed for 50% inhibition of ^{125}I-IgG binding to anti-human F(ab')$_2$. Seven different MS brains and six different non-MS brains were sampled in nine experiments. The amount of protein needed for 50% inhibition was less than 25 μg/ml in 7 of 9 MS brain samples as contrasted to 3 of 12 non-MS brain samples. Some MS and non-MS brains were used more than once. This was to see if different WM areas of the same brain contained similar amounts of cell-bound Ig. Equivalent quantities of Ig were eluted from different areas of MS and non-MS brain tested more than once (data not shown).

At a concentration of 350 μg/ml, myelin basic protein did not significantly inhibit the ability of unlabelled IgG to compete with labelled 7S IgG for rabbit anti-human F(ab')$_2$ (Figure 2).

The amount of unlabelled IgG necessary to provide 50% inhibition of ^{125}I-IgG to rabbit anti-human F(ab')$_2$ ranged from 150-250

Table 1. Protein concentration of material obtained by washing
          human brain with PBS and acetic acid.

μg Protein/ml

PBS Wash	Normal Brain 1	Normal Brain 2	Normal Brain 1
1	363	667	587
2	171	165	416
3	117	138	197
4	90	76	187
5	76	65	114

Acid Eluate

1	1098	886	1485
2	1111	1153	1549
3	1455	1884	1527

ng/ml. On the other hand, 2000 ng/ml of IgA and 7000 ng/ml of
IgM were necessary to provide 50% inhibition of labelled IgG to
anti-human F(ab')$_2$ (Figure 3). This indicates that IgG is the
primary protein in our brain eluates because huge amounts of IgA
or IgM would be needed for 50% inhibition.

Figure 4 demonstrates the influence of various pHs on the
elution of Ig from MS and non-MS brain. After repeated PBS
washings, three consecutive washes at various pHs in the range
of 2.2 to 11.6 were applied to both MS and control brain. At
each pH, the amount of eluted material necessary to inhibit binding of ^{125}I-IgG to anti-human F(ab')$_2$ was less for MS than non-
MS brain. In the first eluate obtained at pHs 5.2 and 8.5, the
greatest difference between MS and non-MS brain was seen.

DISCUSSION

These studies indicate that repeated washing of human brain
results in rapid removal of equivalent quantities of protein from
both MS and control brain tissue. Serial PBS washings decreased
protein concentration in brain tissue to a low level, and subsequent acetic acid washings led to an increase in protein concentration that was again equivalent in both MS and control brains. The
critical finding, however, was that the amount of Ig in MS brain
after elution with acetic acid was significantly greater than that
in control brains when seven MS brains were compared with six
non-MS brains. The finding that different WM areas from the same
MS brain or the same non-MS brain contained similar amounts of cel
bound Ig confirms the reproducibility of the technique described.

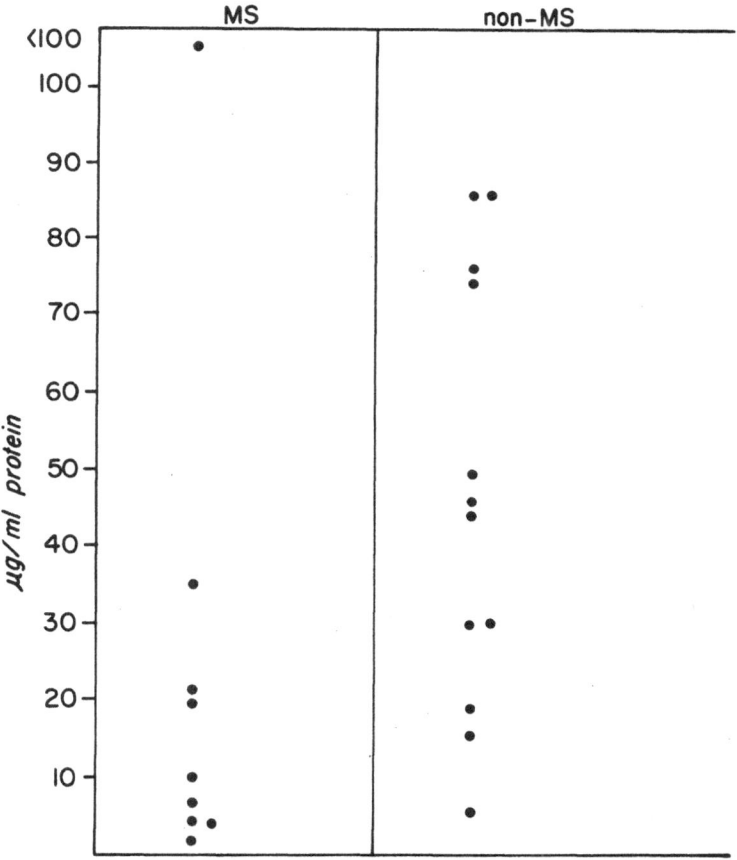

Figure 1. Protein concentrations of eluates from human brain needed for 50% inhibition of ^{125}I-IgG binding to anti-human F(ab')$_2$.

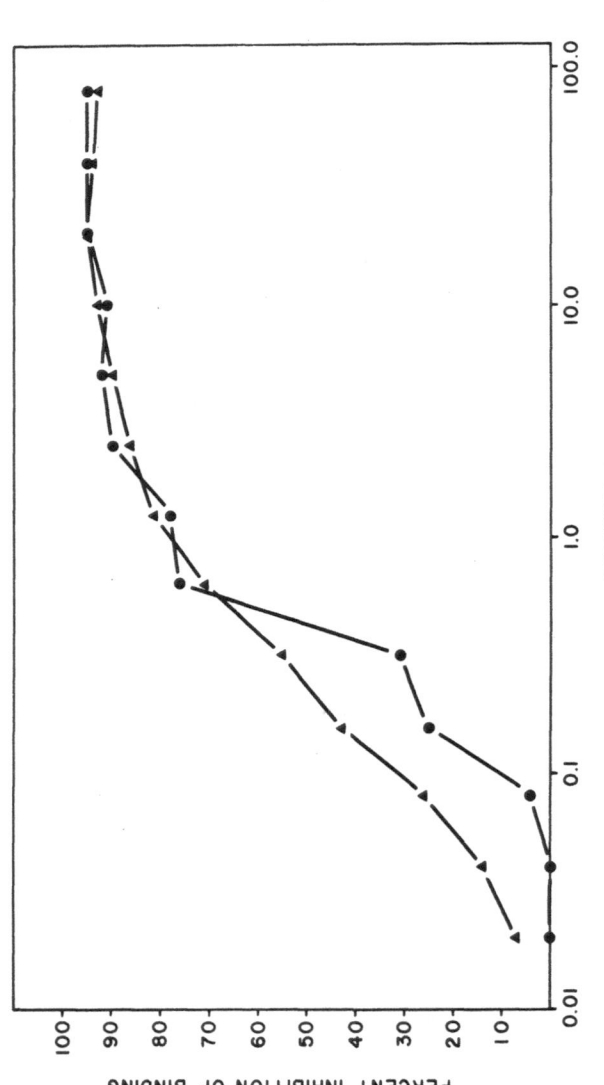

Figure 2. Inhibition of binding of ^{125}I-7S IgG to anti-human F(ab')$_2$ in the presence (●) and absence (▲) of human myelin basic protein (350 μg/ml).

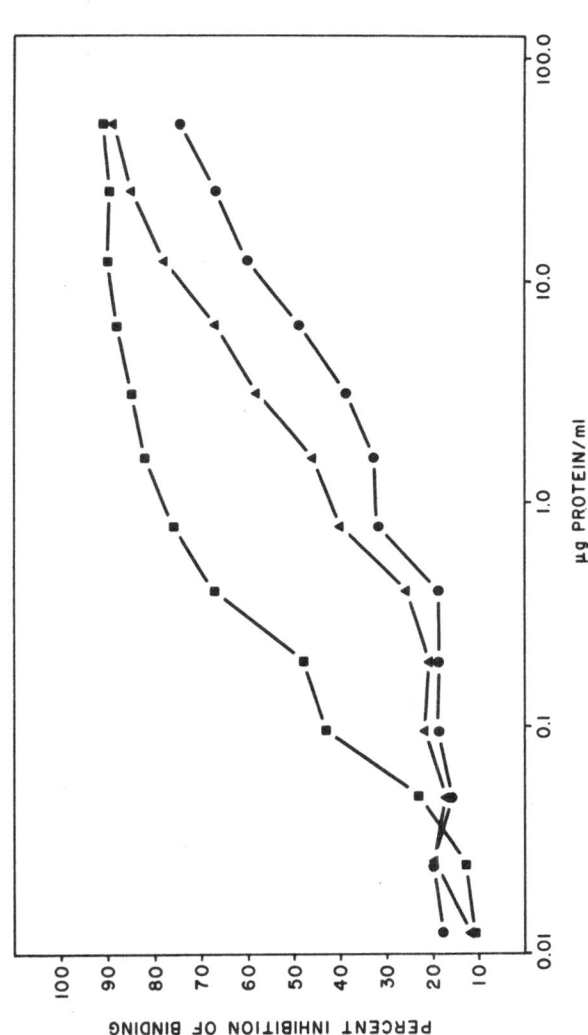

Figure 3. Inhibition of binding of ^{125}I-7S IgG to anti-human F(ab')$_2$ by IgG ■; IgA ▲; and IgM ●.

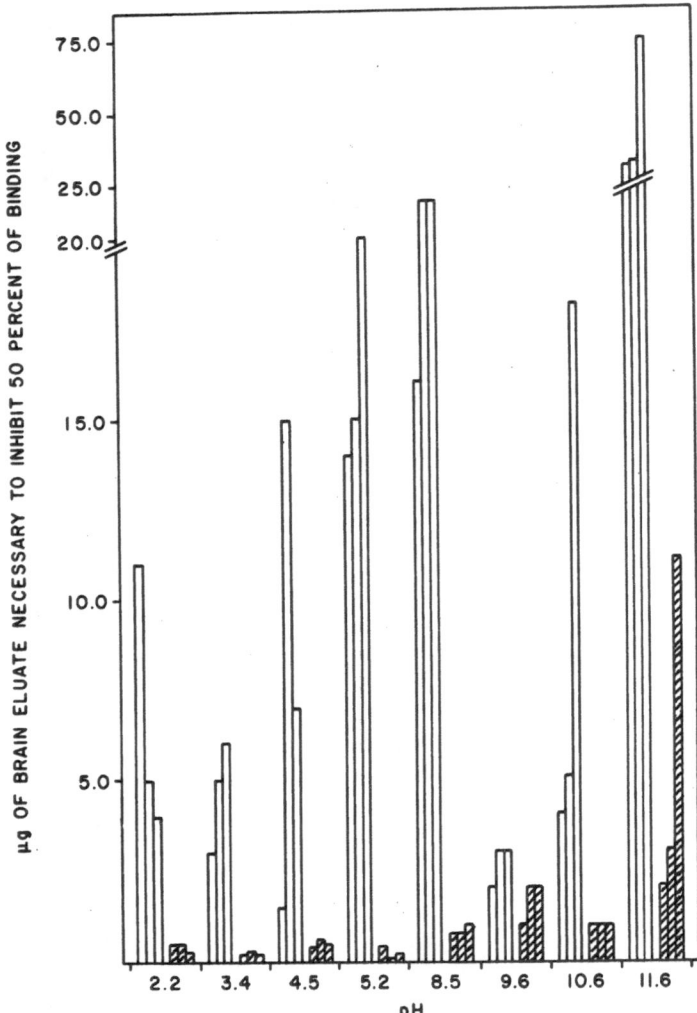

Figure 4. Protein concentrations needed for 50% inhibition of
^{125}I-IgG binding to anti-human F(ab')$_2$. Material was obtained
from three consecutive elutions of human brain at pHs ranging
from 2.2 to 11.6. MS brain ▨. Normal brain ▭.

In the standard competition assay 150-250 ng/ml of unlabelled IgG was necessary to give 50% inhibition of binding of labelled IgG to anti-human $F(ab')_2$, whereas much larger quantities of IgA (2000 ng/ml) and IgM (7000 ng/ml) were necessary for 50% inhibition. This indicates that the primary protein in our brain eluates is IgG because relatively small quantities of the eluate were able to achieve 50% inhibition of binding. Moreover, the finding that the addition to unlabelled IgG of myelin basic protein at a concentration of 350 μg/ml did not significantly alter the inhibition curve indicates that the assay is detecting competing IgG and not "sticky" basic protein. This is important since myelin basic protein is well known to be extracted from human brain under acid conditions (10). However, further, more direct studies are needed to determine the exact composition of the eluted material.

The elution of cell-bound Ig from MS brain in these studies cannot be emphasized too strongly. There have been two prior attempts to extract Ig from MS brain. Link's technique for preparation of water-soluble brain protein was homogenization at 4°C of thawed brain tissue in 0.25 M sucrose (4). No attempt was made to remove serum proteins from brain tissue before homogenization. Vandvik removed oligoclonal IgG from an MS brain extract after absorption with measles antigen (5). Unfortunately, the details for concentrating the brain extract plaque material from the MS patient were not reported.

The spectrum of cell-bound Ig contained in eluted material remains to be determined. Antibody to whole brain, myelin, basic protein, oligodendrocyte surface antigen, and a number of viruses have long been suspected of being part of the IgG found in MS CSF. Elution of this quantity of protein will facilitate immunochemical and biological characterization of the material. Comparison of the Ig eluted from MS brain with the IgG found in the CSF of the same and different MS patients can also be undertaken. Refinements in the elution procedure may enhance the amount stability of protein extracted. Preliminary experiments in this study already indicate that at a pH close to neutrality (pH 5.2 and 8.5) the widest discrepancy between MS and normal brain, as determined by elution of Ig, occurs. The pHs are likely to be less harsh to eluted protein and are easier to neutralize immediately after elution thus preserving antibody integrity (14).

ACKNOWLEDGEMENTS

This study was supported by Public Health Service research grant NS 11036, National Institute of Neurological Diseases and Stroke, and by a grant from the National Multiple Sclerosis Society.

The authors wish to thank Mary Devlin, Mary Wellish, Vincent Palusci, and Mark Erikson for their expert technical assistance, Barbara Cohen for her editorial assistance, and Barbara Tillman for her help in the preparation of the manuscript.

REFERENCES

1. Simpson, J.F., Tourtellotte, W.W. and Kokmen E. et al. (1969). Fluorescent protein tracing in multiple sclerosis brain tissue. Arch. Neurol. 20:373-377.
2. Lumsden, C.E. (1971). The immunogenesis of the multiple sclerosis plaque. Brain Res. 28, 365-390.
3. Esiri, M.M. (1977). Immunoglobulin-containing cells in multiple-sclerosis plaques. Lancet ii:478-480.
4. Link, H. (1972). Oligoclonal immunoglobulin G in multiple sclerosis brains. J. Neurol. Sci. 16:103-114.
5. Vandvik, B., Norrby, E., Nordal, H.J. and Degre, M. (1976). Oligoclonal measles virus-specific IgG antibodies isolated from cerebrospinal fluids, brain extracts, and sera from patients with subacute sclerosing panencephalitis and multiple sclerosis. Scand. J. Immunol. 5:979-992.
6. Gilden, D.H., Devlin, M. and Wroblewska, Z. (1978). A technique for the elution of cell-surface antibody from human brain tissue. Ann. Neurol. 3:403-405.
7. Gilden, D.H. and Tachovsky, T. Immunoglobulin elution from multiple sclerosis brain. Submitted for publication.
8. Marks, N., Grynbaum, A. and Lajtha, A. (1973). Pentapeptide (Pepstatin) inhibition of brain acid proteinase. Sci. 181: 949-951.
9. Lowry, O.H., Rosebrough, N.J., Farr, A.L. and Randall, R.J. (1951). Protein measurement with the Folin phenol reagent. J. Biol. Chem. 193:265-275.
10. Eylar, E.H., Salk, J., Beveridge, G.C. and Brown, L.V. (1969). Experimental allergic encephalomyelitis: an encephalitogenic basic protein from bovine myelin. Arch. Biochem. Biophys. 132:34-48.
11. Oshiro, Y. and Eylar, E.H. (1970). Allergic encephalomyelitis. Preparation of the encephalitogenic basic protein from bovine brain. Arch. Biochem. Biophys. 138:392-398.
12. McConahey, P.J. and Dixon, F.J. (1966). A method of trace iodination of proteins for immunologic studies. Int. Arch. Allergy Appl. Immunol. 29:185-189.
13. Rosenthal, J.D., Hayashi, K. and Notkins, A.L. (1973). Comparison of direct and indirect solid-phase microradioimmuno-assays for the detection of viral antigens and anti-viral antibody. Appl. Micro. 25:567-573.
14. Ruoslahti, E. (1976). "Antigen-antibody interaction, antibody affinity, and dissociation of immune complexes". Scand. J. Immunol. Suppl. 3:3-7.

INTERACTIONS OF VACCINIA VIRUS WITH THE MYELIN MEMBRANE

A.J.Steck
Department of Neurology, University Hospital Center,
Lausanne, Switzerland

R. Tschannen and R. Schäfer
Department of Structure, Biocentrum Basel University,
Basel, Switzerland

Vaccinia virus belongs to a group of viruses associated with post-infectious encephalomyelitis, a condition which shows similarities with the one of experimental allergic encephalomyelitis, though the mechanism for this is poorly understood (1).

It has been suggested that direct viral effects as well as immunological factors have a role in the pathogenesis of virus induced demyelination. We have recently demonstrated as an in vitro model for a specific interaction of vaccinia virus cores with myelin membranes that the myelin basic protein was phosphorylated by the protein kinase located in the viral core (2). In the present paper we present evidence suggesting that purified vaccinia virus which was grown in mouse brain contains myelin basic protein.

Mice were injected intracranially with the neurotropic strain of vaccinia virus (WR). The animals which received $10^4 - 10^8$ p. f.u. died between the third and the sixth day whereas the animals which received 10^2 p.f.u. survived. After determination of virus p.f.u. in brain homogenate of dead animals it turned out that an optimal virus replication occurred in the mouse brain with an inoculum of 10^4 p.f.u. A gradual increase of titer was also found over three passages with an increase of almost 200 times over the first passage. The amount of virus produced in mouse brain after the third passage (2.5×10^9 p.f.u. / mouse brain) served as a basis to purify vaccinia virus from mouse brain in a milligram range.

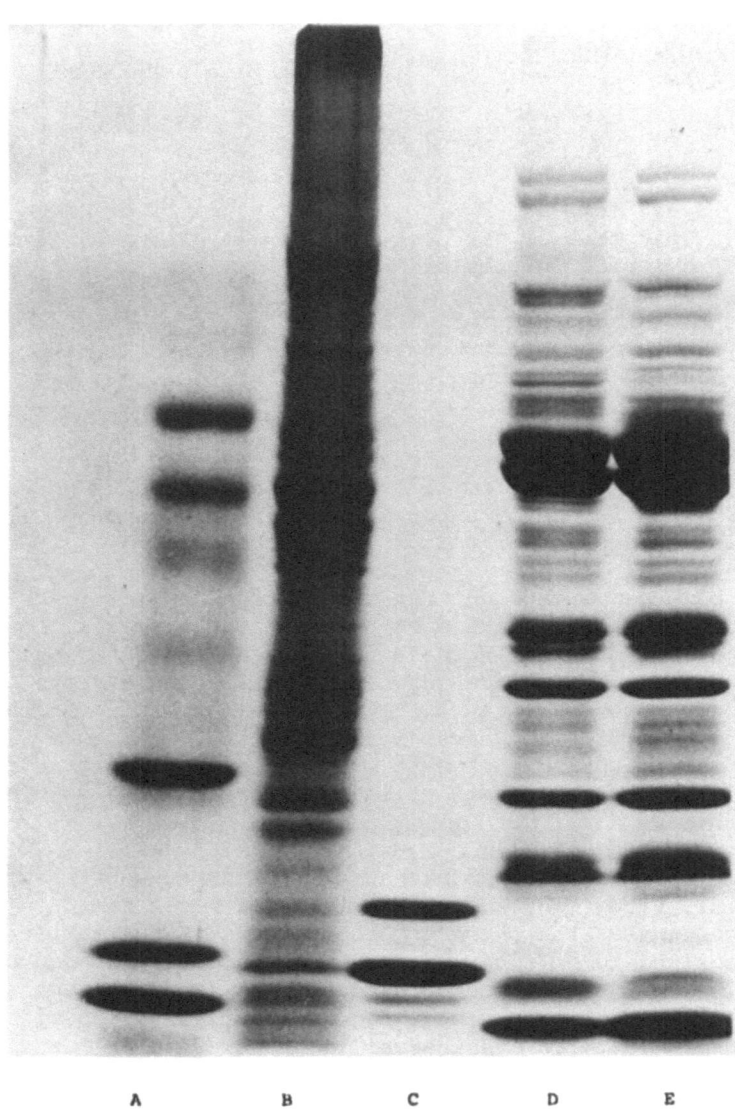

Figure 1

Figure 1 (see p.494)

Polyacrylamide gel electrophoresis of purified vaccinia virus from mouse brain and fibroblasts.

Electrophoresis on 7.5-15% polyacrylamide slab gels in the presence of sodium dodecyl sulfate. Myelin was purified from pooled mouse brain according to Norton (5) and myelin basic protein according to Oshiro et al. (6).
(A-E from left to right)
A : marker proteins : cytochrome C (MW = 12.400), myoglobin (MW = 17.800), chymotrypsinogen A (MW = 25.000), ovalbumin (MW = 45.000), albumin (MW = 67.000), immunoglobulin G (MW = 80.000 in the presence of 2-mercaptoethanol).
B : vaccinia virus grown in mouse brain.
C : myelin basic protein purified from mouse brain (the two main bands represent the two species of myelin basic protein present in mouse brain).
D : vaccinia virus grown on fibroblasts and mixed with mouse brain homogenate.
E : vaccinia virus grown on fibroblasts.

Table 1

Displacement of I^{125}-labeled myelin basic protein from its antibody by unlabeled myelin basic protein

Preparation	$\%^{125}I$-basic protein bound to antibody
dissociated virus grown on fibroblasts	62
dissociated virus grown on fibroblasts and mixed with mouse brain homogenate	63
undissociated virus grown on mouse brain	54
dissociated virus grown on mouse brain	30
unlabeled myelin basic protein	35
control (I^{125}myelin basic protein)	61

The preparation of antisera and the radioimmunoassay with myelin basic protein in the range of nanograms were carried out as described by Cohen et al. (7) with slight modifications.

Virus was purified by a combination of the procedures described by Dales et al. (3) and Joklik (4). As controls, virus grown on fibroblasts and virus grown on fibroblasts and mixed with mouse brain homogenate were purified by the same procedure. These three different virus preparations were analysed by polyacrylamide slab gel electrophoresis in the presence of sodium dodecyl sulfate (Fig. 1). Virus grown on fibroblasts and virus grown on fibroblasts and mixed with mouse brain homogenate contained an identical polypeptide composition whereas virus grown in mouse brain was different but clearly included polypeptide bands which migrate with the same mobility as purified myelin basic proteins. The identification of these polypeptides in the virus which comigrated with myelin basic proteins was performed by radioimmunoassay.

The three different virus preparations described above were dissociated in the presence of 2% sodium deoxycholate and 2% Triton X-100 and incubated for 5 minutes at 90°C for use in the radioimmunoassay (Table 1). Dissociated vaccinia virus grown on fibroblasts and dissociated virus grown on fibroblasts and mixed before purification with mouse brain homogenate did not contain myelin basic protein whereas dissociated virus which was grown in mouse brain contained myelin basic protein. Undissociated virus which was grown in mouse brain showed a much smaller displacement of I^{125}- labeled myelin basic protein when compared with dissociated virus. This supports the assumption that the myelin basic protein is incorporated into the virions and not merely absorbed on its surface.

Regarding the pathogenic mechanisms during postinfectious encephalomyelitis we draw the following conclusions. The virus is known to have a high affinity to mesenchymal cells, the place of rapid multiplication and the semi-permissivity of some glial cells is expressed by the presence of the myelin basic protein in the virus. This acute infection is accompanied by an inflammatory reaction consisting of a perivascular accumulation of mononuclear cells, mostly lymphocytes and macrophages. The overall impact of these inflammatory cells is rather complex but the resulting clearance of the virus containing myelin basic protein by macrophages may then allow the presentation of the myelin basic protein in an immunogenic form to T lymphocytes. In preliminary experiments we found that virus grown and isolated from mouse brains, inactivated by UV-irradiation, and injected intravenously into mice in the absence of Freund's adjuvant induced a disease which was clinically similar to the experimental allergic encephalomyelitis induced with myelin basic protein in Freund's adjuvant.

In conclusion the available evidence suggests an association of vaccinia virus with the myelin membrane after intracranial injection and supports the concept that this membrane might be modified following a viral infection. The possibility that the virus may also act on the immune system to amplify the autoimmune response as an adjuvant is an intriguing problem which merits further investigation.

ACKNOWLEDGEMENTS

This research was supported by grant 3.574.075 from the Swiss National Science Foundation and a fund from the Swiss Multiple Sclerosis Society.

REFERENCES

1. Harter, D.H. and Choppin, P.W. In Rowland L.P. (ed) Immunological disorders of the nervous system. Baltimore, The Williams and Wilkins Company, 1971, pp. 342-355.
2. Steck, A.J., Siegrist, P., Herschkowitz, N. and Schäfer, R. 1976. Nature 263 : 436-438.
3. Dales, S. and Mosbach, E.H. 1968. Virology 35 : 564-583.
4. Joklik, W.K. 1962. Virology 18 : 9-18.
5. Norton, W.T. 1971. Adv. in Exp. Med. and Biol. 13 : 327-337.
6. Oshiro, Y. and Eylar, E.M. 1970. Arch. Biochem. Biophys. 138 : 392-396.
7. Cohen, S.R., McKhann, G.M. and Guarnieri, M. 1975. J. Neurochem. 25 : 371-376.

FUNCTIONAL IMPAIRMENT OF NEURONAL MODEL CELLS INDUCED BY

PERSISTENT VIRAL INFECTION

M. Halbach and K. Koschel

Institute of Virology and Immunology, University of
Würzburg, Würzburg, F.R. Germany

In many neurological diseases where characteristic immunological reactions have been observed, it seems not clear, whether
the immune reactions - directed against viruses and/or host
tissue - are playing the essential role in pathogenesis or are
more or less incidental.

It therefore seems interesting to evaluate the possible
direct pathogenetic action of viruses, which are often found
associated with these neurological diseases and are to some
extent implicated in the development of pathological events.
Candidates for investigation were neurotropic viruses from the
paramyxovirus group like measles virus, SSPE virus and canine
distemper virus (CDV) and rhabdoviruses like rabies virus.

It is well known that paramyxovirus and rhabdovirus particles leave their host cells after multiplication by budding
from the cell membrane. Viral coded proteins are integrated
into the cell membrane detectable by immunofluorescence. It
seemed possible that these viral proteins could induce specific
or unspecific disturbances of the normal microstructure of the
cellular membrane, thus creating the molecular basis for an
impairment of specialized membrane-bound cellular functions.
So we were looking for suitable CNS-derived model cells which
a) had specialized membrane dependent functions which could conveniently be determined by biochemical methods and
b) could become persistently infected with these neurotropic
viruses.

Two virus/cell systems so far were established to study
this hypothesis :

1) C-6 rat glioma cells were chosen because they possess specific membrane receptors for catecholamines : the stimulation
of these   β-adrenergic receptors with noradrenalin or D,L-iso-
proterenol is followed by an activation of the membrane bound
adenylate cyclase resulting in an up to 1000 fold increase in
intracellular cyclic AMP concentrations. These cells were persistently infected with SSPE virus and CDV.
2) Mouse neuroblastoma x rat glioma hybrid cells (line 108 CC15)
created by Amano & Hamprecht, were chosen because they possess
specific membrane receptors for prostaglandines, adenosine, catecholamines, acetylcholine and opiates. The stimulation of
these receptors with their appropriate agonists is followed
by typical shifts of the intracellular cyclic AMP concentrations :
prostaglandines and adenosine cause a characteristical rise
in cyclic AMP concentrations, catecholamines, acetylcholine,
and opiates have a depressing effect on cyclic AMP levels.
This cell line was persistently infected with rabies virus Hep
Flury strain.

     In all systems the viral infection of cells lead to the
development of a chronic, productive viral infection with characteristic time dependent oscillations of the ratio of viral
antigen positive and antigen negative cells in culture. During
the whole observation period of more than 50 passages no differences in cell morphology, viability and growth rate could be
observed between virus infected and uninfected cells. For tests
of membrane dependent cellular functions only cells from culture
phases were employed where the total viral antigen and the membrane integrated viral antigen could be detected in 100 % of
the cells in culture. Moreover, the hybrid cells were used
for biochemical studies only from very low passages at an early
phase of infection (72 hours after virus inoculation) in order
to exclude possible complications sometimes resulting from changes in cell properties during multiple passages.

     In SSPE virus infected C-6 cells the normal rise of intra-
cellular cyclic AMP levels, observed in uninfected cells, is
reduced by approximately 50 %, while the threshold concentration
of catecholamine for receptor stimulation is not changed under
viral influence (fig. 1A, B). This impaired cyclic AMP response
cannot be caused by a rise in membrane permeability for intracellular cyclic AMP as cyclic AMP concentrations in the medium
show no differences between virus infected and uninfected cells.
Experiments to block the cyclic AMP degrading enzyme by 3-iso-
butyl-1-methylxanthine (IBMX) demonstrate that there are no differences in the activity of the specific phosphodiesterase in
infected and uninfected cells. For these reasons the viral
influence can only be directed to the membrane bound receptor/
adenylate cyclase system itself. As this system can be influenced on the receptor level, on the adenylate cyclase level, or

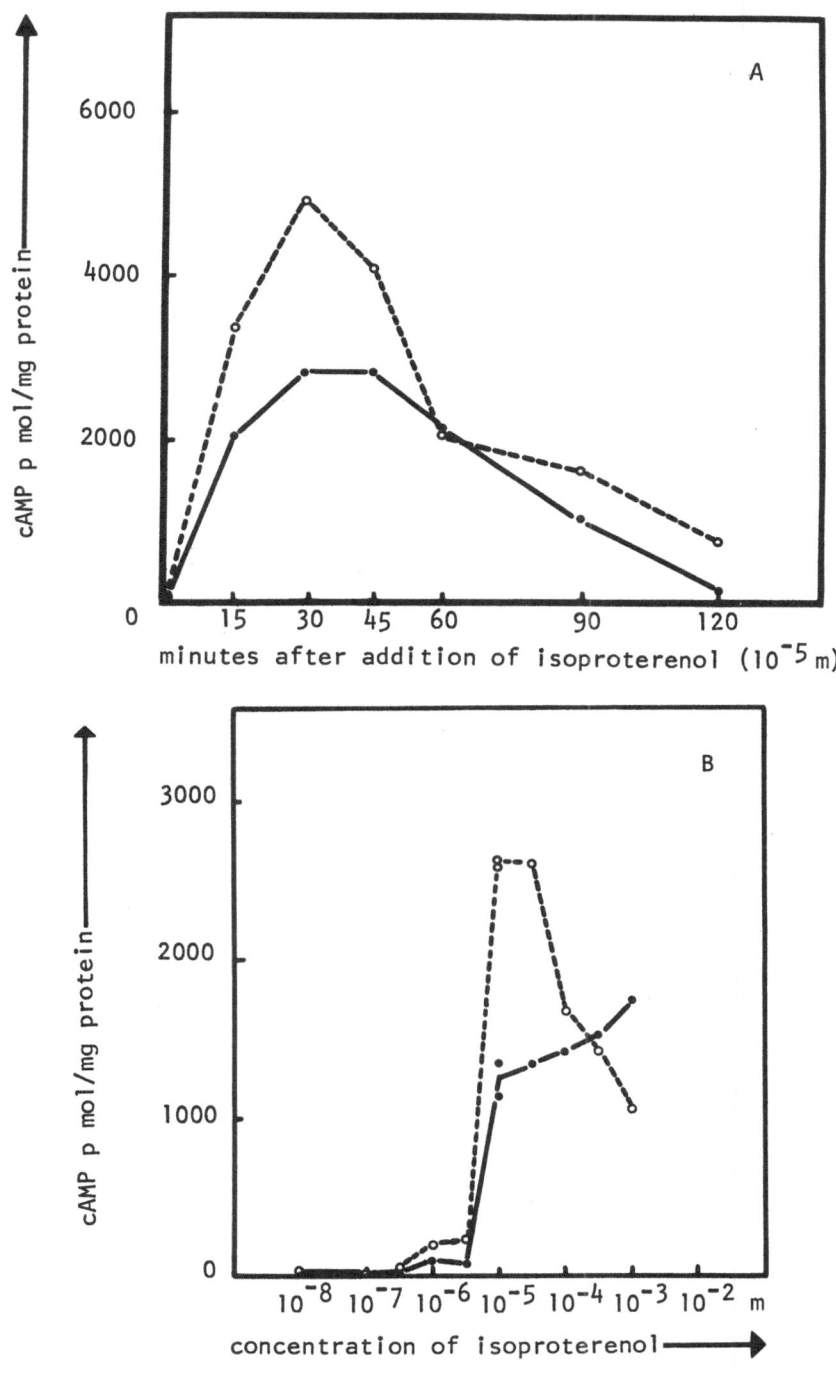

Fig. 1 A & B

Fig. 1 A, B : Intracellular cyclic AMP concentrations after stimulation of C-6 cells with D,L-isoproterenol. Dotted lines :
uninfected cells, Straight lines : SSPE virus infected cells.

on the level of the functional coupling of the receptor to the
enzyme unit we tried to test these parts of the system separately. The adenylate cyclase activity can be determined in membrane preparations under stimulation with fluoride ions. We
observed a considerable loss of enzyme activity in membranes
from virus infected cells as compared to uninfected controls
(fig. 2 A, B), large enough to explain the absolute loss in
cyclic AMP synthesis observed in vivo. From kinetic calculations
it seems probable that this decrease in synthesizing capacity
is due to a loss of catalytic units rather than a decrease in
the activity of the single enzyme molecule (fig. 2c). Whether
membrane receptors for catecholamines are additionally impaired
under viral influence or whether the coupling mechanism is also
influenced has still to be determined.

In the rabies infected neuroblastoma x glioma hybrid cell
line 108 CC15 the cellular response to stimulation of various
receptors monitored by typical shifts of intracellular cyclic
AMP levels was also investigated. Under stimulation with PGE_1
in optimum concentrations the rise of intracellular cyclic AMP
concentrations in infected cells was approximately 50 % of the
levels reached in uninfected cells (fig. 3 A, first two columns).
Addition of IBMX to block the cyclic AMP phosphodiesterase en-
larges the absolute concentrations of cyclic AMP but does not
alter the ratio between the levels in infected and uninfected
cells. Incubations with PGF_2 or adenosine show similar effects.

The situation is somewhat more complicated when the hybrid
cells are incubated with those agonists which have a depressing
effect on cyclic AMP levels. As the cyclic AMP rising and depressing agonists act via different and substance specific receptors on the same adenylate cyclase units available at the
inner side of the cell membrane it is convenient to perform incubations with a cyclic AMP rising and depressing agonist simultaneously. So when hybrid cells are incubated with PGE_1
and catecholamines (Fig. 3 A) the typical depression of cyclic
AMP levels observed in uninfected cells is abolished in rabies
virus infected cells.

Under simultaneous stimulation with PGE_1 and the opiate
methadone (Fig. 3 B) we can observe an in general comparable
viral influence on the cellular response to opiates as seen
with catecholamines. Here as well the cyclic AMP concentrations
of infected cells are not or to a far lower extent depressed

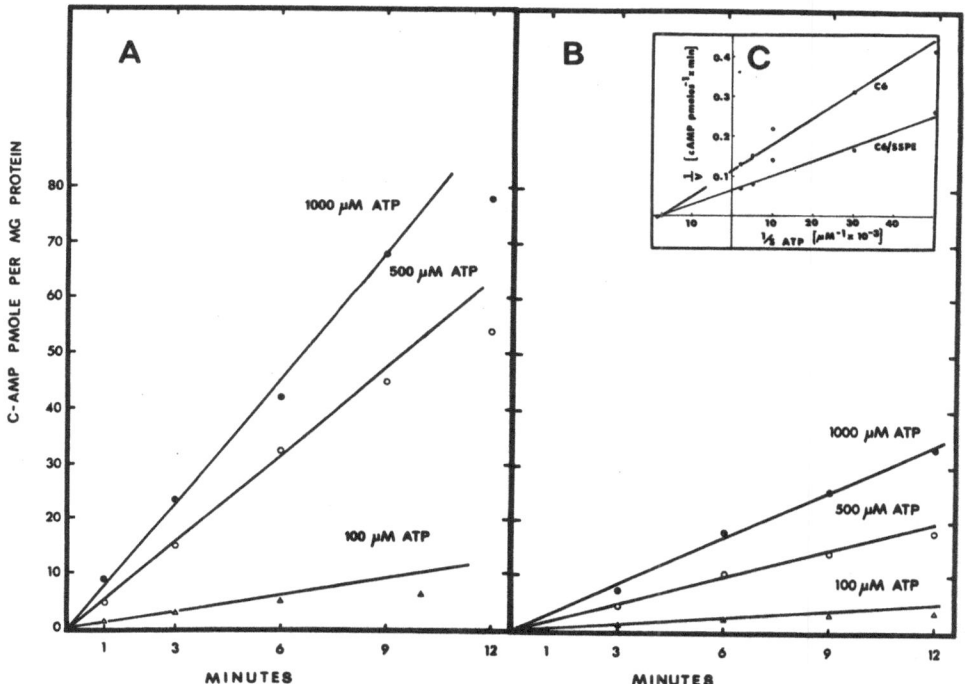

Fig. 2 A, B, C : Adenylate cyclase activity, tested in membrane preparations with fluoride stimulation (10^{-2}M NaF) at different ATP concentrations : A)Uninfected C-6 cells, specific activity 7,6 pMol cyclic AMP x mg protein $^{-1}$ x minute $^{-1}$. B) SSPE virus infected C-6 cells, specific activity 2,85 pMol cyclic AMP x mg protein $^{-1}$ x minute $^{-1}$. C) Lineweaver-Burk plot : Km = 5,7 x 10^{-5} M.

as compared to cyclic AMP levels in uninfected cells.

    A completely different situation has to be noticed under simultaneous stimulation with PGE, and acetylcholine (fig. 3C). The cyclic AMP depression found in uninfected cells under the influence of acetylcholine, can clearly be observed to nearly the same extent in virus infected cells.

    From these findings we can assume a selective viral influence on special membrane receptor functions. Attempts to further clear up the point of viral attack into the membrane bound receptor/adenylate cyclase system have so far not been elucidated in detail. But we can say that in contrary the C-6/SSPE system

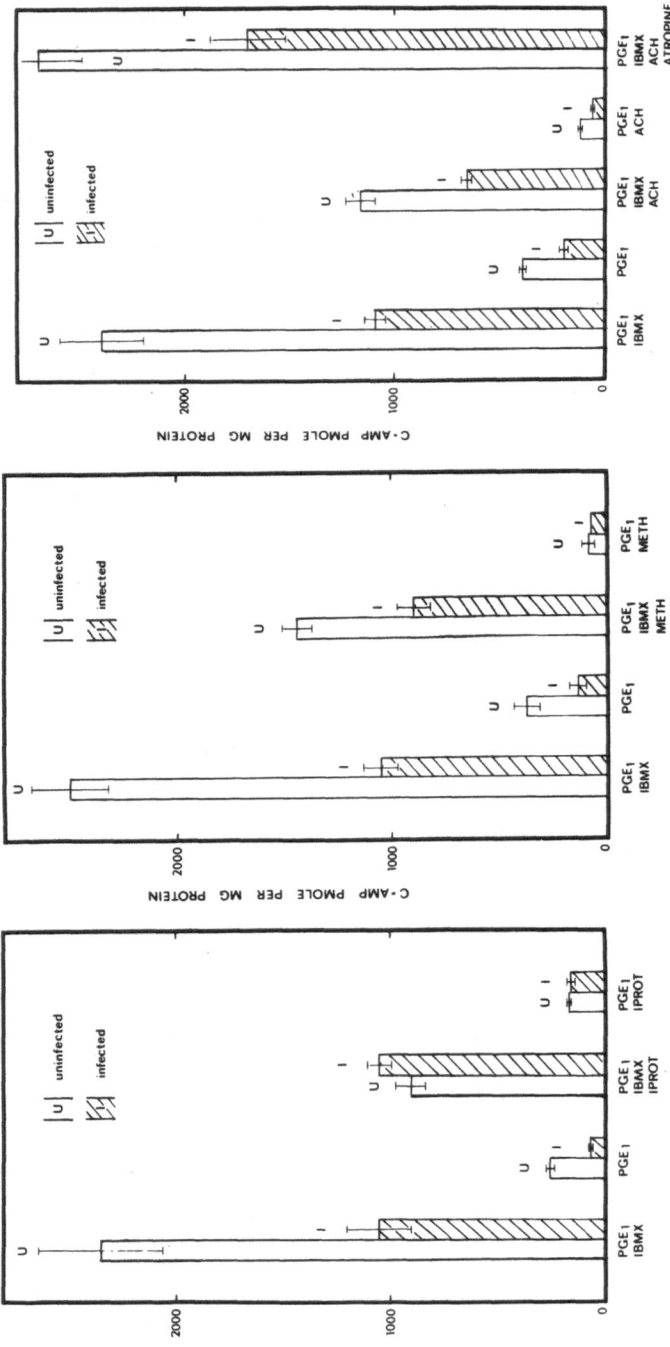

Fig. 3 A, B, C : Intracellular cyclic AMP concentrations after stimulation of 108 CC15 hybrid cells with different receptor binding agonists in the presence and absence of IBMX : A) PGE₁ and isoproterenol; B) PGE₁ and methadone; C) PGE₁ and acetylcholine with atropine control. Agonist concentrations : 2,5 x 10⁻⁵ M PGE₁, 2,5 x 10⁻⁵ M D,L-isoproterenol, 2 x 10⁻⁴ M methadone, 10⁻⁵ M acetylcholine, 10⁻³ M IBMX. Clear columns : uninfected cells, full columns : rabies virus infected cells.

in rabies virus infected 108 CC15 cells the virus induced functional lesion must be associated to the receptor sides or the coupling of receptors to the adenylate cyclase units, as the fluoride stimulated adenylate cyclase activities, determined in membrane preparations, show no differences between virus infected and uninfected cells. Definite results can only be obtained by direct determination of the number of specific receptor sides and their binding affinity for their appropriate agonists in virus infected cells.

It is well known that certain viral infections can persist in host cells for long periods without detectable morphological alterations. At least in our model systems there is - without additional immunological reactions - a considerable impairment of higher cell functions, which are not vitally important for the single cell but are absolutely essential for intercellular functions in the central nervous system.

Many examples from the field of hormone research have clearly demonstrated that already less important changes in receptor mediated cyclic AMP synthesis than we have observed in virus infected cells of our systems are able to cause severe physiological dysfunction of the adequate cellular response to target cells. If we consider that this mode of subtle but effective viral action on nervous tissue membrane functions could not only have some influence on neurotransmitter action but as a consequence directly on bioelectric functions in the CNS, it seems reasonable to look for such possible pathogenetic mechanisms in neurological diseases where immunological reactions and morphological alterations - as it is often observed - do not match the severe clinical illness.

REFERENCES

1. A.G. Gilman and M. Nirenberg, Proc. Natl. Acad. Sci. U.S.A. 68, 2165 (1971).
2. B. Hamprecht, Int. Rev. Cytol. 49, 99-170 (1977).

ACTIVE T CELLS IN BLOOD AND CSF IN MS AND CONTROLS

S. Kam-Hansen

Department of Neurology, University Hospital,
Linköping, Sweden

SUMMARY

Using a modification of the active rosette test of Wybran
and Fudenberg, significantly lower percentages of active T cells
were found in CSF compared with blood in MS and in optic neuritis, while the reverse was found in acute aseptic meningitis.
The active T cell count of CSF may reflect involvement of cellular immunity in CNS disorders.

INTRODUCTION

The finding of elevated T and decreased B lymphocytes (4),
and of non-reactivity on mitogen stimulation of CSF compared with
blood lymphocytes (5), indicate changes in lymphocyte function
within the CNS in MS. For further evaluation of cellular immune
competence in MS, the active rosette test described by Wybran and
Fudenberg (8) was used in the present investigation.

MATERIALS AND METHODS

Fifteen patients with clinically definite MS, 8 with optic
neuritis (ON) and 19 with acute aseptic meningitis were investigated for active T cells in blood and CSF, 8 healthy controls
for active T cells in blood only.

A modification of the active rosette test was used, requiring only 50×10^3 lymphocytes (3). A sheep red blood cell (SRBC)
to lymphocyte ratio of 30:1 was used.

RESULTS

    Fig 1 shows that CSF lymphocytes from MS and ON patients gave significantly ($p < 0.001$; t-test) lower mean percentages of active T cell rosettes compared with blood lymphocytes. In contrast, patients with aseptic meningitis displayed significantly ($p < 0.001$) higher active T cell values in CSF compared with blood.

    The mean percentage of active T cell rosettes in blood in the 3 groups did not differ significantly. In 8 healthy controls hitherto investigated, the mean value of active T cells in blood was 44.4 (range 28.0 - 60.5).

DISCUSSION

    The consistently low active T cell rosettes obtained with MS CSF lymphocytes using a SRBC to lymphocyte ratio of 30:1

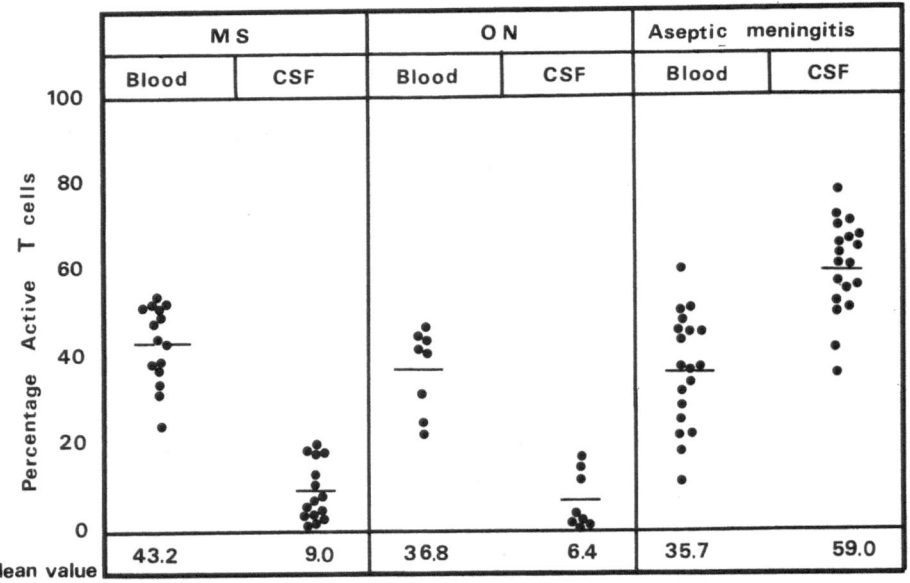

Fig. 1. Percentage of active T cells in multiple sclerosis, optic neuritis and aseptic meningitis.

are in agreement with previous findings with a SRBC to lymphocyte ratio of 175:1 (3). It is not known whether this abnormality is secondary to an accumulation of active T cells within and around plaques, or a consequence of a primary defect in cellular immunity. The elevated active T cell count in CSF in aseptic meningitis may reflect the adequate immune response against viral antigen within the meninges.

Normal numbers of active T cells in MS patients' blood have been described previously (1, 2, 3). The derangement in cell-mediated immuno-competence as reflected by low numbers of active T cells in MS and ON patients seems, therefore, to be confined to the CNS, in the same way as abnormalities in the humoral immune response as manifested by the occurrence in CSF (6) and brain tissue (7) of oligoclonal immunoglobulins.

ACKNOWLEDGEMENT

This work has been supported by the Swedish Medical Research Council (Project No. 3381).

REFERENCES

1. Goust, J.M., Chenais, F., Carnes, J.E., Hames, C.G., Fudenberg, H.H. and Hogan, E.L., Abnormal T cell subpopulations and circulating immune complexes in the Guillain-Barré syndrome and multiple sclerosis, Neurology 28, 421-425 (1978).
2. Hashim, G.A., Lee, D.H., Pierce, J.C., Braun, C.W. and Fitzpatrick, H.F., Myelin basic protein-stimulated rosette-forming T cells in multiple sclerosis, Neurochem. Research 3, 37-48 (1978).
3. Kam-Hansen, S., Reduced number of active T cells in cerebrospinal fluid in multiple sclerosis, Neurology, submitted for publication (1978).
4. Kam-Hansen, S., Frydén, A. and Link, H., B and T cells in cerebrospinal fluid and blood in multiple sclerosis and acute mumps meningitis, Acta Neurol. Scand., in press (1978).
5. Kam-Hansen, S., Frydén, A., Link, H. and Möller, E., Reduced in vitro response of CSF lymphocytes to mitogen stimulation in multiple sclerosis. Manuscript.
6. Link, H., Immunoglobulin G and low molecular weight proteins in human cerebrospinal fluid : Chemical and immunological characterization with special reference to multiple sclerosis, Acta Neurol. Scand. 43, Suppl. 28, 1-136 (1967).
7. Link, H., Oligoclonal immunoglobulin G in multiple sclerosis brains, J. Neurol. Sci. 16, 103-114 (1972).
8. Wybran, J. and Fudenberg, H.H., Thymus-derived rosette-forming

cells in various human disease states : Cancer, lymphoma, bacterial and viral infections, and other diseases, J. Clin. Invest. 52, 1026–1032 (1973).

ISOLATION AND CHARACTERIZATION OF THE T CELL RECEPTOR FOR THE BASIC ENCEPHALITOGENIC PROTEIN IN EAE

P. Bartman [+], B.-U.v. Specht [+], J. Eder [x], D. Teitelbaum [o], and W. Brendel [+]

+ Institute for Surgical Research, University of Munich, F.R. Germany; x M.P.I. for Biochemistry, Martinsried, F.R. Germany; o Department of Chemical Immunology, Weizmann Institute of Science, Rehovot, Israel

INTRODUCTION

Experimental allergic encephalomyelitis (EAE) is studied both as a model of human demyelinating diseases and organ-specific T cell dependent autoimmune diseases. It is induced in laboratory animals by injection of myelin basic protein (BE) in complete Freund's adjuvant (CFA) and results in characteristic lesions restricted to the central nervous system.

Recent work of Binz and Wigzell (1) as well as Krawinkel and Rajewsky (2) has given strong evidence that T cells express an antigen recognizing receptor, which does not seem to carry markers of the immunoglobulin constant domain but of the variable part of an Ig molecule. Hapten binding material could be enriched from hapten sensitized T cells using an affinity method originally developed by Kiefer (3).

We wish to report the enrichment of BE binding material from spleen and lymph node cell suspensions of guinea pig strain 13, which had been sensitized with the basic encephalitogenic protein. This purification was performed with regard to the production of an antiserum against the BE specific T cell receptor, which may induce tolerance to EAE by elimination of the appropriate T cell clones. Furthermore, evidence should be obtained about the molecular structure of the receptor and its part in cellular immune response.

511

EXPERIMENTAL PROCEDURES

Inbred guinea pigs strain 2 and 13 (400 - 650 g) were a gift
from the Institut für Biologisch-Medizinisch Forschung, Füllinsdorf, Switzerland. Nylon mesh (obtained from Schweiz. Seidengaze-
fabrik AG) was partially hydrolysed with HCl, succinylated and
activated by formation of a succinimidester. Binding of the basic protein to the activated nylon mesh was performed in 0.2M bo-
rate buffer pH 8.2 and controlled by using 131 I-modified BE.
Discs having a diameter of 2.5 cm and a central hole of 2 mm were
cut out of the nylon mesh and stacked on a shaft with 3 mm teflon
spacers. This was placed into a 50 ml glass column where it could
be rotated at 5rpm.

Basic protein was extracted from bovine spinal cord as described by Hirshfeld et al. (4). Strain 13 guinea pigs were immunized by injecting 10 µg of BE in PBS/CFA, 1 : 2 into each footpad.
The animals were sacrificed after 12 days, spleen and draining
lymph nodes isolated and cell suspensions prepared in RPMI 1640.
These were then incubated with the BE coupled nylon mesh for one
hour at +4°C under gentle stirring. Non binding cells were removed by elution and washing with cold medium. Antigen specific
cells were released from the nylon mesh by shifting the temperature to +25°C and were thus collected for further experiments.
After washing the nylon mesh three times with PBS, antigen binding
material was eluted with 3.5M KSCN in PBS. Analysis of the eluted
material was performed after dialysis and concentration by the
phage inactivation assay (5). Specificity of the assay was shown
by using anti BE antiserum from rabbits and inhibition of the inactivation by free antigen (BE).

RESULTS AND DISCUSSION

Figure 1 shows the analysis of material isolated from the
BE modified nylon mesh by the phage inactivation method. A typical inactivation pattern is obtained which is comparable to that
with rabbit anti BE antiserum. Phage inactivating material was
obtained from lymph node cells as well as spleen cells. To demonstrate that this material is not identical with humoral antibodies produced against the basic protein, absorption with cross-
linked anti guinea pig Ig was performed. No difference in phage
inactivation capacity could be found after the absorption step.
This result gives evidence that the inactivating material is not
identical with common immunoglobulin molecules. Moreover, no inactivation capacity was found in the serum pool of the immunized

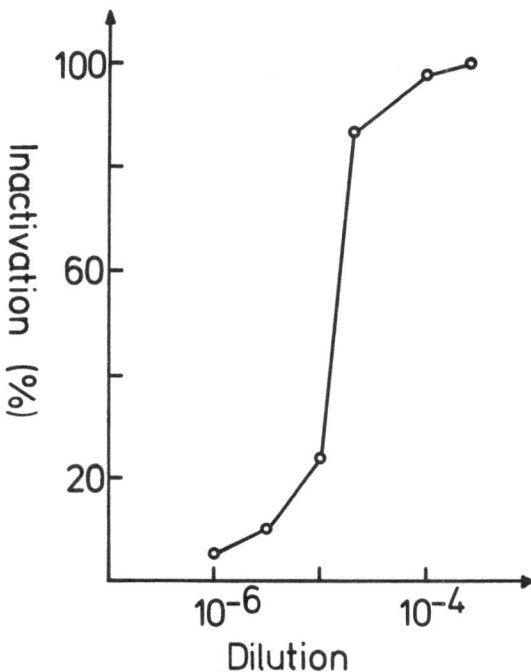

Fig. 1. Phage inactivation assay of material obtained from BE
sensitized lymphocytes of guinea pig strain 13

animals. To exclude the possibility of non specific phage inactivation, ten guinea pigs were immunized with 10 μg of egg albumin and the whole procedure repeated as described for the BE immunized animals. No inactivation of BE modified T4 coliphage
could be obtained, thus ruling out nonspecific interactions.

     In order to analyse if the phage inactivating material is
produced by the modified nylon adherent cells, this cell fraction
was kept in culture for two days. Repeated absorption of these
cells to the affinity column revealed after the appropriate washing steps again phage inactivating material. This demonstrates
that the cells are capable of reproducing the antigen recognizing
factor under culture conditions.

To answer the question of a T cell origin of the inactivating material, the cells were analysed by immunofluorescence and cytotoxicity tests. More than 97% of the specifically bound cells were identified as T cells.

To analyse the molecular weight of the phage inactivating material, samples from ten guinea pigs were concentrated and subjected to SDS polyacrylamide gel electrophoresis in the presence of 50mM β -mercaptoethanol. The migration pattern after staining with Coomassie blue and scanning in a Gilford spectrophotometer is shown in figure 2. One single band is revealed with a molecular weight of 71.000 ± 2.000 daltons.

The presented data demonstrate that T lymphocytes from guinea pigs immunized with BE produce a specific antigen recognizing protein. This was shown not to be identical with common immunoglobulin molecules.

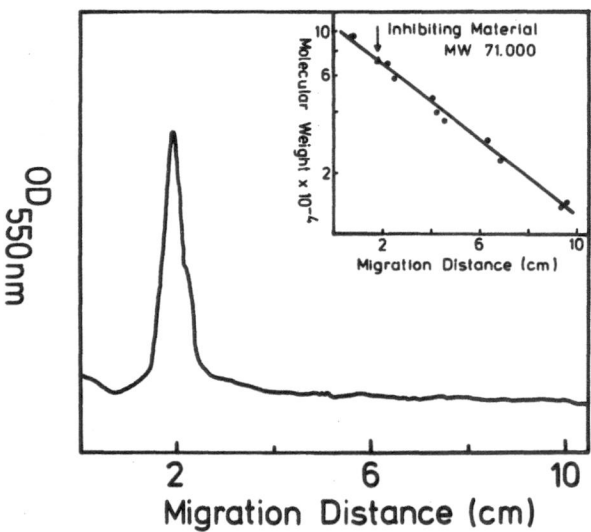

Fig. 2. Profile of phage inactivating material after SDS-PAGE and staining with Coomassie blue. The inset shows the linear relationship between the logarithm of the molecular weight and standard proteins and their migration distance.

ACKNOWLEDGEMENT

We are indebted to the Institut für Biologisch-Medizinische Forschung, Füllinsdorf, Switzerland for a generous gift of guinea pigs strain 2 and 13 and to Miss M. Waltenberger for excellent technical assistance. We thank Dr. E. Holler, Univ. Regensburg, for providing research facilities. This work was supported by the SFB 37 of the Deutsche Forschungsgemeinschaft.

REFERENCES

1. H. Binz and H. Wigzell, Scand. J. Immunol. 5, 559 (1976).
2. U. Krawinkel and K. Rajewsky, Eur. J. Immunol. 6, 529, (1976).
3. H. Kiefer, Eur. J. Immunol. 3, 181, (1973).
4. H. Hirshfeld, D. Teitelbaum, R. Arnon, and M. Sela, FEBS Letters 7, 317 (1970).
5. J. Haimovich and M. Sela, J. Immunol. 97, 338 (1966).

THE INFLUENCE OF THE T IMMUNE SYSTEM ON THE APPEARANCE OF

HOMOGENEOUS IMMUNOGLOBULINS IN MAN AND EXPERIMENTAL ANIMALS

J. Radl

Institute for Experimental Gerontology of the
Organization for Health Research TNO
Rijswijck, The Netherlands

"Benign" disorders of the immune system accompanied by the production of homogeneous immunoglobulins (H-Ig) - paraproteins - are about 100 times more frequent than paraproteinaemias of B cell malignancies. Evaluation of the clinical and laboratory data on these "nonmalignant" paraproteinaemias shows that this group is heterogeneous and that the etiology and the pathogenesis of most of these disorders are still unknown (1,2,3). Their tentative classification is given in Table I. Comparable conditions which have been described in animals are also listed. They serve as useful models for experimental studies on the etiology and the mechanisms of the development of the individual paraproteinaemias. Recent clinical and experimental animal studies have added to our understanding of these mechanisms in at least three of the conditions (mentioned in the table as 1, 2 and 3). Results of the investigations indicated that diminished or impaired T cell functions and not a defect of B cells may be regarded as responsible for the production of H-Ig in these conditions.

Detailed studies in children suffering from various immunodeficiency diseases demonstrated that H-Ig are frequent findings in the serum of patients with Nezelof syndrome, Di George syndrome, Wiskott-Aldrich syndrome and in some cases of severe combined immunodeficiency (SCID) (4,5,6,7). In general, the T cell functions were clearly impaired in the patients showing a paraproteinaemia, while much less severe or no defects of the B cell functions could be demonstrated.

An intriguing finding of multiple transient H-Ig was described in sera of three children with SCID after successful bone marrow

Table I.

Nonmalignant paraproteinaemias in man and in some animal species

Condition	Human	Animal model	Paraproteinaemia
1. Immunodeficiency diseases	Syndrome: Nezelof; DiGeorge; Wiskott-Aldrich; SCID	Thymectomized mice	Often transient
2. Early ontogenesis with excess stimulation	Intrauterine infections	-	Transient
3. Reconstitution of the immune system after bone marrow transplantation	SCID; aplastic anemia, leukemia, pretreatment with an immunosuppressive regimen	Irradiated mice Rh monkeys	Transient
4. Ageing	Idiopathic paraproteinaemia (benign monoclonal gammapathy)	Mice (C57BL)	Persistent, frequency increases with ageing
5. Autoimmune diseases	Chronic cold agglutinin disease; chronic autoimmune liver disease	Mice (NZB)	Autoantibody activity or unknown
6. Subacute and chron. infections; tumors	Reactive paraproteinaemia? Lichen myxedematosus; mycosis fungoides; SSPE; MS	Aleutian mink disease EAE?	Often oligoclonal CSF > S
7. Homogeneous response to polysaccharides	E.g. dextran, levan, bacterial polysaccharides	Rabbits mice	Genetically determined

transplantation treatment (5,8). Later, it became clear that
transient H-Ig are a common finding in serum during the reconstitution
process after bone marrow transplantation. This was also true in
patients with aplastic anemia and leukemia, who received pretreatment with an immunosuppressive regimen (6). Similar results
were obtained in rhesus monkeys which were lethally irradiated
and reconstituted with syngeneic or autologous bone marrow cells
(9). In further experiments, it was shown that these H-Ig were
specific antibodies (10). After immunization of monkeys with 2,4-
dinitrophenol (DNP) substituted rhesus monkey albumin (but not
with human IgA paraprotein), some of the H-Ig appearing during
the restoration period were demonstrated to have an anti-DNP
antibody activity. A gradual transformation of the homogeneous
antibodies into heterogeneous populations of antibodies was
observed as the reconstitution proceeded.

In a similar experimental model (lethally irradiated and
reconstituted mice), B cells were demonstrated to reach their
normal values within 4-6 weeks after irradiation and transplantation
(11,12). In contrast, T cells did not reach their normal values
even 15 weeks after transplantation (12). These results indicated
that the reconstitution is a gradual process in which the T cells
mature more slowly than the B cells; during that time imbalanced
T-B cell interactions may lead to an immune response of restricted
heterogeneity.

A direct correlation between the severity of the T system
impairment and the frequency of H-Ig production was demonstrated
in another experiment (13). Follow-up studies were performed in
three groups of (DBA/2 x C57BL/Rij)F_1 mice which were lethally
irradiated and reconstituted with T cell-depleted bone marrow
cells. A different grade of T system impairment was induced. The
first group consisted of thymectomized mice. Animals of the
second and the third group were submitted to a sham operation
only. Mice of the third group received additionally three injections
of 10^7 corticosteroid-resistant thymocytes in the first week
after transplantation. During the reconstitution period, the
highest frequency of H-Ig occurred in the first group and the
lowest in the third group.

The paraproteins appearing in newborns with congenital
infections (6,7,14) may have an origin similar to that described
in the reconstitution experiments. In both clinical and experimental
animal bone marrow transplantation, it has been shown that the
reconstitution of the immune system follows a pathway that is
similar to normal ontogenesis in several aspects. It seems that,
also in normal development, the B cell functions appear early and
soon express a wide repertoire, while T cell functions mature
later (15,16). In the early stages of ontogenesis, the immune

response shows a restriction in its heterogeneity as compared to
that in a mature individual (17). Therefore, excess stimulation
in such a situation may lead to the appearance of H-Ig antibodies
by similar mechanisms as in the reconstitution experiments.

All of these observations strongly suggest a crucial role of
the T system in the regulation of the immune response heterogeneity. A defect in the helper T cells may restrict numbers of
the responding B cell clones. Due to a deficiency in suppressor T
cells, an overshoot reaction of a restricted number of B cell
clones to thymus dependent but also to some "thymus independent"
antigens (being otherwise under control of T suppressor cells
(18)) can become possible. The role of the individual T cell
subpopulations in the above-mentioned monoclonal or oligoclonal
proliferations can be investigated in the animal models, where a
selective depletion or enrichment of the individual cell subpopulations is possible.

There are some indications that, apart from the first three
groups of our classification scheme, an impairment of the T
immune system may play a pathogenic role also in the next condition,
known as Idiopathic Paraproteinaemia (IP) or Benign Monoclonal
Gammapathy. Here, however, the situation is more complicated.
Recent studies in ageing C57BL/KaLwRij mice (an animal model for
IP) demonstrated that a B cell clone is affected in the final
stage of this immune system disorder (19). Once developed, this
IP is persistent; it is transplantable into young healthy mice by
bone marrow or spleen cells and can be propagated by cell transfers
for two to three generations. A T system impairment may, however,
play an important role in the early stages of the development of
this disorder. This is indicated by the fact that thymectomy
performed in young adult mice but even more clearly thymectomy in
neonatal mice, can substantially increase the frequency of IP
which appear during ageing of these animals (20).

Less is known about the other conditions listed in the
table. However, it is possible that also in these cases a T
system impairment (probably a selective one) may play a role in
their etiology or pathogenesis. More detailed investigations will
be necessary to reveal exactly these immunopathological and other
factors (such as genetic predisposition and the role of antigen
stimulation) in each of the conditions in order to improve our
chances for a correct etiological classification and perhaps for
efficient treatment of these disorders of the immune system.

REFERENCES

1. Waldenström, J.G. Benign monoclonal gammapathies. In:
   Multiple myeloma and related disorders, Vol. 1, p. 247
   Ed. A. Azar and M. Potter, Harper & Row, Hagerstown,
   Md., 1973.

2. Zawadzki, Z.A. and Edwards, G.A. : Nonmyelomatous monoclonal
   immunoglobulins. In: Progress in Clinical Immunology, Vol. 1,
   p. 105. Ed. R.S. Schwartz, Grune & Stratton, New York, 1972.

3. Radl, J.: Immune system disorders in man and in experimental
   models accompanied by the production of homogeneous immunoglobulins - paraproteins. In: Protides of the Biological
   Fluids, Vol. 23, p. 405. Ed. H. Peeters, Pergamon Press,
   Oxford, 1976.

4. Radl, J., Dooren, L.J., Morell, A., Skvaril, F., Vossen, J.M.J.J.
   and Uittenbogaart, C.H. : Immunoglobulins and transient paraproteins in sera of patients with the Wiskott-Aldrich syndrome:
   a follow-up study. Clin. exp. Immunol. 25; 256, 1976.

5. Radl, J. and Berg van den, P.: Transitory appearance of homogeneous immunoglobulins - "paraproteins" - in children with
   severe combined immunodeficiency before and after transplantation
   treatment. In: Protides of the Biological Fluids, Vol. 20,
   p. 263. Ed. H. Peeters, Pergamon Press, Oxford, 1973.

6. Dooren, L.J., Vossen, J.M.J.J. and Radl, J.: unpublished
   results.

7. Hitzig, W.H. and Jako, J.: Monoclonal immunoglobulins in
   children. In: Protides of Biological Fluids, Vol. 18, p. 139.
   Ed. H. Peeters, Pergamon Press, Oxford, 1971.

8. Radl, J., Dooren, L.J., Eijsvoogel, V.P., van Went, J.J. and
   Hijmans, W.: An immunological study during post-transplantation
   follow-up of a case of severe combined immunodeficiency.
   Clin. exp. Immunol., 10, 367, 1972.

9. Radl, J., Berg, P. van den, Voormolen, M., Hendriks, W.D.H. and
   Schaefer, U.W. : Homogeneous immunoglobulins in sera of Rhesus
   monkeys after lethal irradiation and bone marrow transplantation.
   Clin. exp. Immunol. 16; 259, 1974.

10. Berg, P. van den, Radl, J., Löwenberg, B. and Swart, A.C.W. :
    Homogeneous antibodies in lethally irradiated and autologous bone
    marrow reconstituted Rhesus monkeys. Clin. exp. Immunol. 23;
    355, 1976.

11. Nossal, G.J.V. and Pike, B.L.: Differantiation of B lymphocytes
    from stem cell precursors. Microenvironmental aspects of
    immunity. Adv. Exp. Med. Biol. 29; 11, 1973.

12. Rozing, J. and Benner, R.: The recovery of the B cell compartment
    in lethally irradiated and reconstituted mice. Adv. Exp. Med.
    Biol. 66; 203, 1976.

13. Muiswinkel, W.B. van, Radl, J. and Wal, D.J. van der : The
    regulatory influence of the thymus dependent immune system on
    the heterogeneity of immunoglobulins in irradiated and
    reconstituted mice. Adv. Exp. Med. Biol. 66, 617, 1976.

14. Oxelius, V.A.: Monoclonal immunoglobulins in congenital toxo-
    plasmosis. Clin. exp. Immunol. 11; 367, 1972.
15. Chiscon, M.O. and Golub, E.S. : Functional development of the
    interacting cells in the immune response. I. Development of
    T cell and B cell function. J. Immunol. 108; 1379, 1972.
16. Rowlands, D.T. Jr., Blakeslee, D. and Augala, E.: Acquired
    immunity in opossum (Didelphis Virginiana) embryos.
    J. Immunol. 112; 2148, 1974.
17. Goidl, E.A. and Siskind, G.W. : Ontogeny of B lymphocyte
    function. I. Restricted heterogeneity of the antibody response
    of B lymphocytes from neonatal and fetal mice. J. exp. Med.
    140; 1285, 1974.
18. Rotter, V. and Trainin, N. : Thymus cell population exerting
    a regulatory function in the immune response of mice to
    Polyvinyl Pyrrolidone. Cell. Immunol. 13; 76, 1974.
19. Radl, J., Glopper, E. de, Schuit, H.R.E. and Zurcher, C. :
    Idiopathic paraproteinaemia.II. Transplantation of the
    paraprotein producing clone from old to young C57BL/KaLwRij
    mice. In preparation.
20. Radl, J., Glopper, E. de, Berg, P. van den, Zwieten, M.J. van:
    Idiopathic paraproteinaemia.IV. Increased frequency of the
    paraproteinemia in thymectomized C57BL/KaLwRij mice. In
    preparation.

REGULATORY INTERACTIONS BETWEEN CELLS IN IMMUNE RESPONSES

H. Valdimarsson and G. Agnarsdottir

Department of Immunology and Department of Virology
St. Mary's Hospital Medical School and Hammersmith
Hospital, London, U.K.

INTRODUCTION

Most naturally occurring immune responses involve interactions between different types of leukocytes. A few of these
interactions, and the cell types involved, are listed in Table I.
They apply at all levels of the immune response but here we are
mainly concerned with the regulatory aspects of these interactions
in relation to antibody production. The mechanisms involved,
although intensively studied by many groups in recent years, are
still incompletely understood. Most of the available information
is derived from studies on mice. There is, however, no a priori
reason to believe that fundamental differences exist between mice
and other mammalian species in this respect. Indeed, the limited
data obtained from other species, including man, indicate that
immune responses are controlled by basically similar mechanisms in
all mammals.

The objective of this paper is to present a fairly elementary
overview of the subject, and only a few references will be cited.
First, some relevant properties of the interacting cells will be
discussed. A few of the main experimental approaches will then
be outlined and the information obtained briefly summarised. One
of several tentative models which, on the basis of available data,
have been proposed for the mechanism of cell cooperation, will then
be presented. Finally we will speculate on the anatomical
requirements of immunoregulatory cell interactions with reference
to the special immunoanatomical features of the brain.

Table I. Examples of cellular cooperation in immune responses

Type of response	Principal cooperating cells
Facilitation of antibody production	MØ[*], T and B cells
Suppression of antibody production	T and B cells (and ? MØ)
Activation of T lymphocyte proliferation	MØ and T cells
Production of delayed hyper-sensitivity	MØ and T cells
Generation of cytotoxic cells	T cell subpopulations
Suppression of delayed hyper-sensitivity	T cell subpopulations
Macrophage "arming" in cytotoxicity	T cells and MØ
Antibody dependent cell mediated cytotoxicity	T, B and K cells

[*]MØ = macrophages

B AND T LYMPHOCYTES

The differentiation of B and T lymphocytes from lymphoid stem cells does not require external antigens, but their maturation into antibody producing plasma cells or effector T cells is dependent both on antigen stimulation and interaction with other cells.

B Cells

Although antibody production is undoubtedly the principal function of B cells, it should not be forgotten that they are also capable of producing large amounts of other important substances such as MIF, LIF and interferon.

Subclasses of B cells have hitherto been defined in terms of the immunoglobulin type expressed on their surface membrane.

Table II. Various stages of B cell maturation in mice

Maturation stage	Membrane immuno-globulin	Principal anatomical compartment	Consequence of antigen experience
Pre-B cells	Absent	Fetal liver and adult bone marrow	Antigen blind
Immature B cells	IgM only	Spleen	Tolerance
Mature virgin B cells	IgM and IgD	Blood, lymph nodes and spleen	Primary (IgM) response
Memory B cells	IgD only	Recirculate	Secondary (IgG or IgA) response
Plasma cells	Absent	Bone marrow or gut	Antigen blind

However, recent observations summarised in Table II suggest that, although individual B cells are programmed to synthesise only one type of antibody specificity during their life span, they may sequentially produce different immunoglobulin classes during the various stages of their maturation (1,2).

The B precursor cells have cytoplasmic IgM but lack detectable surface immunoglobulin and are therefore antigen blind. These cells develop into immature B cells which express only IgM on their surface and tend to become unresponsive (tolerant) if they are exposed to antigen.   In the mouse these immature B cells populate the spleen where in addition to their IgM they also acquire surface IgD.   These IgM^+IgD^+ cells are found in the blood and lymph nodes as well as in the spleen.   They are fully differentiated and respond to antigen stimulation either by becoming IgM producing plasma cells (primary response) or maturing further into $IgM^- IgD^+$ B cells.   The latter recirculate as antigen primed memory B cells which on further antigenic challenge settle down in the bone marrow or gut mucosa to become IgG or IgA producing plasma cells (secondary response).

Table III.   Tentative functional classification of T cell
             types in mice

T cell responsible for	Symbol	Ly phenotype	Probable role
Overall control	T_I	Ly 1,2,3	Precursor and/or regulators for T_H & T_S
B cell help	T_{HB}	Ly 1	Help B cells to produce antibodies
Tc cell help	T_{HC}	Ly 1	Help cytotoxic T cells to kill
Delayed hyper-sensitivity	T_{DH}	Ly 1	Memory cells for DH responses
Cytotoxicity	Tc	Ly 2,3	Kill certain abnormal cells
Suppression	Ts	Ly 2,3	Inhibit most B and T cell response

T Cells

The great majority of the lymphocytes which re-circulate
through blood, tissues, lymph nodes and the thoracic duct are T-
cells.   A wide variety of functions have been attributed to these
cells (Table III) and they have been divided into many subpopulations according to differences in surface characteristics and
other properties which will not be elaborated upon here.   However,
in the mouse, it has recently been demonstrated that certain
surface components (the so called Ly antigens) are markers for
distinct functional properties of T cell subpopulations and we
will come back to this, later.   Although markers corresponding to
the Ly antigens in the mouse have not yet been identified in man,
recent work (3) suggests that certain surface components such as
the TH_1 antigen may also be used to distinguish functional subpopulation in man.   (Table IV)

CELLULAR INTERACTIONS AND IMMUNOREGULATION

Studies on regulatory cell interactions began in the late
sixties when it was convincingly demonstrated that T lymphocytes,

Table IV. Tentative functional classification of T cells in man

Cells responsible for	Symbol	TH1 surface antigen	Fc receptors	
			γ	μ
B suppression	T_S	O	+	+ or O
B cell help	T_H	+	O	+
Ag. ind. proliferation	TsAg	O	NT*	NT
MLC reaction	T_{MLC}	+	NT	NT
MIF production	T_{MIF}	+	NT	NT
LMF production	T_{LMF}	+	NT	NT
CML reaction	T_{CML}	+ or O	NT	NT

*NT = Not Tested

though themselves not capable of manufacturing antibodies, were required for helping B lymphocytes to produce antibodies to certain antigens   (T help) (4).   More recently it has been demonstrated that this T-B cell cooperation has a negative counterpart in that T cells can also suppress or tolerise B cells (T suppression) (5).

It is now known that all aspects of immune responses involve regulatory interactions or signals between different cells.   The complexity of these interactions is only just beginning to be understood.   They serve to initiate, suppress or otherwise regulate and stabilise immune reactivity according to requirements dictated by the amount, type and localization of the antigen challenge.

Moreover, recent observations indicate that cell membrane components which are products of genes belonging to the Major Histocompatibility Complex play a critical role in these regulatory interactions.   This has of course wide-ranging biological implications which are currently being studied by many groups (6).

Before reviewing some of the cardinal features of T-B lymphocyte interactions, it might be helpful to recall very briefly a few relevant properties of antigens and immunogens and also to describe some assay models which have been most widely used for analysing these phenomena.

Antigens and Immunogens

Substances are generally not immunogenic unless their molecular weight is more than 5,000 daltons. They must also be accessible and suitably presented to antigen reactive cells and they must be foreign to the animal in that they were not present during the early stages of its lymphocyte differentiation.

Strictly speaking, the term 'antigen' only refers to the ability of a substance to combine with an antibody. Thus, substances such as haptens which are too small to be immunogenic in their own right can, nevertheless, act as antigens by reacting with and blocking specific combining sites on antibodies.

All immunogenic molecules have several or many antigen determinants (epitopes) and a hapten can, of course, be made immunogenic if it is coupled to a large molecule such as protein where it forms a new antigen determinant. The immunogenic molecule is now called a hapten-carrier conjugate.

Antigens and T Cell Help in Antibody Production

Substances which can stimulate antibody production in the absence of T cells are called T independent antigens. However, most naturally occurring antigens are T dependent because they require help from T cells for stimulating B cells to antibody

Table V. Different features of T independent and T dependent antigens

	T independent antigens	T dependent antigens
Identical epitopes per molecule:	Several or many	None or few
Predominant antibody type in secondary response :	IgM	IgG and IgA
Require macrophages:	Probably not	Yes
Act as polyclonal B cell mitogens:	Yes	No

production.   Table V. summarises the main features which
distinguish these two types of antigens.

Each T independent antigen molecule is composed of many
identical antigen determinants, while each T dependent antigen
molecule has many but different epitopes.   T independent antigens
can only stimulate IgM antibody production even after repeated
injections, while secondary antibody responses to T dependent
antigens are predominantly of IgG and IgA type.   T dependent
antigens not only require T cells but also macrophages while the
T independent antigens are less dependent on the presence of
macrophages.   Lastly, most T independent antigens are "polyclonal"
B cell mitogens but T dependent substances are only able to
stimulate specifically reactive cells to proliferation.

Table VI.   Some experimental systems for analysing T cell help

Test system	Information gained
1. Thymectomized (or nude) mice	T cells are required for antibody production
2. Adoptive transfer of T cells to irradiated recipients (test-tube mice)	Helper T cells do not themselves produce antibodies
3. Hapten-carriers into intact mice	Secondary response to hapten is carrier specific
4. Hapten-carriers into reconstituted test-tube mice	Secondary response to hapten involves carrier recognition by T cells and hapten recognition by B cells
5. T and B cells separated in culture by a membrane (modified Marbrook culture system)	T cells release both specific and non-specific factors which facilitate antibody production by B cells
6. "T-primed" macrophages co-cultured with B cells	Macrophages can take up specific T cell factors and then help B cells in the absence of T cells

Analytical Systems

Table VI lists some experimental systems which have been used to analyse the mechanisms of T cell help in antibody production and, more recently, similar systems have been used to investigate T cell suppression.

Mechanisms of T-B Cell Cooperation

Cooperation between T and B cells was first convincingly demonstrated in neonatally thymectomized mice. Such T cell depleted mice failed to produce normal amounts of antibodies to many antigens (T dependent) unless they were reconstituted with syngeneic T cells before immunization (Table VI - 1). Further studies showed that the transferred T cells did not, themselves, produce antibodies but acted by facilitating antibody production by the recipient's own B cells (Table VI - 2). The nature of this cooperation was further elucidated by using hapten-carrier conjugates. Thus intact mice which had been sensitized to certain hapten-carrier combinations could only produce a secondary anti-hapten response if they were reinjected with the hapten coupled to the original carrier molecule (Table VII).

Moreover, since secondary anti-NIP responses did not appear in mice injected with both the hapten (NIP) and the carrier (BSA) determinants, if each was present on separate molecules (last line of Table VII), the cooperation had to involve recognition of the two determinants on a single antigenic molecule.

Furthermore, NIP-BSA conjugates were injected into irradiated recipients of two cell populations, one obtained from mice primed

Table VII. Carrier specificity of secondary anti-hapten responses

NIP-BSA primed mice challenged with:	Secondary anti-NIP responses
NIP-BSA	+
NIP-CG	O
DNP-BSA	O
NIP-CG and DNP-BSA	O

Table VIII.   Cooperation involves carrier recognition by T cells

Mice reconstituted with cells separately primed to:	Anti-NIP response to NIP-BSA
NIP-CG	O
BSA	O
NIP-CG + BSA	+
NIP-CG (anti-Thy 1 and C'treated) + BSA	+
BSA (anti-Thy 1 and C'treated) + NIP-CG	O

to BSA and the other from mice primed to NIP.   The anti-NIP response failed to appear in these recipients if T cells were selectively removed from the cell population obtained from the BSA sensitized donors while removal of T cells from the hapten sensitized population did not affect the anti-NIP response (Table VIII).   This demonstrates that the cells recognising the carrier determinants are T cells while the immunogenic activity of the hapten determinant does not involve hapten recognition by T cells.

More recently, it has been demonstrated that T and B cells can cooperate in a secondary antibody response in vitro when they are separated from each other by a cell-impermeable membrane indicating that B cells are helped by soluble factors released from the T cells   (Fig. 1).

Both specific and non-specific helper factors have been observed and Table IX summarizes experiments with hapten-carrier conjugates in this system (7).   The T cells only produce helper factors if they have been primed to the carrier present in the culture system.   The last line in Table IX shows that washed macrophages which have been exposed to KLH stimulated T_{KLH} cells can provide B cell help in the absence of T cells indicating that the T cell factors can be taken up by macrophages.

In another series of in vitro experiments (8) it was demonstrated that T cells could help B cells provided that the antigen to which the T cells were primed was present during the secondary response (Table X).   Thus, stimulation of T_{KLH} cells with KLH helped B cells to produce antibodies against SRBC.

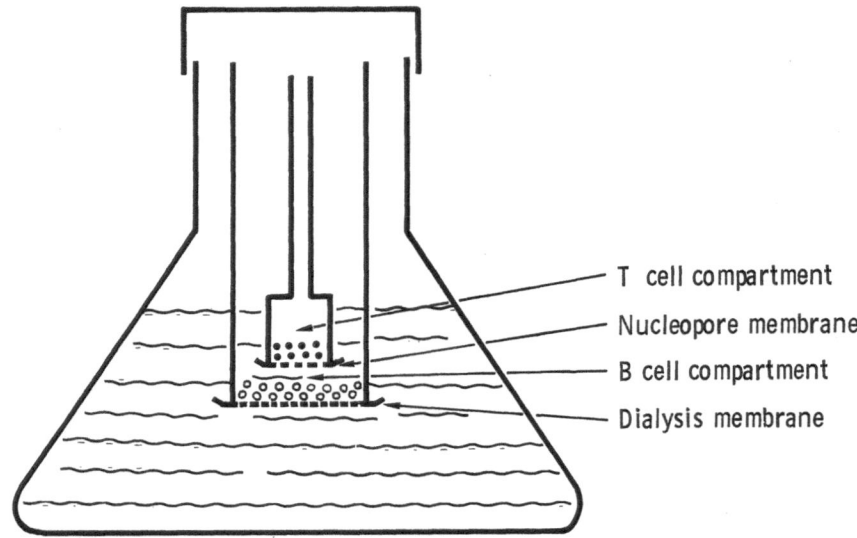

Fig. 1   Modified Marbrook culture system for analysing cell interaction in vitro. T cells are kept in the upper compartment, B cells (and MØ) in the lower, and antigens in both.
Plaque forming cells enumerated after 4-5 days culture.

Table IX.   Hapten-carrier analysis of cell cooperation in vitro

Cells in:		Response (PFC) to DNP-KLH in lower chamber*
Upper chamber	Lower chamber	
No cells	T_{KLH} + B_{DNP}**	+
T_{KLH}	B_{DNP}	+
T_{KLH}	B_{DNP} + anti-Thy 1 + C'	+
T (not primed)	B_{DNP}	O
T_{FGG}	B_{DNP}	O
No cells	B_{DNP} + MØ (T_{KLH} exposed)	+

* DNP-KLH and MØ present in both chambers

** T_{KLH} = KLH-primed T cells; B_{DNP} = DNP-primed B cells; etc.

Table X. Analysis of cell cooperation in vitro

Upper chamber	Lower chamber	Response (PFC) to SRBC*
No cells	T_{KLH} + B_{SRBC}**	+
T_{KLH}	B_{SRBC}	+
T_{DRBC}***	B_{SRBC}	O
No cells	B_{SRBC} + ($M\emptyset_{SRBC}$)	+
No cells	B_{SRBC} + ($M\emptyset_{KLH}$)	O

*   SRBC and KLH present in both chambers
** B_{SRBC} = B cells primed with sheep red cells, etc.
*** T_{DRBC} = T cells primed with donkey red cells

This suggests nonspecific T cell help since it is not likely that KLH and SRBC share antigenic determinants (second line in Table X). However, in contrast to T_{SRBC} exposed macrophages, washed macrophages which had been exposed to T_{KLH}, stimulated with KLH, could not provide the help in the absence of T cells suggesting that the macrophages could only take up the specific T cell factors (last two lines in Table X).

Suppressor T Cells

One of the first observations leading to the discovery of suppressor T cells was that specific unresponsiveness to SRBC could be transferred to normal non-tolerant mice by giving them T cells from syngeneic mice which had been made tolerant to SRBC (9). The phenomenon was called infective tolerance.

Another simple demonstration of T cell mediated inhibition of antibody production is summarized in Table XI (10). In this experiment, DNP-OVA primed spleen cells were transferred to non-immunized mice. The recipient mice were then injected with a very small dose of the hapten-carrier conjugate which did not give rise to a significant anti-DNP response in recipients with an intact immune system. However, recipients which were irradiated prior to the cell transfer produced a strong anti-hapten response and a similar response was observed in recipients which had been selectively depleted of their own T cells.

Table XI. The effect of T cell depletion on adoptive
           antibody response

Recipient treatment	Anti-DNP response to DNP-OVA
None	O
400 R, day -1	++
*AT$_x$ + 0.20 ml ATS, day -9	+

*AT$_x$ = Adult thymectomy, ATS = Anti-thymocyte serum

The transfer of the primed cells in this experiment would
correspond to a strong sensitization of the recipients and the
findings therefore indicate that in normal mice, T cells are
present which reduce the response to a subsequent antigenic
challenge. The experiment thus suggests a physiological
regulatory role for suppressor T cells in animals with intact
immune system.

It is now clear that a variety of immune responses can be
regulated by suppressor T cells and both specific and nonspecific
mechanisms are probably involved. The normal physiological role
of suppressor T cells has not yet been fully elucidated but it
seems likely that they are involved in maintaining self tolerance
and preventing excessive antibody and cell mediated immune
responses when antigen persists in the body. Deficiency of
suppressor T cells has been demonstrated in mice with autoimmune
disorders and the manifestation of their disease can be delayed
by giving them syngeneic T cells from healthy animals. Con-
versely, T cells in some human patients with hypogammaglobulinaemia have been found to inhibit pokeweed mitogen induced
maturation of B cells into antibody producing plasma cells in vitro.
It has, moreover, been suggested that malignant proliferation of
immunocytes may sometimes be due to suppressor cell failure.

As mentioned earlier, three types of T cells can now be
defined in the mouse depending on the types of Ly antigens
expressed in their surface membrane. These Ly antigens are
particularly interesting because they can be used to identify and
separate different functional subpopulations of T cells as
indicated in Table XII.

It is obvious that manipulation of the immunoregulatory
balance between helper and suppressor T cells could be beneficial
in a variety of clinical conditions but this can only be seriously

Table XII.   Surface markers for functional T cell
subclasses in mice

Ly phenotype	% of adult T cells	Principal function
Ly 1	30	Helper activity, delayed hypersensitivity
Ly 2,3	10	Cytotoxicity, suppressor activity
Ly 1,2,3	50	? Generation of suppressor cells, regulatory function

considered when these cells have been more fully characterized in
health and disease.

Hypothetical Model for Cellular Interactions
in Antibody Production

The way in which T cell help operates is beginning to be
understood but the mechanisms of T cell suppression are still
unknown.

Fig. 2 presents one of several tentative models which have
been suggested for T cell help and a few mechanisms which have
been proposed for T cell suppression are also indicated.   Regarding the helper mechanisms, the model is in our view largely consistent with available information, and we are not aware of any
widely accepted experimental data which make it untenable.   It
does not however, indicate the requirement for shared histocompatibility determinants between the interacting cells, and it
is probably over simplified in several other respects.   Most
carrier molecules have for instance more than one antigen
determinant.

The model proposes that macrophages play a central role in
the interaction.   Thus, the hapten-carrier is initially presented
by macrophages to carrier reactive T helper cells.   The activated
T cells release their carrier specific receptors complexed with
the hapten-carrier conjugates.   The presence of acceptors for
complexed helper T cell factors in the surface membrane of macrophages (cp. complexed IgG antibodies) then enables these cells to

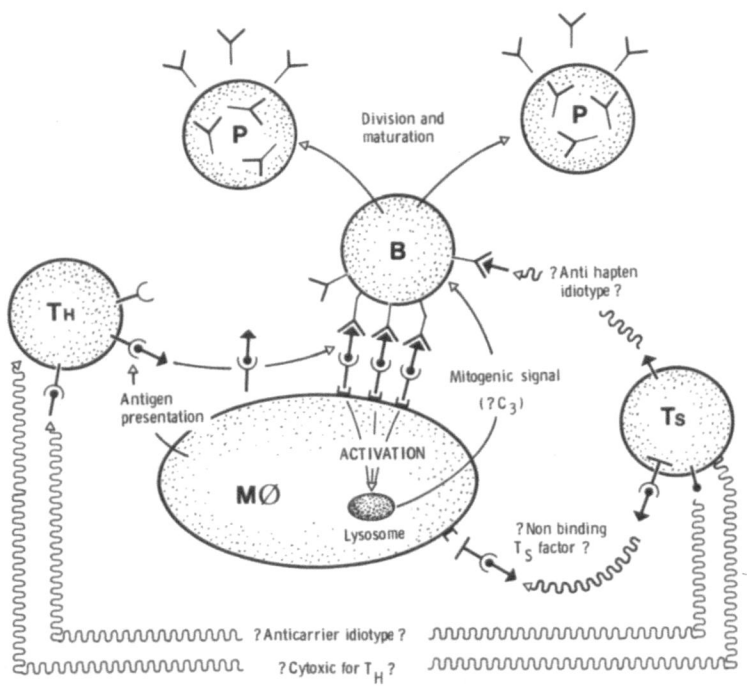

Fig. 2   HYPOTHETICAL MODEL FOR CELLULAR INTERACTIONS IN ANTIBODY
         PRODUCTION

The mechanisms of the positive interaction (straight arrows) are
better understood than the suppressor mechanisms (spiral arrows)
which are entirely speculative.

MØ: Macrophage;   B: Hapten specific B cell; T_H Helper T cell;
      T_S: Suppressor T cell;   P: Plasma cells

→   : Hypothetical antigen with one hapten and one carrier
        epitope

Y   : Hapten specific receptor or antibody

C   : Carrier specific helper T cell receptor or factor

C   : Hypothetical suppressor T cell receptor or factor

•→   : Hypothetical Ts anti carrier idiotype factor

→   : Hypothetical Ts anti hapten idiotype factor

[: Macrophage membrane acceptor for helper T cell factors

focus the hapten determinants onto the surface of hapten specific
B cells (first signal).   At the same time the complexed T cell
factors probably stimulate the macrophage to release lysosomal
enzymes which either directly or indirectly, by activating the
third complement component (C3), act as mitogen for B cells which
divide and thereby mature into antibody producing plasma cells
(second signal).   This short ranging mitogenic signal, although
nonspecific, will selectively activate hapten specific B cells
because they are attached to the macrophages through bridges made
of the antigen and the T cell factor.

At least three types of mechanisms have been postulated for
T suppressor cells (Fig. 2).   First, they might be cytotoxic
either to the T helper cells or B cells.   Secondly, they could
inhibit antibody production to T dependent antigens by expressing
idiotype specificity against either the carrier receptors on the
helper cells or the hapten receptor on the B cells.   Finally, if
macrophages do not have membrane acceptor for the T suppressor
factor, antibody production would be regulated through competition
between helper and suppressor factors for carrier determinants.

ANATOMICAL REQUIREMENTS OF REGULATORY CELL
INTERACTIONS AND DIVERSIFICATION OF ANTIBODY RESPONSES

The magnitude and regulation of an antibody response is
dependent on many factors including the nature, amount and mode of
presentation of the immunogen, the availability of specific B
cells and the balance of regulatory signals from helper and
suppressor T cells.

The heterogeneity of an antibody response to a particular
immunogen is determined in part by the diversity of its antigen
determinants and in part by the class and receptor diversity of
antigen reactive lymphocytes which can be recruited from the
circulating pool to the site of the antigen challenge.   Thus,
under optimal conditions, a single immunogen can give rise to
antibodies which are widely heterogeneous with respect to both the
variable and the constant parts of the antibody molecule, the
latter reflecting the involvement of different B cell subsets in
various stages of maturation.

The generation of vigorous, diverse and controlled antibody
responses therefore requires a device which can trap immunogens,
present them in a suitably concentrated form to a large number of
recirculating lymphocytes and at the same time provide a structural
framework for interaction between different types of antigen
interested cells.   It seems reasonable to assume that lymph nodes
have evolved to meet these requirements.   First, phagocytic and

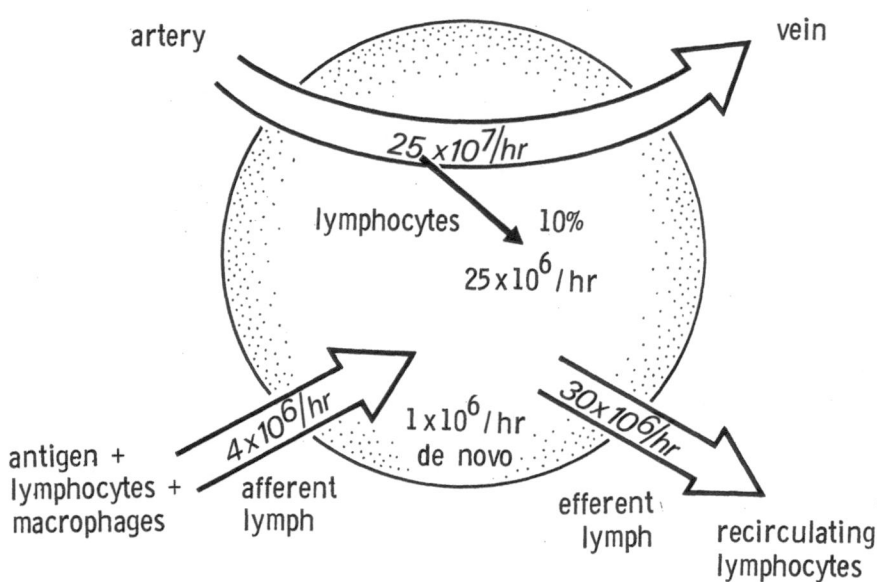

Fig. 3   Hourly lymphocyte turn over in a single resting lymph
         node.   Approximately 4 x 10^6 cells, mainly MØ and T cells,
         arrive via six or more afferent lymphatics, 25 x 10^6 T and
         B cells extravasate through postcapillary venules and
         1 x 10^6 are produced de novo.   30 x 10^6 T and B cells
         leave the node via its single efferent lymphatic, but this
         number can increase at least ten fold after antigen
         stimulation.

reticulo-endothelial cells in lymph nodes trap antigens from interstitial fluid, and the convergence of their afferent lymphatics acts
to concentrate antigens which would otherwise be diluted by
diffusion throughout the body.   Second, postcapillary venules in
lymph nodes are the major exit routes of recirculating lymphocytes
from the blood.   Different types of lymphocytes, mixing as they
migrate through the lymph node stroma towards its efferent lymphatic, are exposed to antigens which may have been trapped by the
lymph node.   At the same time they can interact with each other
and with macrophages presenting the antigen determinants.

     Fig. 3 illustrates schematically the extent of the lymphocyte
traffic from blood to lymph in a resting lymph node.   Approximately
10% of the lymphocytes which enter a lymph node via the bloodstream
extravasate, and this ratio is probably much higher during antigen

stimulation.   Thus, the lymphocyte efflux from a resting lymph node is approximately 30 x 10^6/hr but it can increase at least tenfold after antigen challenge (11).   Moreover, localization of antigen on the inner surface of the high endothelial cells lining the postcapillary lymph node venules probably promotes a selective extravasation of lymphocytes which can recognize the antigen (12, 13).   Superficially lymph nodes may perhaps be likened to shopping centres which keep large stocks and wide selections of goods (antigens).   These centres are therefore normally visited by very many potential customers (lymphocytes) with heterogeneous buying interests.   At the same time any new item of goods is effectively advertised and displayed to attract selectively a variety of different customers who are all interested in the new product.   All this gives rise to a vigorous business activity, both in terms of quantity and heterogeneity of goods being sold.

The brain does not have an effective lymphatic drainage system and as discussed later, immune responses in this organ might therefore be expected to be impaired with respect to magnitude, control and diversity.

REFERENCES

1. Scher I., Ahmed A., Sharrow S.O. and Paul W.E.   (1977), In Cooper M.D. and Dayton D.H. (Eds.), Development of Host Defences. p. 55. The Raven Press, New York.

2. Vitetta E.S., Cambier J., Spiva D., Kettman J.R. and Uhr J.W. (1977), In Cooper M.D. and Dayton D.H. (Eds.), Development of Host Defences. p. 75. The Raven Press, New York.

3. Chess L. and Schlossman S.F. (1977) Advanc. Immunol. 25, 213.

4. Miller J.A.F. and Mitchell G.F.   (1968) J. exp. Med. 128 801.

5. Weber G. and Kolsch E.   (1973) Europ. J. Immunol. 3, 767.

6. The Role of Products of the Histocompatibility Gene Complex in Immune Responses. (Katz D.H. and Benacerraf B. Eds.), Academic Press, New York (1976).

7. Feldmann M.   (1972) J. exp. Med. 136, 737.

8. Waldmann H., Munro A.J. and Hunter P. (1973) Europ. J. Immunol. 3, 167.

9. Gershon R.K. (1974) In Cooper M.D. and Warner N.L. (Eds.),
    Contemporary Topics in Immunobiology 3, 1. Plenum Press,
    New York.

10. Janeway C.A. (1978) Transplant. Proc. 10, 355

11. Frost H. (1978) Cell. Immunol. 37, 390.

12. McConnell I., Lachmann P.J. and Hobart M.J. (1974) Nature
    250, 113.

13. Cottier H., Hess M.W. and Keller H.U. (1978) In Symposium
    on lymph and Milieu Interieur. XVII Congress of International
    Society of Haematology, p. 841 (abstract).

INHIBITING FACTOR : GENERAL REVIEW

D. Karcher

Born-Bunge Foundation, Department of Neurochemistry
U.I.A., Wilrijk, Belgium

A factor inhibiting the immunological reaction could explain the simultaneous presence of the virus and the antibodies in subacute sclerosing panencephalitis (SSPE), a persistent viral disease with a hyperimmune reaction.

The inhibiting factors described in the literature are in most instances an α globulin or immunoregulatory α globulin (IRA), present in the serum (6, 9, 11, 12, 14, 24, 26, 27, 28, 39). The active fraction is not species specific and can be found in the sera of rats, cows, rabbits, mice, guinea pigs and man (7, 36). It is suppressive for the immunological process (13), in species of origin and across species lines. Experiments in vitro and in vivo tend to confirm the presence in the serum of such an inhibiting factor regulating the immune process.

IN VITRO

The experimental conditions used to detect an inhibiting factor in vitro are : plaque forming cells (11), rosette formation (11), phagocytosis (11), stimulatory effect of phytohemagglutinin (4, 5), and macrophage immobilisation (5, 7, 9).

a) plaque forming cells (11, 12) : to determine the most suitable conditions in which the inhibiting factor (an α globulin isolated from the serum) can act, the following tests were carried out :

1) either the inhibiting factor is injected 0 to 30 minutes prior to the antigen,
2) or after the foregoing procedure, the antigen is again given 10 days later,

3) or the animals are injected with the antigen, and ten days later with the inhibiting factor, an α -globulin, followed by a
second dose of antigen.

   The inhibiting activity occurs only when the α globulin
is injected shortly prior to the antigen; the plaque formation
is then suppressed.

b) rosette formation (11, 12) : lymphocytes bind sheep red blood
cells (SRBC) to form rosettes.

   Here too the α globulin added prior to the SRBC suppresses
the rosette formation. The α globulin isolated from the serum
added to the medium is 20 to 120 times its normal concentration
in serum (12).

c) phagocytosis (11) : for the inhibiting factor to exert any
activity on phagocytosis, it has to be applied at the latest ten
minutes after the addition of the microorganisms, not 10 to
30 minutes when most are already engulfed (11).

   Washing lymphocytes, which had been incubated with the suppressive factor, before adding the microorganisms, removes the
inhibitory effect, showing that the inhibiting factor seems to
bind relatively weakly to the lymphocyte surface (11).

d) lymphocyte transformation (4, 5, 6) : α globulin can prevent
the stimulatory effects of both phytohemagglutinin and specific
antigen (25, 28). The IRA acts at about the time when activation
of lymphocytes occurs (6).

   The inhibiting factor does not prevent the proliferation
response of the lymphocytes once they are activated by phytohemagglutinin (6).

   Lymphocyte proliferation is observed after washing the
lymphocytes, thus removing the inhibiting effect (6, 7).

e) macrophage immobilisation (5, 7, 9) : the increase in the size
of the macrophage tuft area by exposure to α globulin in addition to the antigen, results from interference with antigen
recognition (5). If IRA was cytotoxic, it would prevent the
macrophages from migrating (9).

   The inhibition of macrophage migration by specific antigen
is apparently reversed by the presence of α globulin, but not
by control proteins (9). Increase of tuft area occurs in a
linear fashion with increasing concentrations of α globulin
(5, 9, 25).

f) immunization : the presence of an inhibiting factor in the
serum capable of suppressing the immune response of spleen cells
culture to SRBC has been demonstrated. Spleen cells are incubated
3 hours with normal serum; then cultured 4 days in vitro with
SRBC, an impairment of the immune response is then observed (39).
However when the spleen cells are washed twice the inhibitory
effect is almost removed. Trypsin treatment also removes the
inhibitory effect (39). In addition, it was demonstrated that
serum of an immunized animal contains higher concentration of
inhibitory activity than does normal serum (39).

                          IN VIVO

     In vivo experiments with animals confirm the observations
made in vitro and show that :

1. a) the immunosuppressive factor in the serum, an α globulin,
   acts upon the earliest events of all observed lymphocyte mediated immune responses(5).

   b) the suppressive factor appears to bind relatively weakly
   to a receptor on the lymphocyte surface (7).

   c) it interferes with the recognition of specific antigen by
   sensitized lymphocytes (9, 14).

   The inhibitory factor when injected at the same time as the
antigen, acts on the inductive phase of antibody synthesis, but
does not affect the established antibody level (7, 27). Given
after antibody production started, the factor is ineffective (27).
However, animals do not produce detectable quantities of antibodies against a different antigen injected later, at a time
when the immunosuppressive activity of the initial IRA should have
gone (7).

   The time relationship of the injection of the inhibiting
factor and the antigen is critical (27). The injection of an
inhibiting factor has either full or no effect on antibody synthesis (27).

   Some (7, 14) claim that most activity occurs when the inhibiting factor is injected 24 hours before the antigen; when injected 4 days before, the effect is reduced to 50%; 7 days before
there is no inhibitory effect. Thus the time span for the inhibiting effect to take place varies according to the assay.

2. A phenomenon observed in graft rejection illustrates again the
role played by the inhibiting factor.

   a) allograft rejection can be suppressed in animals which are
   injected with α globulin (24), there can be reciprocal tole-

rance of none litter mates achieved by the injection of α
globulin (17, 18). Prolonged survival of skin allograft
depressed the formation of circulating antibodies against the
graft (24). It also demonstrated that the suppressive material is not an antibody : after absorbing the antibodies,
the suppressive activity of the serum is maintained (35).
Working with antilymphocyte serum besides the immunosuppression
artifically induced, there appears to be an inhibitory
factor, an α globulin present in the serum (40).

b) <u>in man, raised levels of α_2 globulin</u> have been observed in
the serum of patients undergoing renal graft rejection (7).
The presence of raised levels of α_2 globulins foresees an
unfavorable prognosis for the graft : normal levels indicate
a favourable issue (29). This underlines the fact that the
inhibiting factor needs to act before the immune response is
induced. The time seems to be of major importance, delayed
α globulin production remains ineffective.

Experiments carried out in mice confirm these observations.
When the first injection of the inhibiting factor is given 0-30
minutes after the application of the graft to its bed, 35% of
the grafts survive for 30 days, there was 20% survival for 8
months. If the injection is delayed for a short a time as 4
hours, there was no prolongation of the graft survival (26).
If the inhibiting factor is given 4 hours after grafting instead
of half an hour, the survival of the graft in injected animals
is not different from the grafts in control untreated animals
(26).

<u>The inhibiting factor appears to be concerned with the early
stage of rejection mechanism</u> (7, 26).

Skin grafts, antagonism of DNA synthesis in lymphocyte transformation,inhibition of antibody formation are all assays requiring the presence of T lymphocytes (36). α globulin acts upon
the earliest events of lymphocyte mediated immune response, at
the time of antigen recognition of these cells (5).

3. <u>The part played by the inhibiting factor in animals injected</u>
with an inhibiting factor along <u>with viruses</u> corroborate the
foregoing observations (30). No method was employed rendering
an absolutely positive distinction between the effects of an
inhibitor and those of antibodies in immune sera (30, 32).

A distinction could be achieved by treating the serum with
either :

a) trypsin : one notices the removal of the inhibiting factor
   with trypsin but no inactivation of the specific antibodies (21).

b) or by heating : destruction of the immunoglobulins, inactivation of complement, and retention of the inhibiting factor are observed (30).

The titers of both inhibiting factors and antibodies are individually measured by hemagglutination inhibition after the foregoing procedures.

The mode of action of the inhibitor may be explained as a result of competition for virus between the inhibitor and the immunoglobulin. The hemagglutination inhibition reaction might occur when the affinity of the virus to the inhibitor is greater than the affinity of the cell receptor (33). The comparative testing of serum samples taken before and after immunization, shows close relationship between the capability of the organism to produce specific antibody and the titer of serum inhibitors (30). The most important changes in the inhibitor titer is found on immunization with viral antigen which develop active inhibitors (30). The inhibition of virus multiplication is observed when a sufficient concentration of inhibitor is given to mice either before, at the same time, or shortly after inoculation with virus before it enters cells (21).

The various inhibitors show :

1) different specific activities against different strains of viruses,

2) different modes of interaction with the virus,

3) distinct susceptibility to the action of certain chemicals,

4) variations in the occurrence in sera of different animals (30).

These experiments with animals on inhibitors and antibodies in the course of immunization with viruses may shed light on the problem of slow viral diseases.

SUBACUTE SCLEROSING PANENCEPHALITIS

Subacute sclerosing panencephalitis (SSPE), was defined by Burnet (3) as a condition in which cells differentiated in the thymus, have developed specific tolerance to measles antigen, while the antibody system remains active. This concept supports the findings of coexistence in SSPE of high measles antibody titer and paramyxovirus, and consequently the presence of immunosuppressive or blocking factors in the serum of SSPE (2). The blocking factors are immunosuppressive to a specific cell population, so that antibody producing cells are uncontrolled and are producing high levels of immunoglobulins (40). The immunoglobulin is not likely to be involved in the pathology of the disease, although it is important in the persistence of the infection (40).

The hyperimmunization in SSPE is on a par with high measles antibody titer, and therewith, oligoclonal IgG. This tends to explain the discrepancies (1) between the observations made by various investigators, namely due to :

1) the type of antigen, in this case the components of the para-myxovirus,

2) the assay system used,

3) the stage of the disease,

4) the course of the disease, either subacute or chronic,

5) the clinical treatment,

6) infections other than SSPE virus, or other medical complications.

This allows for the immunological basis of SSPE to be explained by the failure of T lymphocytes to eliminate the measles virus in the presence of antibody response (19), or for the action of an inhibiting factor to take place.

In experiments made in animals with (influenza) viruses, the level of inhibiting factor can vary according to the type of virus injected. A complex might be considered to form between the antigen and the inhibiting factor, in a way competing with the specific immunoglobulins present. This consideration rests partially on the fact that a blocking factor in SSPE inhibits cell mediated immunity in the majority of patients studied :

a) skin test reactions to intradermal antigen (candida, mumps, measles virus) are absent (10, 22),

b) stimulation of lymphocytes by tuberculin purified protein derivative (22), phytohemagglutinin (19, 20, 34, 37, 38), measles and SSPE virus antigen (1),

c) measles vaccine (22),

d) skin allograft is rejected more slowly (11),

e) the ability to block the release of migration inhibitory factor from lymphocytes of both SSPE and measles positive controls (1, 22).

The degree of blocking increases as the disease advances (37, 38). Apparently, the blocking factor is ten times more potent in cerebrospinal fluid (CSF) than in plasma (1, 31).

Normal transformation occurs when SSPE lymphocytes are cultured in the presence of normal plasma. The response was

suppressed significantly in the presence of autologous plasma
(1). In addition, the blocking factor is considered to be
effective in the SSPE lymphocytes' response to SSPE virus (34).

The inhibiting compound contributes to the pathogenesis of
SSPE by preventing effective host response to SSPE virus (34).
There is little doubt that some type of inhibition has to be
taken into account.

PERSONAL INVESTIGATIONS

We were able to demonstrate that SSPE serum IgG's were
absorbed by incubating the measles virus with isolated serum
IgG (23). The antigen antibody reaction was attained with
isolated IgG not with whole serum, working at all times under
identical conditions.

This difference in behaviour between whole serum and purified
IgG from an identical serum specimen has been investigated.
SSPE CSF, however, treated under identical conditions revealed
antibody absorption when incubated with measles virus comparable
to that seen for serum isolated IgG.

A factor inhibiting the antigen antibody reaction was
isolated from the serum according to four different methods (16) :

1) preparative electrophoresis,

2) precipitation with ammonium sulfate, working with the supernatant,

3) isolation from the serum after passage on an ion exchange
   column,

4) heating the serum at 100°C for 10 minutes.

The immunosuppressive effect corresponds to fractions located
in the α globulin region after agar gel electrophoresis.

The different samples obtained were tested as follows :

1) qualitatively, by adding them to the incubation medium prior
   to electrophoresis; no decrease in immunoglobulin concentration was observed;

2) quantitatively, with the help of radioimmunoassay, the inhibiting activity of the different samples was demonstrated.

IgG's isolated from SSPE serum were labelled according to
the method of Greenwood et al. (15). Specific rabbit anti-human

IgG serum were coupled to cellulose CNBr. This insoluble complex
reacts with the labelled antigen after incubation of room temperature. The immunoabsorbent and the total radioactivity (20.000 cpm)
was kept constant. The various preparations of inhibiting
factor were added in serial dilutions to the immunoabsorbent
prior to the labelled SSPE serum IgG's. The decrease in counts per
minute reflected the inhibiting effect on the reaction showing
14 to 92 % inhibition.

Having analyzed more than 200 serum specimens from different
SSPE patients, it became quite clear, that in the great majority
of cases the α_2 globulins are markedly increased (20). The
inhibiting activity in control and multiple sclerosis sera is
less prevalent than in SSPE serum. Differences in inhibiting
effect when dealing with productive and non productive strains
of SSPE viruses of serum from patients affected with either
strains has to be demonstrated. The outcome of these studies
might enable to show some specificity for these reactions. So
far commercially available measles were used in most instances.

The factor inhibiting or blocking the antigen antibody
reaction can even be observed when SSPE serum immunoglobulins
react with rabbit anti SSPE immunoglobulins. This has been
shown with radioimmunoassay (16).

An inhibiting factor or immunoregulatory compound acts in
the inductive phase of antibody synthesis and interferes with the
recognition of specific antigen by sensitized lymphocytes. It
affects also the antigen antibody reaction.

If indeed, these observations are true, in a neurological
disease, such as SSPE, could the immune reaction not play its
role and thereby, immunity fulfil its task after suppression of
the inhibiting effect? Could the abolishing of the inhibiting
factor possibly lead to an amelioration of the neurological
condition?

ACKNOWLEDGEMENT

This study has been supported by grants from the Belgian
National Fund for Medical Scientific Research (grant nr 30033),
the Belgian Ministry of Education and Culture and the "Universitaire Instelling Antwerpen".

REFERENCES

1. A. Ahmed, D.M. Strong, K.W. Sell, G.B. Thurman, R.C. Knudsen, R.W.I. Star Jr., W.R. Grace . Demonstration of a blocking factor in the plasma and spinal fluid of patients with SSPE. J. Exp. Med. 139, 902-924, 1974.

2. J. Allen, J. Oppenheim, J.A. Brody, J. Miller. Labile inhibitor of lymphocyte transformation in plasma from a patient with SSPE. Infec. Immunity 8, 80-82, 1973.

3. F.M. Burnet. Measles as an index of immunological function. Lancet, 2, 610-613, 1968.

4. S.R. Cooperband, H. Bonnevik, K. Schmid, J.A. Mannick. Transformation of human lymphocytes : inhibition by homologous α globulin. Science 159, 1243-1244, 1968.

5. S.R. Cooperband, R.C. Davis, K. Schmid, J.A. Mannick. Competitive blockade of lymphocyte stimulation by serum immuno-regulatory alpha globulin (IRA). Transplant. Proc. 1, 516-523, 1969.

6. S.R. Cooperband, A.M. Badger, R.C. Davis, K. Schmid, J.A. Mannick. The effect of immunoregulatory α globulin upon lymphocytes in vitro. J. Immunol. 109, 154-163, 1972.

7. S.R. Cooperband, R. Nimberg, K. Schmid, J.A. Mannick. Humoral immunosuppressive factors. Transplant. Proc. 8, 225-242, 1976.

8. J.R. David, S. Al-Askari, H.S. Lawrence, L. Thomas. Delayed hypersensitivity in vitro. J. Immunol. 93, 264-273, 1964.

9. R.C. Davis, S.R. Cooperband, J.A. Mannick. The effect of immunoregulatory α globulin (IRA) on antigen mediated macrophage immobilization in vitro. J. Immunol. 106, 755-760, 1971.

10. K.L. Gerson, H.A. Haslam. Subtle immunologic abnormalities in four boys with subacute sclerosing panencephalitis. N. Engl. J. Med. 285, 78-82, 1971.

11. M. Glaser, I. Ofek, D. Nelken. Inhibition of plaque formation, rosette formation and phagocytosis by alpha globulin. Immunology, 23 (2), 205-214, 1972.

12. M. Glaser, I. Cohen, D. Nelken. In vitro inhibition of plaque and rosette formation by α globulin. J. Immunol. 108, 286-288, 1972.

13. M. Glaser, C.C. Ting, R.B. Herberman. In vitro inhibition of cell mediated cytotoxicity against syngeneic friend virus induced leukemia by immunoregulatory α globulin. J. Nat. Cancer Inst. 55, 1477-1479, 1975.

14. A.H. Glasgow, S.R. Cooperband, K. Schmid, J.T. Parker, J.C. Occhino, J.A. Mannick. Inhibition of secondary immune responses by immunoregulatory alpha globulin. Transplant. Proc. 3, 835-837, 1971.

15. F.C. Greenwood, W.M. Hunter, J.S. Glover. The preparation of 131 I labelled human growth hormone of high specific radioactivity. Biochem. J. 89, 114-123, 1963.

16. D. Karcher, M. Noppe, A. Lowenthal. A heat stable serum inhibitor of an antigen antibody reaction of SSPE. J. Neurol.216,

51-56, 1977.

17. B.B. Karim. Ann. NY Acad. Sci. 73, 848, 1958.

18. B.B. Kamrin. Successful skin homografts in mature non-litter-mate rats treated with fractions containing α -globulins. Proc. Soc. Exp. Biol. Med. : 100, 58-61, 1959.

19. A. Klajman, M. Sternbach, L. Ranon, M. Drucker, D. Geminder, N. Sadan. Impaired delayed hypersensitivity in subacute sclerosing panencephalitis. Acta Paediat. Scand. 62, 523-526, 1973.

20. O. Kolar. Measles and subacute sclerosing panencephalitis. Lancet, 2, 1242, 1968.

21. O. Krizanova, V. Rathova. Serum inhibitors of myxovirus. Current topics in microbiology and Immunology, Springer Verlag Berlin Heidelber, New York, Ed. W. Arber Basle. 47, 125-151, 1969.

22. E. Livni, E. Kott, Y. Danon, A. Kuritzky, J. Joshua. Cell mediated immunity in SSPE. Isr. J. Med. Sci. 12, 1183-1188, 1976.

23. A. Lowenthal, D. Karcher. Is multiple sclerosis as subacute sclerosing panencephalitis an hyperimmune disease. Livre Jubilaire Prof. Rylant ULB Brussel 1976, Le coeur et l'esprit, 410-413, 1976.

24. J.A. Mannick, K. Schmid. Prolongation of allograft survival by an alpha globulin isolated from normal blood. Transplantation : 5, 1231-1239, 1967.

25. J.D. Milton. Effect of an immunosuppressive serum α_2 glycoprotein with ribonuclease activity on the proliferation of human lymphocytes in culture. Immunology, 20, 205-212, 1971.

26. J.F. Mowbray. Effect of large doses of an α_2-glycoprotein fraction on the survival of rat skin homografts. Transplantation : 1, 15-20, 1963.

27. J.F. Mowbray. Ability of large doses of an $alpha_2$ plasma protein fraction to inhibit antibody production. Immunology 6, 217-225, 1963.

28. J.F. Mowbray, D.C. Hargrave. Further studies on the preparation of the immunosuppressive $alpha_2$ protein fraction from serum and its assay in mice. Immunology, 11, 413-419, 1966.

29. R.R. Riggio, G.H. Schwartz, K.H. Stenzel, A.L. Rubin. $Alpha_2$ hyperglobulinaemia as a humoral indicator of the homograft reaction. Lancet, ii, 1218-1221, 1968.

30. Z.I. Revnova, P.N. Kosyalov. Inhibitors and antibodies in the course of immunization of animals with viral preparations. Acta Virol. 11: 69-77, 1967.

31. K.W. Sell, G.B. Thurman, A. Ahmed, D.M. Strong. Plasma and spinal fluid blocking factor in SSPE. N. Engl. J. Med. 288, 215-216, 1973.

32. K.F. Shortridge, F. Biddle. A human serum inhibition of adenovirus haemagglutination. Arch. ges. Virusforsch. 25, 148-159, 1968.

33. W. Smith, J.C.N. Westwood. Influenza virus haemagglutination.
    The mechanism of the Francis phenomenon. Brit. J. Exp. Path.
    31, 725-738, 1950.
34. R.W. Steele, D.A. Fuccillo, S.A. Hensen, M.M. Vincent, J.A.
    Bellanti. Specific inhibitory factors of cellular immunity
    in children with subacute sclerosing panencephalitis. J.
    Pediat. 88, 56-62, 1976.
35. J.S.Streilein, D.A. Hart. Serum free culture of hamster
    lymphoid cells and differential inhibition of lipopolysaccha-
    ride stimulation by isologous serum. Infec. Immunity 14,
    463-470, 1976.
36. J. Streilein, D.A. Hart. Role of alpha globulins in nonspe-
    cific regulation of the immune response : possible mechanisms
    for external and internal signals. Fed. Proc. 37, 2042-2044,
    1978.
37. H.M. Swick, W.H. Brooks, Th.L. Roszman, D. Caldwell. A heat
    stable blocking factor in the plasma of patients with sub-
    acute sclerosing panencephalitis. Neurology, 26, 84-88, 1976.
38. H.M. Swick, Host inhibitory or blocking factor in SSPE.
    J. Pediat. Letters to the Editor 89, 518-519, 1976.
39. B. Veit, J.G. Michael. Characterization of an immunosuppres-
    sive factor present in mouse serum. J. Immunol. 111, 341-351,
    1973.
40. D.R. Webb, A. Winkelstein. Immunosuppression and immunopoten-
    tiation. Eds. H.H. Fudenberg, D.P. Stites, J.L. Caldwell,
    J.V. Wells, Longe Medical Publications, Los Altos California
    p. 308, 1978.
41. L.P. Weiner. M.S. Symposium Amsterdam 1977, MS Res. Med. 7/8
    (1976-1977) Bahn Sheltema Holkema Amsterdam. The Dr. Harry
    Weaver Memorial. p. 246.

B LYMPHOCYTE FUNCTION IN SSPE : IS THERE LACK OF SUPPRESSOR CELLS ?

H.W. Kreth, A. Ahmed[+], and V. ter Meulen

Institute of Virology and Immunobiology, University of Würzburg, Würzburg, F.R. Germany, and
[+] Naval Medical Research Institute, Bethesda, U.S.A.

INTRODUCTION

A characteristic feature of subacute sclerosing panencephalitis (SSPE) are elevated levels of measles antibodies in serum and CSF. These antibodies seem to be produced in myeloma-like quantities amounting to almost 10-20 % of total serum IgG (4). Biochemical and immunological studies have further revealed antibody activity to be associated with gammaglobulin bands of restricted heterogeneity implicating a limited number of antibody-producing clones at a given time (7, 8). While all these data support a concept of prolonged hyperimmunization , the mechanisms leading to humoral hyperimmunity in SSPE are not understood.

Under normal conditions, antibody production is subject to a number of feed-back mechanisms. For instance, free antibody might compete with membrane-bound receptors for antigen or mask antigenic sites. Furthermore, antigen-antibody complexes might block Fc receptors on B cells, activate suppressor cells and lead to the production of anti-idiotypic antibodies. The prolonged hyperimmunization could be explained in 2 ways : antigen could be presented to the precursors of antibody-producing cells in a highly immunogenic form thus by-passing normal suppressive forces. Such a possibility could arise if a fraction of T cells or monocytes are persistently infected by SSPE virus. Alternatively, inhibitory signals (e.g. suppressor cells) could be blocked or missing in SSPE due to an inborn or acquired defect of the immune system. Any defect of immunoregulatory functions could have a significant bearing on the pathogenesis of the disease. The high levels of antibodies resulting from such a defect could play a major role

in the immunopathology of the disease as has already been proposed
by several investigators in recent years (1, 2).

In the present investigation, a simple model system was used
to study in vitro immunoglobulin production by peripheral lymphocytes. Surprisingly, the pokeweed mitogen (PWM) induced IgM biosynthesis at the end of a 7-day culture period was found to be strongly
enhanced in SSPE. These preliminary results may suggest a diminished suppressor cell activity.

MATERIALS AND METHODS

Peripheral lymphoid cells (PBL) were obtained from 12 patients
with SSPE and from a random group of 16 healthy children and young
adults. Diagnosis of SSPE had been confirmed by serological,
immunological and electroencephalographic criteria. Patients
marked by an asterisk in Table II and III received Isoprinosine^R
therapy at the time of testing.

PBL were isolated from heparinized venous blood by Ficoll-
Isopaque density centrifugation and washed 7 times (2 x with Hanks'
balanced salt solution and 5 x through fetal calf serum (FCS)) in
order to eliminate serum immunoglobulins. Cultures were set up
according to Waldmann et al (9) at 2×10^6 cells per ml (without
or with 1 % pokeweed mitogen) in HEPES-buffered RPMI 1640 supplemented with 2 mmol glutamine, 50 µg/ml gentamycin and 10 % heat-
inactivated FCS. After a 7-day culture period cells were pelleted
by centrifugation, and the cell-free supernatants stored at − 70°C.
The amount of IgM was determined by a sensitive double antibody
radioimmunoassay.

Lymphocyte subpopulation analysis was carried out on cryopre-
served cells from the same date when cultures were set up for in
vitro IgM induction. T cells were identified by spontaneous rosette formation with neuraminidase-treated sheep red blood cells,
and B cells carrying surface-bound IgM or IgD were detected by
UV light microscopy after staining viable cells with fluorescein-
conjugated specific antisera (Meloy Laboratories). Positive cells
were scored as percentages of total mononuclear cells (lymphocytes
and monocytes). In order to detect viral antigens, cells from
7-day PWM stimulated cultures were spread on microscopic slides
and fixed in acetone for 10 minutes. Smears were then stained by
standard procedures with either a fluorescein-conjugated gammaglobulin preparation derived from a patient with SSPE or with
rabbit anti-measles antibodies followed by a fluoresceinated
goat anti rabbit gammaglobulin reagent. At least 1000 cells
were examined by UV light microscopy.

RESULTS

PWM-Induced IgM Synthesis

Pokeweed mitogen (PWM) was used to induce terminal differentiation of B cells into immunoglobulin-secreting plasmocytes. Pokeweed mitogen is known to stimulate IgM, IgG and IgA production in vitro (9). However, in this study, only the amount of IgM present in the culture media at the end of a 7-day culture period was measured by a sensitive radioimmunoassay.

Cultures prepared with lymphocytes derived from a control group of healthy children and young adults synthesized IgM over a wide range of concentrations (Table 1). The mean geometric titer was 1228 ng IgM per 2×10^6 cells in the absence, and 4850 ng IgM per 2×10^6 cells in the presence of pokeweed mitogen (mean ratio: with PWM/without PWM = 3.9). Exceptionally high ratios (13,9; 20,6; 43,1) which at present could not further be explained were only seen in 3 out of 16 cases with lymphocytes from children 10, 13 and 12 years of age.

Whereas unstimulated SSPE lymphocytes produced levels of IgM comparable to normals (mean geometric titer 774 ng IgM per 2×10^6 cells), a very high response was consistently found after the addition of 1 % PWM (mean geometric titer with PWM : 15900 ng in SSPE versus 4980 ng IgM in controls). It should be noted that in SSPE individual titers and ratios are more evenly distributed as compared to normals.

Some SSPE patients received Isoprinosine[R], a drug with antiviral and immunopotentiating properties, at the time of testing. High IgM synthesis could, however, not be attributed to treatment since titers of IgM were similar before and after drug therapy.

The high response to PWM stimulation seems to be a characteristic and reproducible finding in SSPE. This is demonstrated in Table 3 where cells from 3 patients were repeatedly tested over a period of several months. These cells maintained almost the same level of activity. The IgM produced is probably of polyclonal origin. No attempts were made during this study to detect specific measles antibodies in culture fluids of PWM stimulated SSPE lymphocytes.

Lymphocyte Subpopulations

Peripheral lymphoid cells from SSPE patients and normal controls had similar percentages of T and B cells. The frequencies for T cells were 54 ± 6.8 % in SSPE and 53.9 ± 5.7 % in normals.

TABLE I

IgM BIOSYNTHESIS BY PERIPHERAL LYMPHOCYTES FROM NORMAL CONTROLS.

Donor	Age (years)	Nanograms of IgM per 2 x 10^6 cells		Ratio (with PWM/ without PWM)
		without PWM	with PWM	
1.	22	113	1094	9.7
2.	28	187	541	2.9
3.	1	113	1094	9.7
4.	1	187	540	2.9
5.	10	346	1834	5.3
6.	12	530	824	1.6
7.	10	559	7780	13.9
8.	13	120	2474	20.6
9.	12	116	5004	43.1
10.	8	60	167	2.8
11.	13	90	223	2.5
12.	6	1420	3000	2.1
13.	8	1245	3200	2.6
14.	14	2080	7853	3.8
15.	5	1400	2300	1.6
16.	9	169	232	1.4
Geometric mean titer		1228	4850	

Since the incidence of B cells bearing surface(s) IgG or IgA is very low in human peripheral blood, only B cells carrying IgM or IgD heavy chains were analysed by the fluorescent antibody method. The frequencies of B cells with sIgM or sIgD were 11.8 + 5.2 % and 9.7 + 5.5 % for SSPE patients, as compared to 10.1 + 4.3 % and 9.2 + 3.8 % in normal controls. No correlation was observed between the percentage of B cells with sIgM and the magnitude of the IgM response in individual patients and normals. Sometimes a reverse relationship was found as exemplified for patients $\neq$ 5 and $\neq$ 10 (Table II). Whereas numbers of B^u cells were 22 % and 6.8 % the amounts of IgM produced were 8550 and 32 600 ng in these patients.

Search for Viral Antigens

No specific antigens were detected when acetone-fixed smears of PWM-stimulated SSPE cells were stained for measles antigens and examined by UV light microscopy.

TABLE II

PWM-INDUCED IgM BIOSYNTHESIS BY PERIPHERAL LYMPHOCYTES IN SSPE.

| Patient | Age (years) | Nanograms of IgM per 2 x 10^6 cells | | Ratio (with PWM/ without PWM) |
		without PWM	with PWM	
1.	12	160	6253	39
2.	27	390	12163	31
3.	15	320	7950	25
4.	13	624	9600	15
5.	8	282	8550	30
6.	10	239	7135	30
7. *	14	322	9887	31
8. *	17	884	15500	18
9.	13	134	14844	111
10. *	10	1494	32600	22
11. *	12	680	10666	16
12. *	13	554	4677	8
Geometric mean titer :		774	15900	

* Patients on Isoprinosine^R therapy

TABLE III

IgM PRODUCTION BY SSPE LYMPHOCYTES IN VITRO : REPRODUCIBILITY.

| Patient | Date of testing | Nanograms of IgM per 2 x 10^6 cells | |
		without PWM	with PWM
MR	9/77	230	7200
	10/77 *	180	6950
	5/78 *	79	4608
LE	9/77 *	310	8205
	2/78 *	384	8294
	4/78 *	485	19990
SO	9/77 *	355	9210
	1/78 *	893	9989

* Asterisks indicate treatment with Isoprinosine^R

COMMENTS

It has been shown that PWM-induced B cell differentiation
is dependent on T lymphocytes. Thus, purified human B cells
will not mature into immunoglobulin-secreting plasmocytes unless
syngeneic or allogeneic T cells are added to the test system (3).
Variations of immunoglobulin synthesis in these cultures are not
related to actual numbers of B cells but seem to reflect the functional state of the T cell population. Recently, the T-B cell
interactions in PWM cultures have been further dissected. It is
now possible to subdivide human peripheral T cells into 2 distinct
subpopulations based on their ability to express receptors either
for the Fc part of pentameric IgM (T_μ cells) or the Fc part of
IgG (T γ cells). T_μ cells have been found to promote B cells
proliferation and differentiation while the response is suppressed by T γ cells (6). The magnitude of the IgM response in
SSPE as shown in the present study could thus be interpreted in
terms of an imbalance of T subpopulations with excess helper T
activity and a deficiency (or blocked function)of suppressor T
cells. This interpretation is supported by preliminary studies
using mixtures of SSPE and normal peripheral lymphocytes
(data not shown). Mixtures of cells derived from 2 patients
with SSPE produce a titer of IgM as high as would be expected
from their separate cultures. However, mixing SSPE with normal
cells results in considerably reduced levels of IgM, suggesting
an effect of suppressor cells derived from the normal lymphocyte
donor. If our notion of a diminished suppressor cell activity
is correct, such a deficiency could have an important bearing on
the pathogenesis of the disease. If present at an early stage,
an exaggerated antibody response might well interfere with
elimination of virus-infected host cells by sensitized T lymphocytes and thus facilitate virus persistence. Moreover, clonal
size could be similarly dysregulated resulting in extremely large
pools of memory cells and enhancing the probability for some
precursor cells to escape into the brain and initiate local
antibody synthesis.

ACKNOWLEDEGMENT

Supported by grant ≠ Kr 376/8 from the Deutsche Forschungsgemeinschaft.

REFERENCES

1. Ahmed, A., D.M. Strong, K.W. Sell, G.B. Thurman, R.C. Knudsen,
   R. Wistar, Jr., Gray, W.R. : Demonstration of a blocking factor
   in the plasma and spinal fluid of patients with subacute sclero-

sing panencephalitis. I. Partial characterization. J. exp. Med. 139 : 902, 1974.

2. Joseph B.S., Oldstone, M.B.A. : Immunologic injury in measles virus infection. II. Suppression of immune injury through antigenic modulation. J. exp. Med. 142 : 864, 1975.

3. Keightley, R.G., Cooper, M.D., Lawton, A.R. : The T cell dependence of B cell differentiation induced by Pokeweed mitogen. J. Immunol. 117 : 1538, 1976.

4. Mehta, P.D., A. Kane, H. Thormar : Quantitation of measles virus-specific immunoglobulin in serum, CSF and brain extract from patients with subacute sclerosing panencephalitis. J. Immunol. 118 : 2254, 1977.

5. Moretta, L., M. Ferrarini, M.C. Mingari, A. Moretta, S.R. Webb : Subpopulations of human T cells identified by receptors for immunoglobulins and mitogen responsiveness. J. Immunol. 117 : 2171, 1976.

6. Moretta, L., S.R. Webb, C.E. Grossi, P.M. Lydyard, M.D. Cooper: Functional analysis of two human T-cell subpopulations : help and suppression of B-cell responses by T cells bearing receptors for IgM or IgG. J. exp. Med. 146 : 184, 1977.

7. Strosberg, A.D., Karcher, D., Lowenthal, A. : Structural homogeneity of human subacute sclerosing panencephalitis antibodies. J. Immunol. 115 : 157, 1975.

8. Vandvik, B., Norrby, E., Nordal, H.J., Degré, M. : Oligoclonal measles virus-specific IgG antibodies isolated from cerebrospinal fluids, brain extracts and sera from patients with subacute sclerosing panencephalitis and multiple sclerosis. Scand. J. Immunol. 5 : 979, 1976.

9. Waldmann, T.A., Durm, M., Broder, S., Blackman, M., Blaese, R.M., Strober, W. : Role of suppressor T cells in pathogenesis of common variable hypogammaglobulinaemia. Lancet ii : 609, 1974.

PATHOGENESIS OF THE MS LESION : IMPLICATIONS FOR THERAPY

J.F. Hallpike

Royal Adelaide Hospital, Adelaide, South Australia

INTRODUCTION

Multiple sclerosis (MS) is a multifocal disorder of myelin of the central nervous system (CNS) and the commonest human demyelinating disease. Multiple sclerosis generally runs a relapsing and very chronic course and, in regions where prevalence of this condition is high, MS is as important a cause of neurological disability and socio-economic hardship as stroke or trauma. Research into MS in the last twenty-five years has been an increasingly multidisciplinary venture leading to a considerable measure of understanding of different aspects of pathogenesis and of effects of demyelination. Although the cause of MS remains an enigma, immunological mechanisms are implicated and a rational basis appears to exist for immunosuppressive therapy. With increasing experience of rigorous cytotoxic and immunosuppressive regimes in myelo- and lymphoproliferative diseases affecting the CNS it seems timely to attempt briefly to survey the relevance and limitations of such methods of treatment in MS.

IMMUNOGENESIS OF PLAQUES

Active MS plaques are characterized by cellularity. The significance of perivascular infiltrations of lymphocytes seen in the vicinity of acute and established MS lesions is uncertain and has recently been reviewed (1). Cellular plaques show increased proteolysis and loss of myelin basic protein (6). In-vitro enzymatic degradation of basic encephalitogenic myelin

protein (BP) produces low MS diffusible fragments containing
active encephalitogenic residues (4). Such residues, or the
tryptophan nonapeptide sequence itself, derived from BP, combined with Freund's adjuvant, induce experimental allergic encephalomyelitis (EAE) in guinea pigs. Unsatisfactory features of
this EAE model of MS include the necessity for adjuvant, incon-
spicuous demyelination and the assumption that systemically generated immune cells, antibodies, are responsible for any immunological lesion in MS. Moreover, EAE, as usually produced,
is an acute monophasic disease with a high mortality. However,
chemical studies of the adjuvant (12) indicate that encephalitogenic activity of BP may be modified by complexing with fatty
acids or neural, as opposed to mycobacterial, products.

Species differences exist in encephalitogenic determinants
and a more chronic disease with demyelination can be produced
in monkeys by manipulations such as antigen overloading (5).
The phenomena of EAE suppression, phylogenetic differences and
the adjuvant potential of CNS degradation products now provide
a sounder basis for extrapolating from EAE to the human situation. Ultrastructural evidence of cell-mediated immune damage
of myelin has been expertly reviewed by Lampert (8). In virus-
induced demyelination, the myelin-supporting cells tend to show
early damage (cytolysis) whereas the myelin lamellae are the
target in allergic reactions. Whether the initial injury in MS
affects the oligodendrocyte or the myelin sheath is still unresolved.

The two processes are not mutually exclusive, however, since
viral cytolysis may be associated with cell-mediated demyelination. Evidence for a cell-mediated reaction in MS is conflicting. Although there are, for instance, reports of lymphocyte
transformation and increased production of macrophage migration
inhibition factor in acute MS, other studies have failed to confirm this and deployment of the full range of tests for cellular immunity suggests that the T cell population may be diminished
in acute exacerbations of MS (7). Interpretation of such data
is obviously difficult in the light of the EAE suppression experiments, and the presence of excess antigen may be a factor.
Increased IgG production in MS is on firmer ground. The fact
that CSF IgG may be increased without signs of breakdown of the
blood-brain-barrier (BBB) is now taken as evidence of production
of IgG within the CNS and calculations of CNS IgG production
have been developed by Tourtellotte (15) as a parameter of disease activity and effect of treatment. High concentrations
of IgG also occur in 'normal' white matter as well as in and
around plaques (17).

Oligoclonal IgG electrophoretic patterns in the CSF in MS
are additional evidence of production of immunoglobulins 'be-

hind' the BBB. Although MS is usually regarded as a unique disorder of white matter of the human CNS, overlap between pathological appearances in MS and hypertrophic neuropathy as well
as the occasional concurrence of MS and relapsing polyneuropathy
(14) provide some further support for the relevance of EAE, EAN
to human demyelination. A relationship between histocompatibility determinants (HLA OA3, B7, Dw2) and the prevalence of MS
has now been well documented. The pathological significance
of these linkages is still uncertain but modulation of T-cell
mediated responses to tissue antigens has been suggested.

DIAGNOSIS

     The clinical spectrum of MS is extremely wide and greater
precision in diagnosis and agreement on the classification of
clinical sub-types is requisite for determining effects of treatment and ensuring comparability of results from different centres. While a satisfactory laboratory test for MS has not yet
been devised, the introduction of computer 'averaging' into routine clinical neurophysiological practice has provided the clinician with a powerful means of displaying subclinical conduction defects in the CNS. This aspect has been fully reviewed,
(10, 11) and, from a practical viewpoint, the significance of
routinely measuring visual as well as auditory evoked responses
is that the evidence, thus obtained, of additional CNS pathology
permits more accurate classification of patients. Thus, someone
with a spastic paraparesis,tentatively classified as a possible
or probable MS, may confidently be recategorized as definite
on the basis of unequivocal abnormalities of the visual or brainstem evoked responses. These techniques also have a potential
for obtaining new information about the natural history of the
disease, influence of treatment on central conduction and remyelination which has yet to be exploited.

ASPECTS OF THERAPY

     In the report (13) of the co-operative study of the effects
of short-term ACTH in exacerbations of MS the principal conclusion reached was that, at best, only a marginal advantage accrued
to the actively treated patients. Nevertheless, corticosteroids
continue to be used in short courses for definite relapses and
most neurologists have personal experience (18) of a few patients
with more aggressive types of disease who demonstrate convincing steroid-responsiveness and in whom short-term clinical stability can only be maintained with longer term treatment, often
on an alternate day basis. In acute retrobulbar neuritis, short-
term use of large doses of glucocorticoid, i.e. dexamethasone,
results in rapid improvement in visual acuity in a proportion

of patients with signs of 'papillitis' due to lesions in the
anterior part of the nerve which interfere with flow in the
central retinal vein. The effect of steroids in this special
situation is almost certainly due to reduction of local oedema.
Corticosteroids may also have an effect in limiting release
of lysosomal hydrolases capable of damaging myelin membrane.
Inhibition of lysosomal protease has been successfully employed
to protect animals with EAE from developing paralysis (2).

Experiences with azathioprine; corticosteroids plus cyclophosphamide or cytosine arabinoside; steroids, azathioprine,
ALG and thoracic duct drainage have been reviewed by Liversedge (9). No convincing evidence of clinical benefit has so far
been obtained. Tourtellotte and his colleagues (16) have now
refined the study of such treatment by pointing out that in
order to stand any chance of success the selected regime should
eradicate abnormal CNS IgG production, as judged by daily gross
output, as well as the 'minimonoclonal' CSF patterns. ACTH,
alternate day prednisone, brain irradiation, depress CNS immunoglobulin production.

Clearly, however, the clinical effect of such treatment
in patients with extensive and largely irreversible disease is
likely to be disappointing regardless of changes in IgG synthesis. That is to say, in patients with well established disease,
questions pertaining to remyelination are at least as important
as immunosuppression as regards functional change. The dilemma
facing the clinician, therefore, is to decide at what stage,
in an individual case, intensive immunosuppression might be justified. To take the two extreme situations, neither someone
with a history of a single episode of retrobulbar neuritis or
a bedridden patient with a 20 year history would be regarded
by most sensible clinicians as candidates for intensive chemotherapy.

The situation in MS is different to the malignant disorders
in which intensive immunotherapy and radiotherapy are justified
by the invariably bad prognosis and the demonstrated benefit
of well conducted treatment. Many patients with definite MS
enjoy active, productive lives with little more disability than
occurs in sufferers from a number of other chronic but relatively benign conditions. A literature is developing on CNS side-
effects of systemic and intrathecal (IT) chemotherapy for myelo-
and lymphoproliferative diseases. In a recently studied fatal
case, widespread loss of myelin in the cord and brainstem had
to be attributed to effects of IT methotrexate and radiotherapy
delivered according to a widely employed protocol for the treatment of CNS spread.

Similarity between the pathological appearances in these cases and those induced by CSF barbotage has been stressed (3). The probability is, therefore, that a thin line exists dividing potentially useful immunosuppression on the one hand and toxic effects on myelin or myelin-supporting cells on the other. In addition to defining clinically those patients in whom higher risk forms of treatment might be appropriate, we need to know more about the entry of cytotoxic drugs into the CNS and their neuropathological effects. If the oligodendrocyte is indeed compromised in MS, the effects of cytotoxic drugs and irradiation on this cell need to be better defined. Similarly, until a pathogenic role for CNS IgG is definitely established the rational for concentrated, and potentially harmful, CNS immunotherapy must remain very much in doubt.

CONCLUSION

There is considerable evidence that immune mechanisms, both systemic and within the CNS are implicated in the pathogenesis of MS. To be effective, immunosuppressive therapy must produce lasting depression of CNS as well as peripheral immunoreactivity. Use of evoked responses and HLA typing may help in identifying patients with aggressive disease for whom intensive immunotherapy might have something to offer before irreversible pathological changes occur. Problems of an empirical approach with high risk treatment are stressed. Particular uncertainties are the effect of measures on the oligodendrocyte and the pathological significance of the CNS IgG.

REFERENCES

1. Adams, C.W.M. (1975), J. Neurol. Sci., 25, 165-82.
2. Boehme, D.H., Marks, N. (1978), Fed. Proc., 37, 3, 837.
3. Breuer, A.C. et al. (1977), Cancer, 40, 2817-22.
4. Chao, L.P., Einstein, E.R. (1968), J. Biol. Chem., 243, 6050-55.
5. Eylar, E.H., In Multiple Sclerosis, eds. Wolfgram et al., Academic Press, 1972.
6. Hallpike, J.F. (1972), Prog. Histochem. Cytochem., 3, 179-215.
7. Knight, S.C. (1977), Brit. Med. Bull., 33, 1, 45-9.
8. Lampert, P.W. (1978), Am. J. Path., 91, 176-197.
9. Liversedge, L.A. (1977), Brit. Med. Bull., 33, 1, 78-83.
10. McDonald, W.L. (1975), Multiple Sclerosis Research, HMSO, pp. 1-8.
11. McDonald, W.I., Halliday, A.M. (1977), Brit. Med. Bull., 33, 1, 4-8.

12. Nagai, Y. (1976), Neurology, 26, 45-6.
13. Rose, A.S. (1970), Neurology, 202, 1-59.
14. Schoene, W.C., Carpenter, S., Behan, P.O., Geschwind, N. (1978) Brain, 100, 755-73.
15. Tourtellotte, W. (1970), J. Neurol. Sci., 10, 279-304.
16. Tourtellotte, W., Murphy, K., Brandes, D. (1976), Neurology, 26, 59-61.
17. Tourtellotte, W., Parker, J.A. (1968), Brain Res., 29, 493-522.
18. Walton, J.N. (1975), In Multiple Sclerosis Research, HMSO, p. 264.

IMMUNOLOGIC FACTORS IN THE SUPPRESSION OF EXPERIMENTAL ALLERGIC ENCEPHALOMYELITIS : RELEVENCE TO MULTIPLE SCLEROSIS

E.H. Eylar

Department of Biochemistry, University of Toronto, Toronto, Canada

INTRODUCTION

Numerous autoimmune diseases of both humans and animals have been described over the past few decades, but probably none have received as much attention as experimental allergic encephalo-myelitis (EAE). Progress has been achieved in the study of EAE with the discovery and isolation of the myelin basic protein (BP) antigen (1, 2, 3), determination of its complete amino acid sequence (4), the isolation and synthesis of disease-inducing peptides (5, 6) and clarification of immunopathologic events in EAE (7). Recently new developments have been made in firmly establishing EAE as a cell-mediated autoimmune disease which under appropriate conditions compares closely with multiple sclerosis in humans (8). Horizons have also been extended in our understanding of antigenic and disease-inducing sites of the molecule, and the role of immune cell populations in the induction and suppressing of EAE. The immunogenic sites of the BP molecule responsible for the induction of EAE in several animal species including the monkey, guinea pig, rat and rabbit have recently been reviewed (9). It is now established that EAE is mediated by effector T lymphocytes sensitized to small crucial regions of the BP polypeptide chain. While small peptide fragments are not as potent on a molar basis in inducing EAE as larger peptides containing these regions, they are nonetheless capable of inducing EAE and appear to represent the minimal active sequence. With such an intimate understanding of the disease-inducing regions and the immunologic events in the induction of EAE, it has become a highly attractive model to study immunosuppression as well.

EAE behaves as a classical autoimmune disease since it can
be blocked by prior injection of BP as shown in early studies
(10, 11, 12), or suppressed by BP administered after clinical
signs of EAE have appeared (13). Although antibody has been
suspected to play a role in blocking or suppressing EAE, recent
studies have emphasized suppressor T cells for this role (14, 15).
This report will consider the role of antibody to BP in suppressing
disease in EAE and MS, and data on the antigenic sites of the
molecule. The suppression of EAE with BP in monkeys after clinical
signs have appeared and in appropriate models of EAE in the guinea
pig and mouse will be reviewed with regard to its relevance to
MS. EAE has had a notable resurgence as an appropriate model for
MS (16), and efforts will be made in this report to emphasize
similarities and differences between EAE and MS.

Induction of EAE

With the development of cellular immunology in the past few
years, strong data has now come forth demonstrating that EAE is
induced and mediated solely by T lymphocytes sensitized to BP.
Early work indeed suggested cell-mediated immunity was the causative mechanism in EAE since disease could be transferred with
cells (17), and the delayed hypersensitivity response correlated
with the severity of clinical signs and histologic lesions (3, 18).
More convincing data are presented in Table 1. The encephalitogenic
tryptophan domain (res. 113-121) induces a cell-mediated response
demonstrable in guinea pigs prior to appearance of clinical signs.
As shown by in vitro tests, the sensitized cells also recognize
the tryptophan domain of the intact BP (7).

Susceptibility to EAE appears to be controlled by an Ir-EAE
gene which controls cell-mediated reactivity toward the encephalitogenic determinant as found in studies of different strains of
rats (19). Some of the most impressive data showing that T cells
are absolutely required and are responsible for induction of EAE
comes from work on thymectonized, irradiated rats which were
reconstituted with independent populations of T and B cells (20,
21). Manipulation of the T cells with anti-thymic serum prevents
EAE induction but not anti-BP production in cells previously
sensitized to BP (20). These results, along with suicide experiments (21) which show that loss of antibody forming cells does
not retard EAE induction, offer strong support for the central
role of T lymphocytes (effector cells) in EAE events and the
noninvolvement of antibody to BP.

Encephalitogenic Domains in BP

One of the most striking features of BP - EAE relationship

TABLE 1

SELECTED DATA SHOWING THAT
EAE IS CELL-MEDIATED

1. The tryptophan peptide (res. 113-121) induces EAE in guinea
    pigs and also cell-mediated immunity (MIF, blast transforma-
    tion) which recognizes the intact BP. Antibody is not in-
    duced (7).

2. Susceptibility to EAE in rats is controlled by an autosomal
    dominant gene linked to the major histocompatibility locus
    (20).

3. In passive transfer, of lymphoid cells to thymectomized,
    irradiated rats, depletion of T cells prevented EAE but not
    antibody development (21).

4. In rats reconstituted with normal thymic and bone marrow cells,
    EAE was not produced if specific T cells were first depleted
    (suicide) with BP -^{125}I (22).

is the finding that small peptide fragments derived from the BP
molecule contain the complete information for induction of EAE.
It is even more remarkable that different peptide regions are
active in different species, and three major encephalitogenic
regions (domains) have been discovered to date (see ref. 9 for
a review). Undoubtedly the open expanded conformation of the
BP accounts in part for the localization of immunogenic domains
as part of a small linear sequence of the polypeptide chain rather
than a composite of distal regions in space. It is not so surprising, therefore, that small peptides derived from BP may contain an intact encephalitogenic domain with a conformation and
activity nearly congruent with the same region in the intact BP
molecule (9). In the tedious work of detecting and characterizing
the encephalitogenic domains, one of the most powerful approaches
has been the Merrifield solid state peptide synthesis (5, 27).

     Peptides derived from BP by use of trypsin, pepsin, cathepsin
D (brain and liver) and BNPS-skatole have proven most useful (22,
23, 24) in isolating the immunogenic determinants for cell-mediated
immunity which serve as encephalitogenic domains in different
species. In part, a genetic explanation can account for this
phenomenon; the encephalitogenic response is apparently controlled
by an Ir gene of the major histocompatibility locus (19). For
each species, the regulation emphasizes the cell-mediated response
to one or so encephalitogenic domains of BP. However, cell-mediated responses do occur to other regions of BP but do not lead

to disease (24, 25, 26), perhaps because of discrimination at
the target site (central nervous system).

The encephalitogenic domains, shown as part of the BP sequence in Table 2, comprise short peptide segments of the BP
polypeptide chain : 9 amino acid residues for the guinea pig
and rabbit and 8 residues for the rat. The size of the domains
were established by peptide synthesis, i.e., these represent
essentially the minimum size still having significant activity.
For the monkey, the smallest peptide studied is 13 residues (28)
but the minimum size is likely smaller. In view of the requirement for both haptenic and carrier specificity of an immunogenic
molecule, it is impressive that these peptides themselves elicit
the autoimmune disease, EAE. The data indicate that for the rat
and the guinea pig there is only one major encephalitogenic
determinant, an unusual finding in view of the relatively large
number of immunogenic determinants for cell mediated immunity
existing in the BP molecule (29). In the monkey, one or two minor
determinants may exist in the region 1-89 but they are relatively

TABLE 2

ENCEPHALITOGENIC DOMAINS IN

THE AMINO ACID SEQUENCE OF

THE BOVINE BP

                                        10
N-Ac-Ala-Ala-Gln-Lys-Arg-Pro-Ser-Gln-Arg-Ser-Lys-Tyr-Leu-Ala-
        20   30
Ser-Ala-Ser-Thr-Met-Asp-His-Ala-Arg-His-Gly-Phe-Leu-Pro-Arg-His-
                                40
Arg-Asp-Thr-Gly-Ile-Leu-Asp-Ser-Leu-Gly-Arg-Phe-Phe-Gly-Ser-Asp-
        50   60
Arg-Gly-Ala-Pro-Lys-Arg-Gly-Ser-Gly-Lys-Asp-Gly-His-His-Ala-Ala-
                                70   SER
Arg-THR-THR-HIS-TYR-GLY-SER-LEU-PRO-GLN-LYS-Ala-GLN-(Gly-His)-
        80   90
ARG-PRO-GLN-ASP-GLU-ASN-PRO-VAL-Val-His-Phe-Phe-Lys-Asn-Ile-Val-
                        100   (CH₃)
Thr-Pro-Arg-Thr-Pro-Pro-Pro-Ser-Gln-Gly-Lys-Gly-Arg-Gly-Leu-Ser
110   120
Leu-Ser-Arg-PHE-SER-TRP-GLY-ALA-GLU-GLY-GLN-LYS-Pro-Gly-Phe-Gly-
                    130   140
Tyr-Gly-Gly-Arg-Ala-Ser-Asp-Tyr-Lys-Ser-Ala-His-Lys-Gly-Leu-Lys-
                            150
Gly-His-Asp-Ala-Gln-Gly-Thr-Leu-Ser-Lys-Ile-PHE-LYS-LEU-GLY-GLY
        160   169
ARG-ASP-SER-ARG-SER-GLY-SER-PRO-MET-Ala-Arg-Arg-COOH

weak (23, 30). The major determinant active in the monkey also
appears to be the major determinant active in the rabbit as shown
by peptide synthesis (28, 31). Two minor determinants are also
active in the rabbit however, the tryptophan region (32) and
region 64-73 (33). The peptide defining the latter region has
been synthesized and found to be mildly active (33).

An unusual situation exists for the rat since a sharp
delineation exists in the activity of BP from different species.
The bovine BP is relatively inactive because it contains a Gly-His
dipeptide segment (res. 76-77) in the midst of the determinant;
a segment not found in the guinea pig or rat BP, both of which
are very active (34, 35). However, Hashim and coworkers (35, 36)
have shown that in small peptides of nine residues, even inclusion
of the Gly-His does not greatly reduce activity. Activity is
only lost when Gly-His is present along with a long extension of
the peptide chain at the amino end as in BP itself or large peptides. Presumably the appropriate conformation normally will not
permit the Gly-His segment but greater flexibility must exist in
the smaller peptides so that a conformation compatible with EAE
induction is possible in spite of Gly-His.

The encephalitogenic domains are :

Guinea Pig Phe-Ser-Trp-Gly-Ala-Glu-Gly-Gln-Lys(Arg) (res. 113-121)

Rat   Ser-Gln-Arg-Ser-Gln-Asp-Glu-Asn (res. 74-81)

Monkey   Phe-Lys-Leu-Gly-Gly-Arg-Asp-Ser-Arg-Ser-Gly-Ser-Pro-Hser
            (res. 153-166)

Rabbit   Phe-Lys-Leu-Gly-Gly-Arg-Asp-Ser-Arg (res. 153-161)

They are shown in their appropriate position as part of the
BP molecule in Table 2; they appear to congregate mainly in the
central and carboxyl region of the polypeptide chain. Of most
interest is the monkey domain since this region could be important
in human diseases in which the BP may be implicated.

Antibody to BP

In studies of EAE nearly all of the data indicate that antibody to BP correlates neither with the onset nor the severity of
the disease (37, 38, 39). Antibody to BP may be important, however,
by serving to protect or inhibit against the disease. It is
instructive as well to understand the immune response to the BP
molecule in order to further characterize this protein and seek
a better understanding of natural antigens. It should be noted
that while BP is very encephalitogenic and readily able to elicit
cell mediated immunity, it is poorly antigenic for antibody induction. In one study using 44 rabbits, only 3 animals developed

anti-BP. Generally, repeated injections of large doses of BP
with relatively large quantities of mycobacterium induce anti-BP;
complexes with negatively charged materials such as albumin or
DNA (40) are also more effective immunogens than BP alone.

There is abundant evidence that suggests that EAE is not
mediated by antibody to BP and that antibody may protect
against development of EAE :

a) Antibody to BP is nontoxic - When animals such as rabbits,
rats, guinea pigs, sheep or goats are hyperimmunized with BP in
incomplete adjuvant, circulating antibody to BP may be elicited.
The anti-BP serum does not lead to pathology in the experimental
animal (3, 41, 42) nor does it transfer pathology. Thus it can
be concluded that circulating Ab to BP produced by hyperimmunization is not toxic per se.

b) Antibody to BP in EAE - The clinical and histologic signs of
EAE can be elicited easily in most guinea pigs when BP is administered in CPA at 5-15 μg (3), a level of BP that does not usually
induce antibody. Even at 100 ug of BP, where the acute fatal
paralytic disease observed at lower dosages is still seen, detectable amounts of antibody to BP are rarely observed (37). If the
amount of BP is increased to 0.5 mg and the mycobacteria increased
to 2.5 mg respectively in the sensitizing dose, circulating
antibody does appear simultaneously with disease onset (43). In
rats also, antibody to BP can be induced independently of disease
and vice versa (39). In rabbits, antibody to BP was only detected
in 45% of the rabbits developing EAE, and in over 50% of the
animals which showed no clinical signs of EAE, antibody to BP
was found (42).

These data show that antibody to BP is not an important
factor in the induction or maintenance of clinical or histologic
signs characterizing EAE in guinea pigs, rats, or rabbits.
Additionally, antibody is produced in animals not developing EAE
and thus is not exclusively associated with disease-inducing
mechanisms.

c) Cell-bound antibody - It was found that when EAE was induced
with low levels of BP (less than 50 μg), plasma cell types which
bound to BP-peroxidase complexes were not observed (38). With
higher levels of BP as the sensitizing dose, however, such cells
are found. These results are fully consistent with studies on
antibody levels and EAE since they reveal that neither antibody
nor antibody-forming cells which bind BP are observed when
animals are sensitized with low levels of BP, yet full clinical
and histologic signs of EAE are seen in most guinea pigs.

d) EAE in immunosuppressed animals - In rats deprived of antibody-
producing cells it was found that EAE was induced as readily as

in untreated animals, but in those rats which were irradiated and deprived of thymic cells, development of EAE was greatly limited (44).

In chickens neonatally bursectomized and irradiated and thus incapable of antibody production, EAE developed in response to chicken BP much more severely and rapidly than in normal chickens (Eylar, E., unpublished data).

Taken together, the above data strongly suggest that EAE is not mediated by antibody to BP, and that such antibody per se is not pathogenic. Even immunogenic peptides, obtained from chymotryptic hydrolysis of BP, protect guinea pigs from EAE (45). These studies are complemented with experiments which show that EAE is mediated by T lymphocytes sensitized to discreet disease-inducing sites of the BP molecule (7). Thus EAE can be considered a model autoimmune disease induced and maintained by cell-mediated immunity to BP whereas the role of antibody is probably protective, and not a significant factor in disease induction.

Antigenic Sites in BP

There are many variables to keep in mind in a study of antigenic sites in the BP molecule. Some of these variables include the type of assay (46), the species of BP, the type of antibody, the species of test animal, and the state of the antigen, i.e., purified, complexed, or part of myelin. Most of the experiments discussed here were performed by immunization of rabbits with bovine BP, and then measuring the ability of peptides from BP to complete or inhibit the reaction of antibody with BP either by radioimmune procedures or by complement fixation.

As shown in Table 3, specific localization of antigenic sites in BP has not been accomplished. Peptides 1-42 or 1-89, obtained by peptic digestion of BP, are highly reactive and it has been concluded by Whitaker et al. (47) that a major site (Table 4) resides in res. 21-42. A minor site probably exists in res. 1-20 because, while not as active as peptide 1-42 or 1-37, it has significant activity. Interestingly, in several studies it was found that res. 43-89 did not react with anti-BP (23, 32, 47). In studies using BP peptides, obtained by cathepsin D and BNPS-skatol treatment, and rabbit antiserum, it was found that the COOH-terminal region, particularly from 117-169 did not appear as reactive as the NH_2 region (23, 48). However, Whitaker et al. (27) found that peptide 89-169 was quite active and based on the reactivity of peptides 116-169 and 89-159 (Table 4) it appears that at least one major and one minor site may reside in the carboxyl region.

TABLE 3

ANTIGENIC SITES OF BP DETERMINED
WITH RABBIT ANTI-BP

PEPTIDE	METHOD	RESULTS
1-42 or 1-89	Complement fixation (CF) Radioimmune assay (RI)	Highly active in both tests
1-37	CF	Quite active but not as
1-20	CF	much as 1-42 or 1-89
44-89	CF, RI	not active
89-169	CF	Highly active
89-115	CF	Much lower
116-169	CF	Much lower

TABLE 4

ANTIGENIC SITES OF BP[*]

Antibody Source	Major Sites	Minor Sites	Not Reactive
Rabbit	21-42 116-169	1-20 89-115	37-88
Rat and Guinea pig	1-115 (89-115) 89-169	116-169	
Rat and Sheep			37-88

[*] Data from Whitaker et al. (47), Kies, (41) and Eylar et al. (32).

    It is apparent that discrete small antigenic sites of BP
have not as yet been pinpointed. Because of the relatively open
conformation of the BP molecule it might be presumed that many
antigenic sites should exist in BP. Studies with synthetic polypeptides have indicated that antigenic sites may comprise only
5-7 amino acids of the polypeptide chain; several such sites
might exist in the res. 21-42 of BP for example. Moreover, it
has been shown that at least 7-10 immunogenic sites for cell-mediated
immunity exist in BP as shown by reaction of cells sensitized to

BP with in vitro tests such as migration inhibition factor (MIF) and lymphoblastic transformation (LTF) etc. (26). Some of these sites also function as disease-inducing sites, that is, cells sensitized to these regions are pathogenic and lead to EAE as discussed in section 2. An interesting question is whether some of these sites are also antigenic sites as well. It is obvious that some differences exist between antigenic sites and cell-mediated sites since peptide 43–89, which induces EAE in rabbits, does not react with antibody to BP (Table 4); the nonapeptide (res. 113–121) which induces EAE in guinea pigs does not induce antibody formation (7).

Studies have also been carried out with anti-BP prepared in guinea pigs, rats and sheep. In the guinea pig, a hyperimmune schedule was used for priming which involved several injections of BP in IFA; finally a single injection of BP in CFA was given (49). It should be noted that guinea pig BP and peptide therefrom were used in these studies (49). With this procedure it was found that unique antibody (not cross reacting) was formed which reacted with three different regions of BP (Table 4). However, if peptides were used for sensitization in CFA following the priming step, then the antigenic sites in 1–88 and 116–169 failed to elicit antibody formation; only peptide 89–169 effectively induced antibody formation.

Driscoll et al. (49) also induced antibody to guinea pig BP by using one injection of BP with 2.5 mg mycobacteria in the CFA (compared to 0.1 mg used above). Here, also, the three antigenic regions were found as in the previous experiments, but the peptides themselves were also effective inducers of antibody in contrast to the priming procedure. These results show similarities to the rabbit anti-BP, in that antigenic regions are found in the terminal regions, but additionally the guinea pig anti-BP shows an antigenic site within res. 89–116.

Studies (41) have also been performed with rat anti-guinea pig BP in which the sensitizing antigen was guinea pig cord or BP. The results obtained were similar regardless of the antigen used, and were similar to those found with rabbit anti-BP. Thus it appears in all cases, whether rabbit, guinea pig, or rat, that major antigenic site appears in the regions 1–88. A less active region is localized in 116–169, but in guinea pigs an antigenic site is also found in 89–115. Definite confirmation of an antigenic site in the carboxyl half of the BP molecule comes from the finding that rabbit anti-monkey BP gave a strong reaction with the rat BP but only very weakly with the small rat BP in which residues 117–156 are deleted (40). Thus the carboxyl region likely contains an antigenic determinant (s) found with monkey BP, in agreement with other studies.

One of the most interesting regions is localized in peptide
43-89, a region that has a major encephalitogenic (cell-mediated)
site active in the rat (50) and a minor region for the rabbit (33).
Early studies all showed that rabbit, rat, and sheep anti-BP did
not react with peptide 43-89. Recently, however, Whitaker et al.
(51) prepared antibody to this peptide and found that it did not
cross react with BP. These data strongly suggest that the peptide
region in the intact BP molecule has a different conformation
than in the isolated peptide. Thus antibody to this region in
intact BP or intact peptide does not cross react and vice versa.
These results emphasize an important point in studies of antigenic
sites. It is assumed that the peptides used to assess binding
sites by competition with BP for antibody have nearly the same
conformation as the peptide region in the intact BP. Obviously
this is not the case for res. 43-89. Thus all studies summarized
in Table 4 must be considered rough approximations since little
information is available on the conformation of peptide regions
in the isolated peptide as compared to the intact BP. One peptide
might approach closely its conformation in the intact BP and be
an accurate indicator of antibody binding, whereas another, like
peptide 43-89 may digress considerably, and thus lead to misinter-
pretation. It can be assumed, however, that if peptides like
1-89, 1-115 or 89-169 (Table 4) compete effectively with anti-BP,
then major antigenic sites exist in that peptide. Even the best
peptides, however, are much less potent than intact BP in their
binding to antibody since molar ratios of peptide to BP at 50%
inhibition are all greater than 3 (47).

These data also emphasize that lack of reactivity of a peptide
with anti-BP does not mean that it is not antigenic. This point
should be stressed; it was not considered of great importance in
studies of immunogenic sites active in cell-mediated immunity
since many studies had achieved notable success in localizing
peptide regions that both induced disease and were active in
tests for cell-mediated immunity.

It must be recalled as well that presumably conformational
differences between a peptide and the same region of an intact
protein do not pose as great a problem in studies of cell-mediated
immunity as with antibody; cells sensitized to denatured proteins
may react equally well with the native protein in contrast to
antibody-protein interaction (52). Thus we suspect that antigenic
sites in BP may be more numerous than previously believed, but
the precise number is not known. Lysozyme and myoglobin each
have 5 antigenic sites as shown by the elegant work of Atassi
and coworkers (53, 54). These proteins are approximately the
same size as the BP, but are quite compact compared to the
asymmetric BP shape. BP is not a highly antigenic molecule (40),
and thus may not contain a large number of antigenic sites in
spite of its unfolded conformation.

BP and Anti-BP in Spinal Fluid

In sheep which were injected with CNS tissue in CFA, several developed EAE, and concomitantly with appearance of clinical signs, both free antibody (to BP) and antibody-bound BP were found in the spinal fluid (55). The antibody appears to be derived from the serum, and was present as well in animals not developing EAE. These data further confirm that anti-BP is not responsible for the induction and continuity of pathology in EAE. Such antibody is not found in patients with active MS, according to this study (55), but in both EAE and MS the BP appears in the spinal fluid (56).

With regard to BP in spinal fluid in MS, significant quantities (12-15 mg per ml) have been found by radioimmune assay during acute attack, but only rarely occurs in the CSF in other diseases. Whitaker (57) has found 3.4 - 15.4 mg per ml of peptide 43-88 in MS spinal fluid, a highly significant level of peptide. Detected by antibody elicited peptide 43-88 in the radioimmune assay, the peptide appears only during acute phase and was only found in 6 of 117 controls. It is known (58) that BP is degraded during active demyelination in the course of MS by acid protease (cathepsin D); peptide 43-88 is a prominant product of such proteolysis (23, 59). It is intriguing to contemplate if the BP or peptide 43-88 in the CSF plays a role in either the perpetuation or suppression of the human disease. Within limits, the presence of BP and the peptide could have diagnostic value.

Antibody to BP in MS

Over the years there have been many studies searching for anti-BP activity in MS patients based on the role of BP in EAE. These studies for the most part have failed to detect meaningful antibody levels to BP in MS. The advent of new immunologic techniques, however, has stimulated further search for antibody to BP in MS. Some of these techniques are the double antibody radioimmune assay, quantitative microcomplement fixation, and radioimmunoelectrophoresis. These tests parallel one another in general as shown by studies with rabbit and rat antisera to monkey and bovine BP, but minor differences sometimes appear (46). Thus it is important to note the type of test employed and the level of sensitivity in studies of antibody to BP.

A summary of selected studies on the search for antibody to BP in MS patients is shown in Table 5, and reveals an inconsistent pattern. Generally such studies have not found antibody to BP in the serum from MS patients as illustrated by the report of Lisak et al, (60) and McPherson and Carnegie (61). However,

TABLE 5

ANTIBODY IN
MULTIPLE SCLEROSIS

STUDY	METHOD	RESULTS
Gutstein and Cohen (55)	RI assay	No antibody to BP in CSF
Panitch et al. (63)	RI assay	In CSF, mean level of antibody: 5.6 (active disease); 3.9 (remission); 1.9 (controls)
Lisak et al. (60)	Radioimmuno-electrophoresis	No antibody to BP in MS serum
McPherson and Carnegie (61)	Radioimmuno-assay	No antibody to BP in MS serum
Sheremata et al. (62)	Double immunodiffusion	Antibody to BP detected in serum in convalescent but not acute or stable MS.

Sheremata, et al. (62), utilizing a different technique detected
antibody in serum to human BP during convalescence but not during
acute attack or stable MS. It is evident that a definitive
conclusion cannot be drawn concerning the presence of BP antibody
in MS because of the conflicting reports. However, it is possible
that a consistent explanation may emerge from further studies
over a time period. The results from studies of anti-BP in the
CSF are also contradictory. No antibody was found in the CSF
from MS patients in the study by Gutstein and Cohen (55), but in
a preliminary study (63) it was found that significant levels of
antibody to BP appear in the CSF during active disease (Table 5).
This result also contrasts with the results of Sheremata et al.
(62) who found detectable antibody during convalescence but not
during active disease. Moreover, the CSF antibody was not found
in all patients.

The question that arises is why some investigators find
antibody in either serum or CSF from MS patients and others do
not. The double immunodiffusion test used by Sheremata et al.
(62) is less sensitive than radioimmune assay, but these workers
used human BP rather than bovine BP or BP from other species.
It is likely that other factors such as the test itself and its
sensitivity and specificity are important. Additionally, the
antigen source may be important. Also, BP itself is present in
spinal fluid and could therefore be present in trace quantities
in serum as well. The presence of BP could no doubt complicate
the assay for antibody.

a) Oligoclonal IgG - One property of the CSF of MS patients often
seen is the presence of several (three or more) oligoclonal IgG
bands on agar gel electrophoresis. The nature of the antigen to
which the oligoclonal IgG may bind is unknown. In one study (64)
both high levels of antibody to measles virus and oligoclonal
IgG were noted, but unlike the case for SSPE patients where measles antigen absorbs out some of the IgG, the measles virus antigen
did affect the oligoclonal IgG from the CSF of MS patients.

These results contrast with those of Vandvik et al. (65) who
found the IgG1 subclass in measles antibody in a brain extract
from an MS patient. They claimed that the IgG1 restriction is
associated with the occurrence of oligoclonal measles antibodies,
and was not observed in normals, but did occur in SSPE.

Thus it appears that while the presence of oligoclonal IgG
is commonly found in MS and some other neurologic diseases, it is
not certain whether they react with measles or other viral antigens,
and there is no evidence that they react with BP.

b) Immune Complexes - In view of the possible viral aetiology of
MS it is logical to search for immune complexes. The usual method
for measuring immune complexes involves binding with labeled Clq.
The results, however, have been conflicting. Powis et al. (66)
found only a slight increase in serum immune complexes in MS and
optic neuritis compared to normal and neurologic controls, and
no correlation with disease state in MS. Tachovsky et al. (67)
reported circulating immune complexes in 50% of MS patients, and
Jacque et al. (68) reported complexes in 29% of MS cases and none
in controls. Attempts to identify the antigens from the isolated
complexes indicated that BP was not involved, but the complexes
were rich in lipids suggesting that they might be a nonspecific
consequence of tissue destruction. Although Goust et al. (69)
found elevated levels of immune complexes in over 70% of MS patients compared to normal serum, there was no correlation with
the state of the disease. Thus the significance of immune complexes in MS remains controversial and uncertain.

c) Demyelinating factor - A factor which demyelinates CNS cultures
in vitro and is thought to be antibody is found more prominantly
in MS sera than in normal sera (76). Over the years, however,
no definite evidence has been uncovered that shows that the
demyelinating factor plays a role in the disease process. Wolfgram
et al. (71) have reported that antibrain antibody and demyelinating
antibody appear in both MS and control sera, and probably do not
play a significant role in MS. It is now well established from
the work of Seil and coworkers (72) that the demyelinating factor
does not represent anti-BP. Demyelinating factor can be induced
in EAE when whole tissue is used for sensitization but not when
purified BP is used.

TABLE 6

DEMYELINATING FACTOR IN THE MONKEY
DURING INDUCTION AND SUPPRESSION
OF EAE

Antigen	Status of the monkey when serum taken	No. of animals	Demyelinating factor*
Human BP in CFA	Day 10 following sensitization	4	none
Human BP in CFA	When clinical signs of EAE appear	4	none
Human BP in CFA	After suppression with human BP in oil	5	none
Rabbit sciatic nerve myelin	Days 20-40 following sensitization	3	+++

* Demyelinating of rat and mouse CNS cultures in vitro performed
in collaboration with Prof. M. Bornstein.

In Table 6 some data is presented from work in monkeys in
which 5 mg human BP in CFA was injected in order to elicit EAE.
This study clearly shows that BP does not elicit demyelinating
factor either prior to appearance of clinical signs, during
clinical attack, or after suppression of EAE with human BP in
oil. Three of the suppressed animals had circulating antibody
to BP as measured by passive hemagglutination. Thus we conclude
that at no stage during induction or suppression of EAE with
purified BP is demyelinating antibody produced. Only rabbit
sciatic nerve myelin successfully induced demyelinating antibody,
and it is evident that the demyelinating antibody is directed
to some myelin component other than BP, and it has been suggested
that it represents anti-cerebroside antibody (73). Interestingly,
the peripheral nerve myelin induced demyelinating factor to the
CNS culture.

Suppression of EAE with BP

EAE shares a characteristic in common with many other autoimmune diseases in that the disease development can be blocked
or inhibited if BP is administered prior to or in the early stage
of sensitization. It is important to avoid the use of CFA in the
blocking procedure, whereas CFA appears to be an obligatory requirement for induction of EAE when purified BP is used. The
mechanism by which tolerance to EAE is evoked by the blocking

procedure has not been understood, but blocking antibody has been considered a possibility. However, there is now evidence (14, 15) that suppressor T cells may be induced and account for immune tolerance by suppressing the cell-mediated response to BP, the process responsible for EAE.

Among other factors which showed some suppressing activity toward EAE was antilymphocytic globulin (ALG) which retarded the development of EAE significantly if administered early and for an adequate time period (74). However, ALG and various drugs which have been used in studies on the suppression of EAE are generally ineffective on a long term basis; once treatment is stopped, EAE returns. In a recent study on hyperacute EAE in the rat (75), it was found that most drugs including steroids were not effective in delaying EAE development. Some immunosuppressive drugs, however, like cycophosphamide retarded development of clinical signs up to 12 days or so when 12 daily doses of drug were given. Even polyunsaturated fatty acids, perhaps acting through stimulation of prostaglandin synthesis, reportedly retarded and inhibited significantly the course of EAE in the guinea pig if given 7 days and thereafter following sensitization (76). Thus it appears that some agents may temporarily inhibit clinical signs of EAE while they are administered, but seldom elicit long term suppression.

In order to evaluate the effect of BP itself on EAE, we chose conditions closely resembling the clinical conditions of MS patients (13). Rhesus monkeys were selected as test animals; the human BP was used for disease induction and suppression; and . suppression procedures were only begun after definite clinical signs of EAE were observed, usually 13-25 days following sensitization. Notably, the monkey shows signs of EAE not far removed from those of MS patients under acute attack, i.e. ataxia, limb weakness and optic nerve impairment. After a period of trial and error, it was found that daily administration of 2 mg of BP given i.m. in mineral oil led to recovery and reversal of the clinical signs, and if maintained for at least two weeks or so, most of the monkeys were returned to a clinically normal state (13). These results appeared remarkable in view of previous unsuccessful attempts to drastically alter the course of EAE with ALG and drugs.

The results, shown in Table 7, reveal that human BP is capable of suppressing EAE; of 20 monkeys sensitized with human BP, only 6 of the monkeys died following suppressive treatment. Generally it was found that approximately 80% of the monkeys recovered to an essentially normal state regardless of which species of BP was used for induction or suppression; EAE induced by human or monkey BP was suppressed by human, monkey or bovine BP. These data show that BP from these species are equally

TABLE 7

Suppression of EAE in rhesus monkeys

Inducing BP	No. of Animals	Suppressing BP	No. dead	No. Recovered
Human	20	Human	6	14
Human	6	Bovine	1	5
Human HNB	4	Human HNB	0	4
Monkey	7	Monkey	2	5
Monkey	4	Human	1	3
Monkey	5	Bovine	1	4
Peptide T	2	Peptide T	0	2
Monkey	3	Peptide T	1	2
TOTAL	51		12	39

EAE was induced with 5 mg BP (emulsified in Difco H37 Ra Freund's adjuvant) given in two 0.1-ml injections in the footpad. Peptide T (2mg) was also used. Suppressive treatment began with i.m. injection of 10 mg Al protein in saline emulsified in mineral oil (1:1) when the animal first showed clear clinical signs of disease such as limb weakness, paralysis, ataxia, etc. Subsequently, one injection per day of 2 mg BP was given for 16 days. Also, penicillin G (100,000 units/day) was given, and in most cases, animals were fed twice daily with 20 cc of AB-dextrose solution.

potent in inducing or suppressing disease. Histologic examination
of brain and spinal cord of suppressed monkeys after 3-4 months
showed virtually no infiltration of inflammatory cells. After
1 month, however, a considerable number of mononuclear cells
were seen but fewer than normal found in a typical case of EAE.

It should be noted that in control monkeys, in which histone
or saline was used for suppression, mortality was 100%, occurring
1-4 days following appearance of severe clinical signs. For
induction of EAE, 5 mg of BP in CFA was used in order to achieve
disease in 100% of the monkeys injected. Normal monkeys were
also given large daily doses of BP in oil, at least 10 fold
greater than used in suppression. In no case were clinical or
histologic signs of EAE induced, or any other evidence of pathology (Table 8).

In those cases of suppressive treatment with BP in which
the animal eventually died, most of the animals survived for 1-2
weeks or more. In these cases there was a relatively high number
of animals that developed blindness. Notably, all monkeys with
EAE examined showed severe demyelination and cellular infiltration in the optic nerve. It is possible that in those animals
developing blindness the course of the disease is more severe
and suppressive treatment therefore less effective. However,
in two cases where complete blindness was established, the suppressed animals eventually recovered their vision after several
weeks. This was one of the most dramatic instances of recovery
and reversal of the pathologic process. In at least 7 other
cases, slow recovery of function was observed where limb paralysis
was involved. Use of an arm or leg, once severely paralyzed,
was slowly recovered over a period of weeks or months. These
data indicate that the demyelinating process, which is probably
responsible for the major pathology, can be reversed and nerves
remyelinated with return of function.

The data in Table 7 also show that there is probably little
difference in the sequence of the disease-inducing site of BP
from various species capable of inducing EAE in monkey since
all were equally active. The major encephalitogenic site for
the monkey is in the COOH-terminal (28, 77), which also constitutes
a minor site for the rabbit (31). Importantly, peptide T
(res. 116-169), the 56 residue fragment containing the encephalitogenic site, also suppresses EAE in monkeys induced either with
intact BP or peptide T. These results further support the role
of the carboxyl region of BP as the major encephalitogenic site
and are compatible with results of Driscoll et al. (78), who
found for guinea pigs that the tryptophan region, the disease-
inducing site, serves best for blocking particularly as part of
a large peptide. Minor encephalitogenic determinants for the
monkey possibly appear in the amino acid-terminal region (23)

TABLE 8

Administration of BP to monkeys

No. of animals	Protein injected	No. dead	No. with signs of EAE
4	Human BP (150 mg total, 10 mg daily)	0	0
3	Monkey BP (30 mg total)	0	0
3	Bovine BP (150 mg total, 10 mg daily)	0	0

The protein (in mineral oil) was given daily intramuscularly. No clinical or histologic evidence of EAE was found.

and possibly in the 43-89 region of BP (30). These minor determinants probably do not play a significant role in the induction
of EAE in the monkey; if they did, peptide T would probably not
have suppressed so effectively.

a) Critical period - One of the most important findings of these
studies is that the suppressive treatment must be extended over
a critical period of 12-18 days in order to achieve permanent
suppression (13). Optimal treatment requires administration of
12 mg BP per day over the critical period. Usually the clinical
signs abate daily over the first week of suppression, but if the
suppressive treatment is stopped at any time during the critical
period, at day 10 for example, the clinical state of the monkey
rapidly deteriorates after a delay of 2-3 days or so, until death,or
then the monkey usually recovers. Thus a type of EAE involving
exacerbation - remission episodes can be introduced by stopping
the suppressive treatment prior to completion of the critical
period, and resuppression. In one case, a monkey was successfully
suppressed three times in this type of experiment. Even the
administration of suppressive doses of BP on an alternate day
basis was not as effective as on a daily basis. Larger doses,
30 mg compared to 2 mg per day, were not noticably superior in
suppressing the disease.

Once the critical period was exceeded, the monkeys showed
no further signs of EAE even after several years, and thus appeared
permanently suppressed. These results suggest that during the
critical period, administration of antigen leads to inactivation
of the sensitized lymphocytes mediating the disease; the critical
period representing the time required to reduce the clone of
effector cells below a threshold level. This interpretation
is based on the large body of data asserting the major role
played by cell-mediated phenomena in EAE (7). It is compatible
with the effect of anti-lymphocytic globulin in temporarily
blocking development of EAE, and with the finding that a minimum
number of sensitized cells are necessary for the passive transfer
of EAE in rats (79).

In order to test the state of the immune response after
suppressive treatment, six recovered animals were rechallenged
in the usual way to induce EAE (Table 9). The results show that
in all six animals tested, not only did EAE develop, but it
developed more rapidly and severely than in the initial induction.
The average time of appearance of severe signs (limb weakness,
paralysis, ataxia, etc.) on rechallenge was 8 days, only a third
of the average time of 24 days originally found. Again, however,
the BP and peptide T effectively suppressed the rechallenged
animals in three out of four cases. Freund's adjuvant itself is
not a reinducing agent. This experiment shows that the animal,
while appearing normal after suppressive treatment, is left with

TABLE 9

Induction of clinical EAE in fully suppressed (clinically normal) monkeys

Monkey	Original day of clinical signs *	Day of rechallenge +	Reinducing challenge antigen	Day of clinical signs ##	Resuppressive protein in IFA	Survival
1	14	245	CFA	None	None	Yes
2	14	244	BP + CFA	10	None	No
3	24	71	BP + CFA	7	Histone	No
4	23	44	BP + CFA	7	BP	No
5	31	24	BP + CFA	7	BP	Yes
6	24	50	BP + CFA	7	Peptide T	Yes
7	21	39	BP + CFA	10	BP	Yes

* No. of days after initial challenge.

+ No. of days after last suppressive dose.

No. of days after second challenge.

The suppressed animals were injected with monkey BP as required to induce EAE. Monkey 1 was rechallenged with adjuvant only. Monkeys 2-7 all developed very severe clinical signs after rechallenge. Attempts to resuppress and reverse the course of disease after expression of clinical signs were successful in monkeys 5, 6 and 7.

greater potential to develop EAE than initially. Immunologically, it appears that after suppression there are more memory cells capable of forming clones of T cells sensitized to the BP. Apparently these cells pose no danger unless the animal is rechallenged since EAE does not develop spontaneously in those animals suppressed past the critical period.

b) Mechanism - What is the mechanism of suppression of EAE by the BP after clinical signs develop? The possibility that blocking antibody was responsible for suppressing of the course of EAE did not appear feasible since antibody was detected in only 30% of the monkeys tested after suppression had been achieved. Moreover, the monkeys often showed improvement in 24-48 hrs., a period possibly too short for significant antibody production to begin. Recently, a more reasonable explanation has come to light. In a study on EAE in the mouse, suppressor cells were found which prevented development of EAE (14). In adoptive transfer experiments, lymphoid cells recruited from mice sensitized to BP in oil after 9-40 days, inhibited the development of EAE in recipient mice. The suppressor cells were derived from bone marrow or spleen, were specific for BP-sensitized cells, and were abolished by anti-Thy serum. Not only did the suppressor cells block development of EAE, but the cell-mediated response (MIF) was also reduced. These results offer a reasonable explanation for the suppression of EAE observed in the monkeys.

Based on the suppression studies in mice and monkeys events in the induction and suppression of EAE are proposed in Table 10. It is now well established that injection of BP in CFA leads to sensitized effector cells which migrate to the CNS and mediate the disease (7). Recently, Traugott et al. (80) found that the decrease of early T cells (high affinity rosetting cells) in the serum of guinea pigs with EAE coincided with the appearance of such cells in the CNS. It appears reasonable to propose in the monkey, as in the mice, that the suppressive treatment of daily injections of BP in oil leads to production of suppressor T cells. Thus the critical period can be explained as the period during which the suppressor T cells, which destroy the clone of effector cells and eventually lead to permanent suppression, must be maintained by daily injection of BP in oil. This phenomenon requires about 14-18 days, presumably in order to reduce the number of effector cells below an active threshold level. However, memory cells remain, as shown by the ease of rechallenge. This interpretation is agreeable with studies (81) showing that memory cells are indeed induced during the course of EAE in the rat. These cells were detected because, when activated by Con A, their ability to transfer EAE is greatly enhanced.

TABLE 10

PROPOSED EVENTS IN INDUCTION
AND SUPPRESSION OF EAE IN MONKEYS

1. Injection of BP with complete Freund's adjuvant <u>induces
   sensitized T cells</u>

2. <u>Effector cells</u> sensitized to BP migrate to the CNS where they
   release mediators such as MIF, etc.

3. After 5 days, <u>histologic lesions</u> appear in the CNS; after
   12-25 days, <u>clinical signs</u> of EAE

4. Suppression initiated when clinical signs appear; <u>inject BP
   in oil i.m.</u>

5. <u>Suppressor T cells</u> recruited from bone marrow and spleen

6. During 2 week <u>critical period</u>, clone of effector cells
   destroyed by suppressor cells

7. Disease course <u>permanently reversed</u> in the suppressed animal;
   histologic lesions disappear after 2-3 months; <u>memory cells</u>
   remain.

Suppression of EAE with Synthetic Polypeptides

    There are other approaches to the suppression of EAE based
on the BP model; in these cases synthetic polypeptide analogues
have been used whose structure is analogous to the tryptophan
region of BP. In these approaches synthetic peptide analogues
were sought which were nonencephalitogenic but yet suppressive.
Hashim et al. (82) addressed the problem by the synthesis of 20
residue peptide (Phe-Ser-Trp-Gln-Lys)$_4$ referred to as peptide
S42, based on the reasoning that the pentapeptide, Phe-Ser-Trp-
Gln-Lys, gave a strong delayed skin reaction in animals sensitized
to BP, yet was not encephalitogenic.

    As shown in Table 11, where peptide S42 was given daily (4mg/
day) for 10 days following the appearance of hind leg paralysis in
guinea pigs sensitized with bovine BP, nearly all of the animals
recovered whereas none of the control animals survived. Apparently
the suppressed animals were completely refractory to any further
signs of disease. Following suppressive treatment, neither antibody nor cells sensitized to BP were found. These results suggest that peptide S42 is capable of initiating events leading to
the destruction of effector cells (sensitized to BP) which mediate
the disease. In its suppressor activity, peptide S42 behaves
similar to BP itself, and is an analogue of the tryptophan region,
the disease-inducing site active in the guinea pig. Presumably

TABLE 11

SUPPRESSION OF EAE WITH SYNTHETIC
POLYPEPTIDES

Material	Cross Reactivity with BP	Treatment	Results
S42 in guinea pig	Cell-mediated (skin test; rosettes)	4mg daily for 10 days after clinical signs	6 out of 7 animal recovered
Cop I in guinea pig	Cell-mediated (skin test; LBT test)	1mg 3x before clinical signs	22% EAE; controls 63%
rabbit	"	8mg 3x before clinical signs	19% EAE; controls 70%
monkey		15 injections after clinical signs (10-100mg per injection)	1 out 2 recovered fully

immunologic recognition of S42 leads to cross recognition of cells
sensitized for the tryptophan region of BP. These results indicate a potential for synthetic peptides in the design of nonencephalitogenic polypeptides capable of suppressing an immunopathologic response.

The other approach, used by Teitelbaum et al. (83, 84) has
utilized a large random copolymer (MW 23,000) of alanine, glutamic
acid, lysine, and tyrosine, referred to as Cop I. When this
material was given to guinea pigs or rabbits following sensitization, a significant number of animals appeared to be protected
(Table 11). In a contrary report (78), however, Cop I was not
effective in blocking EAE development in the guinea pig. In one
out of 2 monkeys (69), Cop I was found to suppress the course
of EAE when given in 15 doses varying in amount from 100 to 10 mg
Cop I. This last report is of particular interest because it
implies that Cop I has the ability to retard EAE in primates and
could therefore have relevance to MS. More extensive studies
need be performed, however, before definite conclusions can be
made. Although the synthetic polymers appear to suppress the
course of EAE, it is highly unlikely that they could be as effective as BP itself. From 5-50 fold more Cop I was used in the
monkey studies compared to BP and it does not appear as effective.
Clearly, however, both S42 and Cop I cross react with BP both in
vivo and in vitro tests for cell-mediated immunity (Table 11),
and it is quite likely, therefore, that they work via the same

mechanism for suppression as BP, probably by suppressor T cell
stimulation. Since Cop I is a random copolymer it may cross
react with several determinants on the BP molecule (85). The
S42 peptide, however, may not be as effective in suppressing
EAE in animals other than guinea pigs since it is modelled after
the tryptophan region which is not disease-inducing in monkeys
or rats. The main virtue of the synthetic polypeptides is that
they are nonencephalitogenic; however, BP appears equally safe
since it is not encephalitogenic when given without mycobacteria.
Moreover, it has been shown (78) that blocking of EAE in guinea
pigs is best achieved where peptides have the encephalitogenic
tryptophan domain intact. Thus in considering the extension of
suppressing studies based on the EAE data to clinical trials in
MS, the synthetic polypeptides may be inferior to BP itself both
in suppressing potency and specificity.

                              Relevance to MS

     Over the past three years, evidence has appeared which sug-
gests that the EAE model may be much closer to MS than previously
believed. A chronic guinea pig model for MS has been evolved by
Raine and Stone (8, 16) which mimics the human disease both clinically and morphologically. Whereas EAE is usually an acute monophasic, severe, and often fatal condition (7), the chronic form
as induced in juvenile strain 13 guinea pigs, has an 8-12 week
latent period, and may persist up to 2 years with occasional
episodes of exacerbation (8, 16). It shares additionally with
some forms of MS a protracted and progressive course, large
demyelinated plaques, is age dependent, and shows genetic predisposition. This chronic form of EAE, therefore, offers a more
suitable and accessible approach to MS and renews confidence in
the EAE model as it relates to MS.

     One of most striking uses of the chronic EAE model was the
recent study of suppression with BP (86). In the 5 intervening
weeks following sensitization but prior to appearance of clinical
signs, a total of 1.4 mg of BP in IFA was given in a series of
10 injections. This suppressive course was remarkably effective
in preventing development of EAE; no clinical signs were found
and no large CNS lesions. Histology revealed only marginal
disease and remyelinated axons. Even rechallenge, unlike the
situation in the monkey, failed to elicit signs of EAE. What is
most significant, however, is that the animals were sensitized
with spinal cord material rather than purified BP. Thus it can
be concluded that the chronic relapsing form of EAE, induced
with spinal cord, is markedly suppressed in nearly all animals
with BP. Thus whatever other immunologic responses which may
arise from components in the spinal cord other than BP, such as
demyelinating factor, they are clearly irrelevent to EAE. Addi-

tionally, the time course level of T lymphocyte populations, in which T cell levels fell during relapse, remained low during early suppressive doses, then rose to normal levels.

The successful suppression of EAE in the monkey and chronic EAE in the guinea pig (induced with spinal cord) with bovine BP offers a compelling and encouraging approach to MS, and should now be seriously evaluated as a potential therapy in the human disease. EAE in the monkey has many clinical and histologic characteristics of early MS, and the chronic guinea pig model mimics MS so closely that the suppressive data urges a logical extension to MS. Both of these studies provide a protocol for a clinical approach to MS, and the guinea pig model now provides a strong rationale as well. Moreover, the findings of Sheremata et al. (87, 88, 89) that effector cells sensitized to the carboxyl region of BP appear prior to and during exacerbation in MS, provides a strong rationale for suppressive treatment on MS patients using BP. If indeed, the effector cells are responsible for early lesions in MS as they are in EAE, then the suppressive treatment could lead to promising results. In this regard, some encouraging results have come from immunosuppressive studies on MS patients using drugs and anti-lymphocytic globulin (90). However, if suppressor T cells are playing a role in the suppression events, then the BP offers a far superior and safer approach than general immunosuppression. The advantage of BP suppression is that only the target cells (effectors) mediating the disease are affected.

a) Clinical trials in MS - There have been a variety of studies on MS patients whose aim was to suppress or retard the course of the disease. Table 12 contains a number of representative studies but is not a complete listing of all such studies. Most of these are based on an immunosuppressive approach and have used ACTH, antilymphocytic globulin, immunosuppressive drugs such as cyclophosphamide, azathiaprine or combinations of these agents. Most of the studies showed no benefit to the MS patients. The study with linoleic acid of Bates et al. (95) is also based theoretically in part on immunosuppression. It has been shown the polyunsaturated fatty acids given continuously after day 7 following sensitization for EAE leads to substantial suppression of the disease (76). Presumably this effect is based on the synthesis of prostaglandin, perhaps secreted by suppressor T cells, which inactivate the effector T cells (sensitized to BP) which mediate the disease. However, the polyunsaturated fatty acids had no discernable influence in MS. The fatty acids are not suppressive if given prior to day 7, and since timing is critical in EAE, perhaps the timing is also critical in MS.

The use of Cop I random polypeptide is also an approach based partly on immunosuppression in view of its cross reactivity with

TABLE 12

CLINICAL STUDIES ON MS PATIENTS

Method	Duration	Patients	Reference	Results
Basic protein (5mg/week)	3-11 months	35	Gonsette et al. (91)(1977)	no influence
Basic protein (5-25mg/week)	up to 3 years		Campbell (92) (1973)	subjective improvement
Anti-lymphocytic globulin; prednisone	1 year	14	Lance et al. (90)(1975)	minor improvement
Anti-lymphocytic globulin; ACTH	14-28 days	10	Kastruckoff et al. (99)(1978)	short term benefit but not long term
Cop I polypeptide	3 weeks - 5 months	4	Abramsky et al. (97)(1976)	minor benefit
Cyclophosphamide (4-5 mg/kg)	10 days	6	Drachman et al. (96)(1975)	no influence
Polyunsaturated fatty acids	2 years	152	Bates et al. (95)(1975)	no influence (chronic progressive)
Transfer factor	13 months	16	Fog et al. (98) (1978)	no influence
ACTH	1 year		Rose et al. (93)(1970)	no benefit
Azathiaprine	13 months	13	Wilkerson et al. (94) (1973)	no benefit

BP shown by tests for cell-mediated immunity. Two of four MS patients showed minor improvement in their vision and speech capacity (97).

Efforts to produce immunoenhancement are reflected in the transfer factor studies (98). The rationale is based on the possibility that MS may be mediated by a virus. Since studies have shown that cell mediated immunity to measles and other viruses may be diminished in MS, transfer factor was administered in order to augment cell-mediated immunity and thus retard the disease process. One of the main problems with this study, which

was unsuccessful in retarding the disease course, is the question
of donors. Apparently blood lymphocytes from a general population
pool were used, and no effort was made to evaluate cell mediated
immunity to viruses. Moreover, since the "MS" virus is unknown,
the question arises about which virus should be designated.

While none of the studies to date have been truly encouraging,
the use of antilymphocytic globulin has produced some minor
although temporary improvement. These studies are important
because they suggest that suppressing rather than enhancing the
immune processes may retard the course of the disease. They
further suggest that immune mechanisms may mediate the pathology
in MS, and that cell-mediated immunity to viruses, which might
be adversely affected by such treatment, is not an important
factor. However, intensive immunosuppressive treatment may have
long range side effects such as an increased susceptibility to
cancer.

b) Potential use of BP in MS - A solid groundwork has now been
established that compells serious consideration of the use of BP
in the attempt to suppress the course of MS as it has EAE in the
monkey. The reasoning can be presented as follows :

1. BP markedly suppresses development of chronic relapsing EAE
   in juvenile guinea pigs, a close animal model of MS where
   disease is induced with spinal cord.

2. BP suppresses EAE in monkeys even after severe clinical signs
   have appeared.

3. BP induces suppressor T cells in mice and rats that block and
   suppress EAE in adoptive transfer experiments.

4. Effector T lymphocytes sensitized to BP, which mediate events
   in EAE, appear in MS patients prior to and during exacerbation.

5. Immunosuppressive treatment with ALG and Cop I appear to offer
   minor improvement in some cases of MS, an indication that suppression of some immune cell population may be beneficial.

6. Use of BP in MS patients has proven safe in two studies (91,
   92). Based on the monkey experiments, the dosage and timing
   of BP administration is crucial to successful suppression;
   much higher doses given daily should be more appropriate.

SUMMARY

In the last few years, EAE has proven to be a useful animal
model for analyzing immunopathologic mechanisms. The BP appears
to contain several antigenic sites which bind specific hyperimmune
antibody, but antibody to BP appears to play no role in the disease
course in EAE and MS either in induction or suppression. The

suppression of EAE in monkeys is accomplished using BP in oil
which presumably induces a population of suppressor T cells which
destroy the clone of effector cells. A critical period of 14-
18 days is required during which BP must be administered regularly
in order to perpetuate suppressive events. A population of
memory cells is also induced as shown by the more rapid and severe
form of EAE occurring on challenge with BP in suppressed animals.
There is now a formidable body of data that supports the use of
BP for clinical attempts to suppress the course of MS based on
the monkey experiments. BP appears as potentially the safest
and most potent agent for immunosuppression in MS when compared
to immunosuppressive drugs and nonencephalitogenic synthetic
polypeptides such as peptide S42 or Cop I.

REFERENCES

1. Nakao, A., Davis, W.J., and Roboz-Einstein, E., Basic proteins
   from the acidic extract of bovine spinal cord. I. Isolation
   and characterization. Biochim. Biophys. Acta. 130, 163-170,
   1966.
2. Kies, M., Murphy, J.B., and Alvord, E.C. Jr., Fractionation
   of guinea pig brain proteins with encephalitogenic activity.
   Fed. Proc. 19, 207, 1960.
3. Eylar, E.H., Salk, J., Beveridge, G.C. and Brown, L.V., Experimental allergic encephalomyelitis basic protein from bovine
   myelin. Arch. Biochem. Biophys. 132, 34-38, 1969.
4. Eylar, E.H., Brostoff, S., Hashim, G., Caccam, J., and Burnett,
   P., Basic A1 protein of the myelin membrane. The complete
   amino acid sequence. J. Biol. Chem. 246, 5770-5784, 1971.
5. Eylar, E.H., Caccam, J., Jackson, J., Westall, F., and Robinson,
   A.P., Experimental allergic encephalomyelitis : synthesis of
   disease-inducing site of the basic protein. Science 168,
   1220-1223, 1970.
6. Westall, F.C., Robinson, A.R., Caccam, J., Jackson, J., and
   Eylar, E.H., Essential chemical requirements for induction of
   allergic encephalomyelitis. Nature 229, 22-24, 1971.
7. Eylar, E.H., EAE and multiple sclerosis, in Multiple Sclerosis,
   Wolfgram, F., Ellison, G., Stevens, J., and Andrews, N., Eds.,
   Academic Press, New York, 1972.
8. Raine, C.S., and Stone, S.H., Animal Model for Multiple Sclerosis. N.Y. State J. Med. Sept., 1693-1696, 1977.
9. Eylar, E.H., Peptides and Autoimmune Disease in "Immunobiology
   of Proteins and Peptides, I,"(Stavitsky, M. and Stavitsky, A.,
   Eds.) Plenum Pub. Corp., p. 259-281, 1978.
10. Alvord, E.C.Jr., Shaw, C.M., Hruby, S. and Kies, M., Encephali-
    togen-induced inhibition of experimental allergic encephalo-
    myelitis : prevention, suppression and therapy. Ann. NY.
    Acad. Sci. 122, 333-345, 1965.
11. Cunningham, V.R., and Field, E.J., Experimental allergic encepha-

lomyelitis : protection experiments with encephalitogenic factor and tubercule fractions. Ann. NY. Acad. Sci. 122, 346-355, 1965.

12. Roboz-Einstein, E., Sejtey, J., Davis, W.J., and Rauch, H.C., Protective action of the encephalitogen in experimental allergic encephalomyelitis. Immunochem. 5, 567-575, 1968.

13. Eylar, E.H., Jackson, J., Rothenberg, B., and Brostoff, S., Suppression of the immune response : reversal of the disease state with antigen in allergic encephalomyelitis. Nature, 236, 74-76, 1972.

14. Bernard, C.C.A., Suppressor T cells prevent experimental auto-immune encephalomyelitis in mice. Clin. Exp. Immunol.29, 100-109, 1977.

15. Swierkosz, J.E., and Swanborg, R.H., Suppressor cell control of unresponsiveness to experimental allergic encephalomyelitis. J. Immunol. 115, 631-633, 1975.

16. Raine, C., Snyder, D.H., Valsamis, M.P., and Stone, S.H., Chronic experimental allergic encephalomyelitis in inbred guinea pigs. An ultrastructural study, Lab. Invest. 31, 369, 1974.

17. Paterson, P.Y., Transfer of allergic encephalomyelitis in rats by means of lymph node cells. J. Exp. Med. , 111, 119-136, 1960.

18. Alvord, E.C.Jr., Shaw, C.M., Hruby, S., and Kies, W., Encepha-litogen-induced inhibition of experimental allergic encepha-lomyelitis : prevention, suppression, and therapy. Ann. NY. Acad. Sci., 122, 333-345, 1965.

19. Williams, R.M., and Moore, M.J., Linkage of susceptibility to experimental allergic encephalomyelitis to the major histocom-patibility locus in the rat. J. Exp. Med. 138, 775-783, 1973.

20. Ortiz-Ortiz, L., Nakamura, R.M., and Weigle, W.O., T cell requirement for experimental allergic encephalomyelitis induc-tion in the rat. J. Immunol. 117 (2), 576-579, 1976.

21. Ortiz-Ortiz, L., and Weigle, W.O., Cellular events in the in-duction of experimental allergic encephalomyelitis in rats. J. Exp. Med. 144, 604-616, 1976.

22. Hashim, G., and Eylar, E.H., Allergic encephalomyelitis : isolation and characterization of encephalitogenic peptides from the basic protein of bovine spinal cord. Arch. Biochem. Biophys. 129, 645-654, 1969a.

23. Brostoff, S., Reuter, W., Hichens, M., and Eylar, E.H., Spe-cific cleavage of the Al protein from myelin with cathepsin D. J. Biol. Chem. 249, 559-567, 1974.

24. Burnett, P.R., and Eylar, E.H., Allergic encephalomyelitis. Oxidation and cleavage of the single tryptophan residue of the Al protein from bovine and human myelin. J. Biol. Chem. 246, 3425-3431, 1971.

25. Spitler, L., von Muller, C., Fudenburg, H.H., and Eylar, E.H., Experimental allergic encephalomyelitis : dissociation of cellular immunity to brain protein and disease production.

J. Exp. Med. 136, 156-174, 1972.

26. Bergstrand, H., Localization of the antigenic determinants on bovine encephalitogenic protein. Further studies with the macrophage migration inhibition assay in guinea pigs. Immunochem. 10, 611, 1973.

27. Hashim, G., Carvalho, E., and Sharpe, R., Definition and synthesis of the essential amino acid sequence for EAE in Lewis rats. J. Immunol. 121, 665-670, 1978.

28. Karkhanis, Y.D., Carlo, J., Brostoff, S., and Eylar, E.H., Allergic encephalomyelitis isolation of an encephalitogenic peptide in the monkey. J. Biol. Chem. 250, 1718-1722, 1975.

29. Bergstrand, H., and Kallen, B., Further studies on Antigenic regions of bovine encephalitogenic protein with the lymph node cell transformation test in rabbits. Neurobiol. 4, 328-336, 1974.

30. Kibler, R.F., Re, P.K., McKneally, S., and Shapira, R., Biological activity of an encephalitogenic fragment in the monkey. J. Biol. Chem. 247, 969-972, 1972.

31. Westall, F.C., and Thompson, M., An encephalitogenic region for rabbits. Immunochem. 15, 189-191, 1978.

32. Eylar, E.H., Westall, F.C., Brostoff, S., Allergic encephalomyelitis : an encephalitogenic peptide derived from the basic protein of myelin. J. Biol. Chem. 246, 3418-3424, 1971.

33. Shapira, R., Chou, F.C.-H., McKneally, S., Urban, E., and Kibler, R., Biological activity and synthesis of an encephalitogenic determinant. Science, 173, 736-738, 1971.

34. Martenson, R.E., Nomura, K., Levine, S., and Sowinski, R., Experimental allergic encephalomyelitis in the Lewis rat : further delineation of active sites in guinea pig and bovine myelin basic proteins. J. Immunol. 118, 1280, 1977.

35. Hashim, G., Experimental allergic encephalomyelitis in Lewis rats : chemical synthesis or disease-inducing determinant. Science, 196, 1219, 1977.

36. Hashim, G., Sharpe, R., and Carvalho, E., EAE : sequestered encephalitogenic determinant in the bovine myelin basic protein. J. Neurochem. in press 1979.

37. Lisak, R.P., Heinze, R.G., Kies, M., and Alvord, E.C.Jr., Antibodies to encephalitogenic basic protein in experimental allergic encephalomyelitis. Proc. Soc. Exp. Biol. Med. 130, 814-818, 1969.

38. Gonatas, N.K., Gonatas, J.O., Steibler, A., Lisak, R., Suzuki, J., and Martenson, R.E., The significance of circulating and cell-bound antibodies in experimental allergic encephalomyelitis. Am. J. Pathol. 76, 529-544, 1974.

39. Day, E.D., and Pitts, O.M., The antibody response to myelin basic protein (BP) in Lewis rats : The effect of time, dosage of BP, and dosage of Mycobacterium butyricum. J. Immunol. 113, 1958-1967, 1974.

40. Whitaker, J.N., The antigenicity of myelin encephalitogenic protein : production of antibodies to encephalitogenic protein

with deoxyribonucleic acid- encephalitogenic protein complexes. J. Immunol. 114, 823-828, 1975.

41. Kies, M., Immunology of myelin basic protein. The Nervous System, Donald B. Tower, Ed. Vol. 1 : The Basic Neurosciences. Raven Press, New York, 1975.

42. Kibler, R.F., and Barnes, A.E., Antibody studies in rabbit encephalomyelitis induced by water-soluble protein fraction of rabbit cord. J. Exp. Med. 116, 807-825, 1962.

43. Kies, M. Driscoll, B.F., Seil, F.J., and Alvord, E.C.Jr., Myelination inhibition factor : Dissociation from induction of experimental allergic encephalomyelitis. Science, 179, 689-690, 1973.

44. Gonatas, N.K., and Howard, J.C., Inhibition of experimental allergic encephalomyelitis in rats severely depleted of T cells. Science, 186, 839-841, 1974.

45. Hashim, G., and Schilling, F.J., Prevention of experimental allergic encephalomyelitis by non-encephalitogenic basic peptides. Arch. Biochem. Biophys. 156, 287-297, 1973a.

46. Whitaker, J.N., and McFarlin, D.E., A comparison of immuno-chemical methods for the detection of antibodies to myelin encephalitogenic protein. Brain Res. 129, 121-128, 1977.

47. Whitaker, J.N., Chou, C-H.J., Chou, C-H.F., and Kibler, R.F., Antigenic determinants of bovine myelin encephalitogenic protein recognized by rabbit antibody to myelin encephalitogenic protein. J. Biol. Chem. 250, 9106-9111, 1975.

48. Burnett, P.R., and Eylar, E.H., Allergic encephalomyelitis. Oxidation and cleavage of the single tryptophan residue of the A1 protein from bovine and human myelin, J. Biol. Chem. 246, 3425-3431, 1971.

49. Driscoll, B.F., Kramer, A.J., and Kies, M., Myelin basic protein : Location of multiple independent antigenic regions. Science, 184, 73-75, 1974.

50. McFarlin, D.E., Blank, S.E., Kibler, R.F., McKneally,S., and Shapira, R., Experimental allergic encephalomyelitis in the rat : Response to the encephalitogenic proteins and peptides. Science 179, 478-480, 1973.

51. Whitaker, J.N., Chou, J., Chou, F., and Kibler, R.F., Molecular internalization of a region of myelin basic protein. J. Exp. Med. 146, 317-331, 1977.

52. Thompson, K., Harris, M., Benjamin, E., Mitchell, G., and Noble, M., Antibody and cell-mediated responses to nature and denatured lysozyme. Nature New Biol. 238, 20, 1972.

53. Atassi, M.Z., and Habeeb, A.F.S.A., The antigenic structure of hen egg-white lysozyme: a model for disulfide-containing proteins. Immunochemistry of Proteins, Volume 2, Edited by M.Z. Atassi, Chapter 4, 1978.

54. M.Z. Atassi, The complete antigenic structure of myoglobin : approaches and conclusions for antigenic structures of proteins. Immunochemistry of Proteins, Volume 2, Editor M.Z. Atassi, Chapter 3, 1978.

55. Gutstein, H.S., and Cohen, S.R., Spinal fluid differences in experimental allergic encephalomyelitis and MS. Science, 199, 301-303, 1978.

56. Cohen, S.R., Herndon, R., McKhann, G.M., Basic protein in spinal fluid. N. Eng. J. Med. 295, 1455, 1976.

57. Whitaker, J.N., Myelin encephalitogenic protein fragments in cerebrospinal fluid of persons with multiple sclerosis. Neurology 27, 911-920, 1977.

58. Einstein, E.R., Csejtey, J., Dala, K.B., et al., Proteolytic activity and basic protein loss in and around multiple sclerosis plaques : Combined biochemical and histochemical observations. J. Neurochem. 19, 653-662, 1972.

59. Marks, N., Benuck, M., Hashim, G., Hydrolysis of myelin basic protein with brain acid proteinase. Biochim. Biophys. Res. Commun. 56, 68-74, 1974.

60. Lisak, R.P., Heinz, R.G., Falk, G.A., and Kies, M., Search for anti-encephalitogen antibody in human demyelinating disease, Neurology, 18, 122-128, 1968.

61. McPherson, T.A., and Carnegie, P.R., Radioimmunoassay with gel filtration for detecting antibody to basic proteins of myelin, J. Lab. Clin. Med. , 72, 824-831, 1968.

62. Sheremata, W., Wood, D., Moscarello, A., and Cosgrove, J., Sensitization to myelin basic protein attacks of MS. J. Neurol. Sci. 36, 165-170, 1978.

63. Panitch, H., Hafler, D., and Johnson, K., Antibodies to myelin basic protein in MS : Clinical correlations, Neurology, 394, 1978.

64. Ammitzboll, T., Clausen, J., and Fog, T., Oligoclonal IgG and measles antibody in CSF of MS patients, Acta. Neurol. Scand. 56, 153-158, 1977.

65. Vandvik, J., Natvig, J., and Norrby, E., IgG subclass restriction of oligoclonal measles virus-specific IgG antibodies in patients with subacute sclerosing panencephalitis and in a patient with MS., Scand. J. Immunol. 6, 651-657, 1977.

66. Powis, P.A., Cuzner, M.L., and Davison, A.N., Serum immune complex in MS. Biochem. Soc. Trans. 5, 1420-1422, 1977; 570th Meeting, Cardiff.

67. Tachovsky, T., Lisak, R., Koprowski, H., Theofilopoulos, A.N., and Dixon, F.J., Lancet, ii, 997-999, 1976.

68. Jacque, C., Davous, P., and Baumann, N., Circulating immune complexes and MS., Lancet, ii, 408, 1977.

69. Goust, J.M., Chenais, F., Carnes, J.E., Hames, C.G., Fudenberg, H.H., Hogan, E.L., Abnormal T cell subpopulations and circulating immune complexes in the Guillain-Barré syndrome and multiple sclerosis. Neurology, 28, 421-425, 1978.

70. Appel, S.H., and Bornstein, M.B., The application of tissue culture to the study of experimental "allergic" encephalomyelitis, Part 2 (Serum factors responsible for demyelination). J. Exp. Med. 119, 303-312, 1964.

71. Wolfgram, F., Myers, L.W., Ellison, G.W., and Sofen, H., Demyelinating antibodies in MS., Neurology, 28, 393, 1978.

72. Seil, F.J., Kies, M.W., and Bacon, M., Neural antigens and induction of myelination inhibition factor. J. Immunol. 114, 630-634, 1975.

73. Fry, J.M., Weissbarth, S., Lehrer, G.M., Cerebroside antibody inhibits sulfatide synthesis and myelination and demyelinates in cord tissue culture. Science 183, 540-542, 1974.

74. Liebowitz, S., Kessof, M., and Kennedy, L., The effect of anti-lymphocytic globulin in EAE. Clin. Exp. Immunol. 3, 735-760, 1968.

75. Levine, S., and Sowinski, R., Suppression of the hyperacute form of experimental allergic encephalomyelitis by drugs. Arch. Int. Pharmacodyn. 230, 309-318, 1977.

76. Meade, C.J., Mertin, J., Sheena, J., Hunt, R., Suppression of EAE with linoleic acid. J. Neurol. Sci. 35, 291, 1978.

77. Eylar, E.H., Brostoff, S., Jackson, J., and Carter, H., Allergic encephalomyelitis in monkeys induced by a peptide from the A1 protein. Proc. Natl. Acad. Sci. 69, 617-619, 1972.

78. Driscoll, B.F., Kies, M., and Alvord, E.C.Jr., Protection against experimental allergic encephalomyelitis with peptides derived from myelin basic proteins : presence of intact encephalitogenic site is essential. J. Immunol. 117, 110-114, 1976.

79. Whitehouse, D.J., Whitehouse, M.W., and Pearson, C.M., Passive transfer of adjuvant-induced arthritis and allergic encephalo-myelitis in rats using thoracic duct lymphocytes. Nature 224, 1322, 1969.

80. Traugott, U., Stone, S.H., and Raine, C.S., Experimental allergic encephalomyelitis - migration of early T cells from the circulation into the central nervous system. J. Neurol. Sci. 36, 55-61, 1978.

81. Panitch, H.S., and McFarlin, D.E., Experimental allergic encephalomyelitis : enhancement of cell-mediated transfer by concanavallin A. J. Immunol. 119, 1134-1137, 1977.

82. Hashim, G., Sharpe, R.D., Carvalho, E.F., and Stevens, L.E., Suppression and reversal of experimental allergic encephalo-myelitis in guinea pigs with a non-encephalitogenic analogue of the tryptophan region of the myelin basic protein, J. Immunol. 116, 126-130, 1976.

83. Teitelbaum, D., Webb, C., Meshorer, A., Arnon, R., and Sela, M., Suppression by several synthetic polypeptides of experi-mental allergic encephalomyelitis induced in guinea pigs and rabbits with bovine and human basic encephalitogen. Eur. J. Immunol. 3, 273-279, 1972.

84. Teitelbaum, D., Webb, C., Bree, M., Meshorer, A., Arnon, R., and Sela, M., Suppression of experimental allergic encephalo-myelitis in Rhesus monkeys by a synthetic basic copolymer. Clin. Immun. and Immunopath., 3, 256-262, 1974.

85. Webb, C., Teitelbaum, D., Arnon, R., and Sela, M., In vivo and in vitro immunological cross-reactions between basic poly-peptides capable of suppressing experimental allergic encepha-lomyelitis. Eur. J. Immunol. 3, 279-286, 1973.

86. Raine, C.S., Traugott, V., and Stone, S., Chronic relapsing allergic encephalomyelitis suppression and relevance to multiple sclerosis. Science, in press.

87. Sheremata, W., Cosgrove, J., and Eylar, E.H., Multiple Scle-rosis and cell-mediated hypersensitivity to myelin A1 protein, J. Neurol. Sci., 27, 413-425, 1976.

88. Sheremata, W., Cosgrove, J., and Eylar, E.H., Hypersensitivity to myelin protein preceding attacks of MS., Trans. Am. Neurol. Assoc. 99, 55-60, 1974.

89. Sheremata, W., Eylar, E.H., and Cosgrove, J., Multiple Sclerosis: Sensitization to a myelin basic protein fragment (Peptide T) encephalitogenic to primates, J. Neurol. Sci. 32, 255-263, 1977.

90. Lance, E., Kremer, M., Abbosh, J., Jones, V.E., Knight, S., and Medawar, P.B., Intensive immunosuppression in patients with disseminated sclerosis. Clin. Exp. Immunol. 21, 1-12, 1975.

91. Gonsette, R.E., Delmotte, P., and Demonty, L., Failure of basic protein therapy for MS., J. Neurol. 216, 27-31, 1977.

92. Campbell, B., Myelin basic protein administration in MS, Arch. Neurol. 29, 10-14, 1973.

93. Rose, A., Kuzma, J., Kurtzke, J., Namerow, Sibley, W., and Tourtellotte, W., Study in the evaluation of therapy of MS., Neurology (Mineap.) 20, 1-20, 1970.

94. Wilkerson, L.D., Lisak, R.P., Zweiman, B., and Silbergerg, D.H., Antimyelin antibody in MS : no change during immunosuppression. J. Neurol. Neurosurg. Psych., 40, 872-875, 1977.

95. Bates, D., Fawcett, P.R.W., Shaw, D.A., and Weightman, D., Trial of polyunsaturated fatty acids in non-relapsing multiple sclerosis. Brit. Med. J. 8, Oct., 932-933, 1977.

96. Drachman, D.A., Paterson, P.Y., Schmidt, R.T., and Spehlmann, R.F., Cyclophosphamide in exacerbations of MS., J. Neurol. Neurosurg. Psych., 38, 592-597, 1975.

97. Abramsky, O., Teitelbaum, D., and Arnon, R., Effect of a syn-thetic polypeptide (Cop I) on patients with MS and with acute disseminated encephalomyelitis. J. Neurol. Sci. 31, 433-438, 1977.

98. Fog, T., Raum, N.E., Pederson, L., Kam-Hansen, S., and Mellerup, E., Long-term transfer-factor treatment for MS., The Lancet, April 22, 851-853, 1978.

99. Kastrukoff, L.R., McLean, D.R., and McPherson, T.A., Multiple Sclerosis with antithymocyte globulin - A five year follow-up. Can. J. Neurol. Sci. 5 ## 2, 175-178, 1978.

FOUR LABORATORY METHODS FOR THE DIAGNOSIS OF MULTIPLE SCLEROSIS

(MS) : A PROGRAMME FOR TREATMENT AND POSSIBLE PROPHYLAXIS

E.J. Field

M.S. Research Unit, Royal Victoria Infirmary, Newcastle
Upon Tyne, U.K.

INTRODUCTION

The methods here described and the logical handling of MS
which stems from them derive from the inspired and highly fruitful
suggestion made by R.H.S. Thompson in his Jephcott Lecture (1),
and elaborated further in 1973 (2), that MS develops against an
inborn background of mishandling of unsaturated fatty acids.

With these methods the diagnosis of multiple sclerosis can
now be made with a very high degree of assurance. Since a rational treatment of the beginning case is now available (3), valuable
time is lost in awaiting the second episode which transfers the
patient from the "possible" to "probable" category. In addition,
young children born as near relatives into MS families (where their
chances of developing the disease are 5-20 times that in the general
population) can be picked out as candidates for the disease, and
a proposal for prophylactic handling should be given serious
consideration.

The tests so far developed comprise :

a) The MEM-LAD (Macrophage Electrophoretic Mobility – Linoleic
   Acid Depression) test (4, 5, 6).
b) The E-UFA (Erythrocyte-Unsaturated Fatty Acid) test (23).
c) The PGE_2 (Prostaglandins) test (8).
d) The TEEM (Tanned Erythrocyte Electrophoretic Mobility) test
   (9, 10).

Unsaturated fatty acids of the linoleic (LA) and arachidonic
(AA) type make up an important part of the surface membrane of all

601

cells in the body, and the methods depend upon the demonstration
of anomalous make-up of such surface membranes in the case of
lymphocytes and RBC.

DISCUSSION

The study of linoleic and arachidonic acid (LA and AA)
activity in these tests arose from the report by Millar et al.
(3) of the beneficial effect of sunflower seed oil (active principle LA) in reducing the number and severity of attacks of MS
over a two-year double blind trial. It was at first that LA
and AA might act simply as immunosuppressives, but it is now known
that this is not so (11, 12, 13). When gamma linolenate administration is prolonged beyond the point (usually 7-9 months) at
which the positive MS result gives way to a negative (normal)
one, the TEEM-LAD test shows that LA and AA now produce the same
result (50-60 % suppression) as they do in normals and OND, and
no longer the 90-100 % suppression which characterises MS. Gamma
linolenate came into consideration after it was shown that its
effect in vitro in suppressing lymphocyte-antigen interaction
was greater (on a weight for weight basis) than was that of LA
(14). If it does in the body what it does in the test tube, it
should therefore be more effective, as well as pleasanter to
take, and more easily controlled than sunflower seed oil with
respect to dosage of active material. Final proof must, of
course, await clinical trial on a double blind basis of active
ambulant cases of MS, showing recurring episodes.

When gamma linolenate is administered beyond 6-8 months,
the typical slowing with LA or AA is reversed, first with AA,
and then, a month or so later, with LA (13, 15), and the normal
responses are, thereafter, maintained (Table III, see page 153).

After about 21 months (and, curiously, not before) the PGE_2
reaction of MS is converted into the normal response. If medica-
tion is discontinued, the PGE_2 reaction is maintained many more
months than that of gamma linolenate. A curious finding is that
when gamma linolenate is continued for 2-3 years or more the
RBC becomes extremely sensitive to PGE_2 travelling faster in the
presence of even 1.95 pg/ml (and occasionally even .0975 pg/ml) –
a phenomenon which might incidentally be developed as a very sensitive assay for PGE_2 (15). A very few people (some 3 out of
several hundreds tested) have been refractory in some degree to
the usual action of gamma linolenate in altering MS response
to LA and AA, taking one year, 20 months and, on one occasion,
more than 2 years to "convert" in the E-UFA test. The enzymology
behind this phenomenon remains to be studied , but the practical
consequence is that the writer now tests all "MS" subjects before
they begin therapy (partly to assure the diagnosis) and then

again at 6-8 months to make sure they are responders. Clearly, non-responders ought not to go into a clinical trial. Moreover, if a patient presents, as is now unfortunately not uncommon, some 12 months or so after beginning to take Naudicelle (and sometimes with a dubious diagnosis in the first place), it is still possible, despite a normal E-UFA result, to establish the original diagnosis because the PGE_2 reaction still remains that of an MS subject.

It would appear that the effect of LA or gamma linolenate is to alter the abnormal constitution of all cell surface membranes in MS (e.g. lymphocytes, RBC) to normality. If this alteration is a general phenomenon, then it would affect also the oligodendrocyte. Direct evidence for the lymphocyte is offered by the chemical observations of Tsang et al. (16), and indirectly by the MLR (17, 18, 19). If Thompson's suggestion (1) indeed extends to all cells in the body, and all cell surface membranes in MS are abnormally constituted -either biochemically or biophysically (if the distinction can indeed be made in the complexity of the membrane structure), then the oligodendrocyte surface, too, would be included. And it is from this surface that the myelin sheath is made (with the addition of protein - probably secreted by the parent nerve cell). Hence myelin produced by a child with such an inborn anomaly up to the age of 16 years with slow turnover thereafter might be expected to differ from normal and this, indeed, was found years ago (20, 21, 22). Apparently normal myelin away from MS lesions is deficient in UFA. There are criticisms of these findings - chiefly on the grounds (very true) that it is most difficult (especially before formalin fixation) to recognise the limitations of lesions (and many are microscopic). However, the balance (2) would appear to suggest that the difference is real.

Thompson's suggestion that MS develops against a background of an inborn mishandling of UFA is borne out by MS family studies with the MEM-LAD and E-UFA tests (5, 6, 23). The partial anomaly (LA - slow; AA - fast) is predominantly found in females of MS families, which serves to underline that it and it alone, is not sufficient to produce MS. Nor do we indeed know that the full "Thompson's anomaly", leading to slow LA and slow AA in the E-UFA test, is in itself sufficient to lead inevitably to MS. Probably it represents a prepared soil on which MS may develop and several possibilities spring to mind :

a) The abnormally constituted myelin may simply not stand up to "wear and tear", i.e. may undergo patchy, perivascular "abiotrophy". It is fascinating to speculate that the absence of certain reactive sites (as shown by the low MLR) on an oligodendrocyte surface may lead to failure of the wrapped surface which makes up myelin to bind securely (zip fastener effect), and indeed in the early stages of myelin breakdown,

as seen electron-microscopically, there is a loosening of
myelin lamellae.

b) It may be more susceptible to the EAE process- an idea
    supported by the work of Clausen and Møller (24) on the
    susceptibility of young rats to EAE when LA in the diet is
    altered. The neonatal rat brain is very immature, so that
    feeding with UFA can alter its myelin composition.

c) It may constitute a more suitable substratum for the
    establishment of a "slow" infection either by a banal virus
    (like measles), either ab initio or as a sequel to an attack,
    or(less likely) by some specific MS virus.

d) It may be more easily damaged as an innocent bystander when
    any allergic process goes on in the nervous system (25).

                        FORWARD PROGRAMME

     The above argument leads to important pointers for the
prophylactic handling of MS - the real function of a National
Health (rather than Sickness) Service. We know (see review- 14)
that the composition of these brain lipids may be altered (in
young rodents) by feeding appropriate UFA. If the same holds
good for the human, and we convert the cell surface to normal,
then normal myelin will be laid down of a type non-susceptible
to the MS process, whatever its cause(s) may ultimately turn out
to be. Fortunately, we can determine the inborn mishandling UFA
in very young children, and it would seem that screening of all
children at risk (those born into MS families where clinical incidence in near relatives is 5-20 times that in the general population) should be carried out. We have already picked up full MS
results in 3 children in this country, out of 130 examined, and
others in the GDR (7). A properly planned campaign and wise
spending of money may well lead to the virtual elimination of
MS in a generation, before its cause(s) is known - a state of
affairs not unknown in other branches of medicine.

     The geographic distribution of MS with its preponderance in
40°-60° N & S latitudes is a long established "fact" in MS, though
its simplicity may be deceptive (26). Many correlates with the
distribution of MS have been established, some difficult to accord
biological significance. However, amongst the putative geographical predisposing factors (GPF) has been the consumption of milk
(27) and this immediately links with the LA and AA considerations
outlined above. Twomey (28) dismisses a correlation with milk
consumption on the grounds that "MS is extraordinarily rare among
Africans living on their own continent, though milk is an important food in many parts of Africa". Dean (29), like Twomey (28),
fails to appreciate the critical importance of adequate linoleic

acid intake by the child at the critical time when myelination is most intense i.e. up to about 5 years of age and thereafter more slowly to 16 years of age and even beyond (30). It is immaterial that the "Afrikanders of South Africa ... eat ... a diet ... which has quite unusually high level of saturated fat - mutton 3 times a day ... and yet they don't get or very seldom get multiple sclerosis" (Dean loc. cit.). Breast milk is especially rich in fatty acids of long C chain (which are "essential"). Thus Bentivoglio (31) shows that linoleic acid (which he considers "really indispensible") makes up 8.3 % (6.8-10.4 %) of human milk fat against 1.6 % (0.5-2.8 %) cow's milk fat. Linoleic acid is also richer in human milk. In a fuller discussion of the EFA content of human milk Insul and Ahrens (32) conclude that it is approximately seven times that found in cow's milk. The question is, how long does linoleic acid-rich breast feeding go on amongst those groups which appear to have a low incidence of multiple sclerosis and for how long is it maintained in our "advanced" societies ? In tropical areas in general and amongst "primitive" people, breast feeding tends to be prolonged sometimes for years. This will ensure an adequate linoleic acid supply over the critical period and hence good myelin being laid down. Thereafter the intake of saturated animal fat may well be immaterial. It is precisely at the time when myelination is going on most vigorously, and it needs it the most, that the 40°-60° latitude child is deprived of adequate breast milk. If the child is born with "Thompson's anomaly" then conditions must be especially adverse to the laying down of normal myelin. Once the crucial period is over then consumption of cow's milk becomes much less important. In some ways there may be a resemblance to the critical protein needs for proper brain development in the neonate, worked out by Dobbing.

Furthermore, the content of PUFA in the infant's food is a direct reflection of that of the mother's intake. There is also some evidence (33) that cow's milk may contain specific inhibitors of the conversion of linoleic to arachidonic acid.

The naturally useful cis-forms of EFA may well be converted into trans-forms in certain types of milk food processing. Clearly as Dick (34) points out the whole question of infant feeding in relation to propensity to develop MS needs prospective study.

REFERENCES

1. Thompson, R.H.S. (1966) : Proc. roy.Soc. Med. 59, 269.
2. Thompson, R.H.S. (1973) : Biochem. Soc. Symp. 35, 103.
3. Millar, J.H.D., Zilkha, K.J., Langman, M.J.S., Payling-Wright, H., Smith, A.D., Belin, J. and Thompson, R.H.S. (1973) : Brit. med. J. 1, 765.

4. Mertin, J., Shenton, B.K. and Field, E.J. (1973) : Brit. med.
    J. 2, 777.
5. Field, E.J., Shenton, B.K. and Joyce, G. (1974) : Brit. med.
    J. 1, 412.
6. Jenssen, H.L., Meyer-Rienecker, H.J., Köhler, H. and Günther,
    iJ.K. (1976) : Acta. Neurol. Scand. 53, 51.
7. Field, E.J., Meyer-Rienecker, H.J., Shenton, B.K., Jenssen,
    H.L. and Köhler, H. (1977) : J. Neurol. 216, 135.
8. Field, E.J. and Joyce, G. (1977) : IRCS Med. Sci. 5, 158.
9. Jenssen, H.L. and Shenton, B.K. (1975) : Acta. Biol. Germ. 34,
    29.
10. Field, E.J., Joyce, G. and Veitch, K. (1978) : Unpublished.
11. Meyer-Rienecker, H.J., Jenssen, H.L., Köhler, H., Field, E.J.
    and Shenton, B.K. (1976) : Lancet 2, 966.
12. McHugh, M.I., Wilkinson, R., Elliott, R.W., Field, E.J., Dewar,
    P., Hall, R.R., Taylor, R.M.R. and Uldall, P.R. (1977) : Trans-
    plantation 24, 263.
13. Field, E.J. (1977) : In "Multiple Sclerosis : a Critical Con-
    spectus" (ed. E.J. Field). MTP Press, Lancaster, England.
14. Field, E.J. and Shenton, B.K. (1975b) : Acta Neurol. Scand.
    52, 121.
15. Field, E.J. and Joyce, G. (1978) : Europ. Neurol. 17, 67.
16. Tsang, W.M., Belin, J., Monro, J.A., Smith, A.D., Thompson,
    R.H.S., and Zilkha, K.J. (1976) : J. Neurol. Neurosurg. Psychiat.
    39, 767.
17. Källen, B. and Nilsson, O. (1971) : Nature (New Biol.) 229, 91.
18. Källen, B., Low, B. and Nilsson, O. (1975) : Acta Neurol.
    Scand. 51, 184.
19. Field, E.J., Shenton, B.K. and Meyer-Rienecker, H.J. (1976) :
    Acta. Neurol. Scand. 54, 181.
20. Jatzkewitz, H. and Mehl, E. (1962) : Hoppe-Seyler's Z. physiol.
    Chem. 329, 264.
21. Baker, R.W.R., Thompson, R.H.S. and Zilkha, K.J. (1963) :
    Lancet 1, 26.
22. Gerstl, B., Eng, L., Taviststjerna, M.C., Smith, J.K. and Kruse,
    S.D. (1970) : J. Neurochem. 17, 677.
23. Field, E.J., Joyce, G. and Smith, B.M. (1977) : J. Neurol.
    214, 113.
24. Clausen, J. and Møller, J. (1967) : Acta Neurol. Scand. 43,
    375.
25. Humphrey, J.H. and Jacques, R. (1955) : J. Physiol. 128, 9.
26. Kurtske, J.K. (1977) : In " Multiple Sclerosis : a Critical
    Conspectus" (ed. E.J. Field). MTP Press, Lancaster. pp83ff.
27. Agranoff, B.W. and Goldberg, D. (1974) : Lancet 2, 1061.
28. Twomey, J. (1974) : Lancet 2, 1204.
29. Dean, G. (1977) : In "Dr. Harry Weaver Memorial : M.S.
    Symposium Amsterdam", p.251, Bohn, Scheltema and Holkema,
    Amsterdam.
30. Yakovlev, P.I. and Lecours, A.R. (1967) : The myelogenetic
    cycles of regional maturation of the brain. Blackwell Scien-

tific Public., Oxford and Edinburgh.
31. Bentivoglio, G.C. (1961) : Carlo Erba. Foundation Symposium, Milan.
32. Insull, W., Jr., and Ahrens, E.J., Jnr. (1959) : Biochem. J. 72, 27.
33. Cash, R. and Berger, C.K. (1969) : J. Pediat. 74, 717.
34. Dick, G.W.A. (1976): Proc. roy. Soc. Med. 69, 611.

SUPPRESSION OF EXPERIMENTAL ALLERGIC ENCEPHALOMYELITIS WITH A

SYNTHETIC COPOLYMER - RELEVANCE TO MULTIPLE SCLEROSIS

D. Teitelbaum

Department of Chemical Immunology
The Weizmann Institute of Science, Rehovot, Israel

INTRODUCTION

Experimental Allergic Encephalomyelitis (EAE) is an acute neurological autoimmune disease, which serves as a model for human demyelinating diseases including multiple sclerosis (MS). EAE is induced in experimental animals by injection of brain and spinal cord tissues or the basic encephalitogenic protein (BE) isolated thereof. Cellular immune response to BE was demonstrated as the major pathogenic mechanism involved in EAE (1).

Considering the immunological mechanism of EAE, attempts were carried out in several laboratories to suppress the disease in animals challenged with BE, by desensitization procedures using the specific antigens relevant to the system. The course of EAE is known to be modified by administration of BE or related substances such as myelin non-encephalitogenic basic proteins, altered BE, non encephalitogenic degradation products of BE or synthetic peptides These findings may indicate that the site responsible for the immunological inhibition of EAE is not necessarily the site responsible for induction of the disease (1).

In view of these findings that EAE can be suppressed or inhibited not only by the BE but by non encephalitogenic basic proteins of neural origin as well, we have synthetized in our laboratory several random basic copolymers, of amino acid composition approaching to a certain extent, that of the natural encephalitogen, and tested their activity in inducing or suppressing EAE.

ANALYSIS OF THE SUPPRESSIVE EFFECT OF COP 1

The synthetic copolymers were prepared from the N-carboxy-anhydride derivatives of the respective amino acids according to Katchalski & Sela (2). Most of our work has been carried out with a copolymer, denoted Cop 1, composed of L-alanine, L-glutamic acid, L-lysine and L-tyrosine, in a residue molar ratio of 6.0 : 1.9 : 4.7 : 1.0, with an average molecular weight of 23,000. This co-polymer did not exert any encephalitogenic activity when injected into guinea pigs in doses of 10 μg up to 5 mg. On the other hand, it had marked suppressive effect on EAE, when injected either in incomplete Freund's adjuvant or in aqueous saline solution, after initial challenge with a disease-inducing dose of BE. The suppres-sive effect on EAE attained by Cop 1 is of the same order of magni-tude as that of BE. The effect of Cop 1 is specific, since neither an acidic amino acid copolymer, nor unrelated basic pro-teins, had any suppressive action. On the other hand, several pre-parations of Cop 1 showed identical effect (3). Several other polymers related to Cop 1, in which either the glutamic acid was replaced by aspartic acid, or the tyrosine was replaced by trypto-phan or omitted, were also effective in suppressing EAE (4,5).

In dose-response study of the antigen suppression phenomenon, the efficacy of Cop 1 was compared to that of BE, when tested under identical conditions. The results demonstrate that the synthetic material, Cop 1, is at least as effective as the natural encephal-itogen in disease suppression, and that the dose of the encephal-itogenic challenge influenced the suppressive efficacy of Cop 1, as well as that of BE. If the challenging dose was 10 μg BE, effective suppression was obtained with as low dose of 10 μg Cop 1. However, if the challenge was carried out with 100 μg BE, neither Cop 1, nor BE, could suppress the disease (6).

When EAE is induced with whole spinal cord homogenate, rather than the purified BE, additional factors may be involved in the pathogenesis of the disease. The suppression efficacy of Cop 1 under various sensitization conditions with homologous spinal cord was tested in guinea pigs. It was demonstrated that Cop 1 is efficient in disease suppression even when whole spinal cord homogenate is used for induction of EAE.

In view of the known diversity in the response among various susceptible species to different encephalitogenic determinants, and in their susceptibility to BE of various origins, we tested whether the species specificity applies also to the suppressive effect by Cop 1. We have shown that Cop 1 was equally efficient in the suppression of EAE induced in guinea pigs by encephalitogen of either human or bovine origin. Furthermore, suppression of EAE was obtained also in rabbits, mice and in two monkey species, rhesus

monkeys and baboons. It is thus apparent that Cop 1 does not manifest species specificity, neither for the source of the encephalitogen nor for the test animal (4).

The experiments in monkeys have further connotation since,
though concerned with EAE, they may prove relevant to demyelinating diseases in man, both because of the phylogenetic relatedness,
and due to the closer similarity between manifestation of EAE in
primates and the human diseases. We have demonstrated in rhesus
monkeys and in baboons that Cop 1 can suppress EAE when administered
to the animals after the onset of clinical symptoms. Monkeys treated with daily injections of Cop 1 in incomplete Freund's adjuvant
over a period of 15-30 days showed reversal of the disease state
with full recovery. In these monkeys either no histopathological
lesions were detected or only few small foci were observed (7, 8).

IMMUNOLOGICAL MECHANISM INVOLVED IN SUPPRESSION

OF EAE BY COP 1

Bearing in mind that EAE is a disease of autoimmune nature,
and apparently a manifestation of sensitization to BE, we have
tested for immunological cross-reactivity between Cop 1 and BE,
as a possible explanation for the specific suppression of EAE by
Cop 1.

A significant extent of immunological cross-reactivity has
been demonstrated between the basic encephalitogenic protein of
bovine origin and several synthetic amino acid copolymers which
have suppressive effect on experimental allergic encephalomyelitis.
This cross-reactivity has been conclusively established on the
cellular level, both in vivo by means of delayed hypersensitivity
skin tests and in vitro using transformation of sensitized lymphocytes, as measured by incorporation of radioactive thymidine.
Definite cross-reactivity was observed between the basic encephalitogen and all the synthetic copolymers which were shown effective
in suppression of EAE, whereas ineffective copolymers or unrelated
proteins did not show any cross-reactivity (9). Furthermore D-Cop
1, composed of amino acids of all D-configuration, failed to suppress EAE, thus lending evidence to the hypothesis that immunological mechanisms are involved in the suppressive phenomenon (5).

To understand more the mechanism by which Cop 1 operates, we
have employed our recently developed in vitro system for sensitization of lymphocytes to BE. This system involves incubation of
normal lymphocytes on syngeneic macrophage monolayers after their
prior pulse with BE. In this system, the presence of soluble BE
during the primary lymphocyte-macrophage interaction can block
recognition to BE (10). We have demonstrated that soluble Cop 1

can similarly block the in vitro sensitization to BE (11). It is
feasible therefore that the mechanism of action of Cop 1 might be
via specific blocking of BE-sensitized lymphoid cells.

RELEVANCE TO MULTIPLE SCLEROSIS

The quest for therapeutic means to multiple sclerosis, is
still one of the major problems of modern medicine. In view of the
relatedness between the human demyelinating diseases and EAE, and
the benificial effect of Cop 1 in the treatment of EAE, a preliminary limited trial was conducted on 3 ADE and 4 MS patients (12).
Under the treatment, the ADE patients recovered completely within
3 weeks, but 1 of 2 control cases treated with steroids showed
complete recovery as well. The MS patients did not show any
significant change in their motor function; however, 2 of them
showed some improvement in vision and speech capacity. It is too
early to conclude whether this improvement is related to the treatment. No side effect was observed in any of the patients treated
with Cop 1.

Although it is difficult to draw conclusions from this trial,
its results, and our findings that Cop 1 has no general immunosuppressive activity (4) and it has no toxic effects when tested
in mice, rats, rabbits, or dogs, renders it suitable for further
clinical trial.

REFERENCES

1. Paterson, P.Y. in Textbook of Immunopathology Vol. 1.,
   Ed. P.A. Miescher and H.J. Muller-Eberhard, Grune & Statton
   Inc., N.Y. p. 701 (1976).
2. Katchalski, E. and Sela, M. Adv. Protein Chem. 13, 243 (1958).
3. Teitelbaum, D., Meshorer, A., Hirshfeld, T., Arnon, R. and
   Sela, M. Eur. J. Immunol. 1, 242 (1971).
4. Teitelbaum, D., Webb, C., Meshorer, A., Arnon, R. and Sela, M.
   Eur. J. Immunol. 3, 273 (1973).
5. Webb,C., Teitelbaum, D., Herz, A., Arnon, R. and Sela, M.
   Immunochemistry 13, 333 (1976).
6. Sela, M., Teitelbaum, D., and Arnon, R. in First Symposium on
   Organ Specific Autoimmunity, Cremona, Italy. Ed. P.A. Miescher,
   Schwabe & Co. A.G. Publishers, Basel/Stutgart, 1978.
7. Teitelbaum, D., Webb, C., Bree, M., Meshorer, A., Arnon, R. and
   Sela, M. Clin. Immunol. Immunopath. 3, 256 (1974).
8. Teitelbaum, D., Meshorer, A. and Arnon, R. Israel J. Med. Sci.
   13, 1038 (1977).
9. Webb, C., Teitelbaum, D., Arnon, R. and Sela, M. Eur·J. Immunol.
   3, 270 (1973).

10. Steinman, L., Cohen, I.R., Teitelbaum, D. and Arnon, R., Nature 265 (1977).
11. Teitelbaum, D. and Bently, C., 12th Int. Leukocyte Culture Conference, 1978.
12. Abramsky, O., Teitelbaum, D. and Arnon, R. J. Neurol. Sci. 31, 443 (1977).

INTRATHECAL METHOTREXATE IN MULTIPLE SCLEROSIS

R. Dominguez, N. Chamoles and M. Somoza

Neurological Service, "J.M. Ramos Mejia" Hospital, and
Laboratory of Neurochemistry, Buenos Aires, Argentina

In several studies it was found that 80 % of patients with
clinically definite multiple sclerosis (MS), showed an increased
CSF IgG with a pattern of restricted heterogeneity (1, 2). The
oligoclonal bands seem to be unique for each patient and remarkably stable for a long time (3). The unchanged oligoclonal
band pattern occuring in the CSF studies, suggests that the same
clones of immunocompetent cells persist in the central nervous
tissue for long periods (4).

The aim of this study was to determine the effect of the
intrathecal methotrexate (IM) therapy on the CSF proteins of
patients with MS. We limited time of treatment due to the possibility of development of a toxic encephalopathy (5).

MATERIAL AND METHODS

Two groups of patients with definite MS, in whom deterioration had not been stopped by steroids were treated with I.M.
This drug was initially given weekly in a dose of 10-12 mg by
m^2 of body surface. After 3 to 6 weeks of treatment, one or
two intrathecal injections were done monthly. Dexamethasone
(0.2 mg/kg/day), was instituted during 48 hs after IM. Haemato-
logical and neurological examinations were performed in each
patient before IM lumbar administration. The four patients of
group A showed an increased CSF IgG with an oligoclonal pattern.
The control group B was composed by three MS cases with normal
CSF protein findings.

CSF and serum samples were obtained both prior to the treatment and at the end of it. Total protein assays, immunochemical determination of albumin, IgG and agar gel electrophoresis of concentrated CSF proteins were then carried out. Total protein, albumin and IgG were determined in the serum specimens.

NEUROLOGICAL COMPLICATIONS ARISING DURING TREATMENT

In four instances the appearence of CSF hypotensia syndrome was observed. In case 1, a meningeal syndrome occurred after the 1st IM injection. In three cases we found a mildly impaired vision, only for a transient period. They recovered completely and spontaneously without requiring any specific treatment nor discontinuing the IM injection. In one patient this trouble was unilateral : the sight acuteness decreased to 7/10 after the 3rd IM injection. This sign disappeared within 3 weeks. In 2 cases the visual affection was bilateral, decreasing the sight acuteness in both of them up to 6/10. In one case the trouble appeared after the 2nd injection, and in the other after the 3rd one. The relapse took place between the 2nd and 4th week after the onset. This visual alteration would be due to the toxic action of the IM on the desmyelinized optic nerves (6). One of the patients that had shown a visual complication also developed a systemic delirium after the 3rd IM injection. This trouble disappeared after one month of psychopharmachological treatment.

RESULTS

The abnormal intrathecal IgG concentration decreased in all the 4 cases of group A. In 3 of them, the reduction was very important, and in two of them the IgG index returned to the normal range. In the 4th patient, the decrease, eventhough still present, was considerably less outstanding. The restricted heterogeneity of the CSF gamma globulins studied with agar gel electrophoresis disappeared in one case, and decreased in two other patients. In the last case of A group the abnormal electrophoresis did not show any important modification.

In the 3 cases of the control group, CSF proteins did not show any alterations after the IM., likewise no changes were noted in concentrations of total proteins, in IgG levels nor in the electrophoretic pattern.

The treatment with intrathecal lumbar methotrexate decreases the abnormal CSF IgG concentration.

The relationship between the CSF proteins changes and the clinical parameters will be followed in a longitudinal study.

Case N°		1	2	3	4	5	6	7
AGE years		38	36	24	22	33	28	24
SEX		M	M	F	F	M	M	F
EVOLUTION years		1	5	6	5	13	4	12
RELAPSES		0	5	4	2	10	2	10
IM mg		120	90	90	90	90	90	45
CSF IgG mg/l	Basal	105	93	77	36	17	19	19
	Final	22	22	47	33	15	24	20
SERUM IgG g/l	Basal	14	14	10	9	16	12	11
	Final	13	12	13	8	12	13	12
CSF ALBUMIN mg/l	Basal	200	175	110	89	98	122	161
	Final	110	118	116	96	100	135	140
SERUM ALBUMIN g/l	Basal	40	38	33	35	40	41	46
	Final	41	36	34	36	36	43	44
IgG	Basal	1.46	1.36	2.20	1.52	0.43	0.52	0.49
INDEX	Final	0.62	0.56	1.03	1.43	0.45	0.58	0.51
OLIGOCLO-NAL PATTERN	Basal	+ +	+ +	+ +	+ +	0	0	0
	Final	+	0	+	+ +			

Normal IgG INDEX : 0.30 to 0.65

REFERENCES

1. Lowenthal, A., van Sande, M., Karcher, D. : The differential diagnosis of neurological diseases by fractionating electrophoretically the CSF gamma globulins. J. Neurochem. 6 : 51-56, 1960.
2. Johnson, K.P., Nelson, B.J. : Multiple Sclerosis : diagnostic usefulness of cerebrospinal fluid. Ann. Neurol. 2 : 425-431, 1977.
3. Olsson, J.E., Link, H. : Immunoglobulin abnormalities in

multiple sclerosis. Arch. Neurol. 28 : 392-399, 1973.

4. Prineas, J.W., Wright, R.G. : Macrophages, Lymphocytes, and
   Plasma cells in the Perivascular Compartment in Chronic
   Multiple Sclerosis. Lab. Invest. 38 : 409-421, 1978.

5. Norrell, H., Wilson, C.B., Slagel, D.E. et al. : Leukoencepha-
   lopathy following the administration of methotrexate into the
   cerebrospinal fluid in the treatment of primary brain tumors.
   Cancer 33 : 923-932, 1974.

REMISSIONS AND EXACERBATIONS DURING CYCLOPHOSPHAMIDE AND STEROID THERAPY IN A CASE OF NEUROMYELITIS OPTICA

M.C. Perez, W.K.T. Wong and F. Enrile-Bacsal

Section of Neurology, Department of Medicine,
University of the Philippines, Manila, Philippines

On the possibility that multiple sclerosis is an autoimmune disorder, various immunosuppressive modes of treatment have been tried with conflicting results.

The difficulty in assessing the effect of drugs is that the clinical recovery arising from the natural body repair-mechanisms may be falsely ascribed to the drug tested. Furthermore, the disease may be more extensive than clinically manifest as demonstrated by changes in visually evoked potentials (1, 2), C.T. Scans (3, 4, 5), and subsequent necropsy reports (6). In order to avoid this confusion it is suggested that the achievement of a stable remission or the prevention of an exacerbation should be used as the main criterion in gauging the efficacity of the drug.

Based on our experience in myasthenia gravis, (7) wherein we were able to produce stable remissions employing long term cyclophosphamide and prednisone therapy (10 of 15 patients are now asymptomatic and no longer on any medications for a period ranging from 7 to 44 months), we propose the following model: (Fig.)1.

There is an uncontrolled IgG synthesis in the active clinical state by B lymphocytes with the aid of helper T cells. For as long as this system is suppressed, the patients remain well. Reducing the load of B cells producing IgG such as thoracic duct lymph drainage (8), or removing the IgG by plasmapheresis (9, 10), temporarily improves the patients. However, on withdrawing or reducing prednisone, (11) or azathioprine (12) an exacerbation occurs. In the case of cyclophosphamide, however, if given on a long term basis (18-33months), a stable remission may be

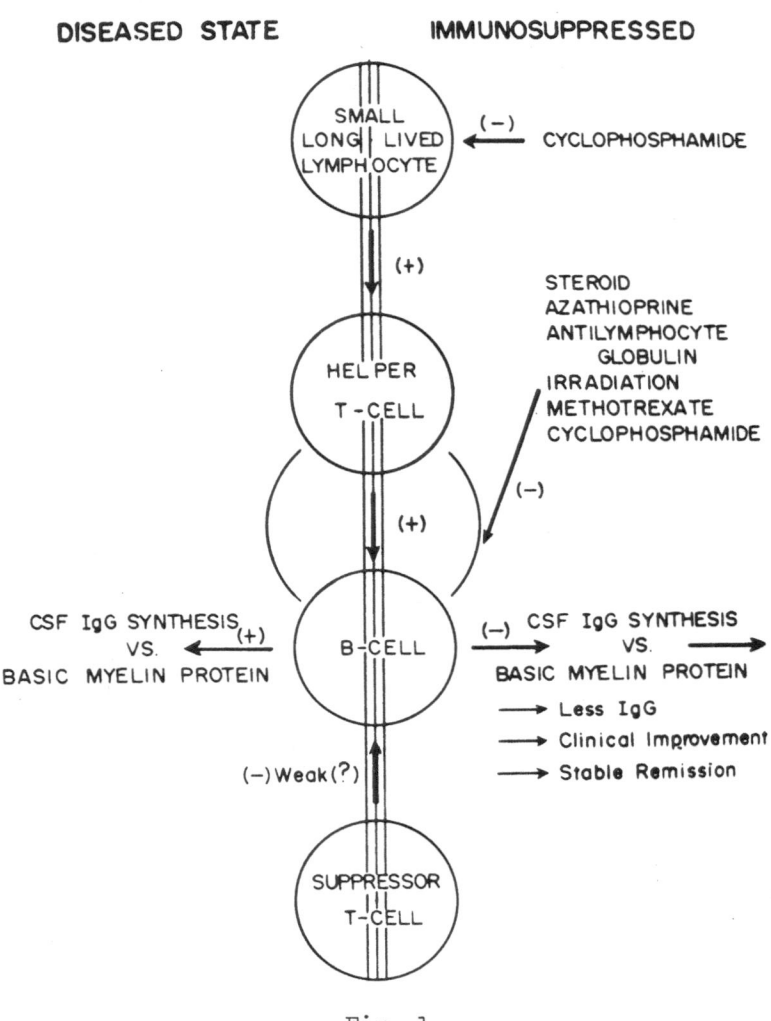

Fig. 1

achieved. It is postulated that in addition to suppressing the
system directly responsible for the production of IgG, cyclophosphamide destroys a "perpetuator cell", perhaps a small long lived
lymphocyte that can direct a B cell-helper T cell system to start
producing IgG the moment prednisone or azathioprine is stopped.
Since this cell is long lived, it is susceptible to cyclophosphamide
during the infrequent periods it undergoes mitosis.

If indeed multiple sclerosis is an autoimmune disorder, and
if our model proposed for myasthenia gravis would also apply, then
we would expect that long term cyclophosphamide and prednisone
administration may reduce or prevent the occurrence of exacerbations.

CASE REPORT

R.C., 21-year-old, female, of mixed parentage (Chinese father,
Filipino mother) first complained of vomiting and vertigo in
November 15, 1976. She developed nasal twang and dysphagia within
a week. Her symptoms gradually cleared.

A month later, in December, 1976, over a period of 1 week
(Dec. 19 - Dec. 28, 1976) she had a progressive course consisting
of vertigo, poor balance on sitting and walking, general weakness
and numbness of the face and left arm. Urinary bladder was distended.
Examination revealed an alert, coherent female with coarse horizontal
nystagmus to either side,more to the left. There was hypalgesia
of both sides of the face and on the left arm. The right nasolabial
fold was smoother. Visual fields were full. Optic disc margins
were blurred but vision remained intact. Vibration and position
senses were intact. There was ataxia on finger to nose on the left
and bilateral ataxia on heel to knee to shin. There was dishing on
both hands. There was mild right hemiparesis, hyperactive deep
tendon reflexes with a right sided preponderance. Plantar responses
were extensor bilaterally. CSF was normal.

She received 2 doses of ACTH and methyl prednisone but she
left the hospital against medical advice and apparently improved
outside, being able to ambulate fairly well.

She was readmitted 2 weeks after discharge for generalized
convulsions. On admission she was in marked respiratory distress,
cyanotic, incoherent and lethargic. She recovered and was again
able to ambulate on discharge after staying in the hospital for
28 days.

On the 4th month after onset she developed a progressive
numbness and weakness of the extremities and bladder distension.
These symptoms evolved in a period of 2 days.

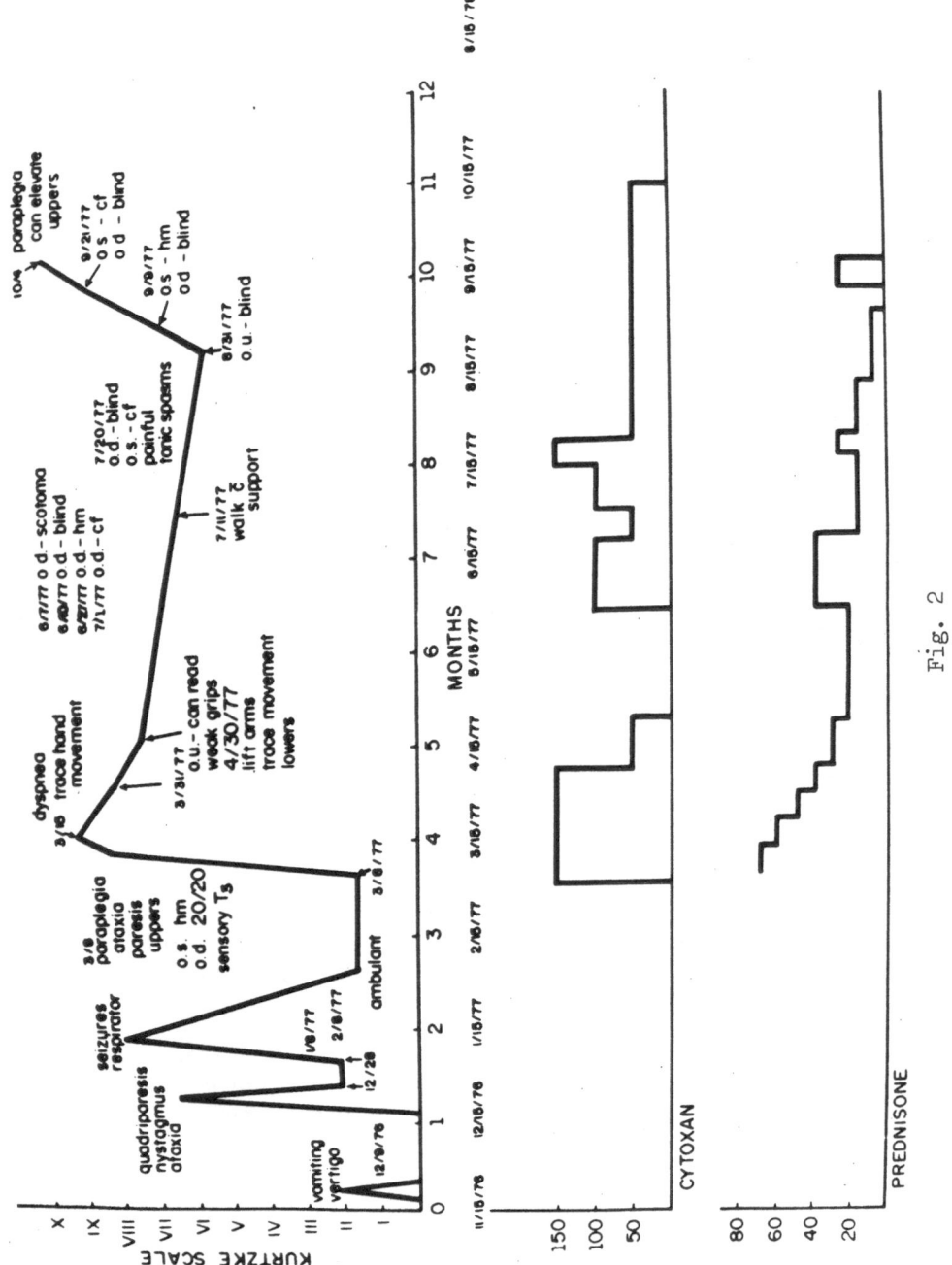

Fig. 2

On examination, she had blurring of the margins of both optic
discs, more on the left with diminished visual acuity on the left
(H.M.). She was paraplegic with a distended bladder, bilateral
extensor plantar response and ankle clonus, paresis and ataxia of
the upper extremities. Intrinsic hand muscles were weak and
atrophic. Sensation was intact.

It was during this confinement that the patient was under our
continuous care for seven and a half months. (Fig. 2). She was
started on simultaneous cyclophosphamide and prednisone treatment
on March 8, 1977. Initial dose of cyclophosphamide was 150 mgs./day.
Prednisone was given at 80 mgs./day.

A case of multiple sclerosis (neuromyelitis optica or Devic's
disease) is presented which during immunosuppressive therapy
utilizing cyclophosphamide and prednisone improved starting at the
second to third week of treatment. Despite the continuous immunosuppressive treatment, the patient developed perhaps 2 or 3 exacerbations with incomplete improvement in between.

REFERENCES

1. Halliday, A.M., McDonald, W.Z., and Mushin, J. Brit. Med. J.
   4:661-664, 1973.
2. McAlpine, D., Lumsden, C.E., and Acheson, E.D. Multiple sclerosis: A reappraisal 2nd ed. p. 81-307, Churchill Livingstone
   Edinburgh.(1965).
3. Davis, D.O., and Pressman, B.D. Radiol. Clin. N. Amer. 12:
   297-313, 1974.
4. Warren, K.G., Bill, M.J., Paty, D.W., et al. Can. J. Neurol.
   Sci. 3:211-216, 1975.
5. Aita, J.F., Bennett, D.R., Anderson, R.E. and Ziter, F. Neurology 28:251-255, 1978.
6. Ghatak, N.R., Hirano, A., Liztmaer, H., and Zweiman, M.M.
   Arch. Neurol. 30:484-486, 1974.
7. Perez, M.C., Mercado-Danguilan, C.G., Bagabaldo, Z.G., Buot,
   W.L. Stable remission achieved with long term cyclophosphamide
   therapy in myasthenia gravis. 1978 unpublished.
8. Tindall, S.C., Peters, B.H., Caverly, J.R., et al. Arch. Neurol.
   29:202-203, 1973.
9. Dau, P., et al. N. Engl. J. Med. 297:1134-1140, 1977.
10. Newsom-Davis, J., Pinching, A.J., Vincent, A., Wilson, S.G. :
    Neurology 28:266-272, 1978.
11. Mann, J.D., Johns, T.R., Joseph, B.S., et al. Neurology 22:
    400, 1972.
12. Matell, G., Bergstrom, K.F., Hammarstrom, L., et al. Ann. NY
    Acad. Sci. 274:659, 1976.

INTRATHECAL ADMINISTRATION OF INTERFERON IN MS PATIENTS ?

D. Ververken, H. Carton and A. Billiau

Rega Institute, Department of Human Biology, University of Leuven, Leuven, Belgium and A.Z. St. Rafaël, Department of Neurology, Leuven, Belgium

Interferons are glycoproteins elaborated by cells in defense against viral infection : cells exposed to interferon have a reduced ability to replicate viruses. In recent years techniques have been developed to produce large quantities of interferons which are active on human cells (1, 2). Although the cost of production is still prohibitive, clinical trials in various viral diseases are now being performed (3). Although the etiology of multiple sclerosis (MS) is still unknown, many workers speculate that chronic viral infection is one of the causal factors involved.

In experimental models and in human volunteers the administration of interferon prior to virus inoculation or during the incubation period has been shown to provide partial protection against acute virus infections (for a review, see ref. 3). In contrast, interferon has been found unable to alter the course of acute infections when given after the appearance of clinical symptoms. Therefore, it can be questioned whether interferon can be expected to be of any use in a chronic condition such as MS. However, cells (4, 5) as well as intact animals (6) which are chronically infected by viruses and which do not produce endogenous interferon have been found to respond favorably to the antiviral effect of interferon. Thus the possibility for interferon to influence the course of MS cannot a priori be excluded.

In this perspective, we treated three MS patients showing a chronic progressive course with fibroblast interferon prepared and purified as described earlier (3, 7). Each patient was given intramuscularly 0.05×10^6 units/kg body weight on alternate days during 2 weeks. One MS patient received in addition one intramuscular injection of 0.3×10^6 units/kg body weight while a catheter was placed in the dural sac and CSF samples were taken at different intervals during 24 hours. No effect on the course of the disease was noted after follow-up periods ranging from 9 to 18 months. Even after a dose as high as 0.3×10^6 units/kg body weight, only low titers of antiviral activity (20 units/ml) were found in the serum and no detectable interferon could be recovered from the spinal fluid. This corresponds well to the earlier finding of Emödi et al. (8) who used leukocyte interferon (appr. 1×10^6 units/kg) in an SSPE patient and failed to recover interferon from the liquor. In monkeys, Habif and Cantell (9) had to use intramuscular doses of approximately 6×10^6 units/kg to obtain low titers in the liquor.

From this it would seem that the intramuscular route is inadequate if one assumes that an effect on MS would require measurable levels of interferon in the CNS. Therefore we explored the possibility to administer interferon intrathecally. Monkeys receiving a single dose of 0.4×10^6 units/kg did not show inadvertent reactions; high concentrations of the interferon (2000 units/ml) were reached in liquor samples taken 2 hr after injection; interferon (1000 units/ml) was also found in the serum. Autopsies performed after 10 days failed to reveal pathologic reactions in the arachnoids, the spinal cord or brain.

Intrathecal injections (1×10^6 units) of fibroblast interferon were also given to a patient with Creutzfeldt-Jakob disease. A liquor sample taken by suboccipal punction 5 hr after lumbar injection contained 3000 units/ml of interferon, indicating that the entire spinal cord and probably the entire CNS was embedded in a high concentration of interferon for several hours. The progression and duration of the disease seemed unaltered, which was not unexpected in view of the negative findings with interferon and interferon inducers in animal model systems using scrapie agent (10, 11). The intrathecal injections did not provoke detectable untoward effects. At autopsy no other changes were seen other than those characteristic for Creutzfeldt-Jakob disease.

From these experiments it appears that intrathecal administration of fibroblast interferon is a safe procedure and offers the only chance to deliver exogenous interferon to the CNS. Whether the interferon injected in the spinal fluid does actually reach the nerve cells is an unresolved question which needs further investigation.

REFERENCES

1. Cantell, K. and Hirvonen, S. (1978) J. Gen. Virol., 39, 541-543.

2. De Somer, P., Joniau, M., Edy, V.G. and Billiau, A. (1974) In Vitro, 3, 39-46.

3. Billiau, A. and De Somer, P. (1978) In Interferon and Interferon Inducers. Clinical Applications, D.A. Stringfellow (Ed.), Publ. Marcel Dekker, New York.

4. Billiau, A., Edy, V.G., Sobis, H. and De Somer, P. (1974) Int. J. Cancer, 14, 335-340.

5. Friedman, R.M., Chang, E.H., Ramseur, J.M. and Myers, M.W. (1975) J. Virol., 16, 569-574.

6. DuBuy, H., Baron, S., Uhlendorf, C. and Johnson, M.L. (1973) Infect. Immun., 8, 977-984.

7. Edy, V.G., Braude, I.A., De Clercq, E., Billiau, A. and De Somer, P. (1976) J. Gen. Virol., 33, 517-521.

8. Emödi, G., Just, M., Hernandez, R. and Hirt, H.R. (1975) J. Nat. Cancer Inst., 54, 1045-1049.

9. Habif, D.V., Lipton, R. and Cantell, K. (1975) Proc. Soc. Exp. Biol. Med., 149, 287-289.

10. Field, E.J., Joyce, G and Keith, A. (1969) J. Gen. Virol., 5, 149-150.

11. Worthington, M. (1972) Infect. Immun., 6, 643-645.

RENAL AND SKIN BIOPSY FINDINGS IN AMYOTROPHIC LATERAL SCLEROSIS

J. Lähdevirta, A. Rissanen, Y. Collan, E.J. Jokinen,
J. Palo and O.P. Salo
Third Department of Medicine, Department of Neurology,
Pathology, Bacteriology and Immunology, and Dermatology
University of Helsinki, Helsinki, Finland

SUMMARY

Renal and skin biopsies of seven patients with amyotrophic
lateral sclerosis (ALS) were studied. Light and electron microscopy of renal biopsy specimens showed slight mesangial prominence
in the glomeruli, slight patchy interstitial fibrosis, and chronic
inflammatory changes. Electron microscopy further showed degenerative changes in the glomeruli and arterioles. Immunohistochemical
study showed in two cases traces of immunoglobulins in the mesangial
areas. In skin biopsies no immunoglobulins or complement could be
found in the dermoepidermal junctions. The morphological renal
findings are probably age dependent changes and/or secondary to
tissue damage occurring in this disease. It is concluded that the
role of circulating immune complexes in the pathogenesis of ALS is
still obscure.

INTRODUCTION

Amyotrophic lateral sclerosis (ALS), a progressive neurological
disorder with rapidly progressive atrophy and fasciculation of
somatic musculature, is histologically characterized by anterior-
horn neuron and pyramidal tract damage. The etiology of the disease
is unknown. Several hypotheses have been presented: metabolic dis-
turbance after gastrectomy (1), connection with abnormal insulin
response and glucose tolerance (10,11), heavy metal poisoning,
especially lead (6) and mercury (7,16). Genetic influence has also
been suggested (12,17), but HLA-antigens of ALS patients have shown

no uniform trend (3,14,15,24). Also the viral theory has received much attention. Intracellular inclusions have been described (4) and the transferring of human ALS to monkeys has been claimed (27). However, identical morphological changes in affected monkeys and human ALS could not be found (13). Attempts to demonstrate a transmissible agent were not successful (9). Connection with poliomyelitis virus has been suggested (18,25).

Circulating immune complexes occur in viral diseases and in autoimmune conditions. The findings of Oldstone et al. (20) who found immunoglobulins in renal tissue of ALS-patients, thus suggested viral or autoimmune etiology. However, our preliminary immunohistochemical findings on renal and skin biopsies in ALS did not suggest primary immune complex disease (21). In the present study the renal biopsies were also studied by electron microscopy.

MATERIALS AND METHODS

The material consisted of seven voluntary ALS-patients. The clinical details are presented in Tables 1 and 2. Two patients (case D and F) had advanced atrophy of both upper and lower extremities and also marked bulbar signs. One patient (case E) had very severe bulbar signs and only little changes in the upper extremities. One patient (case G) had very severe atrophy of both upper and lower extremities and needed the respirator because of ventilatory insufficiency. He had never had clear upper motor neuron signs and no bulbar signs, but the rapid progression and typical EMG findings were for ALS diagnosis which was later confirmed in autopsy. These four patients had a far advanced disease with severe symptoms, which

TABLE 1. Clinical data of the ALS patients

Patient	Age	Sex	Initial symptoms	Duration (months)
A	66	F	Lower extr.	10
B	71	F	Lower extr.	11
C	54	F	Lower extr.	14
D	60	M	Upper extr.	20
E	70	F	Bulbar	24
F	60	F	Lower extr.	28
G	55	M	Lower extr.	31

TABLE 2. Neurological signs in the ALS patients

Patient	Muscular atrophy	Fascicu- lations	Bulbar signs	Tendon reflexes	Babinski reflex
A	++	+	+	+++	-
B	+	+	-	+	-
C	+	+	-	++	-
D	++	+	++	+++	-
E	+	+	+++	+	-
F	++	+	++	++	+
G	+++	+	-	+	-

had started 20 to 31 months before biopsy. The other three patients had only mild or moderate symptoms which had started 10 to 14 months prior to biopsy. The latter were biopsied a few days after the diagnosis.

Blood pressure, the number of blood corpuscles and the differential count of leucocytes were normal in all cases. ERS was a little elevated (range 6-47 mm/h). None of the patients had proteinuria or haematuria or changes in urinary sediment. Serum creatinine was normal in all cases. Concentration and acidification capacities of kidneys were normal.

Percutaneous renal biopsy was performed with a Silverman needle (Goldman's modification) and the specimen was divided in chilled Ringer's solution into two portions: one for immunohistochemical study and one for light and electron microscopic study. For electron microscopy the samples were fixed in 3% phosphate buffered glutaraldehyde for 3 hours and kept in sucrose solution thereafter for several days. They were postfixed with 1% osmium tetroxide for 1 hour, dehydrated and embedded in Epon. Sections were cut with glass knives and stained with lead citrate and uranyl acetate. For immunohistochemical study cryostat sections 6 µm thick were stained by the direct technique with FITC-conjugated antibody to IgA, IgG, IgM, C_3, and fibrinogen. Monospecific antisera to α-, γ- and μ-chains and fibrinogen were obtained commercially (Behringwerke AG).

Skin biopsies for immunohistochemical study were taken from clinically healthy skin of the forearm. The specimens were quickly frozen, cut in a cryostat at 4 µm, washed with phosphate buffered

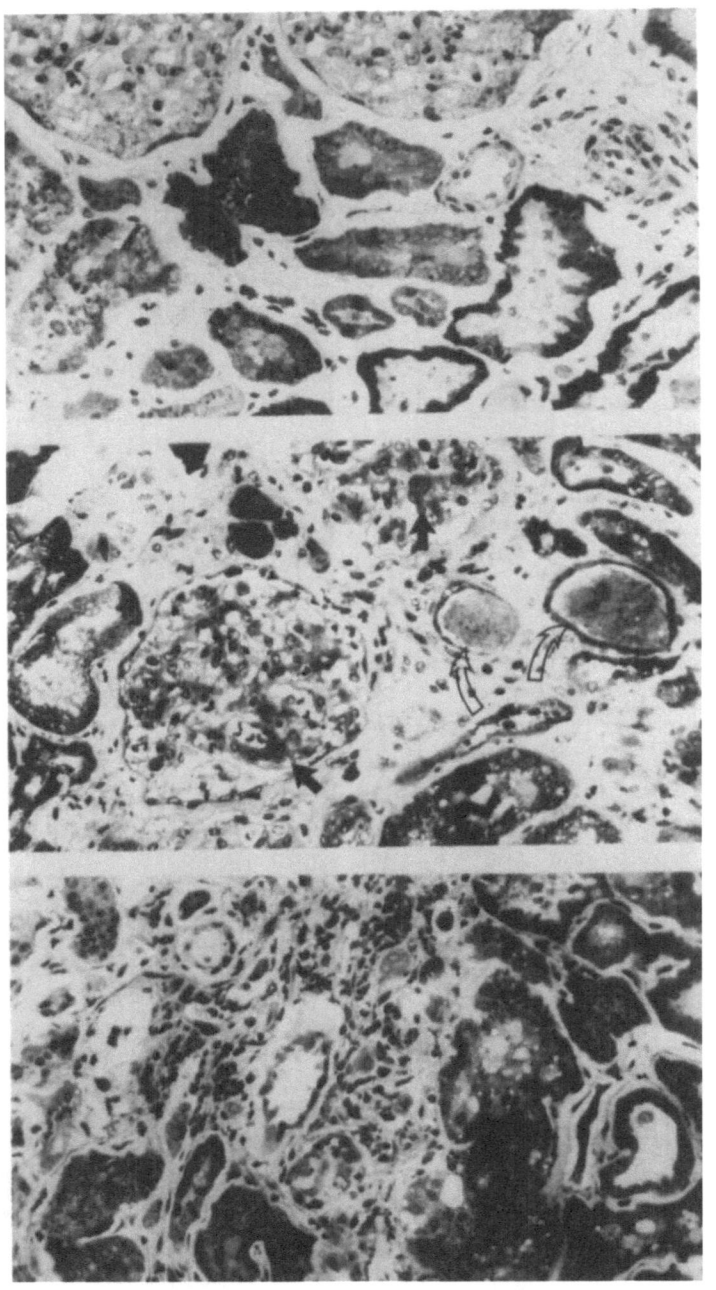

Fig. 1. At right renal cortical tissue from patient E. There is slight interstitial fibrosis but otherwise the findings are normal. In the middle, the biopsy of patient G. Mesangial areas of the glomeruli are more prominent than normal (arrows), interstitial tissue shows fibrosis and a chronic interstitial infiltrate. There are also two distal tubules with a granular cast (arrows). At left interstitial inflammatory changes at the corticomedullary area, in the biopsy of patient E. Epon embedded tissue, methylene blue stain. Magnification 240x.

saline and stained for immunoglobulins and complement with anti-
human globulin conjugate (Baltimore Biological Laboratories,
distributed by Roboz Inc.). The results were read with a Leitz
Orthoplan microscope equipped with epi-illumination, Xenon light
source, two KP 490 excitation filters and an OG 510 barrier filter.

RESULTS

Light microscopy. One µm thick plastic sections were cut and
stained with methylene blue. These showed interstitial chronic
inflammatory changes in places. Also slight interstitial fibrosis
was seen. Glomeruli did not show signs of cell proliferation but
occasionally had mesangial areas more prominent than normal. A
few distal tubules showed hyaline or granular casts (Fig. 1).

Electron microscopy showed increased mesangial matrix material
in many glomeruli, but most glomeruli appeared normal in this respect. Deposits typical of immune complex disease were not seen.
On the other hand there were degenerative changes in the glomeruli
with increased mesangial matrix. These included vesicular debris
and round extracellular particles, membranous convoluted structures and occasional hazy intramembranous deposits. In one patient
"moon craters" were seen in a normal appearing glomerulus (Fig. 2).

Thickened basement membrane was seen around a few proximal
and distal tubules. Granular, vesicular and membranous debris
could be seen in these thickened membranes (Fig. 3). Occasional
distal tubules showed large dark cytosomes (Fig. 4). In one
patient giant mitochondria (26) were seen in the proximal tubules.

The interstitial capillaries appeared normal but the arterioles showed subendothelial granular deposits. In the deposits
smaller vesicles, membranous structures or myelin-like bodies were
occasionally seen. Muscle cells in the walls of the arterioles
were very rich in lipofuscin pigment (Fig. 5). Occasionally the
muscle cells showed huge intracytoplasmic vacuoles in connection
with lipofuscin material (Fig. 6).

Immunohistochemical study of renal biopsies revealed traces
of immunoglobulins and complement in the glomerular mesangium of
only two patients (F and G, Table 3). In skin biopsies neither
immunoglobulins nor complement could be detected in the dermoepidermal junction in any of the cases (Table 3).

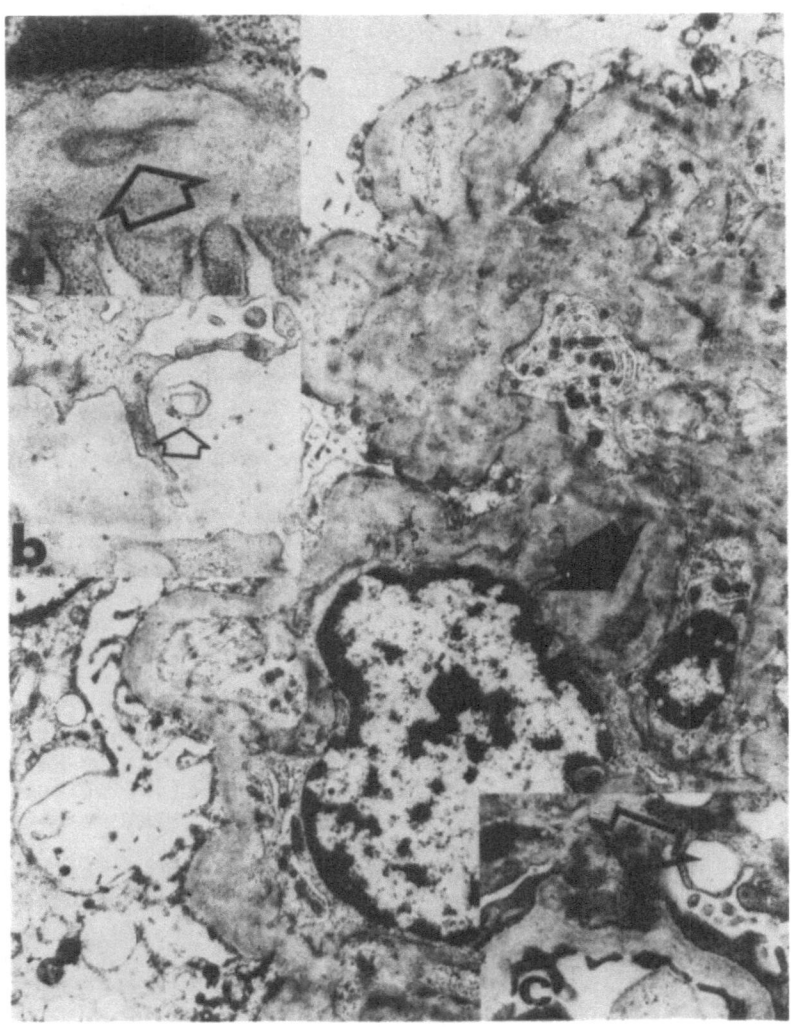

Fig. 2.   Increased glomerular mesangial material in patient G.
The biopsy was fixed in neutral formalin for histological purposes,
which explains distinct condensation of chromatin in the nuclei.
There is a hazy deposit in the mesangium (arrow) but no deposits
in the peripheral basement membrane. Magnification 7,500x.
Insets: a. From patient F.   A hazy deposit (arrow) in the glomerular
basement membrane under an endothelial cell. Magnification 32,600x.
b. From patient F.   Thickened glomerular basement membrane showing
a membranous convoluted structure (arrow).   Magnification 13,000x.
c. From patient E.   A "moon crater" from glomerular periphery
(arrow).   Magnification 12,200x.

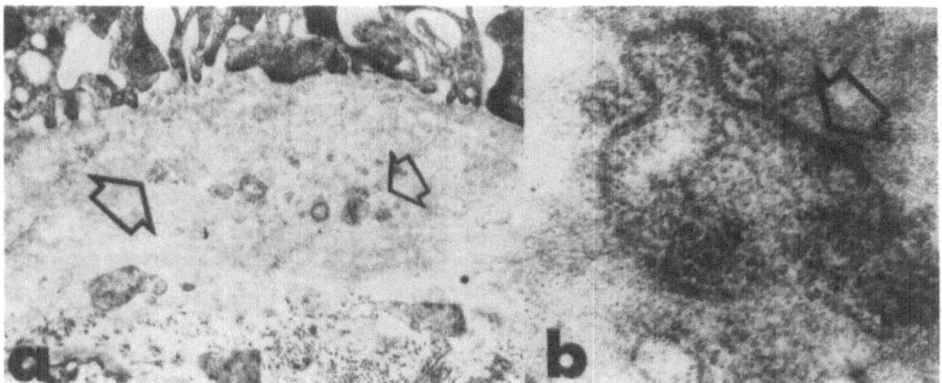

Fig. 3. a. From patient E. Thickened basement membrane of a proximal tubule with intramembranous debris (arrows). Magnification
11,000x. b. From patient F. Granular, vesicular and membranous
debris in the thickened basement membrane. The arrow points at a
structure similar to membranous convoluted structures described by
Bariéty et al. in the glomeruli. Magnification 53,000x.

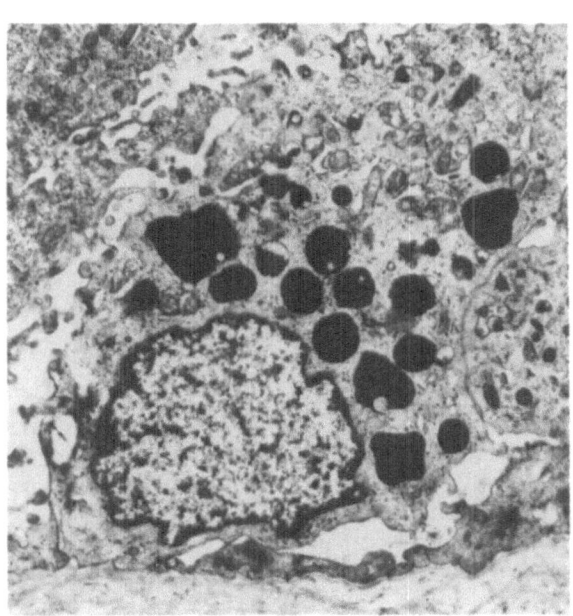

Fig. 4. From patient E. Distal tubule cell with numerous dark
staining cytosomes. Magnification 7,300x.

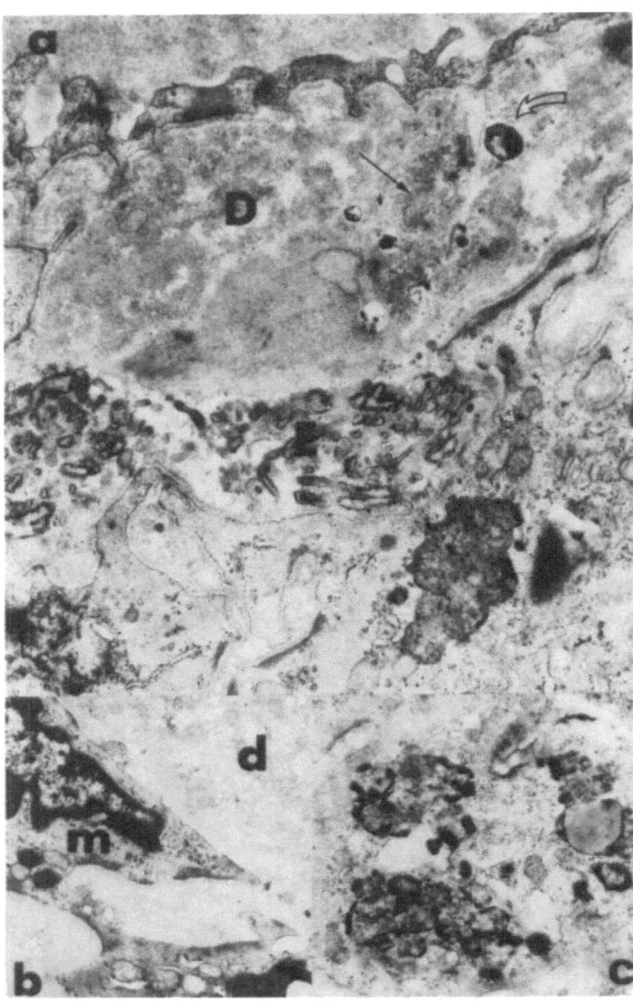

Fig. 5.   a. A renal arteriole in patient C.   Lumen at the top.
At D large subendothelial deposit with finely granular appearance.
In the deposit there are small vesicular structures (small arrow)
and myelin-like bodies (open arrow).   Elastin units at E.   Lots
of lipofuscin material are seen in the cytoplasm of the muscle
cells.   Magnification 13,500x.   b. From patient F.   Vesicular
subendothelial deposit (d) in the wall of an arteriole.
m = muscle cell.   Magnification 9,500x.   c. From patient F.
Lipofuscin pigment in the cytoplasm of a muscle cell.   The pigment
often contained numerous dark clumps that are clearly shown in this
micrograph.   Magnification 11,200x.

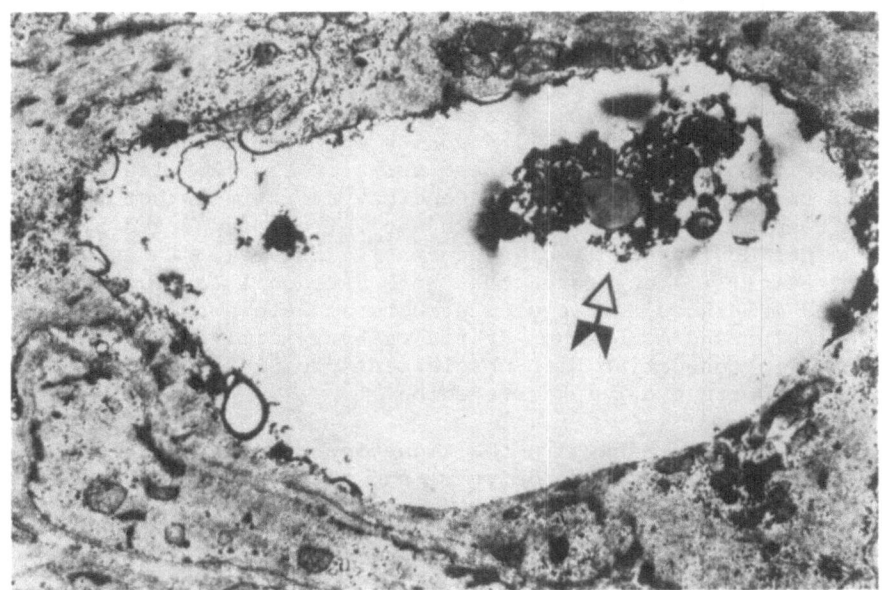

Fig. 6.   A huge cytoplasmic vesicle in a muscle cell of a renal
arteriole in patient C.   Note osmiophilic lipofuscin material
(arrow) in the vesicle which shows that this is not an unstained
lipid vacuole but has mostly watery contents.
Magnification 8,300x.

TABLE 3.   Results of the immunohistochemical investigation

Patient	Kidney	Skin
A	−	−
B	−	−
C	−	−
D	−	−
E	−	−
F	+	−
G	+	−

+ = traces of immunoglobulin and complement in the glomerular
    mesangia

DISCUSSION

The appearance of various kinds of immunological deposits in electron microscopy has been described by Churg and Grishman (5). Deposits typical of classical immune complex diseases were not found in ALS. However, small deposits were found in two patients, one deposit in each, and these are shown in Fig. 2. The appearance of the deposit suggested degenerative origin rather than immune complex disease. This idea was further supported by numerous changes most probably of degenerative nature in the glomeruli. Bariéty et al. (2) suggested that both extracellular round particles, and membranous convoluted structures belong to this category. The vesicular and membranous debris was very similar to what was described in connection with obsolescent glomeruli (19), this further supporting our interpretation.

Degenerative changes in the kidney occur with age. Our patients had a mean age of 62 years and the youngest patient was 54 years old. Superficial cortex may show age-related hyalinisation of the glomeruli and this part of the kidney is usually present in biopsies. So, at least part of the degenerative changes we found appear age-related. On the other hand, all patients showed slight interstitial inflammatory changes. Such changes may accompany age-related changes in the glomeruli. Immunohistochemical study did not suggest active interstitial nephritis.

Finally the arteriolar deposits are not specific because they have been reported in hypertension, systemic sclerosis and also under normal conditions (8,22,23). Because they were prominent and muscle cells of the arterioles also showed changes we would not like to exclude the possibility that the glomerular and interstitial changes we found were originally caused by these changes in the arterioles. This hypothesis, however, does not allow parallel conclusions of nervous system changes in this disease. Our immunohistochemical findings of renal and skin biopsies do not support the role of circulating immune complexes in pathogenesis of ALS. This is in agreement with the electron microscopic study, where no signs of renal immune complex disease was obtained. Also, the morphological study revealed no changes, which could be considered as pathognomonic to ALS.

The conclusion of the present study differs from that of Oldstone et al. (20) who had, however, a greater (27 patients) and thus more representative series of renal biopsies studied by immunohistology. At any case, circulating immune complexes do not regularly occur in ALS.

REFERENCES

1. Ask-Upmark, E. and Meurling, S.: On the presence of a defi-
    ciency factor in the pathogenesis of amyotrophic lateral
    sclerosis. Acta Med. Scand. 152:217-221 (1955).

2. Bariéty, J., Callard, P., Appay, M.D., Grossetete, J. and
    Mandet, Ch.: Ultrastructural study of some frequent and
    poorly known intraglomerular structures. Adv. Nephrol. 3:
    153-172 (1974).

3. Behan, P.O., Dick, H.M. and Durward, W.F.: Histocompatibility
    antigens associated with motor neuron disease. J. Neurol.
    Sci. 32:213-217 (1977).

4. Bunina, T.L.: On intracellular inclusions in familiar ALS.
    Zhur. Nevropatol. i Psikkiat. 62:1293-1299 (1962).

5. Churg, J. and Grishman, E.: Ultrastructure of immune deposits
    in renal glomeruli. Ann. Intern. Med. 76:479-486 (1972).

6. Conradi, S., Ronnevi, L.-O. and Vesterberg, O.: Abnormal
    tissue distribution of lead in amyotrophic lateral sclerosis.
    J. Neurol. Sci. 29:259-265 (1976).

7. Currier, R.D. and Haerer, A.F.: Amyotrophic lateral sclerosis
    and metallic toxins. Arch. Environ. Health 17:712-719 (1968).

8. Fisher, E.R., Perez-Stable, E. and Pardo, V.: Ultrastructural
    studies in hypertension. I. Comparison of renal vascular and
    juxtaglomular cell alterations in essential and renal hyper-
    tension in man. Lab. Invest. 15:1409-1433 (1966).

9. Gibbs, C.J. and Gajdusek, D.C.: Attempts to demonstrate a
    transmissible agent in kuru, amyotrophic lateral sclerosis
    and other subacute and chronic progressive nervous system
    degenerations in man. In: Slow, latent, and temperate virus
    infections. Ed. by Gajdusek, Gibbs and Alpers. NINDB
    Monograph No. 2, pp. 39-48, Bethesda (1965).

10. Gotoh, F., Kitamura, A., Koto, A., Kataoka, K. and Atsuji, H.:
    Abnormal insulin secretion in amyotrophic lateral sclerosis.
    J. Neurol. Sci. 16:201-207 (1972).

11. Gustafson, A. and Störtebecker, P.: Vascular and metabolic
    studies of amyotrophic lateral sclerosis. II. Lipid and
    carbohydrate metabolism. Neurology (Minneap.) 22:528-536
    (1972).

12. Haberlandt, W.F.: Amyotrophische Lateralsklerose. Klinisch-
     pathologische und genetisch-demographische Studie. Gustav
     Fischer Verlag, Stuttgart (1964).

13. Hirano, A.: Pathology of amyotrophic lateral sclerosis. In:
     Slow, latent, and temperate virus infections. Ed. by
     Gajdusek, Gibbs and Alpers. NINDB Monograph No. 2, pp. 23-27,
     Bethesda (1965).

14. Hoffman, P.M., Robbins, D.S., Gibbs, C.J., Gajdusek, D.C.,
     Garruto, R.M. and Terasaki, T.I.: Histocompatibility antigens
     Pardo, V., Fisher, E.R., Perez-Stable, E. and Rodnan, G.P.:
     on Guam. Lancet 2:717 (1977).

15. Jokelainen, M., Lapinleimu, K. and Tiilikainen, A.: Polio
     antibodies and HLA antigens in amyotrophic lateral sclerosis.
     Tissue Antigens 10:259-266 (1977).

16. Kantarjian, A.D.: A syndrome clinically resembling amyotrophic
     lateral sclerosis following chronic mercurialism. Neurology
     (Minneap.) 11:639-644 (1961).

17. Kurland, L.T. and Mulder, D.W.: Epidemiologic investigations
     of amyotrophic lateral sclerosis. Parts I and II. Neurology
     (Minneap.) 5:182-196 and 249-268 (1955).

18. Mulder, D.W., Rosenbaum, R.A. and Layton, D.D.: Late progres-
     sion of poliomyelitis or forme fruste amyotrophic lateral
     sclerosis? Mayo Clin. Proc. 47:756-761 (1972).

19. Nagle, R.B., Kohnen, P.W., Bulger, R.E., Striker, G.E. and
     Benditt, E.P.: Ultrastructure of human renal obsolescent
     glomeruli. Lab. Invest. 21:519-526 (1969).

20. Oldstone, M.B.A., Wilson, C.B., Perrin, L.H. and Norris, F.H.
     Jr.: Evidence for immune-complex formation in patients with
     amyotrophic lateral sclerosis. Lancet 2:169-172 (1976).

21. Palo, J., Rissanen, A., Jokinen, E., Lähdevirta, J. and Salo,
     O.: Kidney and skin biopsy in amyotrophic lateral sclerosis.
     Lancet 1:1270 (1978).

22. Pardo, V., Fisher, E.R., Perez-Stable, E. and Rodnan, G.P.:
     Ultrastructural studies in hypertension. II. Renal vascular
     changes in progressive systemic sclerosis. Lab. Invest. 15:
     1434-1441 (1966).

23. Pardo, V., Perez-Stable, E. and Fisher, E.R.: Ultrastructural
     studies in hypertension. III. Gouty nephropathy. Lab. Invest.
     18:143-150 (1968).

24. Pedersen, L., Platz, P., Jersild, C. and Thomsen, M.: HLA
     (SD and LD) in patients with amyotrophic lateral sclerosis
     (ALS). J. Neurol. Sci. 31:313-318 (1977).

25. Pertschuk, L.P., Cook, A.V., Cupta, J.K., Broome, J.D.,
     Vuletin, J.C., Kim, D.S., Brigati, D.J., Rainford, E.A. and
     Nidsgorski, F.: Jejunal immunopathology in amyotrophic
     lateral sclerosis and multiple sclerosis. Identification of
     viral antigens by immunofluorescence. Lancet 1:1119-1123
     (1977).

26. Suzuki, T., Furusato, M., Takasaki, S. and Ishikawa, E.:
     Giant mitochondria in the epithelial cells of the proximal
     convoluted tubules of diseased human kidneys. Lab. Invest.
     33:578-590 (1975).

27. Zilber, L.A., Bajdakova, Z.L., Gardas, J.A.M., Konovalov, N.V.,
     Bunina, T.L. and Barabadze, E.M.: Study of the etiology of
     the amyotrophic lateral sclerosis. Bull. Wld. Hlth. Org.
     29:449-456 (1963).

SOME MUSCULAR CHANGES IN PATIENTS WITH SCHISTOSOMIASIS

S.E. Mansour

Neuro-Psychiatry Department Alexandria Medical School
Alexandria, Egypt

The clinical observation that patients with Schistosoma mansoni, Schistosoma haematobium or both, present with wasting in the form of either localized or diffuse muscular atrophy and weakness of skeletal muscles, stimulated us to report some of the pathological changes in such a myopathy.

Fifteen schistosomiasis patients ranging in ages from 12 to 40 years (2f and 13m) were examined. Thirteen of the 15 have or have had Schistosoma mansoni infection. Six having active Schistosoma mansoni, and seven giving a history of Schistosoma mansoni. Nine patients have or have had Schistosoma haematobium, with 3 presenting an active infection, and 6 with history of infection. One patient has double infection.

Eleven patients have generalized wasting with weakness of skeletal muscles, especially noticeable in lower limbs, other four have localized wasting and weakness mainly of the shoulder pelvic type. The liver functions in all the patients are normal although 8 have cirrhosis.

Muscle biopsy showed variation in size, with obscuration of striations. Structural changes of hyaline granular or vacuolar types are seen. Nuclei are increased in number and size centrally placed and assumed rows. Some mononuclears solitary or in group are seen inside the fibers. Connective tissue is increased in endomysium and perimysium. In some biopsies these changes are intensified around blood vessels.

Parasite or ova could not be demonstrated in any biopsy.

It is a well known fact that the humoral immunity is disturbed in schistosomal infection, and this mechanism may at least act in part to induce such a myopathy.

IMMUNOLOGICAL DEFICIENCY IN THE DOWN SYNDROME : IMPORTANCE OF

THE AGE FACTOR

B. Tavolato and V. Argentiero

Institute of the Clinic for Nervous and Mental Diseases,
Padova University, Padova, Italy

SUMMARY

Many observations have pointed out an immunological deficiency in Down syndrome. Such deficiency concerns both the B
cells system and the T cells system. Most of such studies have
been done on infants or very young subjects.

With the present report we compare the immunological data
of two groups of Down patients, which are different only for
the age ("young group" with a median age of 21 y. and "adult
group" with a median age of 36 y.).

The two Down groups were subsequently compared with two
corresponding groups of normal individuals.

The immunological abnormalities in Down syndrome appear
to be strongly related to the age of the subjects; the earlier
abnormality probably concerns a deficiency of the T suppressor
subset of cells.

Such data are discussed considering the unusual frequency
of Alzheimer's type dementia in Down subjects.

INTRODUCTION

Many reports pointed out an immunological deficiency in
Down's syndrome. Such deficiency concerns the B cells system :
increased or decreased levels of Ig, presence of autoantibodies
and increased frequency of respiratory infections. The T cells

system is also involved with deficit of the lymphocytes response
to PHA, increased frequency of cancer and leukemia, anergy to
DNCB and ubiquitous antigens which elicit delayed-type hypersensitivity reactions (2, 6, 4, 11).

Such abnormalities have been found mostly in children or
in young subjects. Recently (7) it was observed that the increase
of serum IgG, IgA and IgD levels were present only after the
age of 15 years, while the deficiency of the lymphocytes response to PHA was present only in patients older than 20 years.
However, according to other authors (11) the stimulation index
to PHA in adult patients was similar to controls. Contradictory data have also been presented concerning the number of T cells,
which were found to be decreased (9) as well as increased (11).

From the point of view of the neurologist it is important
to remember that Down patients are affected very early in life
and with an elevated frequency by a dementia which is histologically superimposable to Alzheimer's disease. Several studies
have confirmed that Down patients dying in their thirties, and
occasionally even in their twenties, usually develop senile
plaques although the neurofibrillary tangles tend to appear
somewhat later (10).

More precisely it was observed by Malamud (5) that large
numbers of plaques and tangles were present in all 35 cases
who had died above the age of 40 years.

Therefore adult patients with Down syndrome can be considered as a valid, natural "model" of Alzheimer's disease while
the young patients with trisomy 21 suffer from a condition which
strongly predispose to the development of Alzheimer's disease.

For this reason, and considering also the known immunological deficiencies of old age (i.e. another condition predisposing to Alzheimer type degeneration), we thought it important
to compare the immunological data of the Down patients in the
young and in the adult age.

PATIENTS AND CONTROLS

The Down patients were randomly chosen from an institution
for mentally retarded. The standards of personal hygiene, nu-
trition and medical assistance of the patients were good. The
Down patients were selected according to age and sex. The "young
group" was composed of 12 patients (6 males and 6 females) from
15 to 25 years of age, with a median age of 21. The "adult group"
was comparable to the previous one except for the age which
was from 30 to 46 years, with a median age of 36 years.

The control groups (students and hospital staff) were composed of normal individuals with ages comparable to the Down groups.

METHODS

B Lymphocytes and Complement Functions

Lymphocytes were collected from heparinized blood by centrifugation with "Lymphoprep" (Ficoll-Isopaque).

The EAC rosettes were prepared and enumerated following the method of Bianco et al. (1).

Serum levels of IgG, IgA, IgM, IgD, C3c and C4 were measured by single radial immunodiffusion (tri-partigen plates, Behringwerke, Germany). Serum electrophoresis was done on cellulose acetate and the presence of monoclonal peaks (M-components) was searched by inspection of the pherograms.

Anti-H antibodies were titrated before and 15 days after vaccination with Salmonella antigens (typhidral, Sclavo, Italy). The data are expressed as differences between geometric means.

Serum autoantibodies to thyroid, kidney, liver, pancreas, gastric mucosa and smooth muscle were tested and titrated with indirect immunofluorescence.

The total activity of the serum complement was tested by adding serial dilutions of the serum to a lytic system (sheep erytrocytes plus hemolysin).

T Lymphocytes Functions

The E Rosettes were prepared and enumerated following the method of Gupta and Grieco (3), the E active Rosettes were extimated according to the method of Wybran and Fudenberg (12).

The mitogenic activity of cultured lymphocytes was estimated with and without stimulation by PHA. The results are expressed as stimulation indexes. The stimulation index equalling mean counts per minute with PHA, divided by mean counts per minute without PHA.

Cutaneous sensibilization to di-nitro-chloro-benzene (DNCB) was tested and scored according to the method described by Whittingham et al. (11).

The cutaneous delayed-type hypersensitivity response to 3 ubiquitous antigens-streptokinase-streptodornase (Lederle), candidin (Institute Pasteur) and tubercolin (Sclavo)- were also scored according to routine clinical methods.

RESULTS

In table 1 the B cells and complement functions are summarized. The data of the "young group" is compared with those of the "adult group" both for Down and normal subjects.

TABLE 1

IMMUNOLOGICAL DEFICIENCY IN THE DOWN SYNDROME : IMPORTANCE OF THE AGE FACTOR

B Cells and Complement Functions

Down groups at different ages and normal groups at different ages are compared (^significant difference ($P < 0.05$)).

	Down Youngs N.12 Med.Age 21 y.	Down Adults N.12 Med.Age 36 y.	Normal Youngs N.8 Med.Age 22 y.	Normal Adults N.12 Med.Age 35 y.
EAC Rosette per cent	12^	23	21	27
IgG mg/100 cc.	2257	1940	1097	881
IgA mg/100 cc.	350	302	173	190
IgM mg/100 cc.	151^	203	241	200
IgD I.U./100 cc.	88	79	17	26
Gamma-Globulin per cent	22^	27	18	18
M-Components (presence)	--	--	--	--
Anti-H Antibodies (Title increase)	3.45	5.20		2.30
C3c mg/100 cc.	100	81	85	79
C4 mg/100 cc.	37	33	32	44^
Total complement Activity	16	18	8	9
Autoantibodies (N.pos.)	8	14	--	1
Rheuma Test (N.pos.)	1	3	--	--

It appears that for normal subjects the increase of age from 22 to 35 years is not followed by modifications in the B cells and complement dependent functions, except for a slight increase with age of the C4 concentration.

In the Down groups some differences are instead present: in the "young group" the percent of EAC rosettes and the IgM concentration are lower than in the "adult group". In the latter group an increase of the percent of serum gamma globulin is also present. Such increase is possible related to an observed decrease of serum total protein level in the "adult group".

The increased frequency of autoantibodies in the older Down patients is also noteworthy.

It is quite evident that a very marked dysgammaglobulinemia is already present in the young Down patients and such an alteration will persist for several years. The serum IgM level instead is abnormally low in the Down "young group", but it becomes normal in the Down "adult group". In our opinion the low number of B cells in the Down "young group" is particularly relevant. However such a low number of B cells is capable of producing an amount of IgG and IgA which is more than double the amount of the normal. This means that the single B cell is producing enormous amounts of Ig. Such data are indirectly confirmed also by the higher antibody response after vaccination with Salmonella antigens in both Down groups and particularly in the adult subjects, and by the presence of autoantibodies.

The complement activity is also increased in the Down subjects, although the C3c and C4 components are mostly normal.

In Table 2 the T cells dependent data are reported, comparing the "young group" with the "adult group" both for Down and normal subjects.

It appears that also the T cells system of the normal subjects is unchanged from young to adult age.

In Down patients instead there is an abnormal decrease with the age of the percent of E active rosette and of lymphocytes capacity to become stimulated in presence of PHA. The percentage of E rosette is normal in both groups, thus confirming that the simple enumeration of total T lymphocytes is not expressing the functional capacity of such cells.

The anergy to DNCB is present in both groups of Down patients. Such anergy to DNCB in the "young group" of Down patients is the earliest indication of T cells dysfunction.

TABLE 2

IMMUNOLOGICAL DEFICIENCY IN THE DOWN SYNDROME : IMPORTANCE OF
THE AGE FACTOR

T Cells Functions

Down groups at different ages and normal groups at different
ages are compared

	Down Youngs N.12 Med.Age 21 y.	Down Adults N.12 Med.Age 36 y.	Normal Youngs N.8 Med.Age 22 y.	Normal Adults N.12 Med.Age 35 y.
Lymphocytes/mm^3	2686	2512	2377	2738
E Rosette per cent	72	65	76	80
E Active Rosette per cent	56	43^	49	61
Stimulation Index P.H.A.	167	67^	205	230
D.N.C.B.	--	--	3	2.5
Cutaneous Tests (N.Pos.)				
Tubercolin	3	3	4	2
Candidin	11	9		4
Streptokinase-streptodornase	9	11		7

^significant difference ($P < 0.05$)

     The stimulation index to PHA is in fact lower in the young
Down when confronted to the young normals, but the difference
is not statistically significant.

     In the other group instead we can notice that the mitoge-
nic activity to PHA has fallen only in the Down group.

     The responsiveness to ubiquitous antigens is not substan-
tially compromised in our Down subjects.

DISCUSSION

     The study of the immunological system in Down subjects
at different ages has disclosed some important abnormalities,
which are related to the age.

As reported also by others authors (7) the Down patients
develop before 20 years of age a marked increase of the serum
levels of IgG, IgA and IgD, while the IgM level is below the
normal values. Such dysgammaglobulinemia is marked by the
absence of monoclonal aspects and by the presence of autoantibodies, exceptional in normal individuals at this young age.
Furthermore the elevated serum Ig levels are apparently the
product of a number of B cells lower than normal.

The increase in serum complement activity is possibly a
consequence of the high frequence of infections with elevated
levels of Ig.

At the same moment when such B cell dependent abnormalities
are already very pronounced, the T cell system shows only anergy
to DNCB.

Taking all these abnormalities into account together (i.e.
hypergammaglobulinemia with autoantibodies and selective T cell
deficiency) a defective supressor T cell system has to be considered as the first immunological deficit in Down patients.

The abnormalities concerning the B cell system will persist
and become more evident in the adult Down patients. Particularly relevant is the antibody response to the H antigen of
Salmonella which is markedly increased in Down patients, thus
confirming a deficiency in the supressor T cell system.

In adult Down patients the deficiency of the T cell system becomes also more evident. Low mitotic and effector functions of T lymphocytes are present while the total number of
T cells is still normal.

The immunological abnormalities found in Down's syndrome
have been related by some authors (11) to the poor nutritional
and hygienic conditions of the institutions where the patients
live for long periods.

However controlled studies on Down and others mentally retarded children both living in institutions or both living at
home, have disclosed that the abnormalities of the Ig or of the
T cells dependent functions are present only in the Down patients
(8, 9).

It is not clear if such age related immunological abnormalities have some importance in the development of Alzheimer-Type
alterations in the Down patients.

However, as already stated, the development of senile plaques which is marked by the presence of amyloid fibrils, seems

to take place only in conditions in which immunological abnormalities are present, similar to those found in Down patients.

REFERENCES

1. Bianco C., Patrick R., and W. Nussenzweig : A population of lymphocytes bearing a membrane receptor for antigen-antibody-complement complexes. 1. Separation and characterization. J. Exp. Med. 132 : 702, 1970.
2. Dyggve H., and J. Clausen : The serum immunoglobulin level in Down's syndrome. Develop. Med. Child. Neurol. 12 : 193, 1970.
3. Gupta S., and M. Grieco : Impairment of rosette-forming T lymphocytes in chronic marihuana smokers. N. Engl. J. Med. 291 : 874, 1974.
4. Levin S., Nir E., and B.M. Mogilner : T system immunodeficiency in Down's syndrome. Pediatrics 56 : 123, 1975.
5. Malamud N. : Neuropathology of organic brain syndromes associated with aging. In : Advances in Behavioral Biology. Vol III, Gaitz CM. ed., Plenum Press, New York, 1972.
6. Rigas D., Elsasser P., and F. Hecht : Impaired in vitro response of circulating lymphocytes to phytohemagglutinin in Down's syndrome : Dose-and time-response curves and relation to cellular immunity. Int. Arch. Allergy 39 : 587, 1970.
7. Seger R., Buchinger G. and J. Ströder : On the influence of age on immunity in Down's syndrome. Europ. J. Pediat. 124 : 77, 1977.
8. Srivastava L.M., Agarwal D.P., and H.W. Goedde : The serum immunoglobulin levels in Down's syndrome and other diseases associated with mental disorder. Z. Immun. – Forsh. 150 : 277-280, 1975.
9. Ugazio A., Maccario R., Duse M. and G.R. Burgio : T-lymphocyte deficiency in Down syndrome. Lancet I : 1062, 1977.
10. Wolstenholme G.R.W., and M. O'Connor : Alzheimer's disease and related conditions. Churchill, London, 1970.
11. Whittingham S., Pitt D.B., Sharma D.L.B., and I.R. Mackay : Stress deficiency of the T-lymphocyte system exemplified by Down syndrome. Lancet I : 163, 1977.
12. Wybran J., and H.H. Fudenberg : Thymus-derived rosette-forming cell. N. Engl. J. Med. 288 : 1072, 1973.

CONCLUSIONS

The main topics we would like to quote in our conclusions
are : the oligoclonal reaction in neurological diseases, the
experimental oligoclonal reaction, some of the technical
approaches evoked here, the regulations of the oligoclonal
reaction, the antigens, the immunological problem, the therapeutic
questions.

The Oligoclonal Reaction

The oligoclonal reaction is well accepted, by everybody.
It is a neurological observation discovered in the CSF. It still
remains essential in neurological and fundamental problems. This
reaction is seen in many diseases. During this meeting we discussed mainly MS and SSPE, two diseases provoked probably by conventional viruses. The oligoclonal reaction is not seen in spongiform encephalitis, due to a non conventional agent.

Oligoclonal Reaction in Experimental Hyperimmunisation

Oligoclonal reaction is also seen in experimental hyperimmunisation and leads to the synthesis of homogeneous antibodies. The
homogeneity of the antibodies, at least in SSPE serum, are shown
by κ and λ ratios, aminoacid sequence determination and the definition of idiotypy. Immunochemical studies are still incomplete
but raised some questions as to the existence of a genetic background to the above mentioned disease. This would complicate the
interpretation of the epidemiological data. Should we modify
our views and think of a genetic susceptibility to an agent or to
and immunological process and not anymore to a genetic disease?
Some animals studies seem to indicate it.

Methods

We should also be aware of the fact that the methods used to
confirm the oligoclonal reaction and to identify the fractions
should be improved. Identity between electrophoretic mobilities

does not prove that fractions are identical. Improved methods
will allow a better detection in CSF and serum of the oligoclonal
reaction and more cases and more diseases should be tested.
Recent results showing the oligoclonal reaction in serum of
Guillain-Barré syndrome, or MS give new indications that should
not be overlooked. Oligoclonal fractions may be identified by
their antibody activity. Are they antibodies against one or many
antigens or are they autoimmune antibodies? What is the relative
proportion of the autoimmune antibodies? What is the proportion
of these oligoclonal IgG which possess antibody activities? How
heterogeneous are those bands? We must not neglect the facts
that oligoclonal reactions appear in other fluids, for instance,
serum, synovial fluid and other organs than the nervous system.

Regulation of the Oligoclonal Reaction

Hopeful indications could be found in the interaction between
the T and the B-cells or by the study of factors inhibiting the
immunological reaction. Is the oligoclonal reaction always a
consequence of a hyperimmune process? The discovery in MS sera
of oligoclonal fractions points in that direction. Surely, the
oligoclonal reaction occurs more often than we thought when it
was first described in MS CSF. Can we go as far as to say that
MS and SSPE are generally and mainly immunological diseases?
Should we plan meetings with the internists? Can we accept
that SSPE is only a viral disease or is it also a disease of the
immune system? We should not forget that SSPE can appear during
immunosuppressive treatment and after rubeola infection.
This may open new ways to research.

What can provoke the Oligoclonal Reaction?

Which kind of antigens and how can we define them? We now
saw that visna antigen is variable and that MS patients can still
get measles. What is measles and what is the measles virus?
Are we working with measles antigens that share common immunological characteristics with other proteins? Is the antigen still
complete?

The Immunological Problem

Does the brain or the intrathecal organs modify the immunological reaction as the liver and kidney modify the blood, does the
brain modify the B-lymphocyte or the immunological reaction and
send the immunoglobulins in the CSF and from the CSF in the blood?
Does the myelin have specific immunological properties? Can we
study this immunological reaction of the brain by experimental

processes as EAE in vivo or by in vitro experiments, as in the
experiments with oligodendrocytes and anti-oligodendrocyte sera?
What is the place in fact for EAE and basic protein in our problems?
Would the determination of basic protein give indications for
the physiopathology of MS and SSPE?

Just a last thought : we believe that the study of the oligoclonal reaction opens the door to more basic research in immunology in general, and not only in neurology. The study of homogeneous
antibodies in pathological conditions can lead to the identification of a chemical specificity of these antibodies. Although
antibody aminoacid sequences did not reveal it so far, we must
not forget that in eliciting EAE the chemical specificity of basic
protein rests with a few aminoacids, and that altering in the
hemoglobin molecule, one aminoacid produces a pathological status
in man. Maybe we should also look for small common similarities
in a material with such heterogeneous chemical characteristics
as the IgG.

Treatment

Treatment is still a challenge and we even do not know which
are the biological criteria of therapeutic improvement. We do
not know which way we should choose. Treatment of the virological
disease or of the immunological process or of an inborn error of
metabolism?

These are some of the questions that were raised and discussed during this meeting. As you see we have more questions than
answers. Maybe this meeting helped to put the questions. A
good question may be more helpful than half an answer. We though
that it would be a good thing to put them to you.

A. Lowenthal

DIRECTOR :
A. Lowenthal (Antwerp, Belgium)

SCIENTIFIC COMMITTEE :
J.D. Capra (Dallas, U.S.A.)
D. Karcher (Antwerp, Belgium)
A.D. Strosberg (Brussels, Belgium)

PARTICIPANTS

O. ABRAMSKY	Department of Neurology, Hadassah Hebrew University Hospital, P.O.B. 499, Jerusalem – Israël.
J.M. ADAMS	Department of Pediatrics, UCLA Medical Center, Los Angeles, CA 90024 – U.S.A.
G. AGNARSDOTTIR	Department of Immunology, St. Mary's Hospital Medical School, London W2 IPG – United Kingdom.
M. ALTER	Department of Neurology, Temple University, Philadelphia, PA 19140 – U.S.A.
M. ANDERSSON	Dr. Linds gata 6, 413 25, Gothenburg – Sweden.
E. AUFF	Neurologisches Institut der Universität Wien, Schwarzspanierstrasse 17, A 1090 Wien – Austria.
P. BARTMAN	Am Gries 8, D-8400 Regensburg – F.R. Germany.
A. BESSET	Centre de Pédiatrie, Hôpital de Clocheville, 49 Boulevard Béranger, 37000-Tours – France.
N. BICHARA	Floralienlaan 417, 2600 Berchem-Antwerp – Belgium.
V. BLATON	Klinisch Laboratorium, St. Jansziekenhuis, 8000 Brugge – Belgium.
A. BOEYE	Vrije Universiteit Brussel, Paardenstraat 65, 1640 St. Genesius-Rode – Belgium.
J.D. CAPRA	The University of Texas, Health Science Center at Dallas, 5323 Harry Hines Blvd., Dallas, TX 75235 – U.S.A.

H. CARTON   Department of Neurology, Academisch Ziekenhuis
                      Sint-Rafaël, Kapucijnenvoer 33, 3000 Leuven –
                      Belgium.

N. CHAMOLES   Clinica Stapler, Coronel Diaz 2211, 1425 Buenos
                      Aires – Argentine.

J. CLAUSEN   Neurochemical Institute, Radmansgade 58,
                      DK 2200-Copenhagen – Denmark.

F.B. COCHRAN Jr.   Albert Einstein College of Medicine, 1300
                      Morris Park Avenue, Bronx, NY 10461 – U.S.A.

S.C. COLLIS   Institute For Research On Animal Diseases,
                      Compton, Newbury, RG 16 OQY, Berkshire –
                      United Kingdom.

C.E. COTO   Estado de Israel 4752, 2°A., 1185 Buenos
                      Aires – Argentina.

M.L. CUZNER   Department of Neurochemistry, Institute of
                      Neurology, Queen Square, London WC 1 – United
                      Kingdom.

L.E. DAVIS   Department of Neurology, University New
                      Mexico School of Medicine, Albuquerque, NM
                      87131 – U.S.A.

P. DELMOTTE   Belgisch Nationaal Centrum voor Multiple Scle-
                      rose, Vanheylenstraat 16, 1910 Melsbroek –
                      Belgium.

W. DEN TANDT   Universitaire Instelling Antwerpen, Genetica,
                      Universiteitsplein 1, 2610 Wilrijk – Belgium.

C. DOUTRIAUX   Rue Lepic 102, 75018 Paris – France.

E.R. EINSTEIN   University of California, Institute of Human
                      Development, Tolman Hall, Berkeley, CA 94720 –
                      U.S.A.

R.W. ELSE   Department of Pathology, Royal School of
                      Veterinary Studies, Edinburgh EH9 1QH – United
                      Kingdom.

M.M.A. EL-SAWY   Faculty of Medecine, University of Alexandria,
                      Alexandria – Egypt.

E.H. EYLAR   Playfair Neuroscience Unit, University of
                      Toronto, 1 Spadina Crescent, Toronto, Ontario
                      M5S 2J5 – Canada.

W.C. FERREIRA   Instituto de Higiene e Medecine Tropical, Rua
                      da Junqueira 96, Lisboa 3 – Portugal.

E.J. FIELD   The Royal Victoria Infirmary, Queen Victoria
                      Road, Newcastle upon Tyne NE1 4LP – United
                      Kingdom.

G. FRANCK	Hôpital de Bavière, Boulevard de la Constitution 66, 4020 Liège - Belgium.
A. FRYDEN	Department of Infectious Diseases, University Hospital, S-581 85 Linköping - Sweden.
H. GACOMS	Vorstlaan 310/5, 1160 Brussel - Belgium.
D.C. GAJDUSEK	National Institutes of Health, Laboratory of Central Nervous System Studies, NINCDS, Bg 36, Room 4A15, Bethesda, MD 20014 - U.S.A.
J. GHEUENS	Universitaire Instelling Antwerpen, Neurochemie, Universiteitsplein 1, 2610 Wilrijk - Belgium.
J. GIBBS, Jr.	National Institutes of Health, Laboratory of Central Nervous System Studies, NINCDS, Bg 36, Room 4A15, Bethesda, MD 20014 - U.S.A.
D.H. GILDEN	The Wistar Institute, Thirty-Sixth Street at Spruce, Philadelphia, PA 19104 - U.S.A.
M. GUDNADOTTIR	Department of Microbiology, University of Iceland, Eiriksgata, P.O.B. 855, Reykjavik - Iceland.
G. GULLIKSEN	Department of Psychiatry, Odense University Hospital, DK 5000 Odense C - Denmark.
E. HABER	Cardiac Unit, Massachusetts General Hospital, Boston, Mass. 02114 - U.S.A.
M. HALBACH	Institut für Virologie und Immunbiologie der Universität Würzburg, Versbacher Landstrasse 7, D-8700 Würzburg - F.R. Germany.
J.F. HALLPIKE	Department of Neurology, Royal Adelaide Hospital, Adelaide, S.A. 5000 - Australia.
R. HAMERS	Vrije Universiteit Brussel, Instituut voor Molekulaire Biologie, Paardenstraat 65, 1640 St. Genesius-Rode - Belgium.
S. KAM-HANSEN	Department of Neurology, University Hospital, S-581 85 Linköping - Sweden.
D.S. HODES	Department of Pediatrics, Columbia University, 630 West 168th Street, New York, NY 10032 - U.S.A.
E. HOOGHE-PEETERS	National Institutes of Health, NINCDS, Bg 36 Room 5D04, Bethesda, MD 20014 - U.S.A.
R.W. HORNABROOK	Department of Neurology, Wellington Clinical School of Medicine, Wellington Hospital, Wellington 2 - New Zealand.
G. HUYBRECHTS	Universitaire Instelling Antwerpen, Virologie, Universiteitsplein 1, 2610 Wilrijk - Belgium.

A. ISHAQUE   Playfair Neuroscience Unit, University of
                      Toronto, 1 Spadina Crescent, Toronto, Ontario
                      M5S 2J5 - Canada.

K.P. JOHNSON   Veterans Administration Hospital, 4150 Clement
                      Street, San Francisco, CA 94121 - U.S.A.

M.R.A.F. KANDIL   Department of Neurology, Assiut University
                      Hospital, Assiut - Egypt.

D. KARCHER   Universitaire Instelling Antwerpen, Neurochemie,
                      Universiteitsplein 1, 2610 Wilrijk - Belgium.

W. KRISTOFERITSCH   Neurologische Universitätsklinik, Lazarettgasse
                      14, A-1097 Wien - Austria.

J. LEBAS   Laboratoire de Chimie Biologique, Faculté de
                     Médecine, 1 Place de Verdun, 59045 Lille -
                     France.

N.J. LEGG   Department of Neurology, Hammersmith Hospital,
                     London W 12 OHS - United Kingdom.

G.M. LEHRER   Mount Sinai School of Medecine, 11 East 100th
                     Street, New York, NY 10029 - U.S.A.

J.L. LIESSENS   Interne Geneeskunde, Algemeen Ziekenhuis Middel-
                     heim, Lindendreef 1, 2020 Antwerpen - Belgium.

H. LINK   Department of Neurology, University Hospital,
                     S-581 85 Linköping - Sweden.

D.S. LINTHICUM   The Walter and Eliza Hall Institute of Medical
                     Research, Royal Melbourne Hospital, Victoria
                     3050 - Australia.

A. LOWENTHAL   Universitaire Instelling Antwerpen, Neurochemie,
                     Universiteitsplein 1, 2610 Wilrijk - Belgium.

G.M. McKHANN   Department of Neurology, Johns Hopkins Hospital,
                     Baltimore, MD - U.S.A.

D.L. MADDEN   National Institutes of Health, Infectious
                     Disease Branch, NINCDS, Bg 36, Room 5D06,
                     Bethesda, MD 20014 - U.S.A.

S.E. MANSOUR   Department of Neuro-psychiatry, Alexandria
                     Medical School, Alexandria - Egypt.

J.J. MARTIN   Universitaire Instelling Antwerpen, Neuropatho-
                     logie, Universiteitsplein 1, 2610 Wilrijk -
                     Belgium.

A.R. MASSARO   Clinica Neurologica, Universita Cattolica del
                     Sacro Cuore, Policlinico "A. Gemelli", 00168
                     Roma - Italy.

P. MASSON	Unité de Médecine Expérimentale, 7430 Avenue Hippocrate, 1200 Bruxelles - Belgium.
R. MEDAER	Neurologisch Center-Multiple Sclerose Kliniek, 3583 Overpelt - Belgium.
P.D. MEHTA	Institute for Basic Research in Mental Retardation, 1050 Forest Hill Road, Staten Island, NY 10314 - U.S.A.
Cl. MERTENS	Parkplaats 32, 9820 St. Denijs-Westrem - Belgium.
G.C. MILLSON	Institute for Research on Animal Diseases, Compton, Newbury RG 16 OQY, Berkshire - United Kingdom.
F.F. MILONE	Via Paolo Sarpi 4, 36100 Vicenza - Italy.
M. NOPPE	Universitaire Instelling Antwerpen, Neurochemie, Universiteitsplein 1, 2610 Wilrijk - Belgium.
H. NORDAL	Institute of Immunology and Rheumatology, Rikshospitalet, Oslo 1 - Norway.
E. NORRBY	Department of Virology, Karolinska Institute, SBL. S-105 21 Stockholm - Sweden.
D. NOVICK	Department of Chemical Immunology, Weizmann Institute of Science, P.O.B. 26, Rehovot - Israel.
H. OFFNER	Neurochemical Institute, Rädmandsgade 58, 2200 - Copenhagen N - Denmark.
E. OKAZAKI	Department of Neuropathology, Brain Research Institute, Niigata University, Asahimachi 1, Niigata City 951 - Japan.
T.A. OUT	Centraal Laboratorium van de Bloedtransfusiedienst, Plesmanlaan 125, Amsterdam, The Netherlands.
G. PALLADINI	Università di Roma, Instituto di Biologia Generale della Facoltà di Medicina, Policlinico Umberto 1, 00100-Roma - Italy.
G.L. PALLADINI	Università di Roma, Instituto di Biologia Generale della Facoltà di Medicina, Policlinico Umberto 1, 00100-Roma - Italy.
D.H. PARK	≠ 23 Yueido Seebum apt. ≠ 21, Youngdungpo-ku, Seoul - Korea.
S. PELC	29 rue de Wynants, 1000 Bruxelles - Belgium.
F. PERCEVAULT	Laboratoire Hoechst, 10 rue Clement Marot, 75008 Paris - France.

M.C. PEREZ	Section of Neurology, Department of Medicine, UP-PGH Medical Center, Taft Avenue, Manila – Philippines.
G. PIRE	N.V. Upjohn, 2670 Puurs – Belgium.
P. PLATZ	Tissue Typing Laboratory of Blood Grouping Department, State University Hospital, Blegdamsveg 9, DK-2100 Copenhagen – Denmark.
R. POLAK	Cyriel Buyssestraat 68, 2020 Antwerpen – Belgium.
G.E. QUINONEZ	Universidad de el Salvador, Departemento de Educacion Medica, San Salvador, El Salvador.
J. RADL	Institute for Experimental Gerontology, TNO, 151 Lange Kleiweg, Rijswijk (Z.H.) – The Netherlands.
C.S. RAINE	Department of Pathology, Albert Einstein College of Medicine, 1300 Morris Park Avenue, Bronx, NY 10461 – U.S.A.
R. REINING	Neurologische Klinik, Heidelberger Landstrasse 379, 61 Darmstadt – F.R. Germany.
A. RISSANEN	Department of Neurology, Helsinki University Hospital, Haartmaninkatu 4, 00290 Helsinki 29 – Finland.
L. RÖNNBÄCK	Institute of Neurobiology, University of Göteborg, Fack, S-400 33 Göteborg 33 – Sweden.
B. ROSTRÖM	Department of Neurology, University Hospital, S-581 85 Linköping – Sweden.
S. ROZENBLATT	Department of Virology, Weizmann Institute of Science, P.O.B. 26, Rehovot – Israel.
B. RYBERG	Department of Neurology, University Hospital, S-221 85 Lund – Sweden.
E. SCHULLER	Hôpital de la Salpêtrière, Laboratoire de Neuro-immunologie, 47 Boulevard de l'Hôpital, 75013 Paris – France.
J.L. SEVER	National Institutes of Health, Infectious Diseases Branch, NINCDS, Bg 36, Room 5D-06, Bethesda, MD 20014, U.S.A.
A. SHAKER	Department of Neurology, Mansourah Faculty of Medicine, Mansourah – Egypt.
A. SIDEN	Department of Neurology, Karolinska Hospital, S-104 01 Stockholm – Sweden.

M. SIEGELMAN	University of Texas, Health Science Center at Dallas, 5323 Harry Hines Boulevard, Dallas, TX 75235 - U.S.A.
J. SIMON	Max-Planck-Institut für Psychiatrie, Kraepelinstrasse 2, 8000 München 40 - F.R. Germany.
C. SINDIC	Université Catholique de Louvain, Cliniques universitaires St. Luc, Avenue Hippocrate 10, 1200 Bruxelles - Belgium.
C. SOLHEID	Universitaire Instelling Antwerpen, Neuropathologie, Universiteitsplein 1, 2610 Wilrijk - Belgium.
J. SOTELO	Department of Neurology, The London Hospital, London E1 IBB - United Kingdom.
H. STAUNTON	St. Laurence's Hospital, North Brunswick Street, Dublin 7 - Ireland.
A.J. STECK	Départment de Neurologie, Centre Hospitalier Universitaire Vaudois, 1011 Lausanne - Switzerland.
W. STEVENS	Universitaire Instelling Antwerpen, Immunologie, Universiteitsplein 1, 2610 Wilrijk - Belgium.
H.B. STOKES	6 a Calle 2-48 Zona 1, Guatemala, C.A.
A.D. STROSBERG	Vrije Universiteit Brussel, Instituut voor Molekulaire Biologie, Paardenstraat 65, 1640 St. Genesius-Rode - Belgium.
P. TAVENIER	Klinisch Chemisch Laboratorium, Valeriuskliniek, Valeriusplein 9, Amsterdam Zuid - The Netherlands.
B. TAVOLATO	Clinica delle Malattie Nervose e Mentali dell' Università, Via Giustiniani 5, Padova - Italy.
A.W. TEELKEN	Kliniek voor Neurologie, Rijksuniversiteit, Groningen - The Netherlands.
D. TEITELBAUM	Department of Chemical Immunology, Weizmann Institute of Science, P.O.B. 26, Rehovot, Israel.
I. TEKEOGLU	Pekeler Mah. Karasu Cad., N°64 Adapazari - Turkey.
V. TER MEULEN	Institüt für Virologie und Immunbiologie, Universität Würzburg, Versbacher Landstrasse 7, 8700 Würzburg - F.R. Germany.
L. THIRY	Institut Pasteur du Brabant, Rue du Remorqueur 28, 1040 Bruxelles - Belgium.

R.S.A. TINDALL   Department of Neurology, The University of
                          Texas,Health Science Center at Dallas, 5323
                          Harry Hines Boulevard, Dallas, TX 75235 -
                          U.S.A.

W.W. TOURTELLOTTE   Neurology, Wadsworth Hospital Center, Ve-
                          terans Administration, Welshire and Sawtelle
                          Boulevards, Los Angeles, CA 90073 -
                          U.S.A.

H. VALDIMARSSON   Department of Immunology, St. Mary's Hospital
                          Medical School, London W2 IPG - United Kingdom.

D. VANDEN BERGHE   Universitaire Instelling Antwerpen, Virologie,
                          Universiteitsplein 1, 2610 Wilrijk - Belgium.

B. VANDVIK   Department of Neurology, Ulleval Hospital,
                          Oslo 1 - Norway.

G.J. VAN KAMP   Laboratorium voor Immunochemie, B 343, Acade-
                          misch Ziekenhuis Vrije Universiteit, de
                          Boelelaan 1117, Amsterdam - The Netherlands.

H.K. VAN WALBEEK   Wilhelmina Gasthuis, Eerste Helmersstraat
                          104, Amsterdam - The Netherlands.

J. VAUTHIER   Bt 5621, Rue Américaine 120, 1050 Bruxelles -
                          Belgium.

M. VERMEYLEN   Academisch Ziekenhuis Dijkzigt, Afdeling Neuro-
                          logie, Rotterdam - The Netherlands.

D. VERVERKEN   Celestijnenlaan 71/42, 3030 Heverlee - Belgium.

W.C. WALLEN   National Institutes of Health, Unit on Acute
                          Virol.Diseases, NINCDS, Bg 36, Room 5D-06,
                          Bethesda, MD 20014- U.S.A.

K. WARECKA   Medizinische Hochschule Lübeck, Ratzeburger
                          Allee 160, 2400 Lübeck 1 - F.R. Germany.

M.L. WEIL   Department of Pediatrics, UCLA Medical Center,
                          1000 West Carson Street, Torrance, CA 90509 -
                          U.S.A.

H. WIETHÖLTER   Institut für Hirnforschung der Universität,
                          Calwer Strasse 3, 74 Tübingen - F.R. Germany.

M. YAP HOCK LEONG   Department of Neurology, Tan Tock Seng Hospi-
                          tal, Singapore 1 - Singapore.

V.R. ZURAWSKI   Cardiac Unit, The Massachusetts General Hospi-
                          tal, Boston, Mass. 02114 - U.S.A.

INDEX